Clay and Pounds

Basic Clinical Massage Therapy

Integrating Anatomy and Treatment

Clay and Pounds'

Basic Clinical Massage Therapy

Integrating Anatomy and Treatment

3RD EDITION

Laura Allen, BA, LMBT

David M. Pounds, MA, CMI, FAMI

Photographs by Vicki Overman and Black Horse Studio, Winston-Salem, North Carolina

Illustrations by David M. Pounds, Certified Medical Illustrator

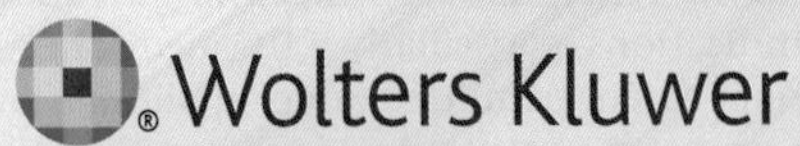

Philadelphia • Baltimore • New York • London
Buenos Aires • Hong Kong • Sydney • Tokyo

Acquisitions Editor: Jay Campbell
Product Development Editor: Linda G. Francis
Editorial Assistant: Tish Rogers
Marketing Manager: Leah Thomson
Production Project Manager: David Orzechowski
Design Coordinator: Joan Wendt
Illustration Coordinator: Jennifer Clements
Manufacturing Coordinator: Margie Orzech
Prepress Vendor: S4Carlisle Publishing Services

Third Edition

9 8 7 6 5 4 3 2 1

Printed in China

Library of Congress Cataloging-in-Publication Data
Allen, Laura (Massage therapist), author.
Clay and Pounds' basic clinical massage therapy : integrating anatomy and treatment / Laura Allen, David M. Pounds ; photographs by Vicki Overman and Black Horse Studio ; illustrations by David M. Pounds. — Third edition.
p. ; cm.
Basic clinical massage therapy
Preceded by Basic clinical massage therapy / James H. Clay, David M. Pounds. 2008.
Includes bibliographical references and index.
ISBN 978-1-4511-8546-1 (alk. paper)
I. Pounds, David M., author, illustrator. II. Clay, James H. Basic clinical massage therapy. Preceded by (work): III. Title. IV. Title: Basic clinical massage therapy.
[DNLM: 1. Massage—methods. WB 537]
RM721
615.8'22—dc23

2015028402

LWW.com

CCS0915

Dedication

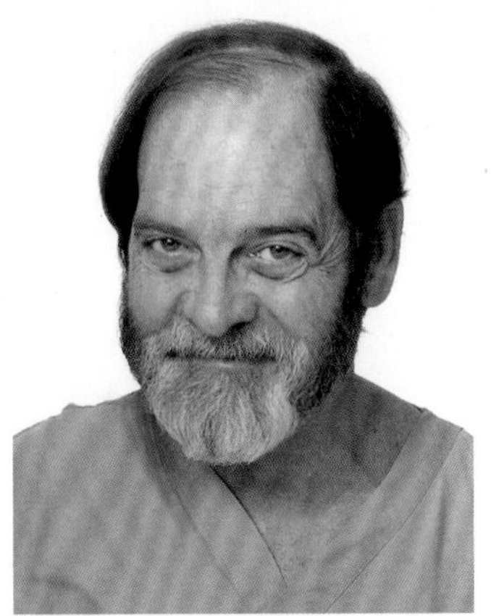

This, the third edition of *Basic Clinical Massage Therapy,* is the first without the direct involvement of original coauthor James ("Doc") Clay. Although he died in 2013, his contribution to this book and its importance to massage therapy are indelible.

Born in Texas and raised in Winston-Salem, North Carolina, Doc took an indirect path to massage therapy. He studied at Duke and Johns Hopkins Universities, earning a master's in mental health. After working in counseling in Germany and Maryland, he returned to North Carolina to study at the Carolina School of Massage, earn his NCTMB certification in the early 1990s, and open a practice in Winston-Salem.

Doc had a passion for the theater and acted in many local productions. His intelligent wit, sense of humor, and love of wordplay (especially the "Anguish Languish" of Howard L. Chace) found expression in this book in such figures as 1-13, 1-26, and the pronunciation guide to "superficialis" (SOUP-or-fishy-Alice), to cite a few examples.

Doc nurtured his vision of what this book could be for more than a year before our paths crossed, and we began to develop the ideas. His open-minded curiosity made him a good collaborator as we did our research, even joining in on an opportunity to do an investigative dissection study of deep back muscles on a human cadaver.

The clarity of purpose he brought to this book is a significant reason why you might find something useful in these pages. Although Doc had many interests and accomplishments, it is of this contribution to your understanding of massage that I believe he was most proud.

This third edition is dedicated to the memory of James H. Clay.

David M. Pounds

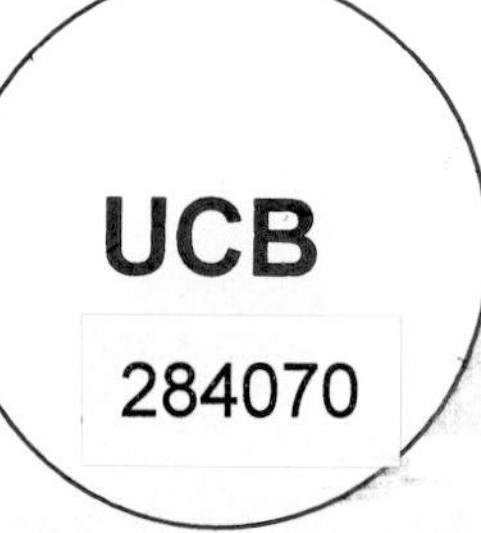

About the Authors

Laura Allen, BA, LMBT

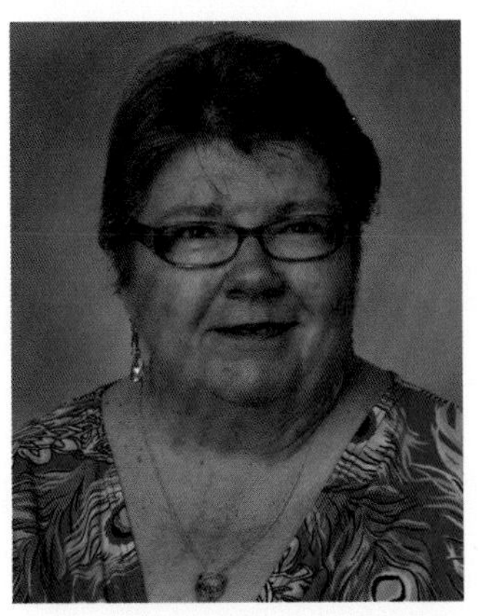

Laura Allen came to massage therapy as a career after spending more than 20 years as a chef and restaurateur. Ready for a change, but not sure what to do, she took a job as the administrator of a massage school. After a few days of seeing clients come into the attached clinic looking stressed and in pain, and seeing them walk out an hour later looking relaxed and feeling better, she decided to attend school herself, earning her massage diploma and a degree in psychology from Shaw University at the same time. Allen also completed a 2,000-hour internship in counseling before deciding that massage therapy was going to be her path. She remained employed at the massage school for 5 years before opening her own clinic in Western North Carolina 13 years ago, where she and her husband, Champ (also a massage therapist), employ a chiropractor, several other massage therapists, and a registered nurse trained in aesthetics.

Allen has had a lifelong love of writing, dating back to writing for the school newspaper and yearbook in middle school. Her first magazine article was published in 1999, and since then, she has had numerous articles published and written over 300 blogs about issues in the massage profession. She is also the author of *Plain & Simple Guide to Therapeutic Massage & Bodywork Examinations* (LWW, third edition to be released in 2016), *One Year to a Successful Massage Therapy Practice* (LWW, 2008), A *Massage Therapist's Guide to Business* (LWW, 2011), and four other self-published titles.

Laura Allen has received numerous honors in the massage profession, including being inducted into the Massage Therapy Hall of Fame in 2011, being named as American Massage Therapist of the Year in 2011, and winning the 2013 Silver Award from the Massage Therapy Foundation for her professional case report on massage therapy for chronic low back pain. She has also received media awards for her writing, and in 2014, she and her husband were jointly presented the Bonnie Prudden Meritorious Service Award.

Allen is the Massage Division Director of Soothing Touch, a position she accepted in 2015. She focuses on writing, teaching continuing education classes nationally and internationally, and writing.

David M. Pounds, MA, CMI, FAMI

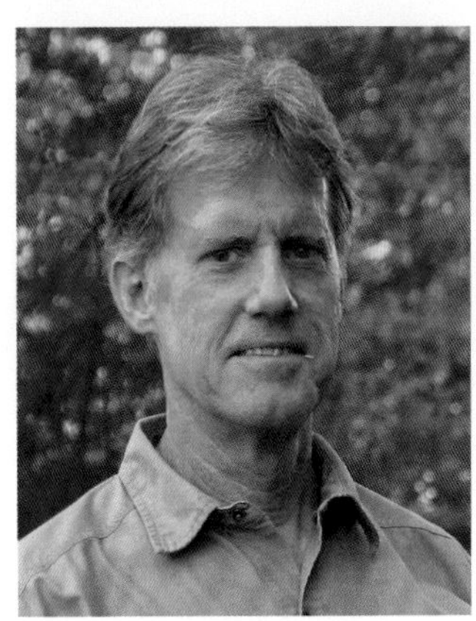

David Pounds has spent his entire professional career in biomedical visualization, communication, and teaching. The fact that he enjoys explaining how the human body works verbally and visually may be part nature and part nurture. His father was a chemical engineer with a second career teaching at Bradley University, and his mother was a fine artist. Early childhood fossil collections and attempted dissection of dead birds evolved to illustrated lab reports and art studio courses in college. He eventually discovered that his interests could be combined in a career as a medical illustrator and instructor.

He currently teaches courses such as "Human Anatomy & Physiology" and "The Biology of Movement" at the University of North Carolina School of the Arts in Winston-Salem, North Carolina, and has been doing so since 1998. He is also owner of D. Pounds Illustration, an independent business providing biomedical illustration and communications nationally for numerous scientific journal publications, textbooks, presentations, and exhibitions.

He earned his BS in biology from Bradley University in Peoria, Illinois. After completing an MA in biomedical communications (medical illustration emphasis) from The University of Texas Southwestern Medical Center (formerly the UT Health Science Center at Dallas), he held a faculty appointment at the Wake Forest School of Medicine (formerly The Bowman Gray School of Medicine) for 16 years.

He has been a Certified Medical Illustrator (CMI) since 1992, when the Board of Certification of Medical Illustrators established the program, and was inducted as a Fellow of The Association of Medical Illustrators (FAMI) in 1989.

Preface

Basic Clinical Massage Therapy: Integrating Anatomy and Treatment, originally written by the late James Clay ("Doc") and David Pounds, with illustrations by David Pounds, was a groundbreaking text when it was first published in 2003. It quickly became a best-selling textbook, and a second edition was published in 2008. The integration of anatomy and clinical applications of massage therapy presented here is a continuum of the original vision of the book: to reach massage therapy students who are ready to refine palpation and assessment skills, increase knowledge of structure and function, and go beyond the techniques of Swedish massage to address complaints of soft tissue pain and dysfunction.

We are delighted to be revising the text for the third edition. We have heard from massage therapy students and instructors that they find the detailed anatomical illustrations, overlaid on photographs of the human body, among the most helpful features of the book, not only as a resource for class, but for educating clients, as well. The third edition has more than 550 full-color images, illustrating the muscles, surrounding tissues, anatomical landmarks, proper draping techniques for each area of the body, the therapist's hand placement, and directional arrows for performing sequences for treating specific muscles. With this edition, we are including small photo guides throughout the text that demonstrate proper draping needed when performing the technique pictured in that area of the body.

Each muscle group is highlighted with name, pronunciation, etymology, overview, comments, actions, attachments, cautions, pain referral zones, other muscles to examine, and description of the sequences used to treat specific muscles and complaints. Icons draw the students' eyes to key information. Case studies and end-of-chapter questions aid students in integrating what they've learned and applying it to the clinical practice of massage therapy.

ELAP

The third edition also provides learning objectives that reflect the knowledge and competencies from *The Core: Entry Level Massage Education Blueprint,* which resulted from the ELAP (Entry-Level Analysis Project), an effort that was supported by all seven national massage organizations. The ELAP seeks to define the knowledge and skills that should be possessed by a graduate of a 625-hour massage therapy program. While there is a great deal of subject matter from the ELAP that is outside the scope of this book, a good portion of the skills and knowledge recommended in the *Blueprint* are included in this edition: the history and evolution of massage; principles of body mechanics; anatomical terminology; structures and functions of the skeletal, nervous, fascial, and muscle systems; assessment forms; interviewing and communication skills in massage and bodywork; positioning and draping guidelines; palpation; session planning; observations of contraindications; physical and ethical cautions; and myofascial and neuromuscular techniques.

When it was announced on social media networks that we were undertaking this project, many school owners and massage instructors immediately responded with "Don't change it!" It's our hope that the changes we have made are for the better. Current research in the areas of trigger points, fascia, and pain science has been incorporated—and will no doubt be updated again in subsequent editions—as old theories are expanded on, refined, or changed altogether. As medical technology advances, so does our knowledge of the human body and how it functions. While there's still plenty of investigation to be done, massage therapy research is a growing body of knowledge.

Online Resources

The following resources are available for students using this book:

- Anatomy flash cards
- Video clips displaying anatomy, physiology, and body mechanics concepts

Readers can find these resources at http://thePoint.lww.com. To access them, just follow the instructions, and use the scratch-off code on the inside cover of this book.

Instructors adopting this book will find the following supportive resources, also on thePoint:

- Image Bank
- Test Generator
- Syllabus
- Lesson Plans

Acknowledgments

For this edition, it was our pleasure to work with Lee Runion and Jennifer Bostic of Black Horse Studio, in Winston-Salem, North Carolina, ably assisted by Griffin Gough in production of the studio photography.

Many thanks to the models for this edition including our model-therapist, Marti Macon (of Marti Macon Massage in Winston-Salem), Alexander Bodine, Courtnee A. Carter, Lilly Nelson, Dean Wilcox, and Steven Williford. Additionally, we'd like to thank the models for the previous editions of this text: Joe Cox, Jack Edmonds, Lindsay Fisher, Amanda Furches, Blakeney Griffin, Sabrina Hertel, Jessica Hightower, Olivia Honeycutt, Erica Jimbo, Sarah Kelly, Jason Kittleberger, Cullen Massenberg, Kate Merritt, Helen Naples, Mike Orsillo, Bronwyn Queen, Nike Roach, Shanta Rudd, Shana Schwarz, Elizabeth Shuler, Emily Sparkman, Matt Swaim, Katie Swords, Joshua Willhite, and Yvonne Truhon.

We are grateful to the reviewers of this edition: Christine Tinner, Lotus Education Institute; Otis S. Watson, WellSpring School of Allied Health; Christopher Moyer; and Ravensara Travillian.

Laura Allen would like to acknowledge her husband Champ for his unwavering support, and Ravensara Travillian, Christopher Moyer, Alice Sanvito, Paul Ingraham, and Bodhi Haraldsson, for teaching her to use research and critical thinking to advance her own study of massage therapy.

David Pounds would like to acknowledge the patient support and assistance of his wife Katheen Pounds, and his parents Arthur M. and Jean T. Pounds for their formative influence and continued, unabashed personal advocacy of this book. He would also like to thank the students and faculty of the UNC School of the Arts for providing a setting where he can hone his teaching skills.

Contents

CHAPTER 1

Approaching Clinical Massage Therapy

LEARNING OBJECTIVES

At the conclusion of this chapter, the learner will be able to:

- Outline the basic history and evolution of massage therapy.
- Describe the place of massage therapy in different disciplines of health care.
- Recall the principles of clinical massage therapy.
- Restate current theories of pain science.
- Explain the structure and function of muscles.
- Identify trigger points, tender points, and release.
- Recognize agonists and antagonists.
- Define fascia and its functions in different areas of the body.
- List different techniques of soft tissue manipulation.
- Select the proper equipment for performing massage.
- Demonstrate proper draping techniques.

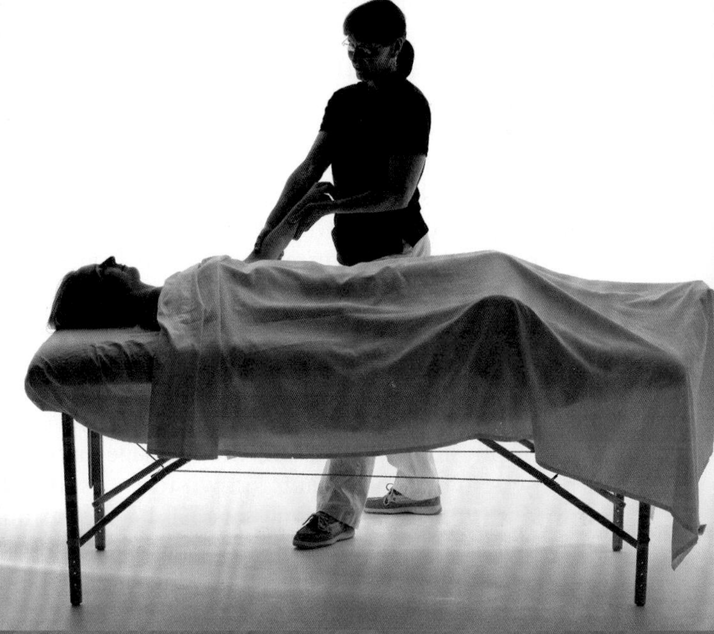

"Is there not such a thing as a diffused bodily pain, extending, radiating out into other parts, which, however, it leaves, to vanish altogether, if the practitioner lays his finger on the precise spot from which it springs? And yet, until that moment, its extension made it seem to us so vague and sinister that, powerless to explain or even to locate it, we imagined that there was no possibility of its being healed."

Marcel Proust, The Remembrance of Things Past (The Guermantes Way, 1920)

Overview

A young girl has pain in her back that does not go away. Her mother has heard from a friend that there is a healer not far away who can get rid of such pain. One day the mother takes the girl to see this healer. The healer asks a few questions; then, rather than giving her something to swallow, the healer places skilled hands on her and presses and rubs in various places. When the healer is finished, the girl's pain is diminished. The mother pays the healer and they leave. A day or two later, the pain is completely gone.

These events may very well have taken place in China in 700 BCE. They could have occurred in Egypt at least as early as 2330 BCE. There is also evidence of massage being used in ancient times in Korea, India, and Mesopotamia. The healer in question could have been Herodicus or his pupil, Hippocrates, in fifth century BCE Greece, or Asclepiades, who brought the practice to Rome in the first century BCE. The story can often be told today, thanks to the rediscovery and development of **clinical massage therapy**, the use of manual manipulation of the soft tissues to relieve specific complaints of pain and dysfunction.

The recorded practice of massage therapy lay dormant in the western world from the decline of Rome until the 18th century, when the Enlightenment fostered renewed interest in exploring the frontiers of medical knowledge. In the early 19th century, Per Henrik Ling developed a system of medical exercises and massage that his followers disseminated throughout the western world in subsequent years. This system profoundly influenced the birth and development of physical therapy, and the massage elements of his system became what is known today as **Swedish massage**. This type of massage has been continuously practiced in health clubs and spas over the past century, but was largely considered a luxury available only to the wealthy and was not generally viewed as a health-related procedure until the gradual resurgence of massage therapy over the last 30 to 40 years.

It has taken many years, but in most states in the United States, massage legislation has now been included in the statutes under various regulatory agencies, some health related, some under other professional boards, or establishing an independent licensing board. There are only a few states left that are not yet regulating massage as a licensed profession, requiring specific hours (which vary in different states) of education in the areas of anatomy, physiology, pathology, kinesiology, professional ethics, theory and practice of massage, and other related subjects.

Not everyone agrees that massage therapy constitutes health care. The proliferation of corporate chain massage schools and massage franchises (and their marketing efforts) has made massage therapy more readily available and affordable to the public, but also sends a mixed message about whether massage is a health care treatment or just another personal service, like getting your hair done. Massage therapy as a profession has had, and continues to have, growing pains.

In conjunction with massage therapy, the term **bodywork** has come into common use. This term arose from two principal sources: first, the psychiatrist Wilhelm Reich, originally a disciple of Freud, postulated the expression of the personality through body structure and formulated an approach to the simultaneous treatment of the body and the emotions. Reich used the term "body armor" to describe the body's reaction to neurosis and believed that palpating and even tickling the body could lead to emotional catharsis and, subsequently, the release of tension in the body. His work has been carried on by Alexander Lowen in the system called bioenergetics. Other practitioners, such as Ron Kurtz, the developer of Hakomi Method, have continued to work along similar lines. While there is evidence to support that massage relieves stress and tension, evidence that massage therapists should be facilitators of emotional catharsis—or that they are even equipped to deal with it should it happen—is very lacking. Although therapists need to understand basic psychological concepts that are inherent in therapeutic relationships, the practice of psychology is outside our scope of practice, unless one is a licensed counselor in addition to being a massage therapist.

Second, Ida Rolf developed a system that she called structural integration, which has come to be called **Rolfing™** in her honor. Her teachings emphasized claims of the restoration of the elasticity and sliding capacity of the fascia, a theory that is still taught today.

The term *bodywork* is now in popular usage, and while many therapists consider themselves heirs and practitioners of both traditions, there are just as many evidence-based, or evidence-informed, as some prefer to say, practitioners who dislike the term, due to the frequent inclusion of energy techniques in the description.

Two other approaches to health care in the last two centuries have also made significant contributions to the formation of clinical massage therapy and bodywork. Osteopathy (see page 3) developed as a medical field that sought to relieve health problems through the manipulation of both joints and soft tissues, and many osteopathic practices overlap with clinical massage therapy. Dr. Leon Chaitow, an osteopath since 1960, has made significant contributions to both osteopathy and massage, including founding and acting as editor-in-chief of the peer-reviewed *Journal of Bodywork and Movement Therapies* and authoring more than 70 books.

In medicine, the late Janet G. Travell and David G. Simons published their authoritative volume in

1992 on the phenomenon of referred pain from **trigger points**, tender points in soft tissue that radiate or refer pain to distant areas. While it is still widely used as a reference, Fred Wolfe, a rheumatologist who worked with Travell and Simons, has since stated that none of the trigger points or treatments suggested for them were validated or tested for reliability and that there were almost no studies cited, just anecdotal evidence—the weakest kind of evidence. Later research, including some personally conducted by Simons, has caused revisions of trigger point theory. A recent study refutes the idea of trigger points as being the cause of myofascial pain syndrome and of chronic widespread pain, stating that the evidence is just not there to support these long-held theories, although there is acknowledgement of trigger points themselves.[1] While clients clearly experience the pain described as trigger points (and tender points) actually exist, but the exact mechanism of how they work has been rehypothesized several times, is still up for discussion, and may continue to evolve for years to come, as more research is conducted. It may be useful to remember that pain, like all sensory experience, does not exist in the periphery but is a construction of our brain. Both conscious and subconscious processing is involved in the experience of pain and that complexity leads to considerable difficulty in understanding cause and effect, as well as producing a wide variation in what individuals may experience. (See section Current Pain Science and Applications in Massage Therapy).

Thus, at a time when many people are looking beyond the traditional medical offerings of pharmacological and surgical intervention, the confluence of these multiple influences has produced the field of clinical massage therapy, which is both one of the oldest and one of the newest health professions.

The Place of Clinical Massage Therapy in Health Care

The complexity of the human organism has led to the evolution of a variety of approaches to the manual treatment of the soft tissues. Other health disciplines take the following approaches to pain and dysfunction:

- ***Traditional western medicine,*** *correctly termed* ***biomedicine***, employs three principal means of treatment: pharmacology, surgery, and referral to an allied therapeutic specialties practitioner. One of the problems with the traditional medical approach to muscular problems is that no medical specialty focuses primarily on muscles, save that of sports medicine—and not everyone is an athlete. Aside from the primary care physician (family practitioner, pediatrician, internist, gynecologist, etc.), a patient with soft-tissue pain or dysfunction is likely to see a neurologist or neurosurgeon (specializing in the nervous system), an orthopedist (specializing in bones), or a rheumatologist (specializing in arthritis and rheumatic diseases of the joints and soft tissues). Depending on the particulars of the case, such a patient is most likely to receive surgery, drugs, or a referral to a physical therapist.

  Perhaps that trend will change. One of the largest research studies to date on the efficacy of massage therapy, a study involving 401 people, compared patients receiving the usual care of drugs and physical therapy to two groups, with one group receiving relaxation massage and another receiving structural massage. The study authors defined structural massage as intended to identify and alleviate musculoskeletal contributors to back pain and allow myofascial, neuromuscular, and other soft tissue techniques and stated that areas of the body treated varied across patients and treatment sessions. Therapists could also recommend a psoas stretch home exercise to enhance and prolong any benefits of structural massage. The two groups receiving massage had much better outcomes in the reduction of pain and increase in function than the group receiving usual care.[2] There was no significant difference in the outcome of the two massage groups; in other words, relaxation massage was found to be as effective for relieving pain as the structural massage.
- ***Osteopathic medicine*** began as an approach to health that focused on the manipulation of bones and joints, nutrition, and natural means of treatment, but has since moved in the direction of biomedicine. Osteopaths in the United States are allowed to prescribe and perform surgery and have the same status as an MD. Osteopathy education in the United States requires 4 years of undergraduate study, another 4 years of osteopathy training, a 1-year internship, and a residency of 2–8 years in length, depending on the specialty. Osteopathy has a heavy focus on the musculoskeletal system. (Osteopathy in countries outside the United States is significantly different in education and practice from American osteopathy, and only in the United States is an osteopathic practitioner considered a physician.) Certain representatives of osteopathy, such as Leon Chaitow and Philip Greenman, have maintained the tradition of examining and treating pain problems through joint manipulation and have had a profound effect on developments in clinical massage therapy.

- ***Chiropractic*** focuses on treatment of the joints, particularly those of the vertebrae. These practitioners attribute pain and other health problems to misalignments of the vertebral joints that impinge on nerve roots, resulting in abnormal functions of the nervous system. Chiropractic has been controversial since its inception; many medical doctors discount chiropractic as being based on scientifically false premises, and many osteopaths view it as a watered-down version of their own discipline. Chiropractors must have 90 hours of undergraduate college, and a 4-year degree in chiropractic, but no internship or residency. There is even a split within the chiropractic community itself, as many chiropractors call for reform of the profession by way of letting go of all scientifically unproven concepts—including the core concept of subluxation.
- ***Physical therapy*** uses physical exercise and movement as a means of restoring healthy function to muscles and joints. Although today physical therapists take advantage of many technological advances, such as hydrotherapy, ultrasound, and electrical stimulation of muscles, their emphasis remains on exercise and movement. While massage is within the scope of practice of physical therapists, it is not usually their focus. Also, physical therapists tend to focus on more severe conditions, such as rehabilitation following surgery, serious injury, or congenital deformities. In recent years, the American Physical Therapy Association made a huge push to raise standards for entry-level education, and the old master of physical therapy degree is being phased out, to be replaced by the minimum requirement of a doctor of physical therapy degree.
- The remaining approach is ***direct manipulation of the soft tissues.*** This approach, while falling within the scope of practice of the practitioners listed above, is especially the domain of the clinical massage therapist and the subject of this book.

Clearly, there are dozens of massage modalities. We have chosen, in this text, to focus on muscle stripping and myofascial release techniques, with the caveat that there's no need to throw out techniques of massage that have been used effectively to address neuromuscular pain just because they may not work in the manner that was originally thought. Trigger point theory, fascia theory, pain science—and the profession of massage therapy itself—are all in a state of evolution, yet during this period of evolution, every day, around the world, massage therapists continue to relieve pain and suffering in practical ways.

The Principles of Clinical Massage Therapy

Clinical massage therapists operate according to certain assumptions that are so self-evident that they might be considered axioms of the field.

1. ***The individual is a whole organism: Everything is connected and related.*** Complex systems are more than the mere sum of their parts; that is, it is essential to see the forest *and* the trees. Although this book is necessarily reductionist to some degree—we cannot understand the whole without knowledge of the parts, and they must be examined in a linear way—the therapist should remember that the part must also be seen in the context of the whole. For example, a client with a sprained ankle will favor the injured leg, causing muscles in the hip and low back to tighten. The resulting imbalance in the back can affect the neck muscles, causing a headache. Treating the neck muscles alone will not solve the problem. As massage therapists, we must remember that the *source* of the pain is not always in the same location as the pain, and that it's important to educate our clients to that effect.
2. ***Shortened muscle tissue can not function optimally.*** Muscle tissue does its work by contracting and, therefore, does not work efficiently if shortened. What we are concerned with as therapists is persistently or pathologically shortened tissue; in other words, tissue that has shortened, in all likelihood for defensive reasons, is unable to function optimally, and resists lengthening.

   A muscle may be shortened actively or passively. Examples of chronic passive shortening are the shortening of biceps brachii when the arm is kept in a sling for a period of healing, and the flexed position of the iliopsoas muscles (hip flexors) in a baby who is not yet standing and walking. Postural misalignment always involves habitual passive shortening of many postural muscles.

   Active shortening, on the other hand, is muscular contraction, and may be either the intentional contraction that is the work of the muscle or defensive contraction representing the muscle's response to a threat such as overload, repetitive motion, or excessive stretch. When a portion of muscle tissue is contracted in this way, it cannot contract further and is unavailable to do the work of the muscle.
3. ***The soft tissues of the body respond to touch.*** One of the most persuasive theories

of the many that seek to explain this is that myofascial pain is caused by a self-perpetuating neuromuscular feedback circuit in which the stimulation of touch interferes, thus restoring normal function. Depending on the choice of technique, manual intervention in the dysfunctional tissues interrupts this feedback process, forcing some change in the neural response and, therefore, in the functioning of the affected tissue itself. This may be akin to skin reddening after rubbing or pressing on it. The physical manipulation of the tissue changes the neural feedback and results in blood vessel dilation. A similar blood flow increase response in muscle may allow it to relax and lengthen (release molecular cross-bridges described later) (see page 6 and 7). The intervention may take the form of **ischemic compression, passive stretching, passive shortening,** or any simultaneous or sequential combination of these.

Clinical massage therapy, and therefore this book, is based firmly on these three principles. The clinical massage therapist is one who approaches persistently shortened soft tissues and attempts to restore their natural, pain-free function through touch, while keeping the whole client in mind.

Current Pain Science and Applications in Massage Therapy

The most widely accepted current definition of pain, from the taxonomy of the International Association of the Study of Pain, is "an unpleasant sensory and emotional experience associated with actual or potential tissue damage, or described in terms of such damage."[3]

The science of pain and the relationship between the brain and the body has been the subject of much study in recent years. Our current understanding of pain recognizes that it is a complex, multifactorial, and highly individual experience. The main approaches of pain science today are the biopsychosocial model and **neuromatrix theory**.

The biopsychosocial model view of pain, theorized by psychiatrist George L. Engel[4] in 1977, is that of a dynamic interaction between the biological, psychological, and social factors that uniquely affect each individual's perception and experience of pain, particularly chronic pain. As massage therapists, that makes immediate sense to us; we often see multiple clients suffering from the same condition, all of whom may have a different physical response to it, and differing attitudes about it.

The concept of a pain "neuromatrix" suggests that perception of pain is simultaneously regulated by multiple influences. The neuromatrix theory was developed by Ronald Melzack[5] and represents an expansion beyond the original **gate control theory** of pain, put forward by Melzack and Patrick Wall[6] in 1962, as the idea that physical pain is not a direct result of activation of pain receptor neurons, but rather its perception is modulated by interaction between different neurons.

In Melzack's[7] own words, "It proposes that the output patterns of the body-self neuromatrix activate perceptual, homeostatic, and behavioral programs after injury, pathology, or chronic stress. Pain, then, is produced by the output of a widely distributed neural network in the brain rather than directly by sensory input evoked by injury, inflammation, or other pathology. The neuromatrix, which is genetically determined and modified by sensory experience, is the primary mechanism that generates the neural pattern that produces pain. Its output pattern is determined by multiple influences, of which the somatic sensory input is only a part, that converge on the neuromatrix."

These two theories are not mutually exclusive, and to paraphrase Melzack, "Good theories are meant to evolve." A current attitude among pain researchers is that effective intervention is dependent upon recognizing the fundamental differences between acute and chronic pain, the effects on and by the neuromatrix upon the biopsychosocial health of the individual, and integrating that knowledge into a comprehensive multidisciplinary therapeutic plan.[8] Hopefully, as more physicians and other health care professionals become aware of the benefits of massage therapy, we will be a part of that multidisciplinary therapeutic plan.

Structure and Function of Muscles

Although we treat muscles as distinct entities for anatomical convenience, we must remember that the neuromuscular system does not activate muscles in that way. The nervous system stimulates portions of contractile tissue to contract in patterns that will produce the desired effect, and this activation usually involves parts of several muscles acting in fine coordination. Few actions recruit all of a muscle, and few actions recruit only one muscle. When we say, for example, that biceps brachii flexes the arm at the elbow, we are making a broad generalization. Depending on the position of the arm when we make the movement, certain portions of biceps brachii will be activated. In addition, portions of brachialis will also contract, as well as portions of certain muscles in the forearm. Depending on the speed and intensity of the movement, the muscle tone in portions of triceps brachii will be recruited to temper the movement and keep it smooth. As the movement occurs, a shift in weight occurs, and parts of muscles throughout the torso and legs respond to maintain balance. Therefore, it is not so much individual muscles that do the work of the body as it is patterns of portions of muscle tissue. To gain an understanding of these broad patterns of muscular action over the whole body, we must first acquaint ourselves with the elemental parts of muscle tissue and how they work.

The Muscle Cell

The contractile protein filaments within a muscle cell that perform the work of the muscle are called **myofilaments.** Two basic types of myofilaments perform the work of the muscle. One type is a bundle of myosin molecules forming the thick **myosin** filament; the other is the thin **actin** filament. The myosin filament has molecular "heads" that extend to attach to specific attractor sites on the adjacent actin filament and bend toward the center of the myosin bundle to bring about contraction. These myosin and actin filaments lie parallel to each other in an overlapping pattern that produces the characteristic striped (striated) appearance of skeletal muscle. Several of these myofilaments together form a **sarcomere,** which is considered the "unit" of contraction in a muscle cell.

A string of **sarcomeres** lined up in sequence form a **myofibril** (muscle thread) (Fig. 1-1). Surrounding and penetrating the myofibrils is a system of microscopic tubes called **transverse tubules** and the **sarcoplasmic reticulum.** These tubules carry the chemical trigger, calcium, necessary to initiate contraction at the molecular level. A muscle cell is composed of many myofibrils.

The expression **"muscle cell"** is equivalent to the expression **"muscle fiber."** The number of muscle cells in the body is believed to remain relatively constant after about age 20; when we strengthen muscles or increase their size and bulk, it is the contractile content, not the number, of the cells or fibers that is changed. Unlike most cells, skeletal muscle cells contain many nuclei scattered along the length of the cell. Multiple nuclei are necessary because muscle cells can be quite long, and their internal needs for synthesis of actin and myosin contractile proteins, for example, must be met by the nuclei throughout that length. Muscle cells are second only to nerve cells in length and can be more than 30 cm long (11 to 12 inches) in some muscles.

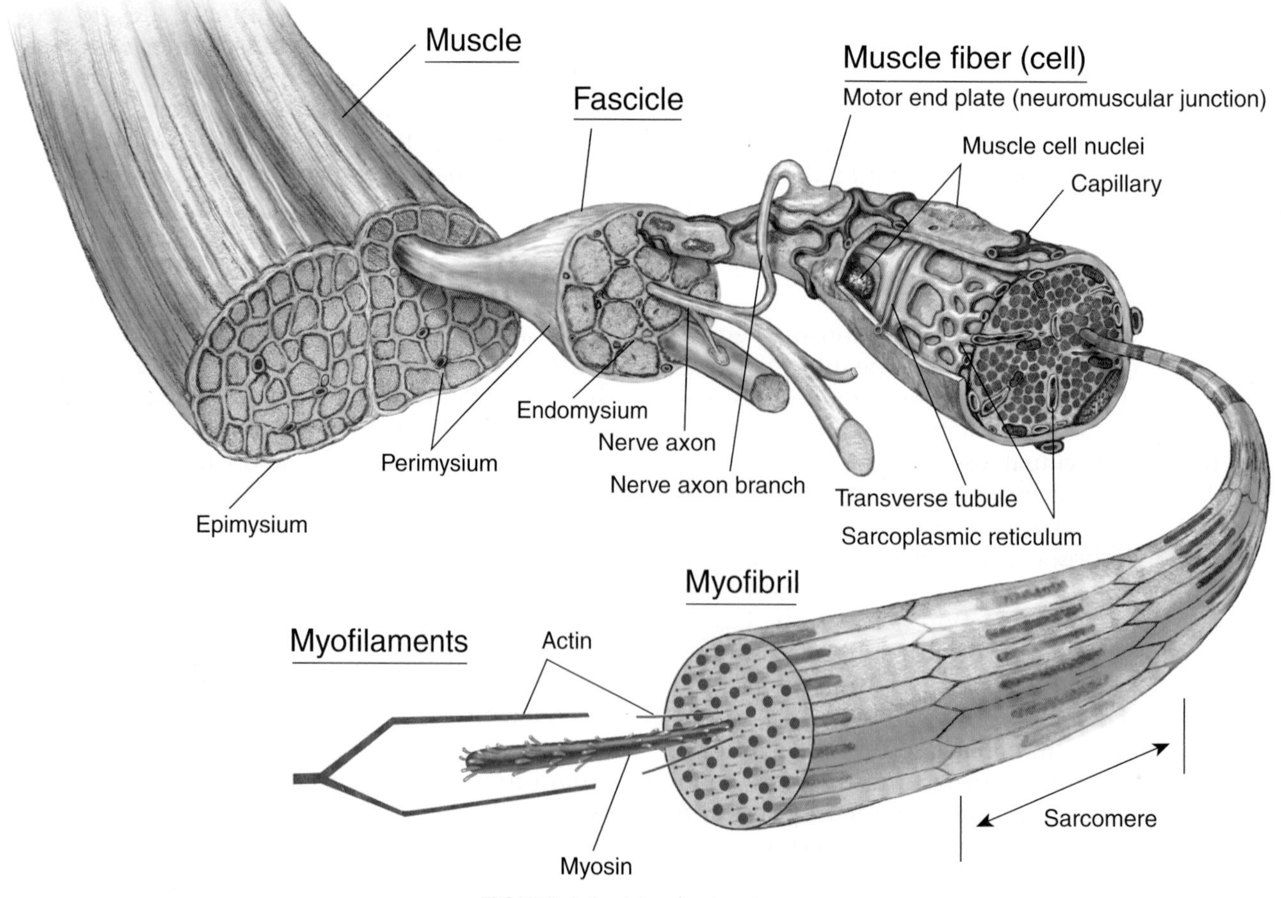

FIGURE 1-1 Muscle structure

The Cross-Bridge Theory

The most commonly accepted theory of muscle function is the **cross-bridge theory**. It attempts to explain the contractile action of muscle tissue—that is, how muscle tissue shortens when stimulated by a motor neuron.

When a nerve impulse excites the neuromuscular junction, calcium is released from the sarcoplasmic reticulum within the muscle cell into the fluid surrounding the myofilaments. This causes a molecular response in which attachment sites on the actin filaments are exposed, attracting "heads" from the myosin filaments, which "bridge" the gap between the filaments, attach themselves to the specific sites on the actin filaments, and bend, propelling the actin filaments into a more deeply overlapped and interlocked position in relation to the myosin filaments. This shortens the sarcomere and, as all the sarcomeres in many muscle cells shorten, contraction occurs in the whole muscle (Fig. 1-2). Muscle tissue is capable of shortening by about 40% of its "resting" length.

When nerve stimulation ceases, the calcium is actively transported back into the sarcoplasmic reticulum, the myosin heads release, and contraction stops. The muscle, however, cannot lengthen on its own. The contractile units (sarcomeres) must be stretched back to their starting position by an outside force, such as the pull of gravity or an opposing muscle, before it can again shorten in contraction.

If you imagine the myosin and actin filaments in fully overlapped position, then you can see how muscle tissue that is shortened in this way can not function effectively.

The Neuromuscular Junction

The point of contact between the nervous system and the muscular system is the **neuromuscular junction. Synapses,** which are the points at which nerve cells communicate chemically with each other, also exist between the motor nerve cell and the muscle and constitute the control mechanism of contraction. Since muscles cover a lot of territory and different parts of them must function in different ways, a nerve made up of many neurons can innervate, or have nerve endings (neuromuscular junctions) with many different locations (many muscle cells) in a whole muscle. Thus, while each muscle cell (fiber) is innervated by only one neuron, each neuron may innervate many muscle cells. A particular neuron and all of the muscle cells that it innervates is known as a **motor unit.** This neuron extends an individual axon branch to each muscle fiber. Each

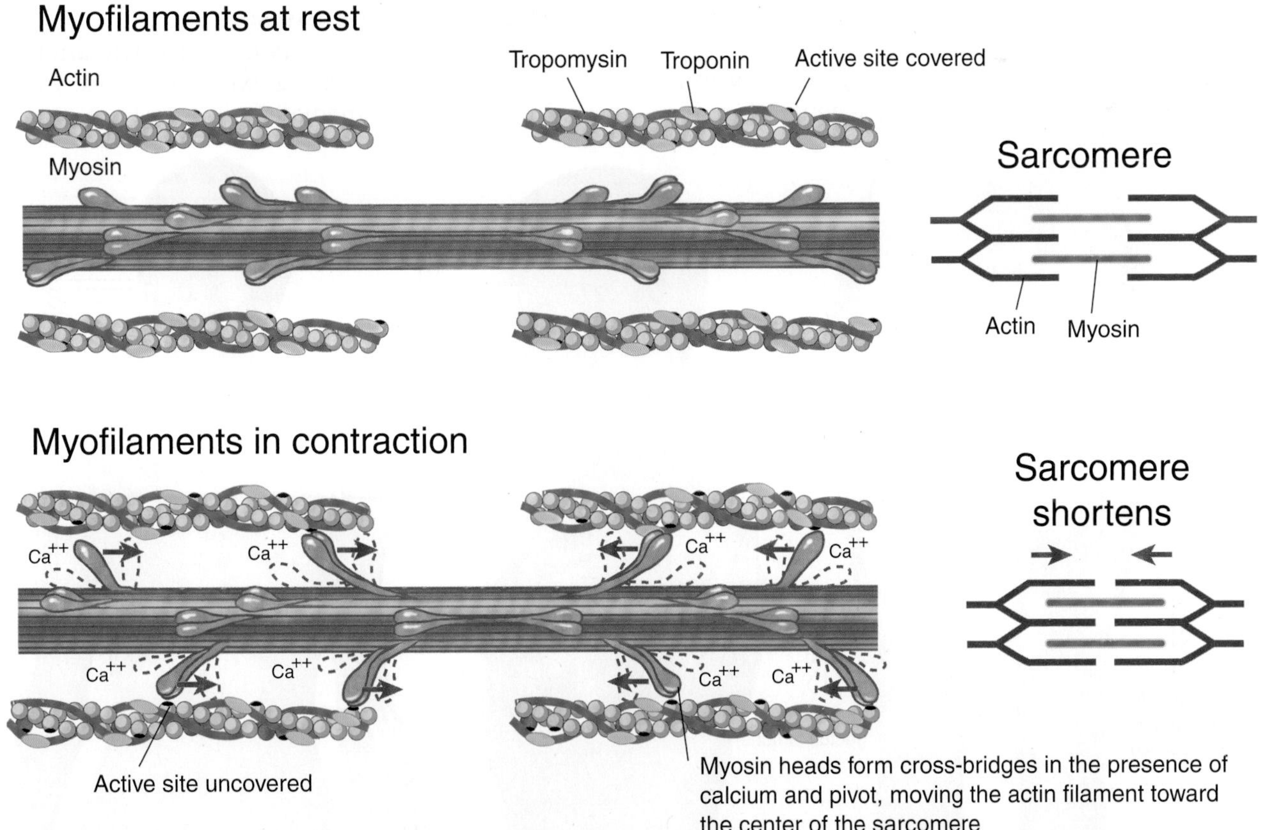

FIGURE 1-2 Cross-bridge theory of muscle contraction

muscle fiber has a single neuromuscular junction, approximately at its middle, composed of a cluster of axon terminals. These are the points at which the impulse to contract is communicated from the nervous system to the muscle. Control of contraction in a whole muscle is achieved by which, and how many, motor units are engaged by the nervous system.

Individual muscles are composed of **fascicles,** or bundles, of muscle cells (fibers). These smaller bundles are held together to form larger bundles and are separated from each other by connective tissue (deep fascia, myofascia).

The energy to power contraction within muscle cells is supplied by a molecule called adenosine triphosphate (ATP). This molecule is derived from the metabolism of glycogen (a form of glucose stored in the muscle) or other calorie sources. When muscle tissue is excited by the nervous system, it **recruits** a number of motor units based on the strength of the excitation. If the excitation and, therefore, the contraction are sustained, then some motor units may experience **exhaustion;** that is, they deplete their supply of ATP. As this occurs, other motor units are recruited to relieve them. As the excitation increases, additional motor units are recruited. A muscle undergoing fatigue and unable to keep up with the demand for ATP may not be able to form new cross-bridges nor break existing ones, becoming paradoxically unable to produce contraction power or to relax and lengthen.

Muscle Architecture

Muscle architecture is the arrangement of muscle fibers relative to the axis of force generation. It is one of the most important aspects of muscle anatomy for massage therapists for two reasons:

1. The arrangement of the muscle fibers determines the kinesiological function of the muscle or that particular part of the muscle.
2. The direction of the fibers in a particular section of a muscle will often determine the direction and type of the work to be done. For these reasons, it is important to learn the architectural characteristics of each muscle.

Muscle fibers may be aligned with the direction or axis of its contraction **(force-generating axis)**, or be arranged at an angle to that axis. The term used to describe the angle of the fibers to the force-generating axis is *pennation*, and muscles fall into several general categories on the basis of the arrangement of its fibers (Fig. 1-3):

- ***Parallel (longitudinal):*** Fibers are parallel to the force-generating axis. (Example: biceps brachii)
- ***Convergent:*** Fibers from a broad attachment converge to a narrow attachment, forming a fan shape. (Example: pectoralis major and gluteal muscles)
- ***Pennate:* Fibers attach obliquely (in a slanting position) to its tendon or force-generating axis, further divided into the following classes:**
  - ***Unipennate:*** Fibers lie at a single angle to the force-generating axis. (Examples: vastus lateralis and medialis)

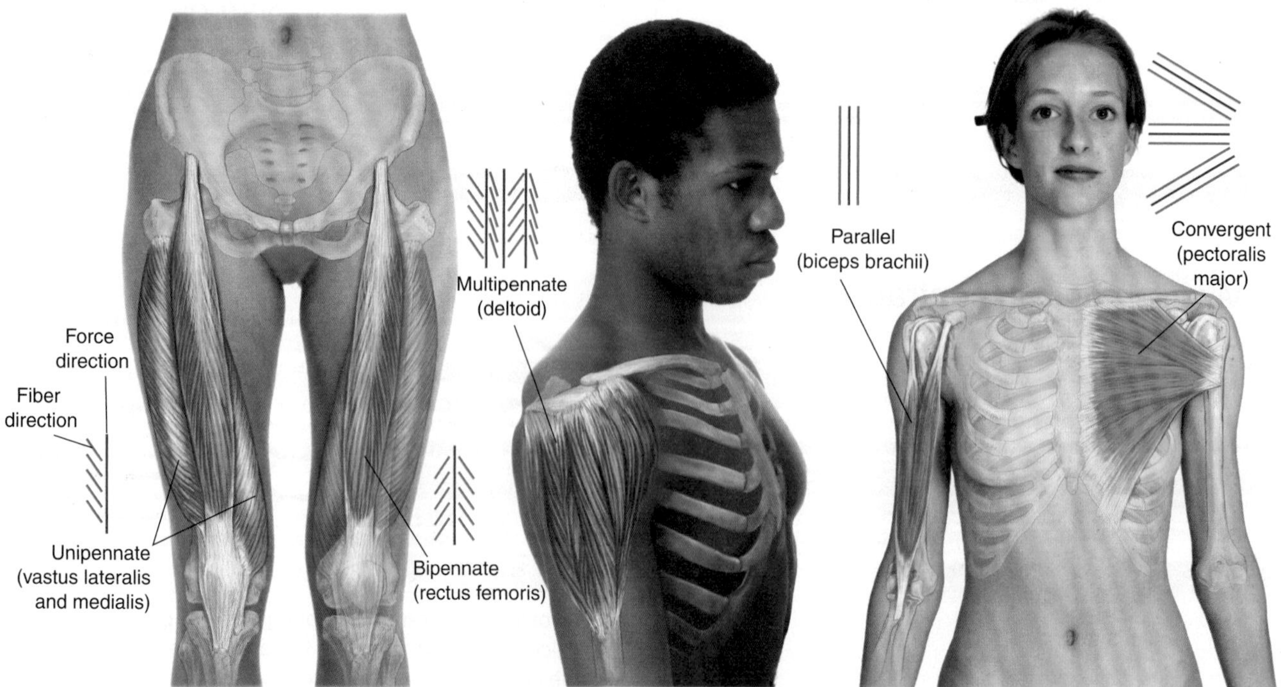

FIGURE 1-3 Muscle architecture

- ***Bipennate:*** Fibers lie at two angles to the force-generating axis. (Example: rectus femoris)
- ***Multipennate:*** Fibers lie at multiple angles to the force-generating axis. (Example: deltoid)

Tender Points, Trigger Points, Release

In palpating clients, you may find points on the body that are tender when pressed. Assuming no other explanation exists for the tenderness, such as bruising or other injury, these points are often called **tender points**. Tender points occur systematically on both sides of the body, but unlike trigger points, tender points are painful only at their location (usually in the insertion zone of the muscle) and do not refer pain to another area. While trigger points have a noticeable mass, tender points do not. Although they are two different things, there may be overlap between tender points and trigger points. In the treatment system called *strain–counterstrain*, or *positional release*, developed by osteopath Lawrence Jones, they are treated by placing the muscle indicated into a passively shortened position until it relaxes and the tender point dissipates.

A myofascial **trigger point** is a point found in a nodule in a taut band of skeletal muscle tissue that is extremely tender and refers or radiates pain in a characteristic pattern. Trigger points may be produced by muscle stress, such as overwork, repetitive motion, or sudden excessive stretch. An **active trigger point** is one that is spontaneously producing referred pain in the client; a **latent trigger point** is one that produces pain only when pressure is applied in palpation. A **primary trigger point** is one that is caused by muscle stress; a **satellite trigger point** is one that is produced secondarily by a primary trigger point.

The term **release** is commonly used by massage therapists to refer to the sensation of softening and lengthening of soft tissue in response to therapy. A trigger point is said to release when its nodule is felt to soften and it ceases referring pain. A muscle is said to release when it relaxes while a therapeutic maneuver is being performed. Fascia is said to release when the therapist feels a softening sensation—but in reality, in this instance we cannot really separate the muscle from the fascia, nor unequivocally state that we have "released the fascia." Although the therapist's sense of release in soft tissue is a subjectively experienced phenomenon that is difficult to describe, it is difficult to miss when you do feel it, and it is a very gratifying feeling for therapist and client alike.

Agonists and Antagonists

For virtually any given skeletal muscle tissue, there will be corresponding muscle tissue that pulls in the opposite direction. Although the actual relationships of such corresponding tissues is complex, we generally refer to muscle pairs as **agonists** and **antagonists,** the agonist being the muscle that is carrying out a motion in question and the antagonist being the muscle that opposes this action. A simple example is biceps brachii (an elbow flexor) and triceps brachii (an elbow extensor), which oppose each other's action at the elbow. **Thus, antagonists produce opposite actions at a given joint**. Under normal conditions, the opposing muscle tone in opposing antagonist muscles can work in a coordinated way to produce a smooth movement in both directions. But that's only part of the picture; many movements require more than one muscle to produce an action. The "helper" muscles, **producing the same action as the agonist muscle at a particular joint**, are known as **synergists.** An example of this synergism is the rectus femoris and vastus lateralis of the quadriceps working together to produce knee extension.

TYPES OF MUSCLE CONTRACTION

Muscles do not always shorten when stimulated by the nervous system. Depending on the amount of force generated in a muscle in relation to the forces resisting its action, muscle length may shorten, lengthen, or remain unchanged.

When a muscle produces **more force** than that of its resistance, **shortening** will occur. This is how we often think of muscle action and it is called **concentric** isotonic **contraction.** For instance, when you pick up an object with your arm, the biceps overcomes the force of gravity and the elbow flexes.

When a muscle produces **less force** that that resisting it, **lengthening** will occur. This is called **eccentric** isotonic **contraction.** In lowering that object back down, the biceps produces less force than gravity, the biceps lengthens and the elbow extends. The biceps just acts like a brake controlling the descent. Note that in eccentric contraction the muscle engaged in control produces a movement in the opposite direction from its "textbook" description.

If you hold that object motionless in the air, the muscle length will not change. This is called **isometric contraction**. In this instance, the biceps produces a **force equal and opposite** the resistance of gravity, and no movement of the elbow occurs. This is how muscles maintain posture or stabilize joints to prevent movement. They cancel out the forces that would move a joint whether that is gravity or an opposing (antagonist) muscle.

We need to be aware of the relationship between muscles and the forces resisting them because it is reflected in clinical problems. A balance in strength between agonists and antagonists may be present in some muscle groups or in some circumstances. But when muscles are weakened, excessively strengthened, or injured, this balance is upset. Imbalances can often occur due to a muscle's responsibility in maintaining posture or position. When we find a problem of any kind in a muscle, it is prudent to examine its synergists and antagonists for they are often affected as well.

Fascia

Fascia is a Latin word meaning "band" or "bandage." It is part of the infrastructure of the body. Fascia both connects and separates many structures of the body. It is the most pervasive type of tissue in the body: it is everywhere, like ivy on old buildings, and yet, it's still somewhat of a mystery. A substantial amount of research into the structure and functions of fascia has been conducted since the first two editions of this book were published, and much of the original thinking about fascia—including whether and how that may be affected by manual therapy—has changed in the interim. There is even disagreement on what constitutes fascia; some doctors, scientists, and bodyworkers include the connective tissues such as tendons, ligaments, and aponeuroses, while many do not include these structures.

The website of the 2012 Fascia Research Congress, the third such gathering of scientists and clinicians devoted to the study of fascia, describes fascia as having been lacking in research for so many years because it is so pervasive and interconnected with the rest of the body that it easily frustrates the common ambition of researchers to divide it into a discrete number of subunits which can be classified and separately described.

Fascia is a type of **connective tissue** that covers everything in the body. It has been assigned different names in different places: around the brain and spinal cord it is the meninges; around bones it is periosteum; around the heart it is pericardium; lining the abdominal cavity it is the peritoneum; and covering the entire body in a layer just under the skin, and enclosing muscles and sections of muscles, it is called subcutaneous fascia. The term *superficial* has been deemed as incorrect and replaced with *subcutaneous* by the Federative International Committee on Anatomical Terminology, but is still commonly (though mistakenly) used. The *Terminologia Anatomica* recommends the use of the term *visceral fascia* in place of *deep fascia*. Fascia serves the following functions:

1. It helps maintain the structural integrity of the body.
2. It contains and compartmentalizes muscles and organs of the body, binding some things together while creating boundaries to keep some structures apart. For example, it bundles muscle cells within a whole muscle or separates groups of whole muscles.
3. Fascia contains and channels body fluids, helping to prevent the spread of infection.
4. It supports capillaries and vessels of the circulatory and lymphatic systems, as well as the ubiquitous branching of the nervous system. This keeps blood vessels and nerves attached to muscle cells during contraction and stretching.
5. It gives rise to new connective tissue. Fascia contains fibroblasts (connective tissue cells) that can specialize as needed to thicken connective tissue, help repair tendons and ligaments, and aid in the formation of scar tissue.

Many fascial therapists firmly believe the healing and restorative functions of fascia can also lead to problems. Their belief is that fascia can form adhesions between structures that should remain free and that it alters the internal structure of muscles with deposits of gristle (fibrosis) that may produce pain and limit movement. Such tissue hardens and contracts with time, becoming increasingly refractory to corrective treatment.

Another problem illustrating that fascia is tough and not as easily movable and/or stretchable as some would like to believe is compartment syndrome, a serious condition that occurs when excessive pressure builds up inside an enclosed space in the body. Compartment syndrome usually results from bleeding or swelling after an injury. The tough walls of fascia cannot easily expand, and compartment pressure rises, preventing adequate blood flow to tissues inside the compartment. Severe tissue damage can result, with loss of body function or even death.

Many therapists feel that fascial distortions and fascial work have an effect over the whole body, including the internal organs. However, we can never be too careful about making claims about what massage can accomplish. Promising a client that we can "get rid of their scar tissue," "break up adhesions," or "release fascial restrictions" of internal organs that lie deep within a body cavity, is just plain irresponsibility. Diagnosing is out of our scope of practice—and how would you *know* that an internal organ is covered in "fascial restrictions?" If one were to work deeply enough to free fascial restrictions between internal organs, one would be working deeply enough to cause trauma to the organ itself.

The pioneer of fascia-centered bodywork was Ida Rolf. Virtually every therapy focused in any way on fascia is grounded in large measure on her theories (which many evidence-based massage therapists disagree with) and her work. Rolf originally theorized that fascia is made up of collagen fibers in a colloidal ground substance that varies in consistency from gel (the solid or semisolid state of a colloidal solution) to sol (the liquid state of a colloidal solution). When energy (such as pressure or friction) is applied to a gel, it moves toward the sol state. Rolf theorized that applying energy manually to the fascia can turn the ground substance from gel to sol and make the direction and distribution of the collagen fibers more elastic and malleable. Rolf theorized that since fascia is continuous throughout the body, the therapist can adjust the "body stocking" of the subcutaneous fascia by releasing restrictions in the deep fascia and breaking up adhesions between fascial layers that restrict free movement of tissues against each other.

However, Ida Rolf,[9] in her later years, stated that her gel/sol theory was incorrect and that she was hopeful that someone in the future would conduct the proper research to find how it actually works. Robert Schleip,[10] one of the organizers of the first Fascia Congress, found that fascia does indeed contain *some* muscle cells that can contract, though slowly and weakly. It has been theorized that the "release" felt by both therapist and client during myofascial release work could be due to the nervous system, or the lengthening of the muscles themselves, rather than any actual "stretching" of the fascia.

While many fascia-based therapists still follow the premise that fascial adhesions exist and can be changed by human hands, there are research results to the contrary . . . and even the question itself is problematic because the definition of "adhesions," as that applies to massage therapy, is not very clear. If we are talking about scar tissue caused by surgery or injury, the possibility that massage is going to change that significantly is not very much. If we are talking about muscles and their surrounding fascia becoming less elastic, and "stuck," as therapists are fond of saying, that's harder to prove, even with all the sophisticated medical technology available today. Fascia is not visible on an MRI, unless it has calcified. In 2005, a video was released by Dr. Jean-Claude Guimberteau,[11] a plastic surgeon, showing a section of in vivo fascia, magnified 25X through the use of fiber optics. The thickness of plantar fascia has been determined with the use of sonographic measurement[12] and measured with ultrasound.[13] Most factual information about fascia, to date, has been gathered through cadaver dissection or experimentation on laboratory rats. Neither, unfortunately, is capable of giving us a true picture of living human fascia. Cadavers start deteriorating at the moment of death and may have been subjected to embalming; rats are not human. The scientific research conducted so far has not proven the existence of fascial adhesions, *at least the subcutaneous kind that massage therapists like to claim can be released by massage*, although this term has been used in the massage profession for many years. In a nutshell, fascia is so tough and strong, that a few moments, or even an hour of "manual therapy," at the level of force that most therapists are capable of working, isn't going to "stretch the fascia." Research *has* shown that the force required to stretch collagen fibers will not "stretch" them until just before they reach the breaking point and that when the pressure is released they resume their original shape.[14]

That doesn't mean giving up the techniques of myofascial release; it just means that it doesn't work in the way it has been explained for many years. All muscle tissue is covered in fascia, so it stands to reason that contracting or stretching a muscle will have *some* effect on the fascia that is helping to hold it in place. The techniques of myofascial release have brought relief to many people, albeit by different mechanisms than have been proposed in the past. Repeat: *there's no need to throw out an effective technique because it works differently than was originally stated.* However, the burden is on us, as manual therapists, to stop passing along misinformation associated with those techniques. There's no need to make claims about what we're doing; the goal is to help relieve pain and help people feel better.

Subcutaneous Fascia

The subcutaneous fascia is also called the hypodermis, tela subcutanea, subcutis, or stratum subcutaneum. It is located directly under the skin and contains cutaneous blood vessels, lymphatic channels and nerves. Although the fascia itself is fibrous tissue, about half of the fat in the body is contained in the spaces between those fibers. This fascia serves to loosely connect the skin to underlying muscle or other tissue so that blood vessels and nerves can traverse the distance without separation damage during movement.

In the skin above (the cutaneous layer), the orientation of the fibers of the connective tissue fibers (collagen) of the dermis follows lines called Langer's lines, or cleavage lines, the direction of which varies from one body area to another (Fig. 1-4). The fibers in a particular region are aligned according to the predominant forces experienced by the tissues in that area of the body to resist those forces. Surgeons often follow these lines in making incisions to minimize scarring.

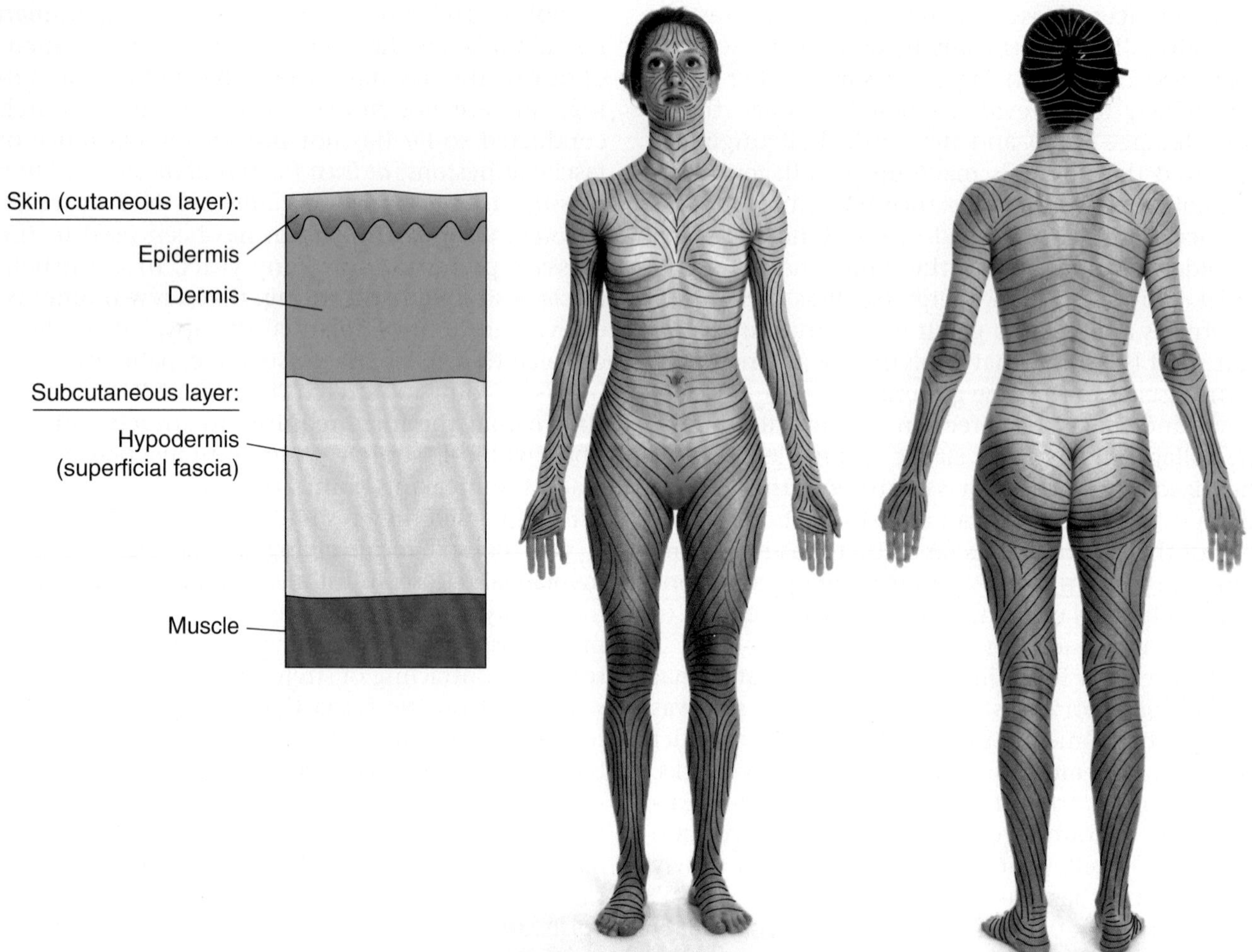

FIGURE 1-4 Tissue layers and Langer's lines (note that the subcutaneous layer varies in thickness throughout the body)

Visceral Fascia

The visceral fascia is all of the fascia that is deep to the subcutaneous fascia, with which it is continuous, albeit distinctly different in structure and purpose. For our purposes, visceral fascia includes the fascia covering a group of muscles, the fascia surrounding the individual muscles (epimysium), the fascia surrounding the fascicles within the muscle (perimysium), and the fascia surrounding the individual muscle fibers (endomysium) (Fig. 1-1). There are many other different subclassifications of fascia, based on location in the body. Each of these layers of deep fascia gives rise to the next deeper layer. Although one of the roles of deep fascia is to restrict the outward (lateral) force of the muscle in contraction to direct and increase contractile force, excessive restriction or limited elasticity is counterproductive.

Types of Myofascial Treatment

Students need to be thoroughly familiar with fascia and its relationship to muscles because in treating muscles, you are treating fascia. Trying to deal with muscle and fascia separately is like trying to deal with a bubble separately from the air inside it. The term *myofascial* is indispensable because muscles and fascia are part and parcel of the same package. Several different approaches to myofascial work can be used:

- **Skin rolling** is a technique in which the tissue is picked up from the surface between the thumbs and fingertips. Both hands are usually used in skin rolling. The purposes of this technique are to increase flexibility and treat tender points (Fig. 1-5).
- **Myofascial release** is a system involving a gentle stretching process, often using two hands to engage muscle and fascia and move with it according to its inclinations, as sensed by the hands (Fig. 1-6).

Directive fascial approaches (Fig. 1-7) include the following:

- **Bindegewebsmassage** (German, *connective tissue massage*) is a directive technique developed by Elisabeth Dicke.

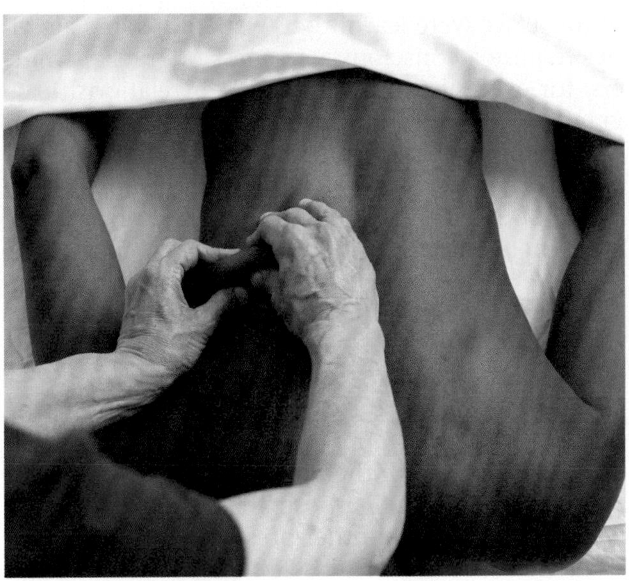

FIGURE 1-5 Skin rolling

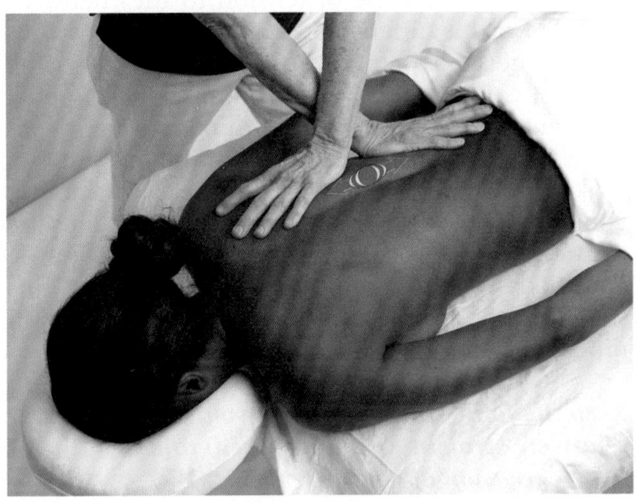

FIGURE 1-6 Myofascial release

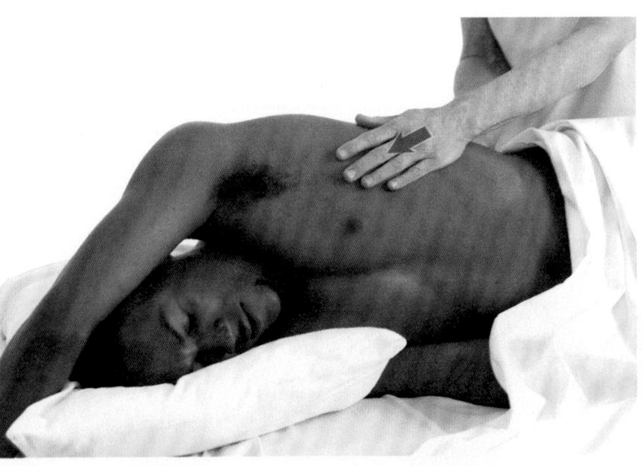

FIGURE 1-7 Directive fascial work

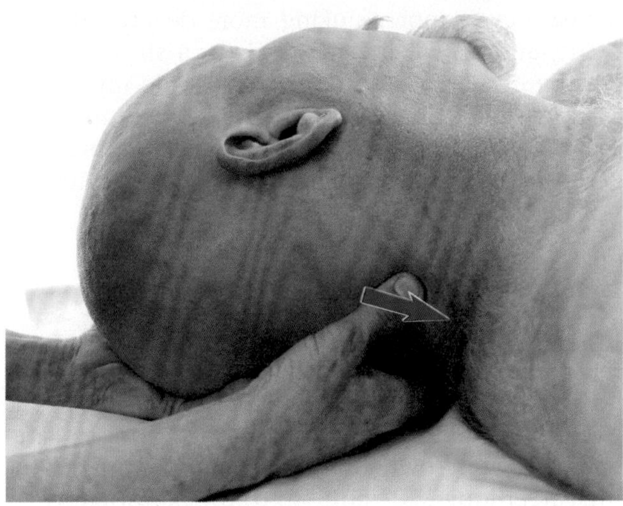

FIGURE 1-8 Neuromuscular therapy

- **Rolfing™, Hellerwork™,** and **CORE™ Myofascial Therapy** are other directive approaches to the reorientation of the fascia. The latter makes a point of working along Langer's lines, whereas the former two do not—and scientific proof that fascia can be "reoriented" is lacking. These descriptions are oversimplifications; therapists interested in learning more about these modalities will need to study them in greater detail. There have been a number of Rolf's former students and collaborators who have split from some part of her theories and/or protocols to create their own variations on her work—the "take what you like and leave the rest" approach.
- **Neuromuscular therapy** is a system of myofascial treatment in which the thumbs are the primary instruments used to engage the myofascial tissue (Fig. 1-8).

Treating the Fascia, Treating the Muscles

Myofascial work is often a helpful precursor to specific muscle treatment as it warms and stimulates the tissue. In the ensuing chapters on treatment, we recommend and describe specific myofascial techniques for the torso, where we feel it is especially important. However, the principles of myofascial treatment are easily transferred to other areas such as the limbs, and their application is helpful over the entire body.

Palpation is a skill that can be learned only by experience. Place your hand lightly on any broad surface of skin, and take a few moments to become aware of the skin. Then allow your pressure to increase slightly, and become aware of the tissue underneath the skin. Gently move the tissue back and forth with your hand, becoming familiar with the feeling of moving layers of tissue—the muscle and its covering of fascia. Now allow your pressure to increase even more, sinking more deeply into the tissue, and visualizing the fascia as a sheath covering the muscle tissue. Whenever you do myofascial work, take the time to engage the tissue in this conscious way. This is primarily *instinctive* and meant to call your attention to the fact that it is there; it's impossible to treat one without the other.

Body Mechanics

Before addressing specific treatment techniques, we must first consider the demands of the therapist's body and the safest and most effective ways to use it.

Body mechanics is the key not only to safeguarding your own body integrity and maintaining career longevity, but also to the performance of effective therapy. It consists entirely of the use of common sense with regard to the placement and movement of weight in relation to gravity. Clients will often ask, "Don't you get tired?" or "Don't your hands hurt?" If you have mastered good body mechanics, the answer will be no.

Just as massage therapy should take a holistic view of the client, the therapist must think of body mechanics in a holistic way. You do not work only with your thumb, your fingers, your hands, or even your body—you work with your whole self. Your approach to body mechanics, even though elements of it focus on a small area, must take your whole person into consideration, from your emotional attitude to the position of your thumb joints.

Weight and gravity are the foremost mechanical considerations in body mechanics. We take gravity so much for granted that we seldom give it much thought, leaving our relationship to it in the hands of unconscious behavior patterns established early in life as we were learning to walk. But some activities require a conscious awareness of gravity. Dancers, for example, must relearn their relationship to gravity. So should massage therapists because our work is largely based on the application of pressure, which is best accomplished through the application of our body weight. Therefore, the first principle of body mechanics is:

Use your body weight, rather than muscle force, to apply pressure.

Using your body weight requires less work. Using muscle strength to apply pressure in massage therapy quickly tires the therapist, particularly the local muscles used for the purpose. In addition, the use of weight applies a smoother pressure, lacking in tension, than the use of muscle force. When muscles sustain a contraction over even short periods of time, the process of recruitment and exhaustion at the tissue level results in an uneven pressure, which communicates a sense of tension to the client. To experience this difference, let someone apply pressure to the same part of your body, using the same point of compression (palm, thumb, knuckles, etc.) with muscle force and then with body weight. Observe the difference in sensation of the pressure.

You do, of course, use your muscles to stabilize your joints. One of the chief functions of muscles in the body is to stabilize joints, and when using your body weight to apply pressure in therapy, this stabilization becomes a key element in the overall process. Therefore,

Keep the joints through which your weight passes relatively straight (but not locked) and avoid hyperextension of your joints (Fig. 1-9).

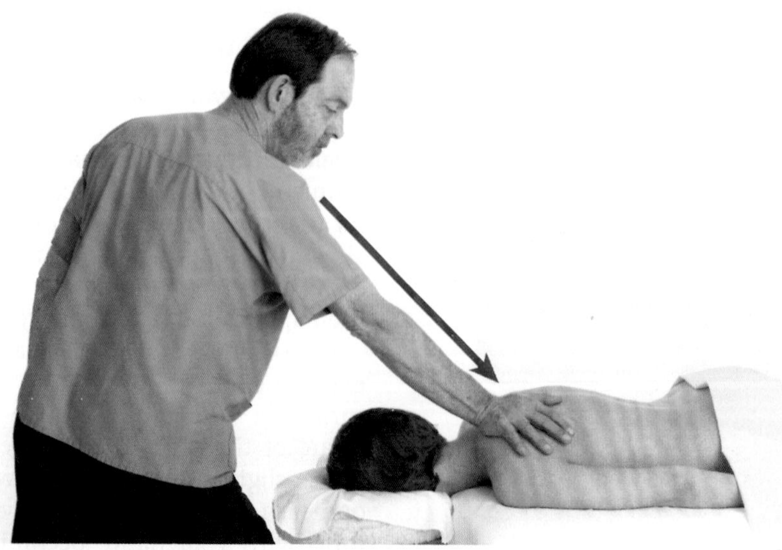

FIGURE 1-9 Avoid hyperextension of joints

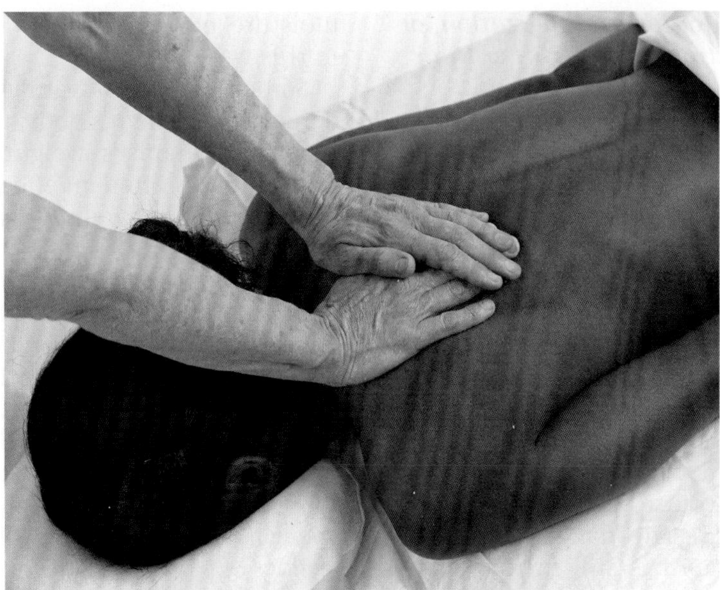

FIGURE 1-10 Supported pressure

If you apply weight through locked joints, then the effect is one of total rigidity, like a solid rod. Although the pressure itself should come from the body weight, the joints should retain the "softness" supplied by muscle stabilization rather than being mechanically locked into place. Hyperextension of joints stresses both the joint itself and the soft tissues that support and stabilize the joint. Use of muscle force in flexing the joint stresses the muscles themselves and communicates tension, as mentioned above. For example, it is known that carpal tunnel syndrome can be caused by repetitive hyperextension of the wrist, but in all likelihood the actual causal factor is the resulting stress on the soft tissues that control and stabilize wrist and finger movement. To avoid the tissue stress and muscle tension of both flexion and hyperextension,

Let your weight pass through as many joints, in a relatively straight line, as feasible.

The weight that applies the pressure should be as much in line with the joints as possible. The weight that is applied to the client's body is the weight of the therapist's torso, whereas the point applying pressure is usually some part of the hand or forearm. By lining up the joints between the torso and point of pressure, you maximize both the stability and "softness" of the pressure. Since the shoulder joint is the primary joint for transmitting weight from the torso to the arm and hand,

Keep your scapula (glenohumeral joint) rotated downward.

If the glenohumeral joint is rotated upward, the weight of the torso has to be communicated to the arm indirectly by pulling downward at the joint. If it is rotated downward, the torso is above and behind the joint and communicates the weight directly through the joints.

Support the body part applying the pressure whenever feasible (Figs. 1-10 and 1-11).

Supporting the thumb or fingertips of one hand with the other has two effects. First, it increases potential pressure, and, second, it stabilizes the joints involved to protect the hands from tissue strain.

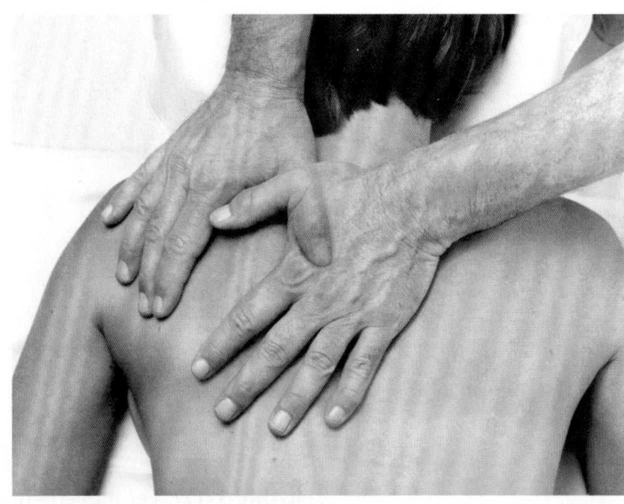

FIGURE 1-11 Supporting the thumb with the hand

Whether using muscles for force, stabilization, or movement, use larger, stronger ones rather than smaller, weaker ones.

For example:

Control your center of gravity with your legs; let movement come from your center of gravity and your legs rather than your arms (Fig. 1-12).

The use of the legs to control the placement and movement of one's weight saves the hands from doing all the work, provides leverage, and allows the weight of the torso to be supported in part by the client's body, and it suggests itself intuitively. The biggest danger, of course, lies in the possible loss of balance (Fig. 1-13). This danger is probably greatest when the therapist is still inexperienced and has not yet learned either the subtleties of body mechanics or the qualities of skin (texture, moisture, etc.) that affect the ability to work safely in this way.

Sometimes it is advantageous to work from underneath the client's body, using the client's, rather than the therapist's, weight to apply pressure. This positioning is often an effective way to work, but it must be applied carefully, as its body mechanics are more challenging.

For example, when working from underneath the neck of a supine client, you should be careful not to hyperextend the thumb. When working from underneath on the abdomen or pelvis of a prone client, the same care should be taken with the fingers. Since more muscles are used in these positions to apply force, and smaller muscles are used to stabilize joints, such work should not be done over an extended period. Also, you will need to be even more conscious than usual of feelings of pain or fatigue in your hands.

Sometimes it is advantageous to let your weight generate force through a part of your body other

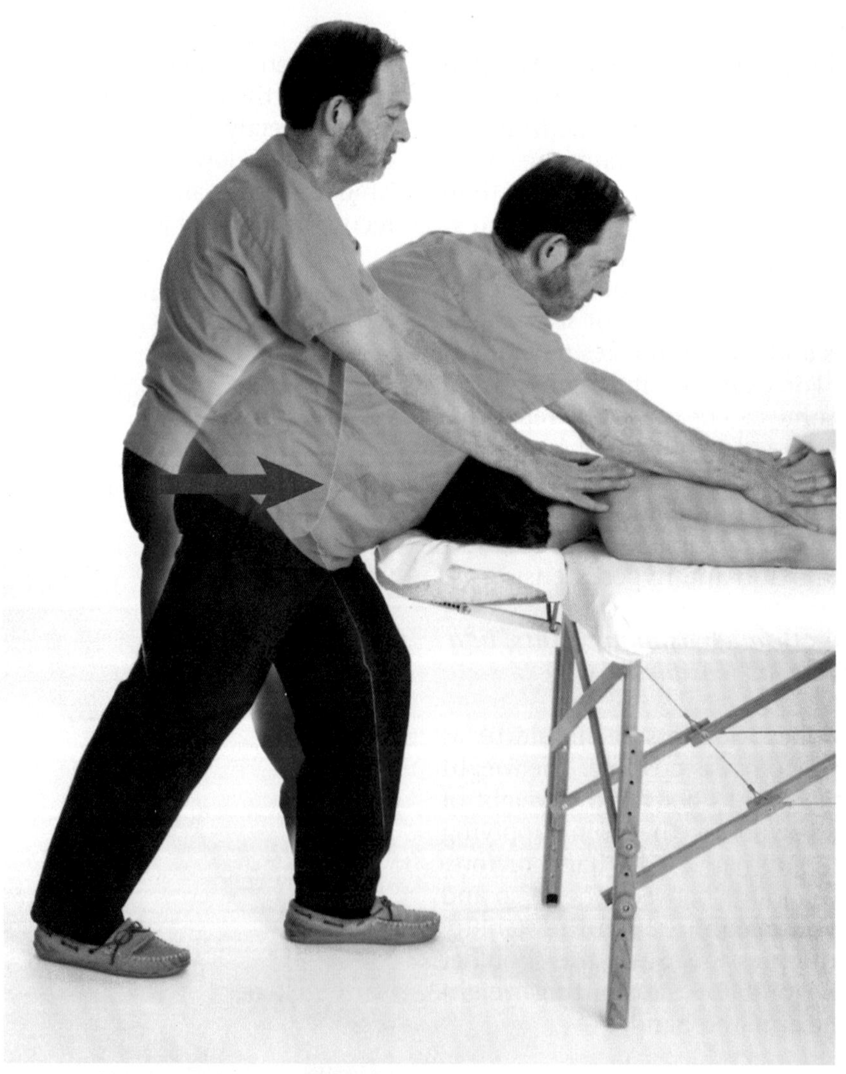

FIGURE 1-12 Let movement come from your center of gravity and your legs rather than your arms

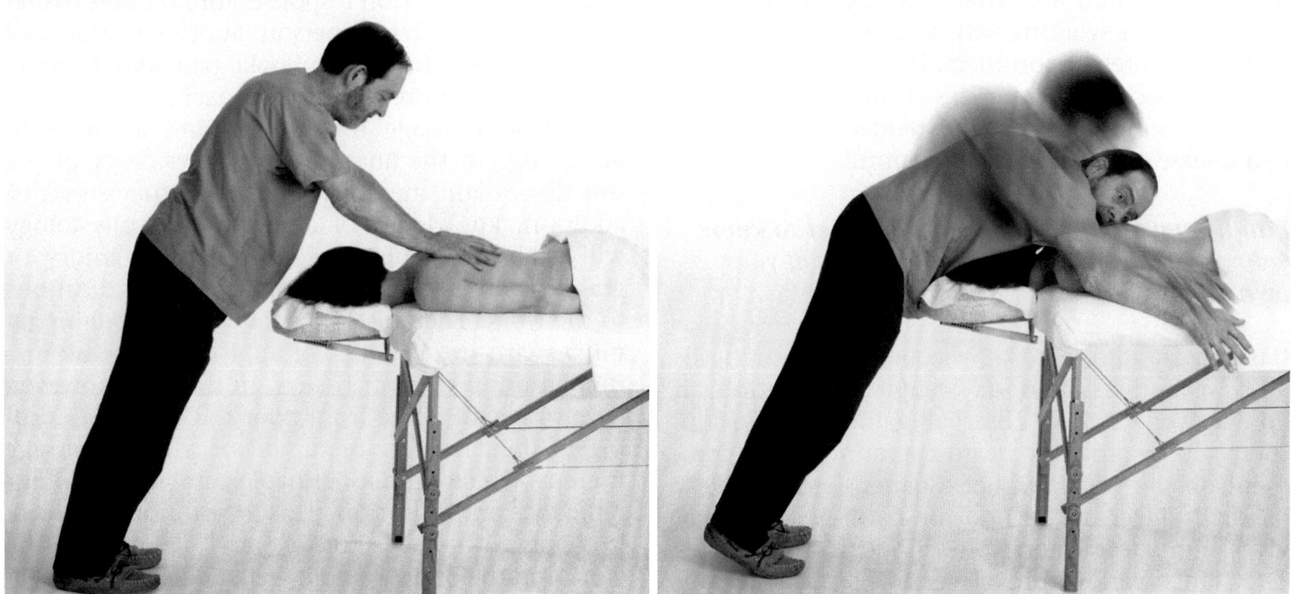

FIGURE 1-13 Comic/tragic consequences of losing your balance

than your shoulder. For example, you can nestle your elbow in your own iliac fossa (just inside your anterior pelvis) and lean into it to transmit force when working on a lateral area on the client's body (Fig. 1-14).

Move into, and out of, pressure slowly.

Slow movement is gentler and less jarring both to the client's tissues (and your own) and to the client's consciousness . . . the slower the movement, the deeper you can work without hurting the client. Moving slowly into and out of pressure also enables you to monitor the feedback of both your own and the client's body. If your work is not to be purely

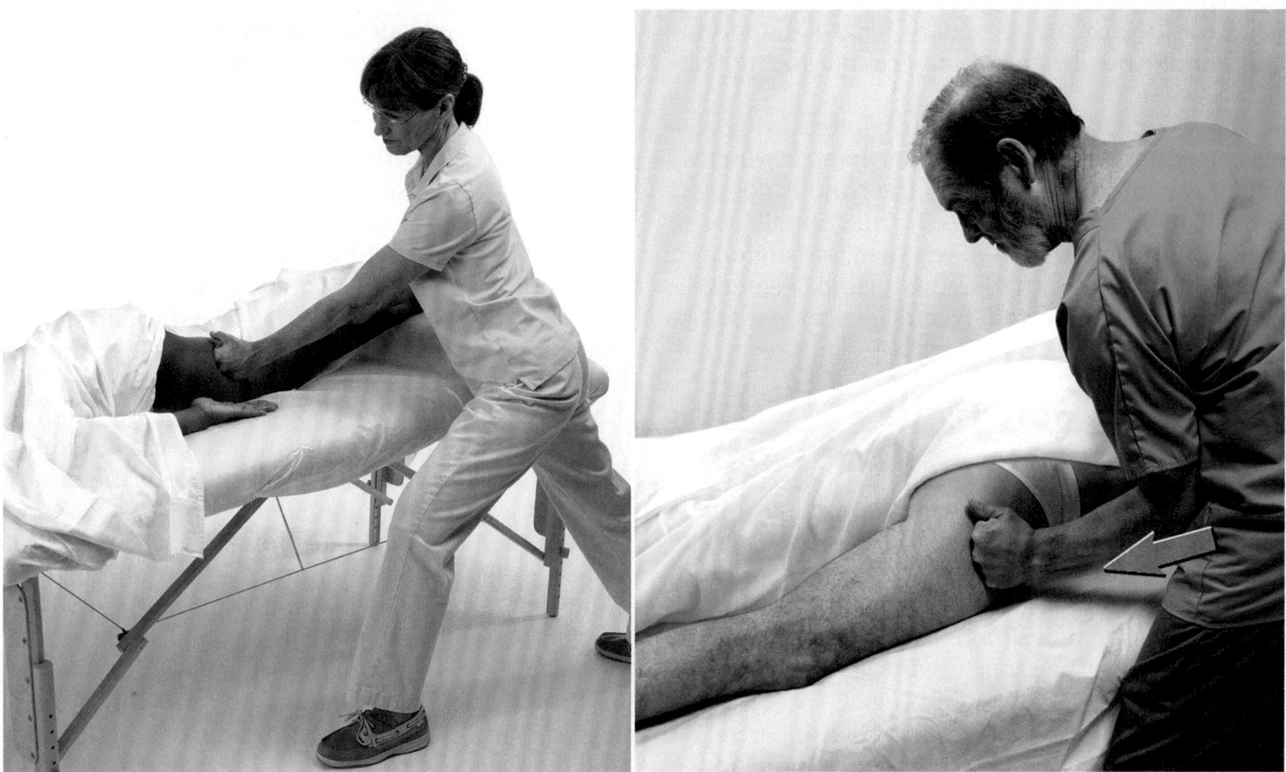

FIGURE 1-14 Transmitting weight through aligned joints or from the pelvis

mechanical, then it is vital that you focus on the tissues you are working with and take time to exert and release pressure on them. In addition, sensitive tissues (especially the muscles of the lumbar region) are often subject to rebound tenderness. The sudden release of pressure can be painful.

Finally, pay attention to your body. Get to know your own body, and use the mechanics of your own body.

It is important to get to know your body, its strengths and weaknesses, and its weight distribution. If you've ever watched a baseball game on television, then you've probably heard the announcers comment on the peculiarity of a batter's stance. Every baseball player has to find the batting stance that gives him the greatest control and hitting power. The stance varies from player to player, and your own application of body mechanics in therapy will be somewhat different from anyone else's, although the same general principles apply.

Although it may seem peripheral to body mechanics proper, one final point that needs to be mentioned here is the use of the secondary hand.

Use your secondary hand mindfully, not casually.

When one is not performing a two-handed stroke or using one hand to support the other, one hand is used to apply pressure or otherwise manipulate tissue. This hand is called the primary hand. Deciding what to do with the secondary hand is important and should not be made in a casual and unconscious way.

The secondary hand is often referred to by shiatsu practitioners as the "mother hand," which is an apt way of thinking of it. If the hand is not used actively to perform some specific function, it can be used to nurture the client. Even then, be careful and conscious of where the hand is placed. Remember to place each hand carefully and consciously before beginning to work.

Varieties of Soft-Tissue Manipulation

Remember the third basic premise of clinical massage therapy: *the soft tissues of the body respond to touch.* The touch may be extremely gentle or quite forceful; it may be moving or still; but touch, for reasons not yet understood, elicits a response from the soft tissues. If the touch is artfully applied, then the response can be one of healing.

The classical strokes used in Swedish, or relaxation, massage are quite effective in inducing a generalized relaxation response from the soft tissues and, thus, in the whole person. But the treatment of specific complaints of myofascial pain and dysfunction require a more specific approach.

Clinical massage therapy requires a thorough knowledge of the anatomy and physiology of the soft tissues and the bones and joints they serve. In addition, knowledge of anatomy and physiology will enable therapists to avoid causing injury or gratuitous pain and to recognize contraindications to the work. Therapists must also be thoroughly familiar with the varieties of approaches to the manipulation of the soft tissues. In the end, however, therapists will range from poor to brilliant according to their mastery of the *art* of clinical massage therapy, which is an indefinable combination of intelligence and intuition. This *art* cannot be forced; it comes with a sense of love and devotion to the work and the desire to do it well, and with time and practice, like learning to speak a foreign language, sing a song, dance, swim, or play tennis. It arrives when your therapy becomes more than the sum of its mechanical parts.

The purpose of this book is not to set forth a series of treatments of various muscles in a mechanical fashion, as one might write a manual for small engine repair. Its purpose is to help the student investigate the possibilities for manipulation of each muscle and explore the responses to such work. Just as each singer must discover, through practice, the optimum control of his or her own vocal chords, clinical massage therapists must continue to explore touching in a variety of ways, constantly evaluating the results of the touch by feeling and observation and feedback from the client—and not just during the "student" period, but throughout their careers.

The purpose of this section is to introduce you to some of the basic ways in which the soft tissues can be touched and manipulated for therapeutic benefit. The approaches and techniques in this section can be applied to a variety of muscles over the whole body. They will be referred to throughout the book as we deal with each specific muscle or muscle group. These techniques are by no means a comprehensive list of possible approaches to tissue manipulation. They are only the most basic techniques. Therapists will expand their repertoire as they study and gain experience.

The intention of the techniques used in clinical massage therapy is to eliminate pain and/or dysfunction in the tissue by inducing persistently contracted tissue to lengthen. The principal difference between the classic strokes used in Swedish massage and the tissue manipulations used in clinical massage therapy is that the former tend to be broader and more general, the latter more concentrated and specific. However, Swedish massage is essential to clinical massage. Using Swedish strokes at the beginning of a clinical massage session, or as a transitional technique when moving from one area of the body to another, serves the multiple purposes of getting the client used to the therapist's touch, helping them to relax, and warming the muscles for receiving deeper work. As a general rule, no matter what part of the body you massage, beginning with a few moments of effleurage strokes, followed by petrissage, and circular palmar friction before moving to the more specific muscle stripping and deep massage, benefits both client and therapist. After you've used deep techniques, applying effleurage, vibration, light percussion, and nerve strokes can help ease the client back into relaxation mode, particularly if the work you did may leave them a little sore.

The Art of Direct Tissue Manipulation: The "Tissue Dialogue"

The key to the art of tissue manipulation is sensitive palpation. Palpation should always be performed initially with the tips of the fingers or thumbs before compressive treatment is begun. One must palpate for the point of resistance in the tissue and then meet it with pressure. Sometimes the resistance will yield only to firm pressure, and sometimes to delicate pressure. *The therapist must gauge the willingness of the tissue to respond and adjust the pressure accordingly.* This mindful sensitivity to the tissue might aptly be called the "tissue dialogue" because the therapist, through palpation, negotiates with the tissue the pressure needed to accomplish release. This "dialogue" is the essence of the art of direct tissue manipulation.

All of these manipulative techniques can be used for both *still compression* and *gliding compression;* in fact, you should find yourself alternating between the two: moving through the tissue, and stopping where the condition of the tissue calls for it. It's also important to "dialogue" with the client. As the therapist on the "giving" end, we can't always accurately judge what the receiver might be experiencing, and each client has a different tolerance for both pain and pressure. Depending on the client's sensitivity to pain and pressure at any given time, pressure that feels fine to one client may be too painful for the next one. If you're asking clients to rate their pain on a scale from 1 to 10, whether that's before, during, or after the session, remember that is a subjective description—what one client considers a "5" may be what the next one considers a "9." Effective client communication is vital, and that includes the therapist's ability to discern nonverbal cues and body language. Some clients will suffer in silence rather than say the pressure is hurting them. Always be alert to any indications of discomfort from the client, and reiterate to them that they shouldn't hesitate to let you know if the pressure feels like too much. It's also important, during the intake interview to discuss with clients the possibility that they may experience soreness for a day or two after deep tissue massage, particularly if it's their first massage experience, and to remind them again postsession and reassure them that it's a normal response. Failing to do so could have the undesirable effect of their thinking you carelessly hurt them or made their original condition worse.

The Tools of the Therapist's Body

Depending on the area and purpose, different body parts of the therapist can be used to manipulate tissue.

THE HEEL OF THE HAND

The heel of the hand, or thenar and hypothenar eminences, can be used to apply a fairly broad compression. It is especially useful when used on larger muscles, such as leg muscles, gluteals, shoulders, or paraspinal muscles. It is also useful over large bony areas, such as the iliac crest. Set in motion, the heel of the hand compresses a relatively wide swath of tissue (Fig. 1-15).

When using the heel of the hand, avoid hyperextension of your wrist. Feel the tissue as you compress it, and be sensitive to tight, hardened areas. Use this information to determine whether another, more localized, stroke should be applied in certain areas.

THE FIST

Another way to apply broad compression is with the closed fist. A particular advantage is the ability to shift between broad compression applied with the full length of the proximal phalanges (the bones of the fingers) and more focused compression with the knuckles (the proximal interphalangeal joints). Again, avoid hyperextension of the wrist. Go slower over hypercontracted areas and negotiate depth of pressure and speed of motion with the tissue Avoid using bone on bone.

THE KNUCKLE(S)

The proximal interphalangeal joints, or knuckles, of the index and middle fingers can also be used for compression. Knuckles are helpful as an alternative to fingertips to avoid constant strain to the fingers and thumbs. The knuckles present a harder and less sensitive compressive surface than the fingertips, thus, the tissue should first be palpated with the

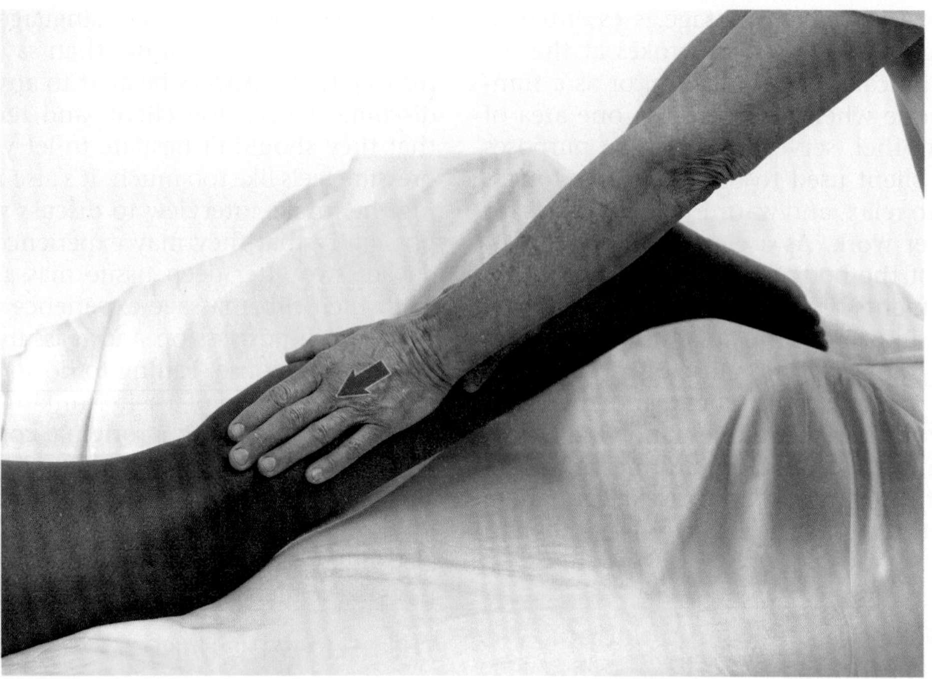

FIGURE 1-15 Moving compression with the heel of the hand

fingers before using a knuckle for compression. In sensitive areas, such as the face, neck, and ribs, fingertips are preferable to knuckles. Avoid using your knuckles on bony areas.

THE THUMB OR FINGERTIPS

Still or gliding compression using the tip of the thumb or finger is ideal for the treatment of small, concentrated areas, such as trigger points or other tender points. It is important to keep body mechanics in mind while applying pressure with the fingers and thumbs, as it can place a tremendous strain on the muscles of the hand and forearm, especially to points deep in the body, and even cause a career-ending injury. It is often wise to support the fingers or thumb with the other hand to help prevent hyperextension of the joints and provide additional pressure. Throughout this book, we will show the use of fingertips and thumbs, sometimes supported, sometimes not. In every case, the practitioner may choose whether to support the thumbs or fingertips according to her or his needs. The directions for muscle stripping in this book are based on using the thumb, but you may choose to use your fingertips, or in some instances, one of the muscle stripping or trigger point tools that now exist for massage therapists.

Remember to line up as many joints in as straight a line ("stacking the joints") as is feasible, and use your body weight, rather than muscular force, whenever possible. When it is not possible to use your body weight, as in approaching posterior neck muscles in the supine client, you should strive to line up several joints and pause and alternate hands frequently.

Although they may be used anywhere on the body, the thumbs and fingertips are used almost exclusively in some areas, such as the face, neck, axilla, abdomen, groin, and any internal work (permitted in only a few states), where the touch must be controlled and sensitive (Fig. 1-16).

THE ELBOW

The elbow–specifically the olecranon process of the ulna (the bony point of the elbow)–is an extremely useful tool for compression (Fig. 1-17). Its use has some caveats:

1. An extraordinary amount of force can be applied with the elbow; therefore, compression should be initiated slowly and applied gradually, with a great deal of attention to the client's responses.
2. The elbow is far less sensitive than the tips of the thumb or fingers. The tissues should be explored first with the fingers, and the elbow used primarily for compression once the need and location for deeper work have been established.
3. Use of the elbow should be avoided in highly sensitive areas, such as the face, neck, and groin, and over any bony areas.

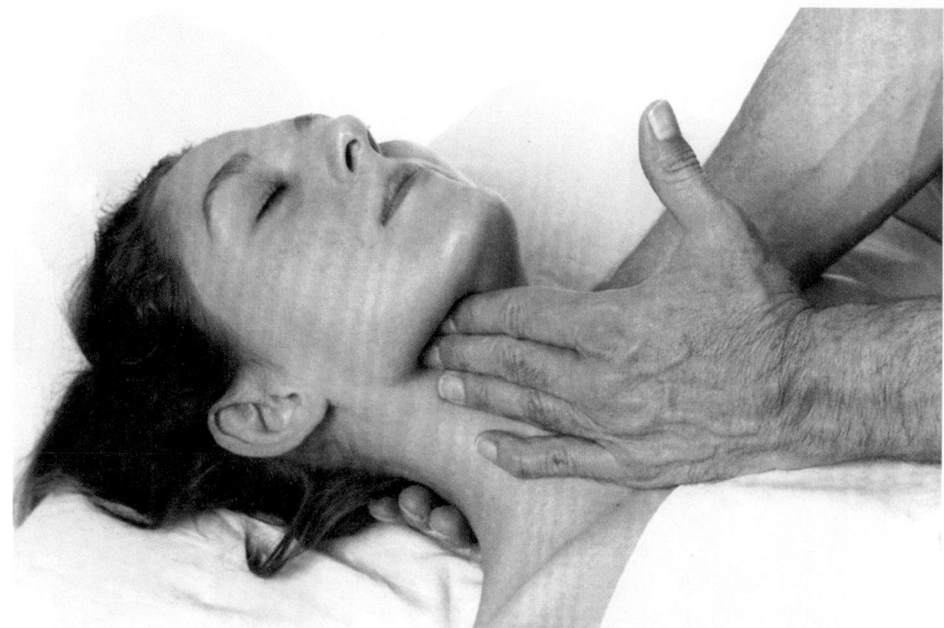

FIGURE 1-16 Use fingertips in sensitive areas

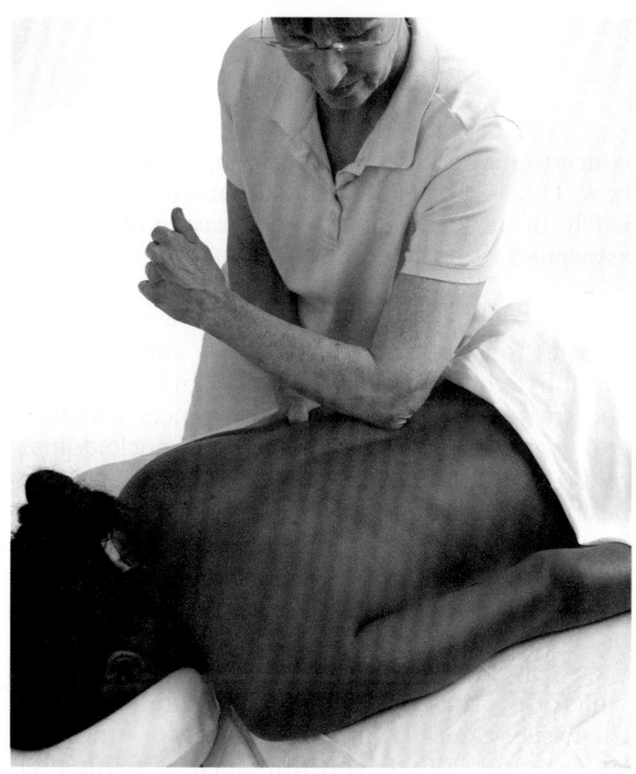

FIGURE 1-17 Using the elbow for compression

THE FOREARM

The ulnar aspect of the forearm provides a broad surface for deep, gliding compression (Fig. 1-18) of long, straight muscles, such as the erector spinae muscles and many muscles of the leg. Like the

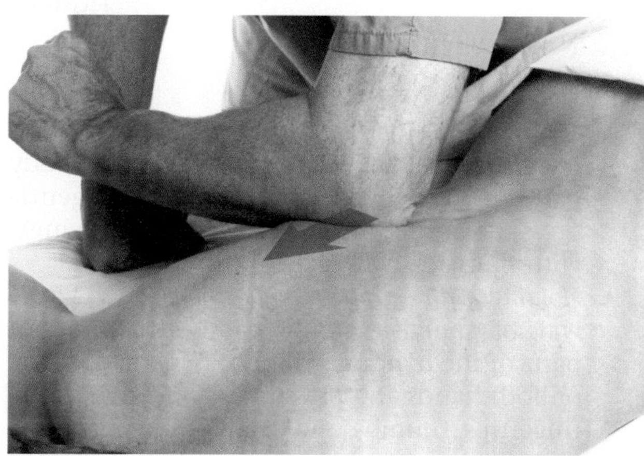

FIGURE 1-18 Using the forearm

elbow, it is comparatively insensitive; palpate the area before treating with the forearm.

Specific Treatment Techniques

HOLDING

The whole hand, or both hands, may be used to hold an area of the body. Several intentions and effects are possible with this approach:

- *Simple holding* can help the client acclimate to the therapist's touch, warm and nurture, and communicate intention. Holding a body part in one or both hands involves a physical warming effect and suggests relaxation to the client (Fig. 1-19).

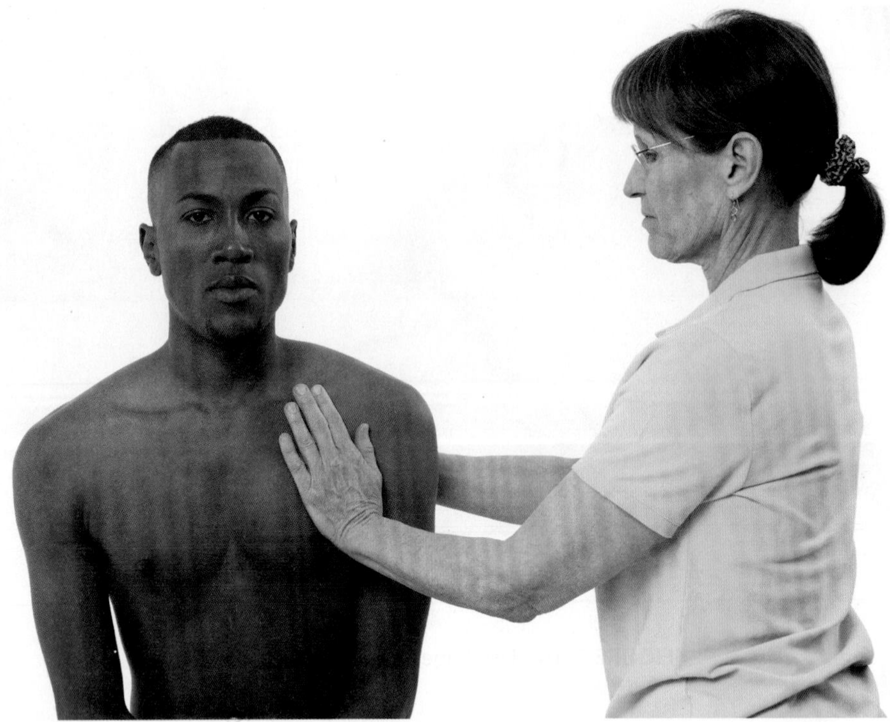

FIGURE 1-19 Holding

- *Intentional holding* suggests change. The body part is held in one or both hands with a gentle pressure in the direction of a desired change, with the slack being taken up as it occurs.
- *Holding with varying compressions* is a gentle way of applying compression with different parts of the hand. The body part is held in one or both hands and pressure is applied with the fingertips, thumbs, and heads of the phalanges and metacarpals, and possibly even squeezed in places, in varying patterns with varying pressure. These varying applications of pressure may also be combined with intentional holding. This "whole hand work" combines suggestion with an element of confusion that allows muscles to be caught "off-guard" and lengthen.

COMPRESSION

Compression consists of pressure exerted perpendicular to the surface of the muscle. Where underlying bone is present, the muscle tissue is compressed against the bone; otherwise, pressure is exerted against the resistance of the deeper structures of the body. Compression may be firm or light, as appropriate and tolerated by the client, and may be applied broadly by the entire hand (Fig. 1-20) or on a concentrated point by the thumb, fingertip, or elbow (Fig. 1-21). Pressure is maintained until release is felt, or until the client reports easing of the pain associated with the point.

PINCER PALPATION/COMPRESSION

Muscles that present a considerable amount of tissue above the surface of the body can be examined and treated very effectively with pincer palpation and compression. Examples are sternocleidomastoid (Fig. 1-22), pectoralis major, the portion of trapezius that lies on top of the shoulder, and the more proximal aspects of the hip adductors.

To perform this technique, grasp the tissue between the thumb and the tips of the first two or three fingers, or the outside of the bent index finger. Each then provides a firm surface against which the other can palpate and compress. Search the tissues carefully for trigger points or other sensitive points. When you find such a point, hold it until you feel it release, and then continue the search.

STRIPPING OR STRIPPING MASSAGE

This technique involves gliding pressure along a muscle, usually from one attachment to the other in the direction of the muscle fiber (Fig. 1-23).

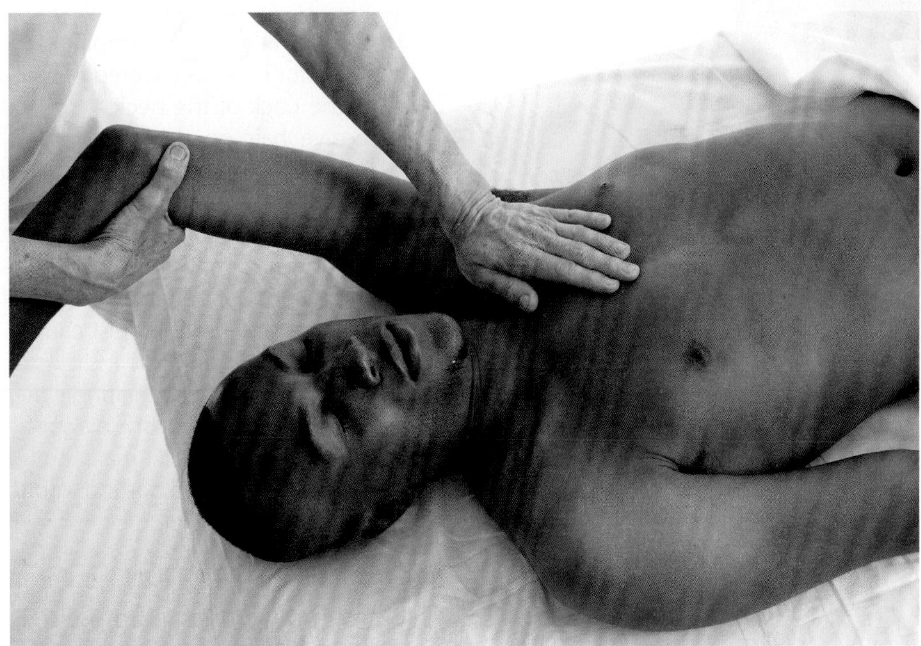

FIGURE 1-20 Broad compression with the hand

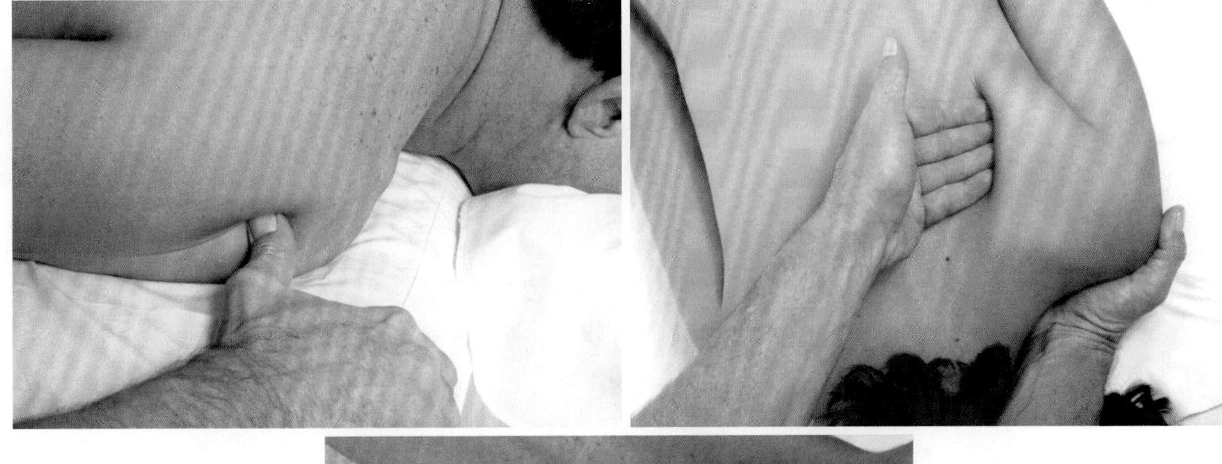

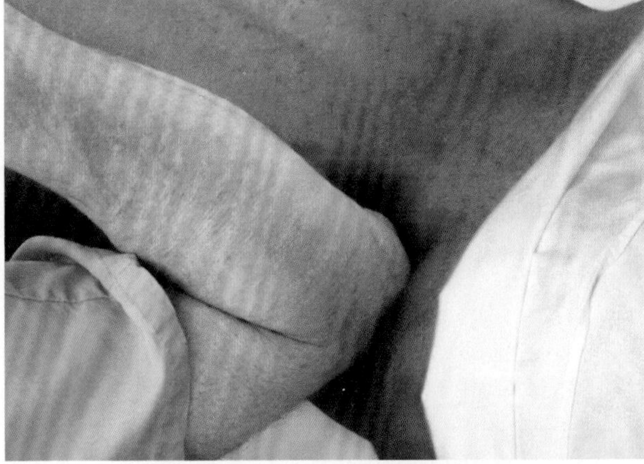

FIGURE 1-21 Focused compression

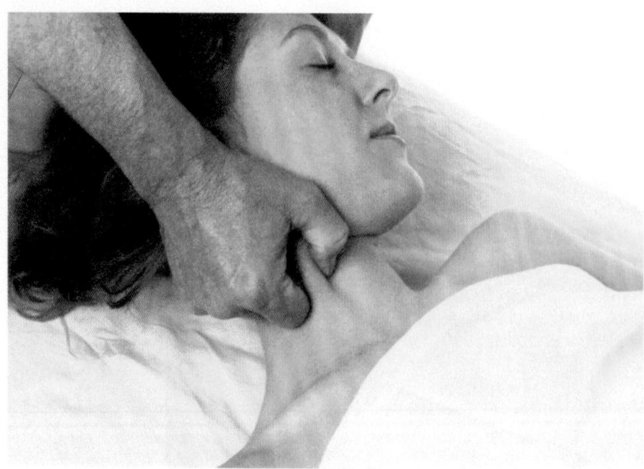

FIGURE 1-22 Pincer compression of sternocleidomastoid

CAUTION Stripping massage is often called for in areas covered in hair, such as the head, or the back of the neck. Also, some men have extensive hair on the chest, back, arms, and legs. Painful pulling of body hair is always a danger with stripping massage in these areas. Ask the client to tell you when such pulling occurs. A *small* amount of lubricant may be helpful. Deep-tissue creams and lotions are generally better for this type of work than are oils; the therapist cannot establish an "anchor" for stripping on a slick surface, so whatever you use, use it very sparingly. Remember to begin the session, or the work in a specific area, with a few moments of Swedish massage techniques to warm the muscles before getting into the deeper work.

CROSS-FIBER FRICTION

Persistently contracted muscle tissue, lesions in tendons or ligaments, and areas of fibrosis can be effectively treated with friction moving the fingertips, thumb, or elbow back and forth across the muscle perpendicular to the fiber (Fig. 1-24). This technique is most frequently performed on or near the attachment. The therapist should always bear in mind that

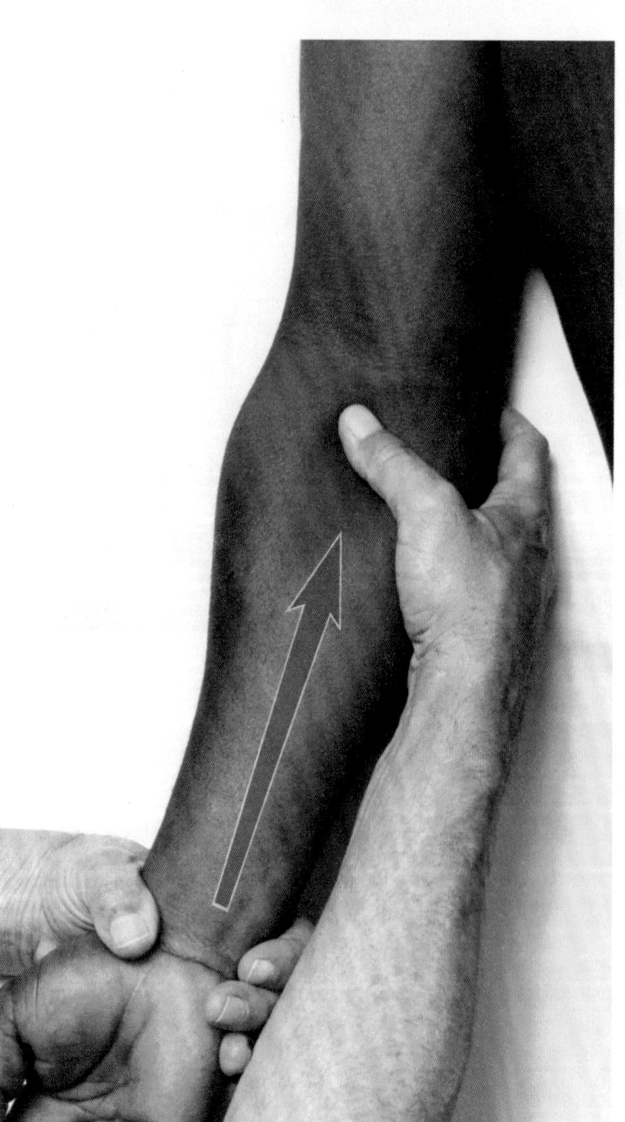

FIGURE 1-23 Stripping, or stripping massage

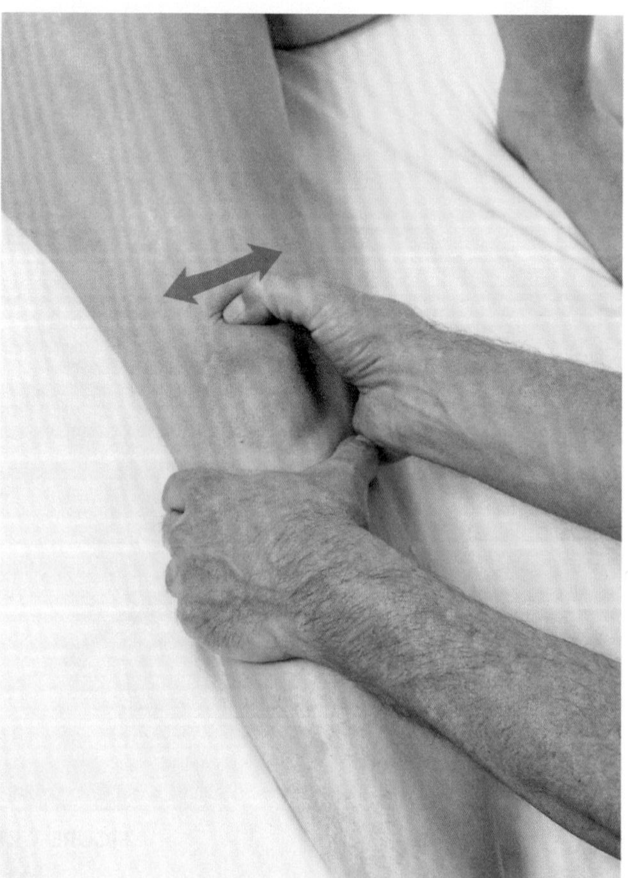

FIGURE 1-24 Cross-fiber friction

in order for the belly of a muscle to relax, the origin and insertion (attachments) must relax as well.

PASSIVE STRETCHING

Although trigger points may be treated directly with any of the above techniques, resolution of them requires passive stretching of the muscle as soon after treatment as possible. The therapist stretches the muscle by moving its attachments away from each other (Fig. 1-25). This technique requires an intimate knowledge of the anatomy of the joints involved and their range of motion.

Approach stretching with care.

Familiarize yourself with the range of motion of each joint, and move into the stretch slowly. Avoid any sudden movements or ballistic stretching. It is very easy to place a client in an uncomfortable position (Fig. 1-26). Postsession, clients may find that it extends the benefits of their massage to do active stretching on their own between sessions.

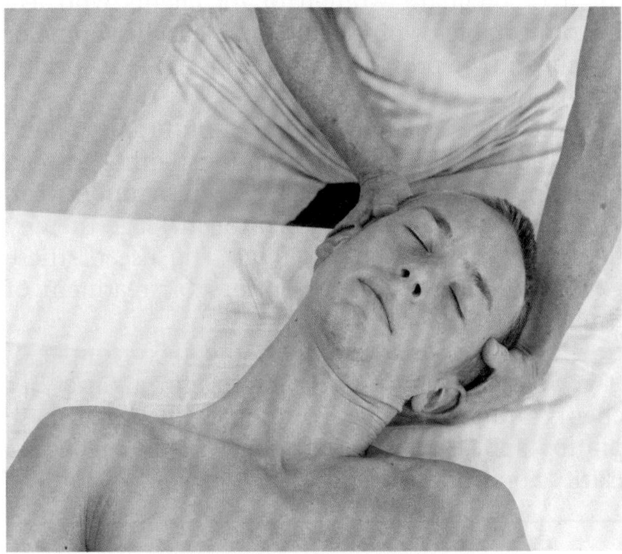

FIGURE 1-25 Passive stretching

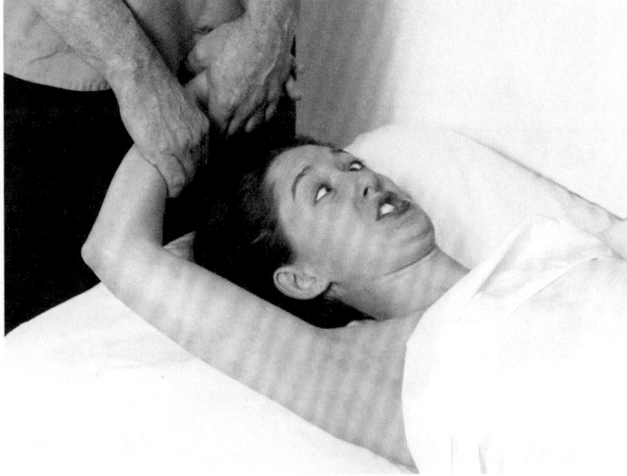

FIGURE 1-26 Unfortunate passive stretching

Most of the manual therapy descriptions in this book are of stripping massage and compression, with a few examples of cross-fiber friction and stretching where such techniques seem particularly appropriate. These descriptions should be taken as examples and starting points, not as an exhaustive repertoire. Each student should experiment with them, as well as with other possibilities not illustrated.

Tables

Students of massage therapy will certainly be familiar with standard massage tables. The most popular tables are portable and can be adjusted in height between clients. Therapists generally set the table height according to their own height and the type of work they plan to do. Clinical massage therapy, however, makes special demands. The optimum table height may vary according to the type of work being done and the size and position of the client. You may use several different treatment approaches in a session, and place the client in several different positions. To accommodate this flexibility in treatment, the ideal solution is an adjustable electric table. A wide variety of such tables are available, either mechanical or pneumatic: prices vary widely as well. These tables are considerably more expensive than a standard portable table, but the investment is well worthwhile, since it enhances both the quality of the work that can be done and the comfort and health of the therapist.

Draping

Most examination and treatment in massage therapy and bodywork require some exposure of the body. Therefore, we need to consider ways of respecting the client's feelings of privacy and modesty, while still accomplishing the therapeutic goal. *Draping* is the term commonly used for the covering of the parts of the client's body that are not being examined or treated. The term originated in the art world, where it referred to the drapery of the subject of a painting or sculpture. In the last century, it came to be used in photography as well, and from that field was adopted by the medical profession.

The codes of ethics and standards of practice of national massage organizations vary somewhat, but all require diligent consideration of the client's feelings of comfort, safety, privacy, and modesty. Although these requirements are clear about the need to consider the client's sense of privacy and modesty, they are not specific in describing precisely what draping is to be used. Therapists, therefore, have the responsibility to determine the best ways to meet these requirements in their own clinical settings with regard to each individual client.

In addition to requirements of professional organizations, therapists must also consider the laws of the jurisdictions in which they practice. In states where massage therapy is licensed, a board normally issues guidelines for the conduct of practitioners. These guidelines often contain more or less specific provisions regarding draping of clients. Some guidelines, for example, specifically permit the temporary uncovering of buttocks or female breasts with the consent of the client in order to apply treatment, whereas others may specifically prohibit such exposure. In states that do not have licensure, laws may exist either at the state or local level that restrict the practitioner's conduct in some way. Therapists must, therefore, take the responsibility for investigating the laws and guidelines that govern their practices. In the handful of states that are still unregulated, there are no laws governing draping—but practicing professionally and ethically mandates that you use proper draping techniques anyway, even if it is not required by law.

Early in the chapter we saw that clinical massage therapy is the result of the coalescence of traditional massage, osteopathic and other techniques, and the bodywork heritage of Wilhelm Reich and Ida Rolf. In traditional massage, the client normally lies prone or supine on a table, with private areas of the body covered by a towel or sheet. Each area is uncovered by the therapist as necessary for treatment. In the bodywork tradition, the emphasis is on the structure of the body as a whole. For that reason, clients are first observed while standing, usually in underwear. Most schools of massage therapy teach conservative, traditional draping techniques and require that these techniques be used when practicing massage therapy in the school setting. As therapists move beyond basic Swedish massage, however, they are likely to need more flexibility in methods of draping to perform the variety of techniques for examination and treatment available to them.

Therefore, depending on the approach, the therapist, the client, and applicable regulations, the client may wear underwear or not, be covered by a sheet or towel, wear an examination gown, or any combination of these choices. With the understanding that both therapists and clients vary widely in their needs, we will present a variety of illustrations of suggested draping for the examination and treatment of each area of the body. We show the basic techniques of draping clients with sheets in supine and prone positions. In conjunction with the technique for draping female breasts for abdominal massage, we show a way of arranging the drape for treating the chest muscles. We also show techniques for draping clients in a side-lying position. This position is well suited for performing certain techniques. It is also appropriate for the general treatment of pregnant women or for clients who feel uncomfortable or physically unable to lie supine or prone, and we provide illustrations for that specific situation.

Some therapists may find it helpful to use an examination gown in some situations, either instead of or in addition to a sheet, towel, or underwear. The most versatile such gown for massage therapy unfastens across each shoulder. The use of these gowns is illustrated as an option for treatment of some areas.

The images below and on the next couple of pages demonstrate proper draping for a variety of clients and techniques. Thumbnail images of these photos appear throughout the text as needed to clarify appropriate draping.

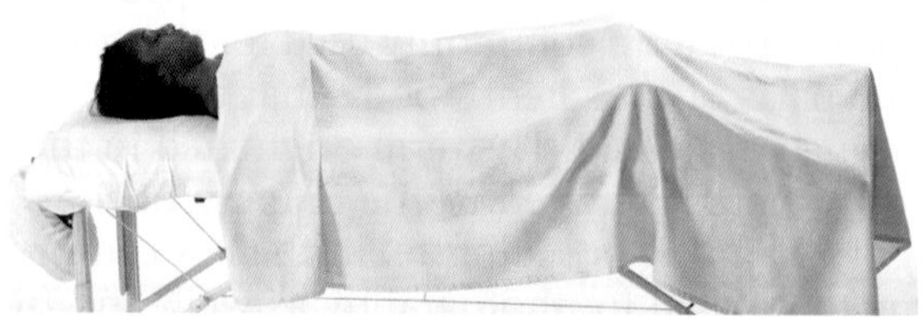

1: Head and neck

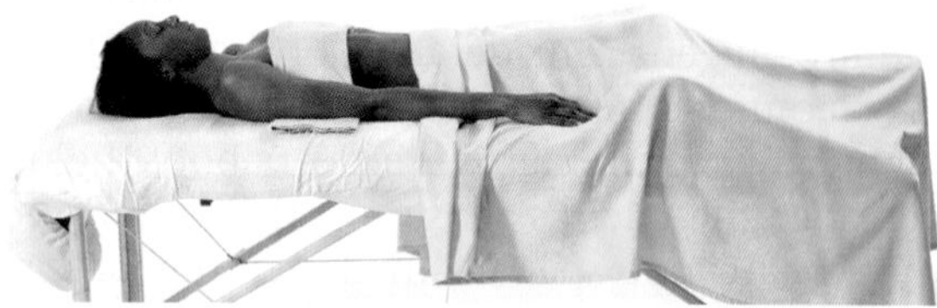

2: Abdomen

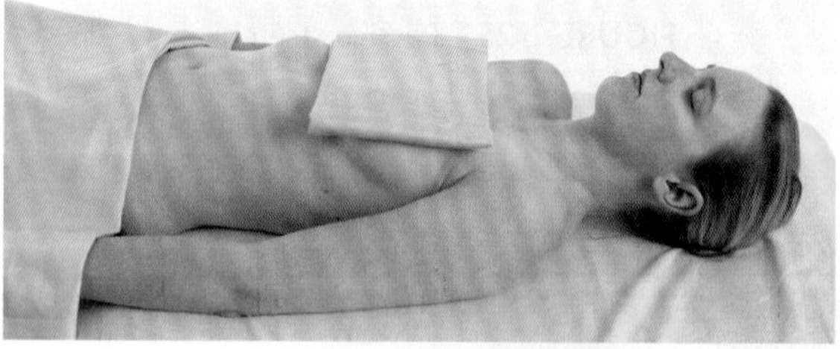

3: Chest muscles

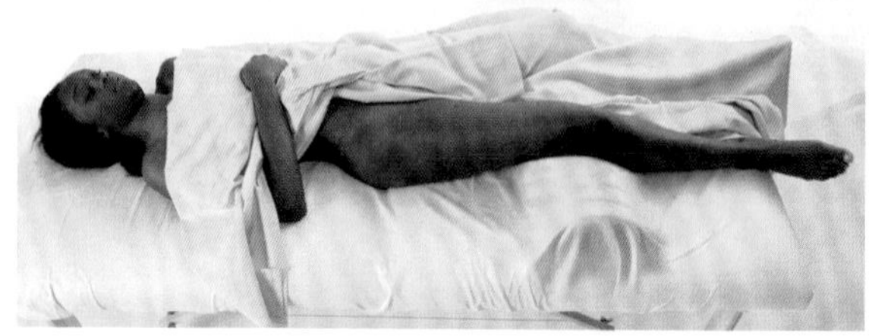

4: Groin and lower abdomen

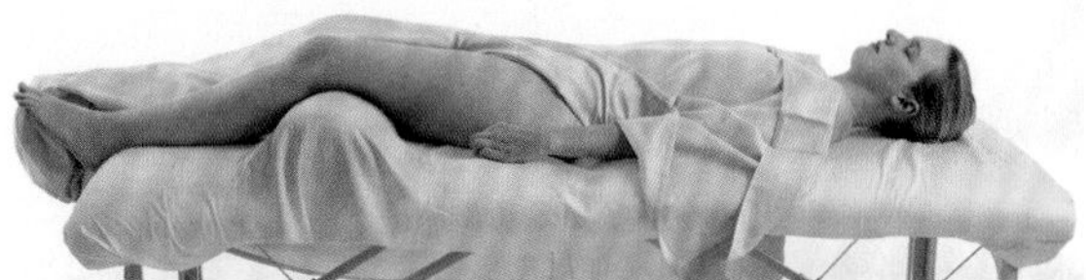

5: Anterior leg

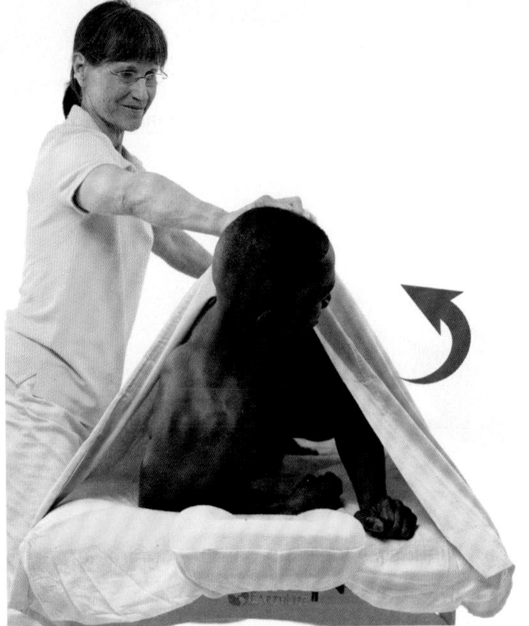

6: Turning the client

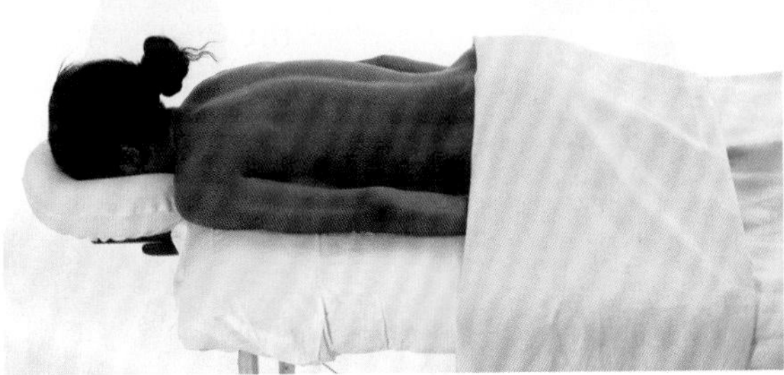

7: Back

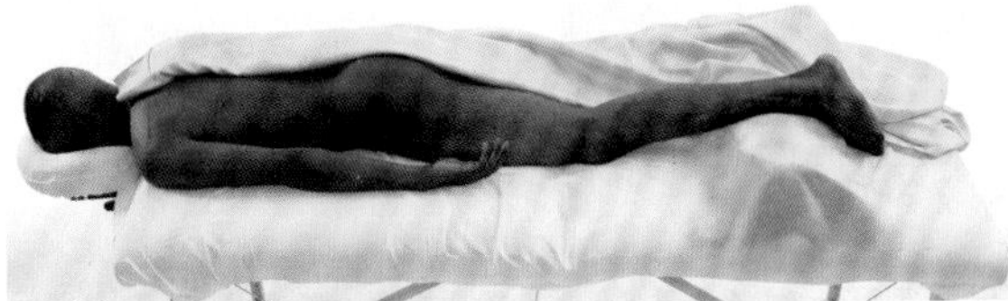

8: Between buttocks

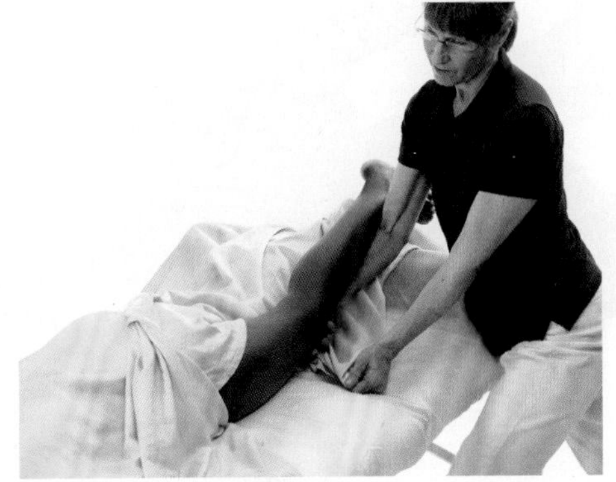

9: Positioning the sheet under the leg

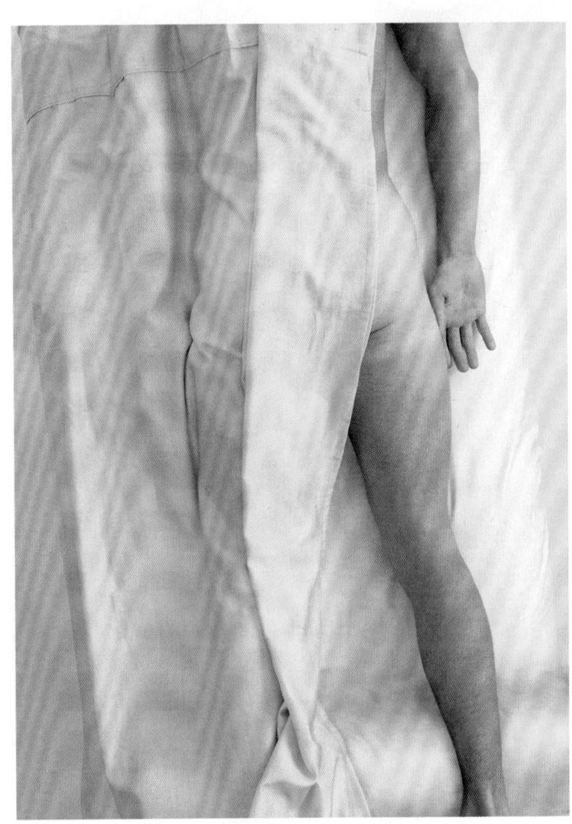

10: Posterior leg and buttock

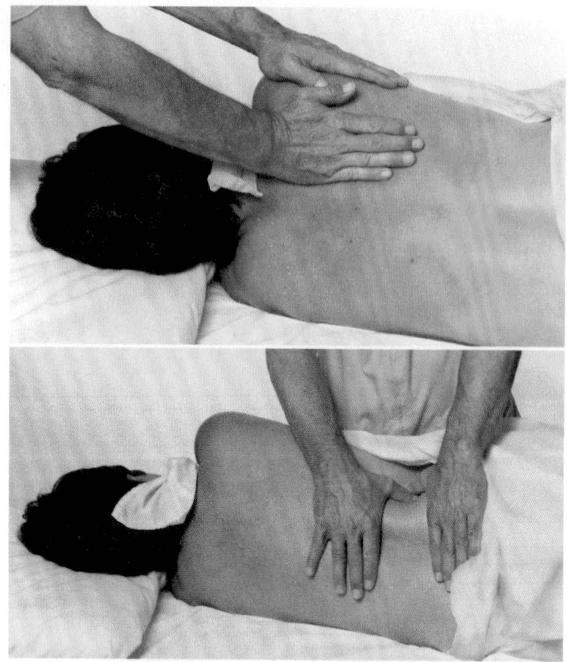

11: Sidelying: shoulder and back (pregnant client)

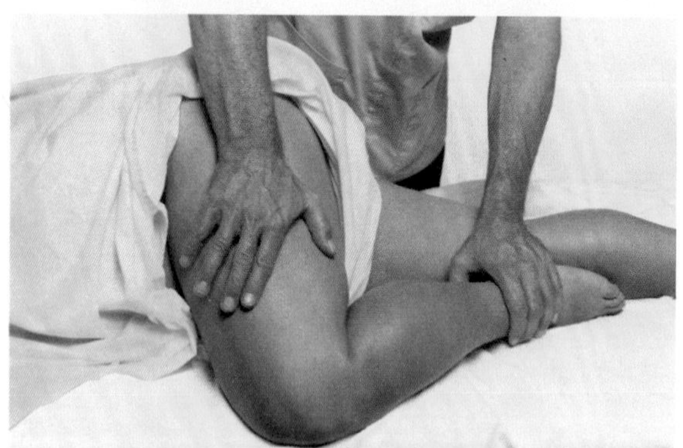

12: Sidelying: thigh (pregnant client)

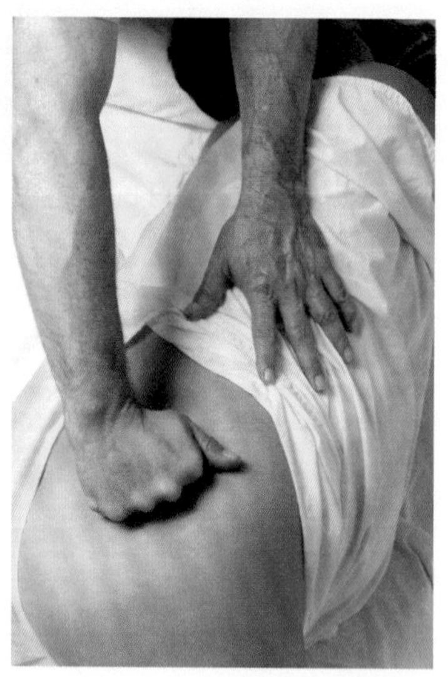

13: Sidelying: buttock (pregnant client)

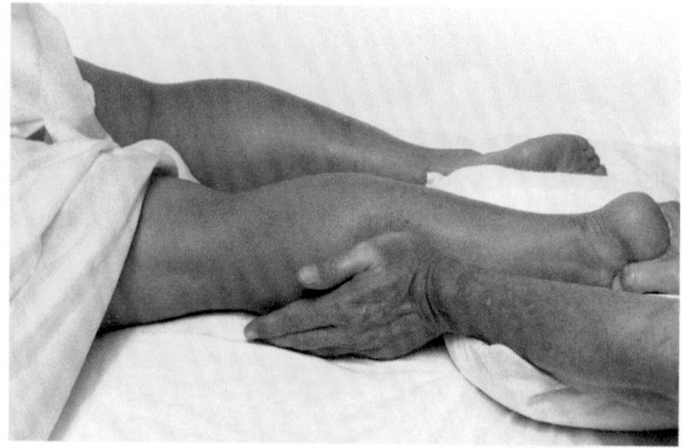

14: Sidelying: lower leg (pregnant client)

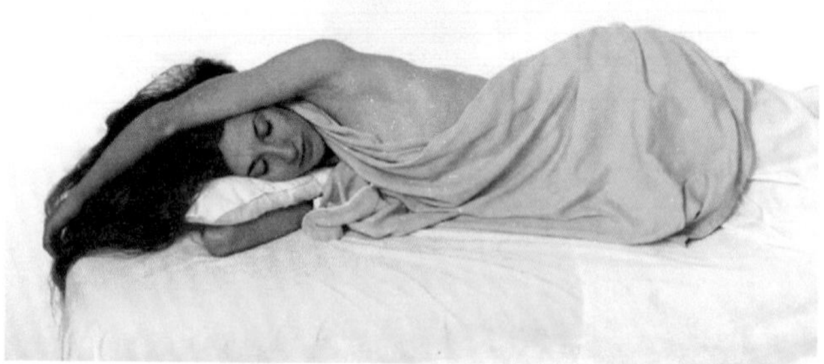

15: Sidelying: shoulder and chest (examination gown)

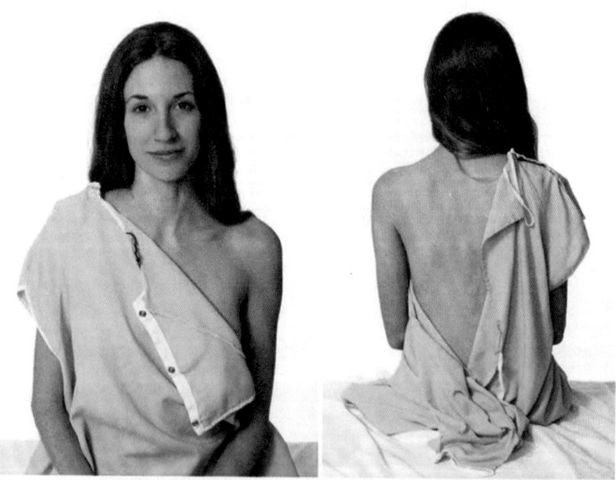

16: Sitting: shoulder and chest (examination gown)

CHAPTER REVIEW

PUTTING THEORY INTO PRACTICE

Use a clean drape for each client. Be careful not to inadvertently touch the client improperly when arranging the drape around the breasts and pelvic areas. Even when applying massage to the breasts or pelvic area, care should be taken to safeguard the client's safety, sense of security, and comfort when draping. Keep it as modest as possible by only exposing what is absolutely necessary to the work.

QUESTIONS FOR REVIEW

1. Compare the tendency, during the evolution of massage, for it to be seen as only accessible to the wealthy, with the view today that is more accessible to everyone as a part of regular health care. How would you describe massage so that a potential client would consider it as part of a regular wellness plan?
2. Choose a condition such as low back pain or other muscular ailment, and list the possible reasons that a physician would choose to prescribe drugs and/or physical therapy instead of massage therapy for treatment. If you were the patient, what would you say to the doctor to persuade him to include massage therapy in your treatment?
3. What are the differences in tender points and trigger points? What are the similarities?
4. List five functions that fascia performs.
5. Why does a client need to be draped? How would you handle a client telling you he/she doesn't want to be draped?

thePoint Additional helpful resources are available at http://thePoint.lww.com.

CHAPTER 2

Approaching Assessment

LEARNING OBJECTIVES

At the conclusion of this chapter, the learner will be able to:

- Describe the components of a clinical assessment.
- List appropriate questions for an intake form and client interview.
- Perform a whole-body assessment.
- Document assessment data.
- Synthesize the findings in order to formulate a treatment plan.
- Effectively communicate with clients.
- Apply the synthesis and subsequent plan to the treatment session(s).
- Effectively communicate with other health care professionals.
- Explain the considerations of working with special populations such as pregnant women, the elderly, and children and adolescents.

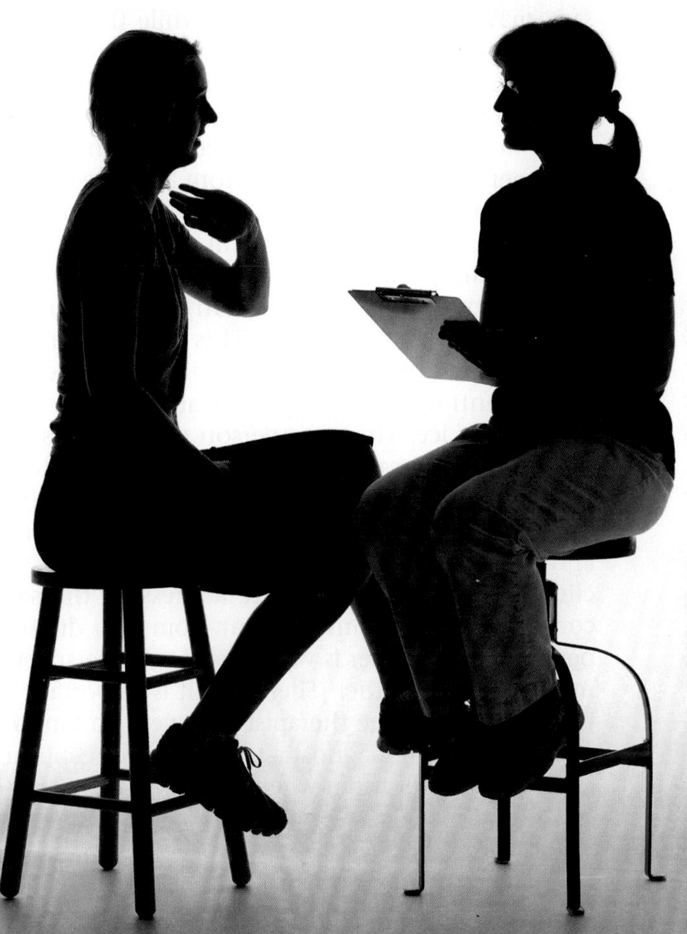

The most important thing in communication is hearing what isn't said.

Peter Drucker

Introduction

The purpose of any system of clinical assessment is to gather information that will allow the therapist to set up a treatment plan that will result in the best outcome for the client, taking into account any pathology, dysfunction, and contraindications to therapy. As this book is about deeper, more intense massage than basic Swedish massage, the therapist has to exercise additional caution concerning contraindications. An example is the client with cancer who may be undergoing radiation or chemotherapy. Whereas a lighter relaxation massage may be fine for them, a deep massage may make them feel worse while they are still receiving treatment. As radiation can cause brittleness of the bones, that should be considered as well.

The term *clinical massage therapy* is more accurate than *medical massage therapy* because clinical massage therapists view the body from a perspective different from that of the physician. We do not treat conditions according to medical diagnostic criteria, but according to clinical massage therapy assessment criteria. For example, a physician might diagnose a patient as having tendinitis. This diagnosis implies an inflammation of a tendon, indicating a prescription for anti-inflammatory medication, rest, and application of ice. The same person might be assessed by a clinical massage therapist as having persistently contracted muscle tissue with referred pain from trigger point activity, indicating deep tissue therapy and trigger point compression. The physician and clinical massage therapist are addressing the same complaint in the same patient from two different perspectives. Neither is wrong, and each perspective may inform the other. Therefore, it is important for the clinical massage therapist to develop a familiarity with medical diagnostic terms and concepts and learn to consider them when assessing the client.

ETHICAL CAUTION

There's a fine line between assessing and diagnosing. Diagnosing is outside the scope of practice of massage therapy, but clients sometimes view massage therapists as medical authorities and will ask questions such as "Do I have carpal tunnel syndrome?" That is not for us to say. An appropriate response might be "Massage therapists are prohibited from diagnosing. You seem to have some of the same issues as some of my other clients that have been diagnosed with that, but you should see your doctor for a diagnosis."

The first priority in relaxation (Swedish) massage is the client's comfort. Within appropriate limits, the wishes and personal preferences of the client take precedence, and the objective is to give the client a pleasant and relaxing experience. The first priority in clinical practice, however, is to offer effective treatment, with all procedures subject to the informed consent of the client. Clear and effective communication is vital. If a client who is in pain and/or experiencing limited range of motion asks for a "light" massage and you feel that deeper work is called for, you definitely should explain your reasoning to them, including the fact that they may feel some discomfort both during and after session. People will sometimes endure a little bit of pain in order to get a lot of relief, but we can't make that decision for the client. Some people may be too sore to tolerate it, and we should never insist on someone going beyond their tolerance level just because we believe that it is therapeutically appropriate.

The first step in treating clients effectively is to correctly identify the areas that need treatment. For this reason, a systematic and intelligent approach to examination and assessment is essential in clinical massage therapy.

Good assessment requires that we look for the following:

- Patterns of misuse
- Postural imbalances
- Shortened postural muscles
- Weakened muscles
- Problems in specific muscles and other soft tissues, such as trigger points, tender points, and areas of persistent shortening
- Restrictions in joints
- Dysfunctional patterns in coordination, balance, gait, respiration

The epigraph to this chapter, "The most important thing in communication is hearing what isn't said," emphasizes the comprehensive nature of effective examination in clinical massage therapy. The body is a system of interdependent elements, and all of those elements must be considered when determining how to solve problems of pain and dysfunction. The body may tell us what the client fails to mention.

The primary methods used to gather information about a client's problem include taking the client's history (both written and oral), observing the client informally, performing a posture analysis, formally observing or measuring certain activities, and manually examining the tissues. Even looking at the wear patterns on a client's shoes can give you important information, such as whether the client is everting or inverting the feet. It is important to remember that examination and assessment do not end in the initial session; it is an ongoing process. This constant reexamination and reassessment is a particular feature of clinical massage therapy, since the hands-on nature of the work involves sensory feedback that regularly informs the direction of treatment.

Client History

Designing a Form for Client Information

Practitioners usually need to gather certain client information for business purposes, such as the client's name, address, phone number, and so on. This information is most easily acquired by having clients fill out a form at the initial visit. It can also be helpful to use the same form to gather information about the client's circumstances and history. The form can serve as a starting point for the gathering of more information in the history interview.

In designing a form, think about what information is best obtained in writing and what information requires a more personal, in-depth exploration. Personal data, family information, occupation, and names of primary health care practitioners (or current specialists) are best acquired on a form. These items are fairly easy to decide on.

It is more difficult to decide, however, what to ask about health history on a form. On the one hand, it is best not to leave all health history to the interview, because it is too easy to digress and overlook important issues. On the other hand, an overly lengthy and complicated history questionnaire may seem tedious and irrelevant. The object is to compose a form that is succinct, yet accounts for most possibilities.

Keep in mind, if it isn't relevant to the therapy, *it doesn't belong on the intake form*. As massage therapists, we need to know the client's contact information and their health data. We need to know medical conditions they are diagnosed with, lest there be any treatment contraindications or cautions for massage. We need to know what medications the client is taking; sometimes the contraindication or caution to treatment is not because of the condition, but because of the drug(s) being used to treat it. We need to know about any recent surgeries, any skin conditions, allergies, or sensitivities they may have, and if there are any areas the client would like for us to avoid touching. Therapists often unintentionally go outside their scope of practice or violate the client's privacy by asking questions that have no bearing on the massage during the intake. For example, it is appropriate to have "stress" as one of the conditions listed on your form that the clients may check off if they are suffering from it. However, when it is presented in the form of a question such as "Does your family (job, relationship) cause you stress?", it becomes invasive and inappropriate. It isn't necessary to the massage for you to know how many children a person has or their ages. It's better to ask if they are a caretaker for anyone. Unless you are filing insurance, taking on a personal injury case on a contingency basis, or obtaining a contact for emergency purposes, you don't need to know information about the person's spouse. There is a fine line between gathering necessary information and being overly inquisitive about their personal life. Asking people to describe their diet is inappropriate, unless you also happen to be educated and licensed as a nutritionist or dietician—and even then, it is none of your business unless the client is visiting you for those services. Asking any questions about their religion, whether or not they have ever suffered any abuse, what their annual salary is ... the list of inappropriate questions just goes on, so repeat: *If it doesn't have any bearing on the massage, you shouldn't be asking..*

In the event you are filing insurance or keeping/filing any electronic records, your forms must be **HIPAA** (Health Insurance Portability Accountability Act) compliant, filed over a secure connection, and the client's personal information and privacy safeguarded—and it should always be safeguarded in any case, even if your type of practice is not subject to HIPAA laws. Complete information about HIPAA is available on the website of the Department of Health and Human Services at http://www.hhs.gov/ocr/privacy/index.html. HIPAA privacy notices and HIPAA-compliant forms may be obtained at any medical supplier and many office supply stores.

In addition to the form itself, clients may be given a drawing of the human form on which they can mark the areas where they are feeling pain or have felt pain recently. On the following sample form, this information is sought in words both on the form itself (Fig. 2-1) and on the accompanying figures (Fig. 2-2). This duplication serves as a double check to make sure all the possibilities are covered. You may find a form that suits your purposes from a massage software or medical supply company. Some of the online scheduling companies that cater to massage therapists provide intake forms.

Another helpful assessment tool is an index called Activities of Daily Living (ADL), commonly used by physicians and insurance companies to find out exactly to what extent a condition is interfering with the client's life. There are copyright-free forms readily available on the Internet for assessing back pain, neck pain, and extremity pain. These cover such activities as working, sleeping, reading, driving, lifting, bending, getting up and down, exercising, and so forth, that can give a detailed insight into what level of pain and dysfunction the client is suffering.

Remember that clients have their own points of view. They may consider the information to be irrelevant that we see as important, and not think to mention it—especially if it is a condition they have lived with for a long time; dysfunction becomes almost commonplace to them. It is our job to collect all the data that we may need for our purposes while clarifying the relevance of these data to the client.

INFORMATION FORM

Name: ______________________ Height __________ Weight __________

Address: ____

Home phone: ________ Work phone: ________ Cell phone: ________ E-mail: ______________

Date of birth: ______________ Sex: M F Living status: Coupled Uncoupled

How did you hear of The Pain and Posture Clinic? ______________________

Emergency contact
Name: ______________________
Relationship: ______________________
Phone: ______________________

History of injuries, illnesses and/or surgeries:

Regular physical activities/sports:

Circle any of the following that you have or have had within the past year:

PAIN: Headaches Back Chest Abdomen Hip Leg
Shoulder Neck Arm Pelvis Groin
Buttock

DISORDERS: Digestion Cramps Seizures Asthma Fibromyalgia/CFS
Scoliosis Depression Anxiety

Other: ____

Present medications: ____

Family or general physician: ____

Specialist: ____

FIGURE 2-1 Intake form

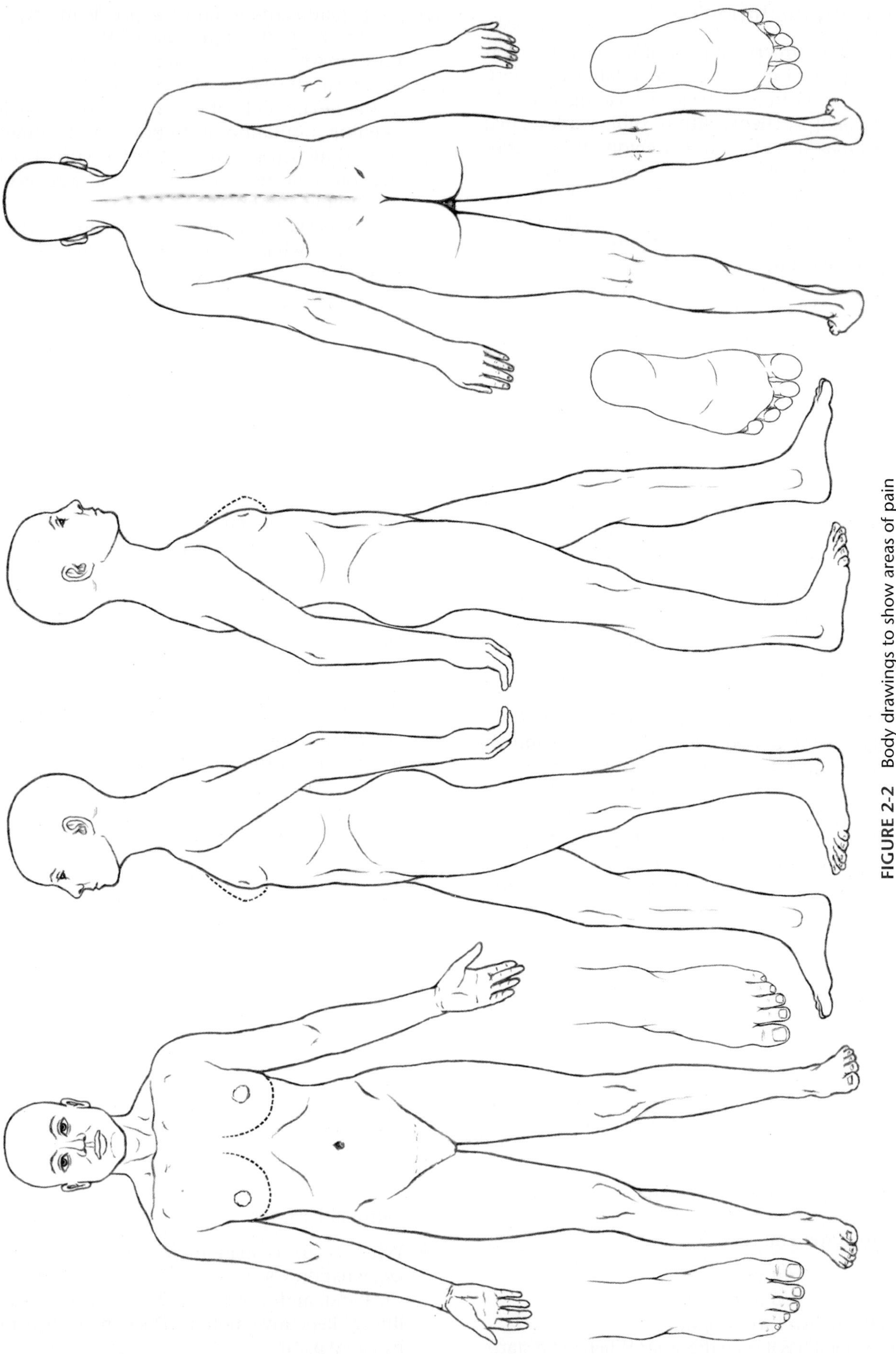

FIGURE 2-2 Body drawings to show areas of pain

Conducting the Interview

Although the primary purpose of the history interview is to gather information and establish rapport, it is also a good time to begin educating your client. For example, clients with possible work-related problems may need to consider ergonomics, repetitive motions, or other problems, such as working at a poorly setup computer station. Some people undertake exercise programs without proper advice. The initial interview provides an opportunity to introduce these issues.

During the interview, you may find yourself "thinking out loud"—that is, sharing your thoughts with the client as the interview progresses. Including clients as you process their information may encourage them to think about their muscular system in a new way. It also builds a team approach to therapy.

Similar to other aspects of the assessment process, the interview has a dual purpose—both holistic and reductionist. On the one hand, you are seeking to build a broad picture of the client and the activities of his or her life to determine what may be causing problems and what kinds of solutions may be most effective. On the other hand, you must remain alert to clues to the cause of the specific complaint. In some cases, the injury may have occurred at a specific time when performing a precise movement (e.g., "I lunged after the ball and felt a sharp pain in my groin"). Most of the time, however, the onset and origin of the presenting problem will be much more vague and will require some detective work on your part. The key to the solution will often lie hidden in the information gathered in the interview.

Ideally, taking a history should be a warm, human encounter, rather than a mechanical process in which the therapist sits with pen poised, reading questions and taking down answers. You should develop the ability to hold a relaxed, conversational interview while also keeping a mental checklist of important areas to cover. In the beginning of your practice, you may want to have a written checklist to consult. This checklist will vary somewhat, of course, from one client and one problem to the next, but the overall territory will remain the same. Above all, do not assume that the client will volunteer important information. Remember that what is important to you may seem trivial to the client. Be thorough—and above all, *listen to the client.*

Your checklist should include the following items.

Presenting Problem:

- What brought you here?
- Where do you hurt?
- What doesn't work right?
- How long has it been this way? When did it start?
- If the pain is the result of a specific injury, exactly how did the injury occur? What physical position were you in when the injury occurred? What was the course of the rest of the day, and of the next couple of days? Describe the pain, swelling, limitation of motion, and treatment (including self-treatment) that occurred over the course of the rest of the day, as well as the days following the injury.
- Have you ever had this problem before? When, and under what circumstances? When was the first time?
- When is the pain worse? When is it better?
- What makes the pain worse? What makes it better? In what physical position does it feel worst and best?
- Have you consulted another health care provider for this issue? Did they perform any diagnostic tests? What did they advise you to do?

Health History:

- How is your general health?
- Have you had any recent illnesses, injuries, surgeries?
- Have you ever had any major illnesses, injuries, surgeries?
- Do you have a history of heart problems or neurologic problems?
- Are you under a doctor's care for any condition? If yes, what condition? Are you taking any medications?
- Are you under the care of a chiropractor, osteopath, naturopath, or any other sort of physician? Any other kind of health professional? Are those visits related to this problem?

Athletic History:

- Do you play any sports or work out? Is there a sporting activity you may have done in the past that you would like to do, or some new activity you would like to undertake, but currently can't due to your physical pain or limitations?

Personal/Family/Social History:

- Are you a caretaker for anyone (spouse, children, parents?)
- Are you under stress?
- Do you have any recreational activities to help with stress relief?

Occupational History:

- What is your occupation? What does it involve—i.e., what do you do all day? How much do you sit, stand, and move about? Is there any heavy lifting? Repetitive motion? Does any work activity cause pain?

- How often do you take breaks, and for how long? What do you do during breaks?
- What types of work have you done in the past?
- Have you ever had any work-related injuries?

Feel free to add to this checklist; your own knowledge and imagination will find questions to ask and leads to pursue that lie beyond these boundaries. You should certainly follow up on any questions in your mind.

Whole-Body Assessment

Most of our clientele is accustomed to thinking in terms of traditional medical approaches. If they present with a specific injury, then they expect the examination and treatment to focus on the injury and its immediately surrounding area. In many cases this expectation may be appropriate: It is certainly possible to suffer an isolated injury at a precise site that can be specifically treated. In most cases, however, a broader approach is needed. After all, the body is all connected, and most local injuries, if left untreated, will eventually affect other parts of the body. For this reason, it is usually appropriate and desirable to evaluate the body as a whole before initiating treatment.

Some clients will refuse such an evaluation and insist on strictly local treatment. The need for informed consent requires that therapists share their assessment of the problem with the client and propose a course of examination and treatment, including possible alternatives. One of the alternatives is, of course, palliative treatment. As long as therapists are honest with clients about what they believe to be the ideal course of action based on the clients' complaints, it is appropriate to work with such clients to alleviate their symptoms on a short-term basis. For such clients, the therapist may perform a more abbreviated interview, confined largely to the circumstances that seem relevant to the chief complaint, and then skip directly to the examination of the area of the presenting problem.

For those clients, however, who agree to pursue a whole-body approach, an examination of posture can be a beneficial part of the assessment. The extent of such an examination can vary according to the skills and judgment of the therapist and the specific situation. A description of the basic requirements for an assessment is presented in the following sections.

Informal Observation

In this first step in the whole-body assessment, the therapist observes the client carefully, beginning with the first encounter in the waiting area. How does the client sit? Stand? Walk? Sit down again in the treatment room? Body language and nonverbal clues can tell us a lot. Notice the change in facial expression as the client gets up and down—do they grimace in pain? Notice if they frequently hold or rub somewhere on their body. The clinical massage therapist should cultivate this observational habit, which can easily be practiced in any public place.

Formal Posture Examination

A thorough, formal examination of body posture should be carried out with the client wearing as little clothing as possible, since it involves not only global observation but fairly precise scrutiny of surface landmarks and their movements. A complete examination is most commonly carried out with clients wearing underwear, but individual therapists can establish their own protocols.

PHOTOGRAPHS

Many therapists take photographs of clients as part of a complete posture examination.

Advantages of this practice include the following:

- The client is able to see what the therapist sees.
- The therapist has access to the photographs in the absence of the client for treatment planning purposes.
- If the therapist has a smartphone or electronic tablet, several inexpensive apps for posture analysis are available. If the client desires, you can e-mail copies to them or send to your computer so they can be printed for the client. *Note: Any photographs should be handled with care in order to avoid compromising client privacy and confidentiality.*
- Photographs taken before and after treatment can provide documentation of changes.

Whether being photographed or observed without photography, clients should be asked to stand in a way that feels reasonably straight, but relaxed and normal, with the hands at the sides. Clients whose hair falls below the shoulders should be asked to push it back for a front view and forward for a back view.

The client should first be photographed full front, full back, left side, and right side. Once the photographs are taken, save them so they can be placed side by side for comparison with photographs taken after the session and/or series of sessions in order to document progress (Figs. 2-3 and 2-4). If the client has **scoliosis**, it is helpful also to take a close-up of the back, from head to coccyx, and photograph the client bending over with arms hanging straight down to document the rotation of the rib cage (Fig. 2-5). It is useful to routinely examine children and early teens in this way for scoliosis. The presence of a **rib hump** (Fig. 2-6) is evidence of the vertebral rotation of **idiopathic scoliosis**, and the parent should be encouraged to consult the child's physician.

Some clients may prefer not to be photographed, or some therapists may choose not to use this technique.

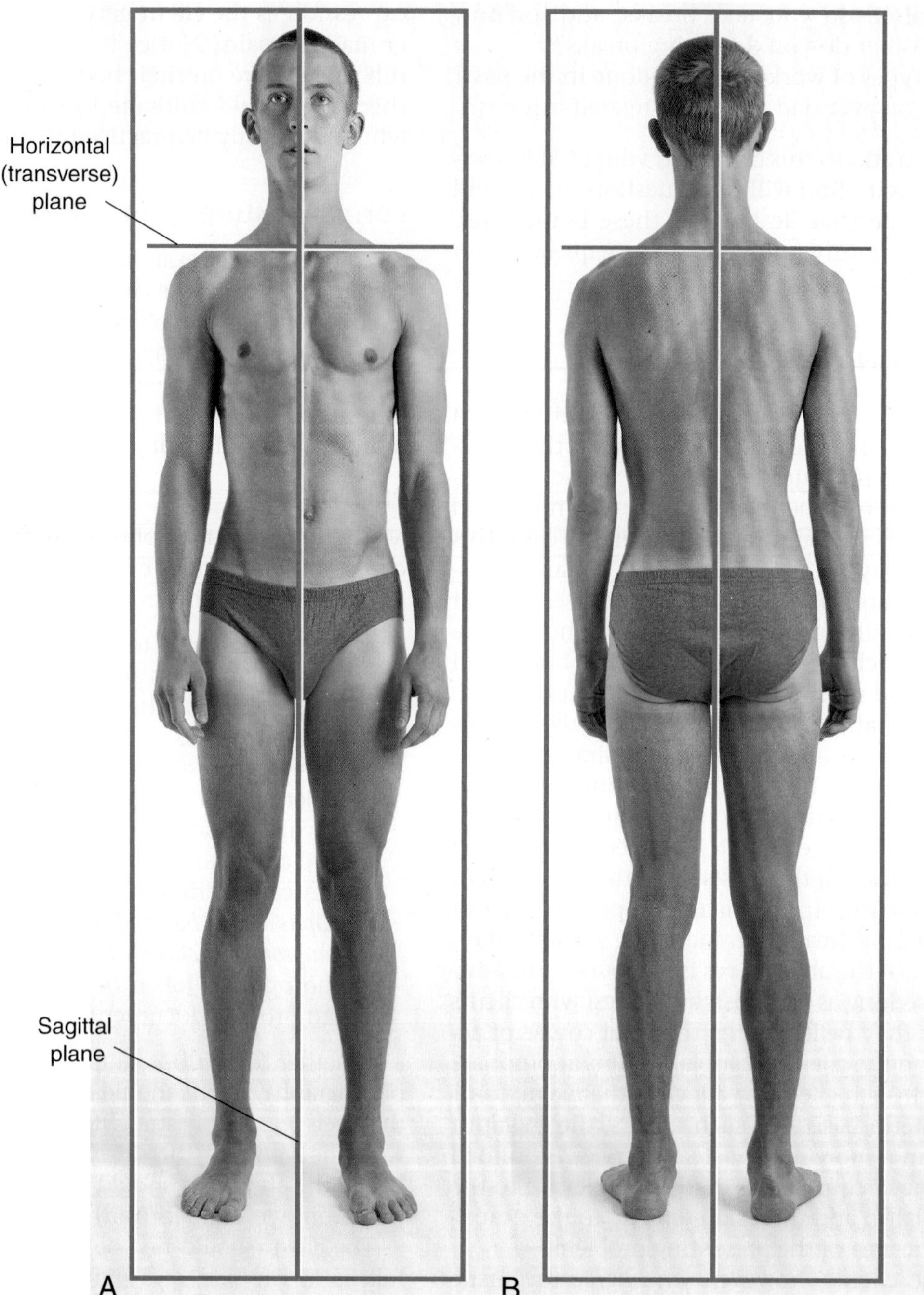

FIGURE 2-3 Posture evaluation: front **(A)** and back **(B)** views with midsagittal and horizontal (transverse) plane

In these cases, the therapist can still observe the client in all of the aforementioned positions.

The goal of asking the client to assume these various positions and stances is to observe the dynamic structure of the body. Even when the client is in a normal resting position, we are actually observing muscles at work. Just as a bird's leg muscles are always working, even in sleep, to keep it on the perch, our muscles must always respond to gravity. The ideal posture of a person standing at rest demands minimal muscle activity to maintain an upright posture. The ideal functioning of the body of a person in motion uses minimal muscle activity to accomplish any task, and will use larger and stronger muscles rather than smaller and weaker ones whenever possible.

BODY ALIGNMENT

While performing a posture analysis, you are bound to notice differences in alignment. No doubt that *some* poor postural habits can cause pain—for example, sitting hunched over a computer for many hours a day when the keyboard and/or monitor is at the wrong

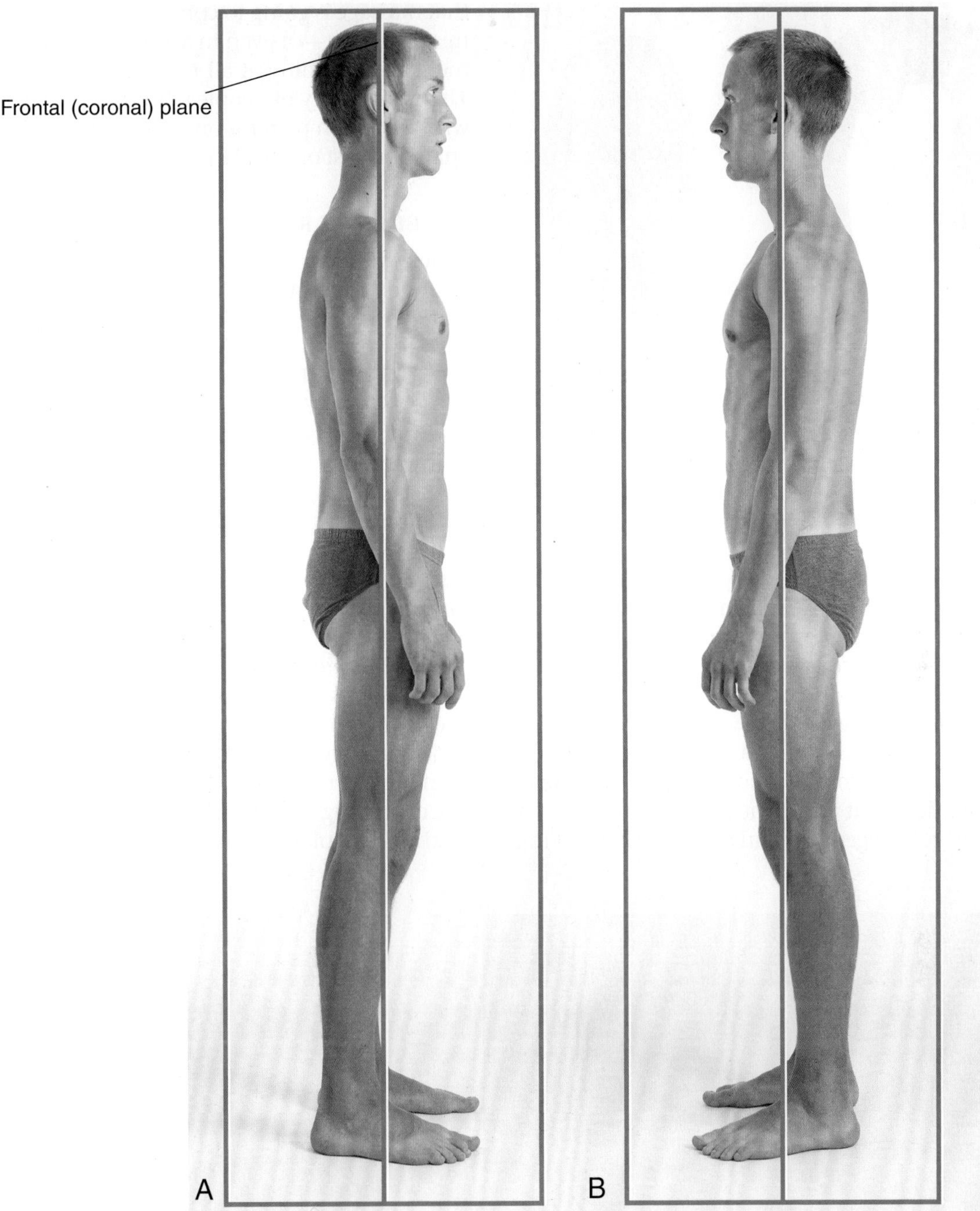

FIGURE 2-4 Posture evaluation: right and left side views with frontal (coronal) midline

height. However, there is plenty of scientific evidence that posture and pain are not as related as has been previously thought. Bad posture, for example, does not *lead* to scoliosis—but scoliosis can certainly affect posture, and may be accompanied by pain—or not.

One epidemiological study that was conducted over a period of 25 years showed that there was no relationship between the asymmetrical posture one had as a teenager (hiked hip, hiked shoulder, and deviation of the spine) and any subsequent back pain or neck pain in later adult years (http://www.ncbi.nlm.nih.gov/pubmed/2938272).

A systematic review of 54 studies concerning posture (sagittal spinal curves) and pain found no evidence of any correlation (http://www.ncbi.nlm.nih.gov/pubmed/19028253). Even when posture is faulty, there is little scientific evidence that it is a hindrance to the flexibility or movement of the subject.

This is not meant to deny that there is *any* correlation between pain and posture, but that this association is neither sufficient nor conclusive to justify our efforts to choreograph people's posture and movement. What we do know for sure is that there is no "ideal" posture, and any posture if maintained for too long

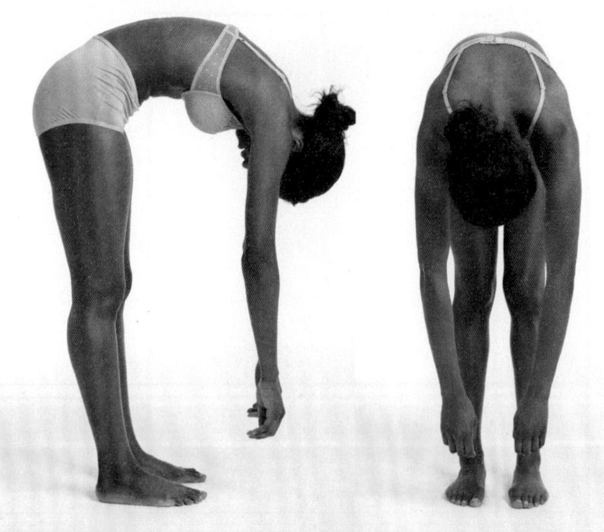

FIGURE 2-5 Scoliosis screening: side and front views

will result in dysfunction, and maybe pain. The key is movement. We may *notice* postural misalignments, and take them into consideration in the context of the whole assessment, but "fixing" them is a task that we may not accomplish. What we *can* accomplish is encouraging clients who sit at a desk all day to stand up and stretch and move, and to replace the telephone/shoulder habit with a headset. We should not let ourselves get bogged down in erroneously thinking that massage is going to correct a curved spine or other misalignment—or even in assuming that the misalignment has anything at all to do with the client's pain. There are plenty of people who have excellent posture who are still in pain for one reason or another. Posture analysis is just one tool in the total assessment toolbox.

THE BODY AT REST

When we observe a client standing at rest, we view the body in relation to certain planes. Although we work with these planes as lines, it is important to remember that they are planes, or we will be deceived.

Looking at the client from the front, the sagittal plane (Fig. 2-3A) is a midline that begins at a point midway between the feet (since that is the resting point for the weight) and passes through the pubic symphysis, the navel, the xiphoid process and manubrium of the sternum, the center of the chin, and the nose. Note any deviation from that line. Also observe the kneecaps and feet. Do they point forward, or does either of them deviate inwardly or outwardly?

Viewing the client from behind, the sagittal plane (Fig. 2-3B) is a line that again begins midway between the feet and passes through the gluteal cleft and the coccyx, straight up through the spinal column, and through the middle of the head.

Comparing these two views can teach you how to think in planes rather than in lines—in other

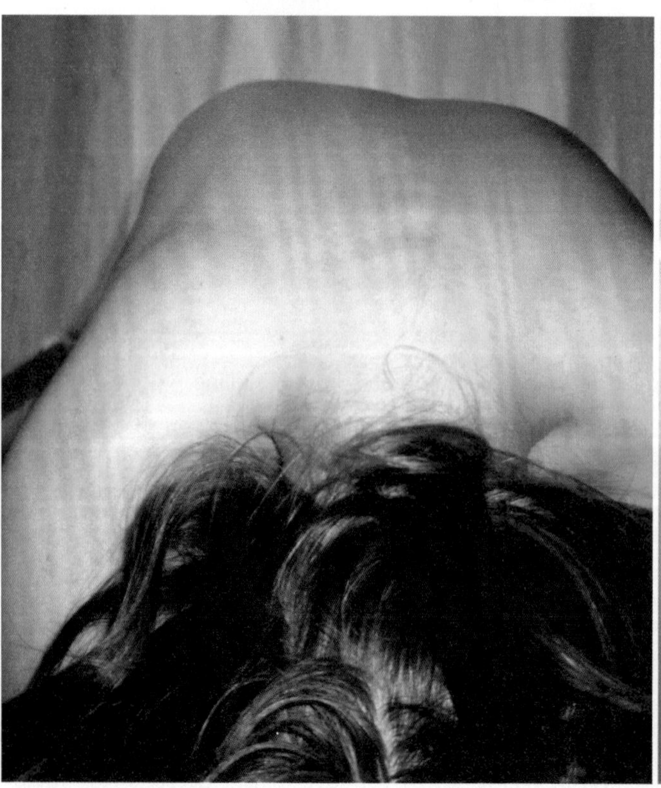

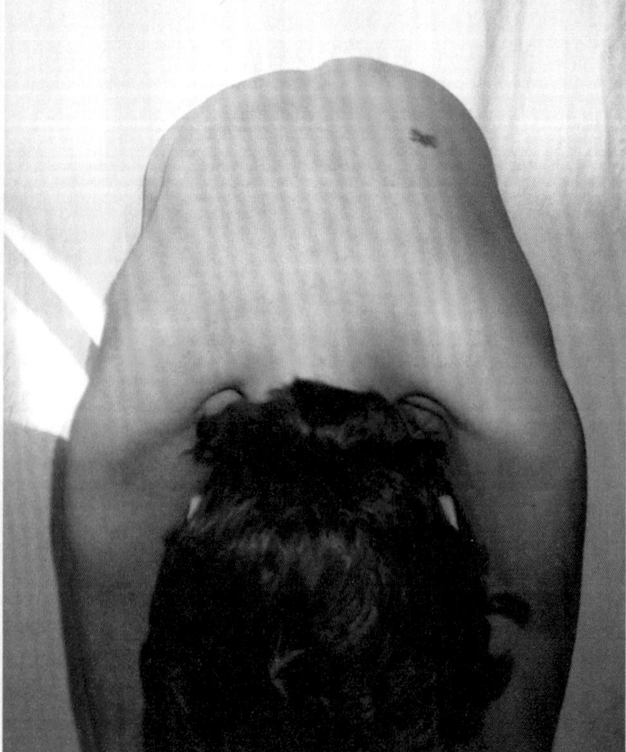

FIGURE 2-6 Rib hump in idiopathic scoliosis

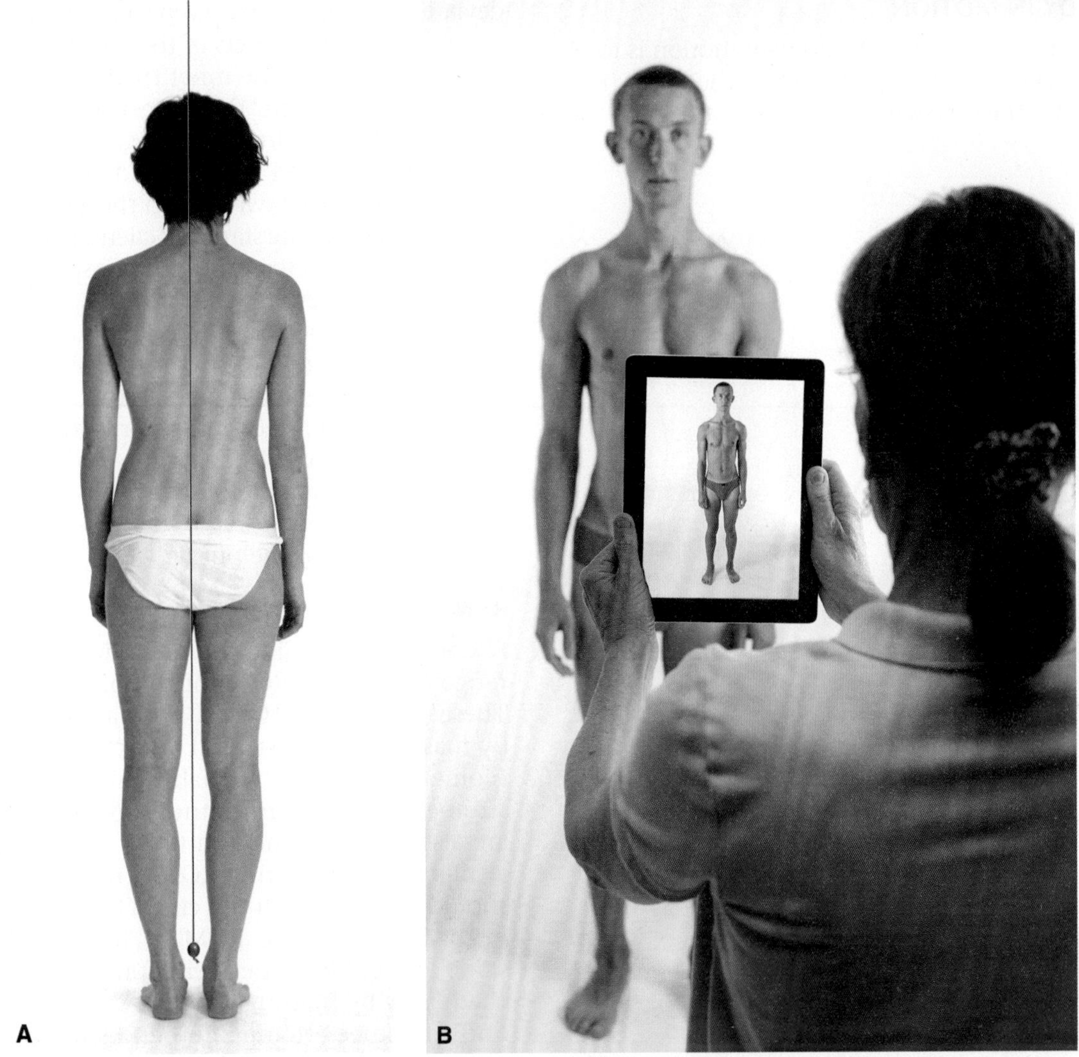

FIGURE 2-7 Assessing posture and alignment using a plumb line (**A**) and an electronic tablet (**B**).

words, how to see a client in a three-dimensional rather than two-dimensional view. Often the upper body of the client appears to lean to one side when viewed from the front, but lean to the opposite side when viewed from behind. This illusion is created by seeing lines rather than planes. In reality, the client's upper body is slightly rotated, placing the landmarks on the torso to one side of the midline in front and to the other side in back.

Viewing the client from each side, the frontal plane (Fig. 2-4) is a line passing just in front of the ankle through the knee, the greater trochanter, the glenohumeral joint of the shoulder, and the ear. Again, note any deviation from this line.

Therapists who do not take photographs or use a computer may find a plumb line and/or posture grid helpful in making these observations. A long string weighted at one end (a 2- or 3-oz fishing sinker works well) can be suspended in a place where the client can stand behind it to be observed. The plumb line gives the therapist a visual reference point for observing postural deviations (Fig. 2-7A). In Figure 2-7B, the therapist is using her electronic tablet to photograph and analyze the client's posture.

In addition to the sagittal and frontal planes, the horizontal plane (Fig. 2-3A) should be considered in relation to the shoulders and hips:

- Are the shoulders level?
- Are the shoulders rotated medially and pulled forward in a slump?
- Is the pelvis tilted to one side or the other?
- Is the pelvis rotated forward?

You may want to make notes of all your observations, particularly if you do not take photographs. *And remember that no individual view is sufficient to yield significant information.* Each view is merely one piece of a three-dimensional puzzle. Merely viewing the body at rest is insufficient to give a full assessment of the client's body. More pieces of the puzzle must be considered.

THE BODY IN MOTION

The first step in assessing the body in motion is to observe the client's gait (Fig. 2-8) from the back, front, and side. Do the legs swing straight forward, or do they deviate from that course, even slightly, along the way? Notice individual aspects of the legs: Is there a medial pulling motion on the inner thigh? Do the kneecaps always point forward? Do the feet point straight ahead throughout the swing of the leg, or are they everted or inverted? Viewed from behind, does the pelvis tilt from side to side or swivel with the gait?

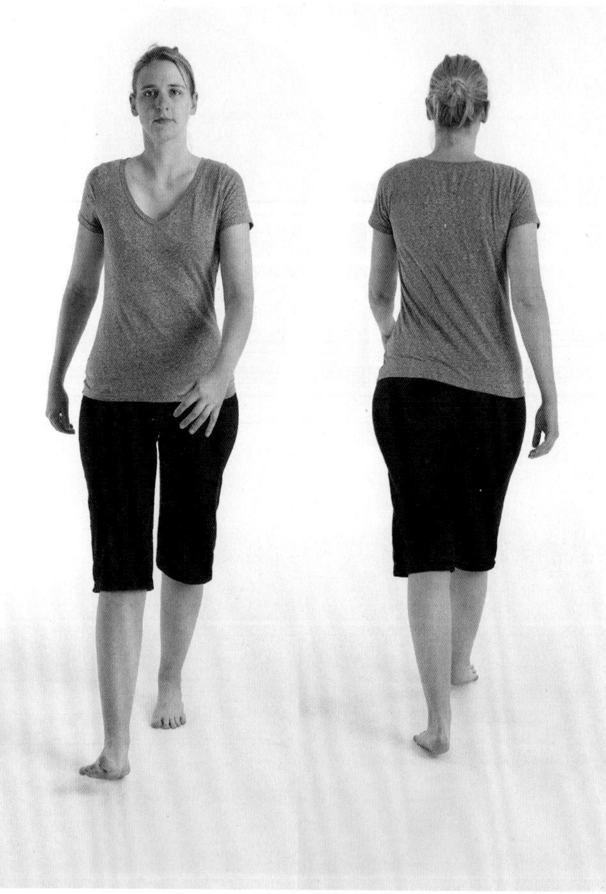

FIGURE 2-8 Gait assessment

Sitting behind the standing client, place your hands on the ilium with your thumbs pressing into the dimples at the posterior superior iliac spines (PSIS). Ask the client to bend forward, and follow the PSIS with your thumbs (Fig. 2-9). Do they remain even, or does one move upward ahead of the other? In other words, does the sacrum rotate during forward bending?

Make notes of all deviations during movement, just as you did for the body at rest. These findings, although not conclusive by themselves, contribute to the solution of the puzzle.

RANGE OF MOTION

A complete examination includes measuring the range of motion (ROM) of the hips and shoulders. These measurements are normally taken visually by massage therapists, but you could also use a goniometer, a widely available and inexpensive instrument for measuring the angles of joints. There are also smart phone and tablet apps that are now available for measuring ROM. These measurements should be made with the client lying supine.

To determine the ROM of the hip (Fig. 2-10), stand at the side of the client at the hip and raise the client's leg by holding it by the calf, fully extended, until the knee attempts to bend slightly to accommodate the stretch of the hamstrings. Measure the angle of the joint in relation to the horizontal plane.

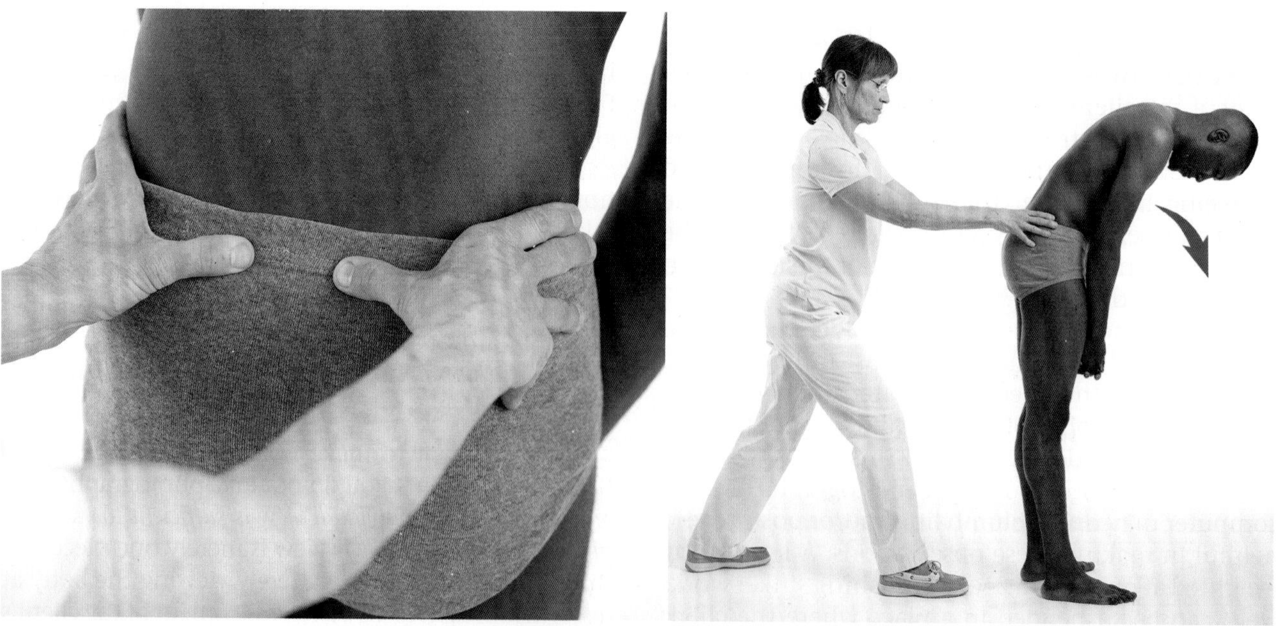

FIGURE 2-9 Examination of PSIS movement

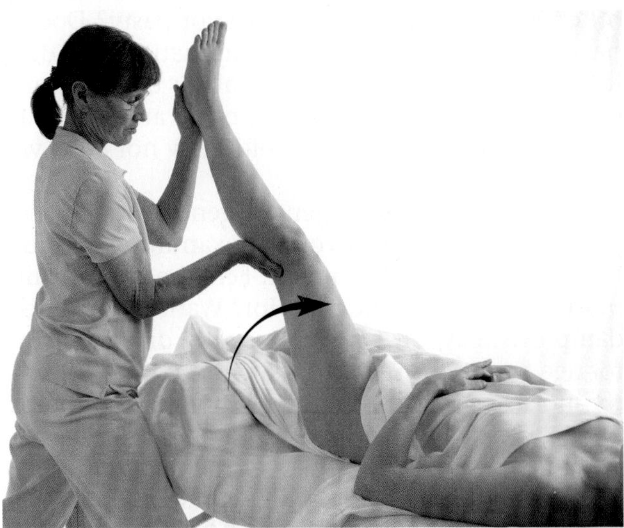

FIGURE 2-10 Evaluation of hip range of motion

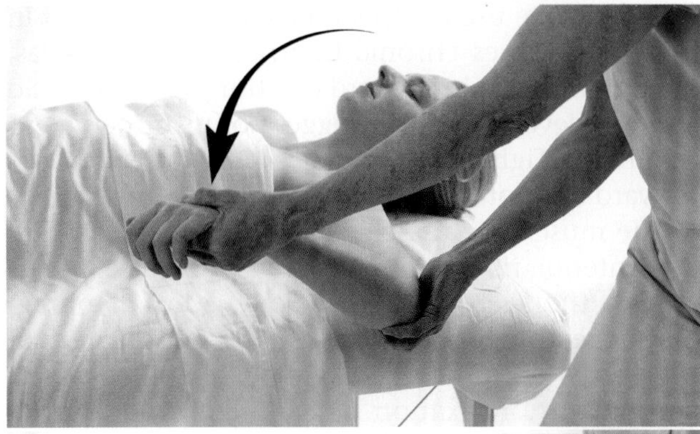

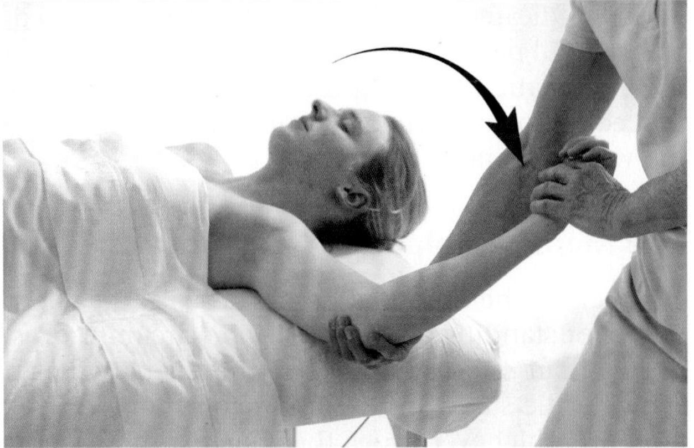

FIGURE 2-11 Evaluation of shoulder range of motion

To determine the ROM of the shoulder (Fig. 2-11), the shoulder should be abducted 90° and the elbow flexed 90°, so that the fingers point to the ceiling. Stand beside the client at the level of the shoulders. Place your hand nearest the head of the client on the shoulder with your fingers lying over the superior border of the scapula. Rotate the forearm toward the table (medial rotation of the shoulder) until it lies flat, or until movement is felt in the scapula. If the forearm does not lie flat without movement of the scapula, the angle should be measured and noted. Then rotate the arm upward (lateral rotation of the shoulder) until it lies flat or movement is felt in the scapula, and again measure and note the angle. Feeling for movement in the scapula is necessary to determine actual *glenohumeral* rotation rather than rotation that may be accommodated by movement of the scapula. The Centers for Disease Control website includes a reference table for normal joint range of motion values at http://www.cdc.gov/ncbddd/jointrom/.

Testing Areas Specific to the Complaint

By carefully noting and analyzing the type and location of discomfort produced by the following combination of tests, the therapist can gain valuable information about the likely nature of the dysfunction. Therefore, the next step in assessment is to test the area or areas specific to the complaint. First, determine the position that best suits this purpose. Usually, the client stands to have the hip joint tested, sits to have the shoulder joint tested, and sits and stands for testing of the knees. More of the area may be accessible when the client is standing or sitting than when the client is lying down, and in these positions you can easily palpate the tissue while the client moves the joint.

Joints should be tested both actively and passively. In active testing, the client moves the joint through its full ROM unassisted, reporting any pain, discomfort, or barriers to movement. In passive testing, the therapist *carefully* moves the joint through the same range, with the client instructed to relax the limb and give control to the therapist. The client should be asked to describe any differences in feeling between active and passive movements.

Then, in whatever position is suitable, the therapist tests active movement of the joint against resistance. The client is instructed to move the limb in a particular direction, while the therapist resists the motion and report any feelings associated with that effort.

Far too many specific tests for soft tissue disorders in particular areas of the body exist to be included in this book. Appendix D lists some excellent references to help you with assessments.

The Breathing Examination

An essential element in assessment is examining the client's breathing technique. Many, if not most, older children and adults have developed the habit of "paradoxical breathing," i.e., expanding and raising the upper rib cage while keeping the abdomen and lower rib cage constricted.

Paradoxical breathing is detrimental to muscle health and posture for a number of reasons.

Inappropriate use of neck and shoulder muscles in breathing causes chronic tightness in those areas, which can result in forward positioning of the head and the development of trigger points or nerve entrapment. Tight chest muscles pull the shoulders forward and rotate the arms internally. Inflexibility in the muscles of the chest and abdomen can pull the anterior rib cage forward and down, exaggerating a thoracic kyphosis. Finally, good diaphragmatic breathing techniques use the full capacity of the lungs, optimize the exchange of blood gases, and enhance relaxation. Therefore, if your examination indicates that the client breathes paradoxically, it will be important to incorporate training in diaphragmatic breathing technique. The complete procedure for assessing and teaching proper breathing will be found in Chapter 4.

The Manual (Palpatory) Examination

This part of the examination begins with the client sitting or standing, according to the circumstances. Throughout the examination, the client will sit, stand, or lie successively supine and prone on the table in whichever order the therapist finds most useful and efficient. It is often best to perform the palpatory examination of the area of complaint before or during the specific testing described above. If the client chooses to be examined and treated only for relief of the specific complaint, then you should limit your palpatory examination to those areas likely to be contributing to it. In any case, finding and treating the immediate source of pain or dysfunction is one of your primary objectives.

You may find it useful to refer to Appendix C in choosing the range of muscles to examine to determine the source of the client's pain. Each muscle description in Part II of this volume presents a list of "Other Muscles to Examine." Do not stop with a single positive finding: A trigger point that reproduces the client's pain may not be the sole source of the problem. Thorough exploration of the muscles in a particular body region will increase the accuracy, efficiency, and effectiveness of your treatment.

Broadly speaking, the palpatory examination has two parts: (1) general assessment of the tissues in each area and (2) precise palpation for taut bands in the muscles, and tender or trigger points. Both parts are continuous and contiguous with therapy: As you treat, you examine. In the initial evaluation, the information you gain through palpation is an essential adjunct to the information you obtain through observations and measurements.

The palpatory examination begins again with observation: Look at the area you are about to examine. Notice its color, especially in comparison with other areas of the body. Is it pale or pasty? Does it have the angry redness of inflammation? Or does it appear gently flushed (as healthy tissue should be), without radical contrast to other areas? Bear in mind that contrasts in skin color may not be as visible on people of color.

Begin with a broad, gentle, general touch. Lay your hand on the area you are examining and just let it rest there for a moment. Feel the temperature of the area. Is it cold? Cool? Hot? Warm? Does it feel damp or sticky, or is it unpleasantly dry? Allowing for age variations, healthy skin should have a subtly moist feeling to it, without dryness, dampness, or stickiness. Allow your hand to press a bit deeper, and move the skin around over the underlying layers. Does it seem rigid, or does it seem loose? Or does it feel firm but mobile, as if connected to the layers underneath but not adhered to them? Draw your finger across the skin, noting whether there is "drag" in the tissue that impedes your motion. Such palpable phenomena at the levels of the epidermis, dermis, and superficial fascia often reflect underlying tissue dysfunction.

Note any marked differences in an area. Differences in temperature and moisture can be signs of sympathetic nervous system activity in response to problems in the underlying tissue. Remember also the classic signs of local inflammation: heat, redness, pain, and swelling. This combination is a contraindication for local massage work.

At this point you can move deeper still, and begin to use your fingers and thumbs in whatever sort of palpation suits the shape of the tissue. You are feeling the muscle tissue, and you want to learn whether it is flabby or firm or hard or contracted. Move your hands, palpating different parts of the muscle to feel for taut bands and knots in the tissue. Ask the client to let you know what areas are tender, ticklish, tingling, numb, or feel in any way "strange." Also be aware of the client's nonverbal responses: clients will not always verbally communicate to you about everything they feel. Be alert to wincing, flinching, face-making, or intakes of breath that indicate that the client is feeling something significant.

You can certainly palpate at this point for trigger points or other sensitive points, but you should also be careful not to press too deeply into trigger points. Arousing them before you are prepared to treat them will only cause needless pain for the client.

Obviously, it is impossible to do a thorough examination for tender points or trigger points over the entire body in a reasonable amount of time. A general assessment of the principal muscles of posture and movement, however, is possible. As you gain experience, you will know the most likely spots to explore more carefully for sensitivity. Also, your awareness of the client's complaint and history will guide your choices about areas to examine more closely.

One rule to remember when examining muscular tissue is to *always examine the antagonists and the synergists*. If a problem is present in a particular muscle, a problem is present in its antagonists and possibly in the synergists as well. This rule is one more reason why a thorough knowledge of anatomy and kinesiology is needed in clinical massage therapy.

The information that you gain from the palpatory examination should be recorded for easy reference. One way to keep this information organized is to design a form similar to the one suggested earlier for clients, with four body views, on which you can make notations according to your own style.

Summation and Detective Work

You now have the following sets of data to work with:

- The chief complaint
- The history
- Informal and formal observations of body posture and movement
- ROM assessment
- Palpatory examination

Table 2-1 shows some questions to ask in your mind, with sources of information about each.

As you think in problem-solving terms, the first question you should consider is,

What is the likelihood that the cause and treatment of this problem lie outside my scope of practice?

This issue is extremely important, both for the client's health and for your own legal protection. Always keep in mind that your assessment may be wrong—and remember, *it is not a diagnosis*.

Although clinical massage therapists should become highly adept at examination and assessment of the musculoskeletal system and work toward mastery of the process, this system is only one aspect of the whole person. Thus, our scope of examination and treatment is necessarily limited. It is always safest to assume that, since we are working within a limited range, our knowledge and awareness may be incomplete. We should never discourage clients from seeking the opinions of other professionals, including their physician. In fact, we should encourage it.

In some cases, the therapist should defer treatment of a client until a physician has evaluated and cleared the client for massage therapy. Such clients include those with internal pain (chest, abdomen, or pelvis) or any client with suspected musculoskeletal injuries such as a dislocated or broken bone or torn muscles, tendons, or ligaments.

Otherwise, the therapist may continue with treatment. When the problem is likely to be myofascial in origin, and direct manipulation of the soft tissue clearly represents no danger to the client, it is normally safe to proceed. The therapist, however, should continue to consider the possibility that other factors may be involved, and be prepared to refer the client at the slightest suspicion that another form of treatment might be called for.

Synthesizing Your Findings

Correctly assessing a client's problem and developing a treatment plan depend on recognizing that problems in the body do not occur in isolation. *A problem anywhere in the musculoskeletal system affects to some degree the integrity of the entire system.* Therefore, you must think simultaneously at both the local and whole-body levels. The longer you are in practice, the more seamless this process will become, because

Table 2-1 Assessment Questions for the Therapist to Consider

Question	Source of Information
What muscles refer pain to the area of complaint?	Charts, your knowledge of referral zones
What muscles seem shortened or contain taut bands?	ROM assessment, palpatory examination, body alignment
Where are tender points or trigger points?	
What are the antagonists of the muscles in the area of complaint?	Presenting complaint, your knowledge of anatomy and kinesiology
If there was a specific injury, what muscles were stretched and what muscles were shortened?	Presenting complaint, your knowledge of anatomy and kinesiology
What muscles are regularly challenged by this client?	Occupational and athletic histories, posture examination
What was the client doing around the time the problem started?	Personal, occupational, and athletic histories
What activities in the client's past could have injured these muscles?	Personal, occupational, and athletic histories
Could this problem be related to a compensation for some other injury?	Health history, observation of movement
Could stress in the client's life be activating a dormant tissue problem?	Personal, athletic, and occupational histories

all the pieces of the puzzle will fit themselves into place as you gather them.

When thinking through muscular problems, keep these two frameworks in mind:

- Think of muscles in terms of groups that work together (synergistically) and consider agonist/antagonist relationships.
- Think of joints as well as muscles, since the primary function of muscles is to move or stabilize joints. Bear in mind that joint *mobilizations* are within the scope of practice of massage therapy, while joint *manipulations* are not. Although our intentions are not directed at bone, muscle origins and insertions are often located near the joints, as are tendons, while ligaments join the bones.

At this point, all of the information you have gathered needs to be synthesized in a view of the whole person. Here is a useful order for considering and synthesizing this information:

- In your observation of the whole body, did you notice profound differences in alignment when comparing one side of the body to the other, and question the client about any postural habits they may have that contributed to that? Add the two side views to let your mind reconstruct what you've seen of the body. Do you see deviations in a single plane, or is there a spiral effect to the deviations that would indicate twisting?
- Consider any measurements you have taken during the range-of-motion test and of postural deviations. Do the measurements support the three-dimensional picture you have built? For example, if the measurements show that the right anterior superior iliac spine (ASIS) is lower than the left in front, but the right PSIS is higher than the left in back, does your picture indicate a spiral effect or twisting of the torso? Does the hip joint have ROM limitations on the higher side or the lower side?
- How does the pain and/or dysfunction reported by the client fit into the picture? Does the pain or restriction occur in an area where muscles appear to be chronically shortened or lengthened? Could the pain be causing compensatory posture or movement? It's important to remember that when there is intense pain on one side, the problem may well be on the other side—compensation could be the culprit.
- Consider your palpatory examination. Where are tender spots, and how do these areas compare with areas of pain reported by the client? Are they in areas where you assessed that the muscles are chronically shortened or lengthened?
- Did you encounter trigger points that reproduce the client's pain?
- Now add the history. What does the client do now, either at work or in recreation, that might affect the problem areas? What about past activities, injuries, surgeries?
- Finally, are there recent stressors that might be causing an already existing problem to surface or worsen?

Communicating with Clients

When the examination is completed, it is time to share your thinking with the client. Since most people are naturally curious, it is a good practice to share your observations with the client throughout the examination. It is annoying to have someone who is examining you say nothing but "Hmmm." Now you can let the client know how the information is coming together for you, what your working assessment is, and what sort of work you propose to do. For example:

"I think that when you sprained your ankle last year, you favored your right leg for a time. That resulted in your left hip muscles working overtime, and may have shortened the muscles supporting your pelvis on the right. Since you're young and in good shape, you didn't feel the effects at first, but your new job pressures have made you tense and lowered your pain threshold, so now those muscles are finally making themselves felt. I'd like to work on your left hip to give you some immediate relief from the pain in your leg, but I think we also need to work on your lower back and abdominal muscles, since they're supporting your pelvis."

ETHICAL CAUTION

Clinical massage therapy sometimes involves working around the pelvis or other sensitive areas such as the breasts and gluteal muscles. Whenever that's going to be the case, that needs to be discussed with the client during the intake process. You would never want to surprise a client with your hand on their pubic bone—an action that could be dreadfully misconstrued as sexual behavior if it has not been discussed with the client. You should always have your clients sign a statement of informed consent—and if you are going to be working in sensitive areas, you want to mention that specifically on the statement. Keep in mind that the client has the right to withdraw that consent at any time during the session, should they begin to feel uncomfortable.

Clients may sometimes question why the examination and proposed treatment wanders so far afield from the specific area of their complaint. For this reason, it is important to educate them about the nature of myofascial pain. This education need not be highly technical. Metaphors are often useful in explaining what seems to be going on. For example, one might describe the relationship of agonists and antagonists as being like two people in bed fighting over the covers, or characterize the gradual spreading of muscle involvement in an injured area as a revolution or a labor dispute.

This educational process is another good reason for documentation such as photographs and recorded measurements. These concrete bits of information support your assessment.

The most important aspect of communication with the client is to establish a relationship in which the client becomes an active and informed participant in the overall process. Although you are the authority (that's why the client consulted you), it is your job as well to help clients become more knowledgeable and take greater responsibility for their own health and well-being.

Applying Your Synthesis to Treatment

Your first responsibility is to give the client relief from the presenting complaint as quickly as is feasible. Therefore, in most cases, begin treatment by eliminating trigger points, tender points, and tightness in the area where the pain is and those areas that appear to be causing it or contributing to it. In Chapters 3 through 10, the pain referral zone is listed for each muscle, as well as a list of other muscles to examine that may refer pain to similar areas.

In the case of multiple trigger points, a **primary trigger point** will be accompanied by **satellite trigger points**. The only way to distinguish them is to treat them and observe the results. Resolving a primary trigger point will eliminate referred pain, while resolving satellite trigger points will not.

Once the presenting problem has been treated and alleviated, it is appropriate to address the issues of poor postural habits and other mitigating factors that are responsible for the client's pain. Although a detailed discussion of postural analysis is beyond the scope of this book, most of the postural habits that result in misalignment and/or myofascial pain are a matter of educating clients by calling the clients' attention to the habits that may be causing the pain, and demonstrating how to make changes to more efficient ways of working. Using good judgment, a thorough knowledge of musculoskeletal anatomy, gaining clinical experience, and additional study and training will round out your skills in this area.

The general order of treatment should proceed:

- From the areas specific to the complaint to the overall body issues
- From superficial to deep
- From general to specific

Communicating with Other Health Professionals

Communicating effectively with other health professionals is important for three reasons:

- It is potentially helpful in the care of specific clients.
- It affects your image as a health professional and helps create the degree of respect (and possibly the number of referrals) you will be accorded in the present and future.
- It affects the image of the bodywork profession as a whole, and will ultimately determine the degree of acceptance we all achieve.

The first requirement in effective professional communication is to master your terminology. On the one hand, do not go out of your way to use the most technical language you can, because it will simply be seen as an attempt to impress. On the other hand, you should know anatomical terms and be able to spell and pronounce them properly, or it will be assumed that you don't know what you're talking about. Keep a medical dictionary handy and use it regularly. If you use a computer, get a medical spell-check program.

Some good policies to follow regularly:

- Ask clients to tell their other health care providers to feel free to contact you.
- With the client's written consent, share your progress notes with their other health care providers to inform them about your assessment and treatment of the client and the results.
- If another health care provider refers a client to you, then write a letter of thanks that includes your report (again, with your client's written consent).

You will find your own style, but two sample reports are included here as examples.

Special Populations

Pregnant Women

Pregnant women can certainly benefit from massage therapy, since the added weight and imbalance in their bodies can cause considerable soft tissue pain, especially in the lower back, hips, and legs. Certain precautions must be taken, however, and special requirements need to be considered.

A pregnant woman may not be able to lie on her stomach after the first trimester, and as the pregnancy progresses, may be uncomfortable lying on her back for any significant period of time. Depending on the area being treated, she may be in a seated position or she may lie on her side. The use of pillows may enable her to feel more comfortable prone or in any position. She should be allowed to arrange these herself (with

Sample 1

Name: Norris A. Rollins

Chief Complaint: pain in neck and left shoulder, radiating into left arm to hand

Treatment Dates: Jan. 23; Feb. 1, 7, 10, 17, 28; March 6, 17

Mr. Rollins was seen on the indicated dates for complaints of pain resulting from an automobile accident in which his car collided with another car while his left arm was resting on the car's windowsill.

He was treated for severe trigger point activity in the scalene muscles, particularly the middle scalene and scalenus minimus, and related spasms and trigger point activity in pectoralis minor, rhomboids, levator scapulae, and rotator cuff muscles. Techniques employed consisted primarily of trigger point compression and deep tissue therapy.

Some temporary relief was achieved, but his problem is complicated by two factors: (1) treatment did not begin until 8 months after his accident and (2) the constant weight of the rib cage on the scalenes continues to irritate the muscles.

Mr. Rollins informs me that he has been told by his physicians that he has nerve damage. I can't comment directly on that, but he has reported that the massage therapy has been helpful, and we believe that improvement can be achieved with additional work on the muscles themselves. This treatment would necessarily be long-term because of the time that has passed since the injury.

your help as needed), as she can determine her needs better than the therapist. Commercial systems are also available, such as the Body Cushion (www.bodycushionstore.com), or the Prego Pillow, available at most massage equipment suppliers, both of which can allow a pregnant woman to lie prone. Any problems can usually be solved in collaboration with the client.

The following guidelines have been established by the American College of Obstetrics and Gynecology. A woman who is experiencing a high-risk pregnancy should obtain a release from her primary care provider before receiving massage. According to the National Institutes of Health, high-risk pregnancy can be due to existing health conditions, age, lifestyle factors, and conditions of pregnancy. High-risk factors include the following:

- The woman has used fertility methods to get pregnant or has had difficulty getting pregnant naturally.
- The woman has miscarried in the first trimester of previous pregnancies.
- The woman has a cardiac or pulmonary disorder (heart or lung problems).
- The woman has been diagnosed with asthma, autoimmune disease, diabetes, epilepsy, HIV/AIDS, kidney disease, or thyroid disease.
- The woman has any history of problems in previous pregnancies.
- The woman is carrying a multiple pregnancy (twins, triplets, etc.).
- The woman is under age 17 or a first-time mother over age 35.

The Elderly

The work described in this book is appropriate for the treatment of older clients, with the following specific cautions:

- Be sure to take a thorough medical history, and be aware of any problems such as stroke, heart disease, blood clots, surgeries, medications, etc.
- Osteoporosis occurs frequently in older adults. Ask about this condition in the client's history. Avoid intense pressure on any bones during therapy.
- Avoid treatment directly over implanted devices, such as pacemakers or electrical implants for pain control.

Avoid treatment directly on and around medications administered by patch; massage could affect the dosage.

- Older people tend to have thinner, less elastic skin that is more apt to tear. Exercise caution in pulling the skin during treatment.

Sample 2

Patient: Esther Megillah

Date of Birth: Aug. 24, 1995

Complaints: Frequent headaches (at least 3 × per week), chronic lower back pain

Observations:

- Left shoulder (acromioclavicular (AC) joint) appears lower than the right.
- Left shoulder blade (inferior angle of scapula) appears lower than the right.
- Left iliac crest appears lower than the right.
- Left ASIS appears lower than the right.
- Left PSIS appears lower than the right.
- Left gluteal fold appears lower than the right.
- Pelvis appears rotated to the right.

Photographs: Photographs show significant rotation of torso from hips counterclockwise (from above). Tightness in chest muscles is indicated by difficulty in raising arms fully overhead and in pulling forward of shoulders, particularly on the right. Lumbar lordosis indicates excessive pelvic rotation, which is confirmed in visual and manual assessments.

Manual Examination: Excessive tenderness found in chest, back, abdomen, buttocks, and legs.

Conclusions: Measurements indicate landmarks on left side to be consistently slightly lower than on right side. Photographs confirm this and indicate rotation of torso and pelvic rotation. Manual examination confirms muscular constriction in legs, abdomen, buttocks, back, and chest.

Recommendations: Neuromuscular and connective tissue therapy is recommended to correct the above imbalances and could eliminate or alleviate headaches and back pain. This procedure is also likely to increase her flexibility for her physical activities.

Children and Adolescents

Adolescent clients may be treated essentially as adults. This work is also appropriate for children, with certain cautions and considerations:

- Most children have not developed a perspective that allows them to deal well with pain or discomfort in treatment. They, therefore, have a lower pain tolerance than adolescents or adults.
- The soft tissues of children tend to be more responsive and resilient than those of adults; so the work usually does not need to be as deep or intense as may be required in adult clients.
- Children tend to be more ticklish than adults, and palpation that elicits pain in adult clients will often elicit ticklishness in children. You will need to learn to distinguish between superficial ticklishness (evoked by light touch) and deep ticklishness (evoked by deep touch). The latter should be seen as equivalent to a pain response in an adult.
- Younger children may not be capable of lying still on the massage table for an hour, and depending on their age and size, there may be less terrain to cover. Shorter sessions may be in order.

Posturally oriented bodywork can be done very effectively with school-age children, depending on their cooperativeness. An ideal time for this work is from the ages of 8 or 9 through puberty. The child is old enough to understand and participate in the work, and it will provide some preventive advantage as the child progresses through the adolescent growth spurt. It may also help the growing child in dealing with body issues at that sensitive age.

ETHICAL CAUTION

Most regulated states have it written into the law that the parent must give informed consent for a minor to have a massage. Additionally, although it may or may not be the law, the best course of action is to have the parent stay in the treatment room with the child. During the course of the massage, you may need to touch a child in an area that he has been warned about as being an inappropriate place to touch. As long as the parent is in the room to explain that it's appropriate in this situation, the child may feel more safe and secure.

The Infirm

We may have opportunities to work with people who are suffering from any number of conditions, such as cancer, Parkinson's disease, multiple sclerosis, posttraumatic stress disorder, arthritis—it's an endless list. Doing a little research on PubMed or the Massage Therapy Foundation's website may give you a clue to any suggested protocols for certain illnesses or conditions. If a client presents with a condition you are unfamiliar with, please take the time to look it up in a pathology book or on a reputable website, such as an online medical encyclopedia. If you're unsure whether or not massage is contraindicated, ask for written consent to check with their physician before performing massage.

Some diseases/conditions may have chronic and acute phases. Avoid massage anytime the client is in an acute phase, and feeling weak or compromised. Remember a good rule of thumb: If the client is in control of the condition, massage is usually safe. If the condition is in control of the client, you need to delay the massage until the client is feeling better. When there is any doubt, it's always best to consult their physician.

CHAPTER REVIEW

PUTTING THEORY INTO PRACTICE

Effective examination and assessment are the keys to good clinical work. Intelligent assessment of the problem is essential to gaining the trust of the client and working with confidence. In the beginning, the process may seem artificial and mechanical, but as you gain experience and self-assurance, it will develop a natural flow. You will master it by touching many bodies, again and again and again, and by using your eyes, hands, and brain to put together coherent concepts of the whole, individual human being. Soon, the dialogue between you and your clients, both physical and verbal, will become as natural to you as breathing.

QUESTIONS FOR REVIEW

1. Why should a clinical assessment be performed, even if the person has a prescription from the doctor for massage?
2. What types of questions are inappropriate to ask when you are taking the client's health history?
3. What factors should you consider when formulating a treatment plan for the client?
4. What should be obtained before performing any work on the client, recognizing that it may be withdrawn at any time?
5. What are the specific considerations of special populations such as pregnant, elderly, or child clients?

thePoint Additional helpful resources are available at http://thePoint.lww.com.

CHAPTER 3

The Head, Face, and Neck

LEARNING OBJECTIVES

At the end of this chapter, the learner will be able to:

- State the correct terminology of the muscles of the head, face, and neck.
- Palpate the muscles of the head, face, and neck.
- Identify their attachments at the origins and insertions.
- Explain the actions of the muscles.
- Describe their pain referral areas.
- Recall related muscles.
- Recognize any endangerment sites and ethical cautions for massage therapy.
- Demonstrate proficiency in manual therapy techniques for muscles of the head, face, and neck.

The Overview of the Region begins on page 62, after the anatomy plates.

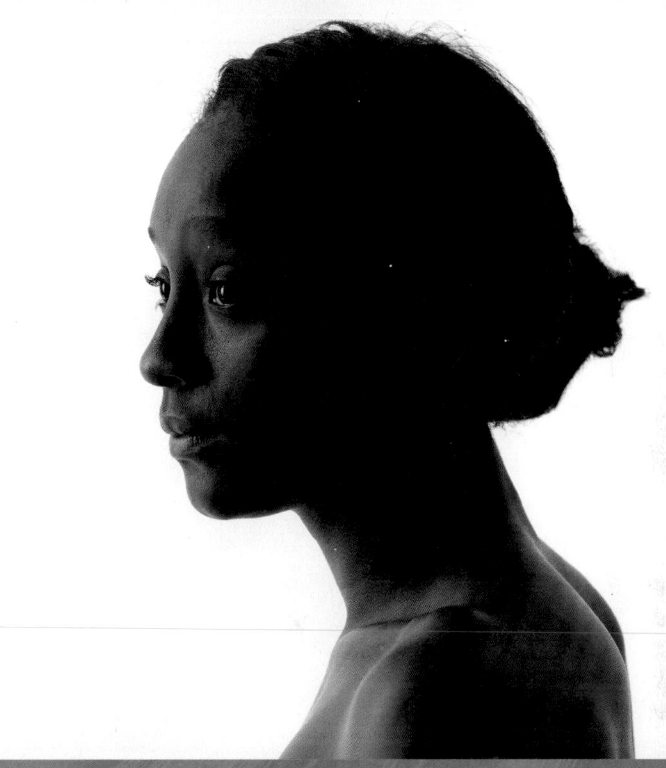

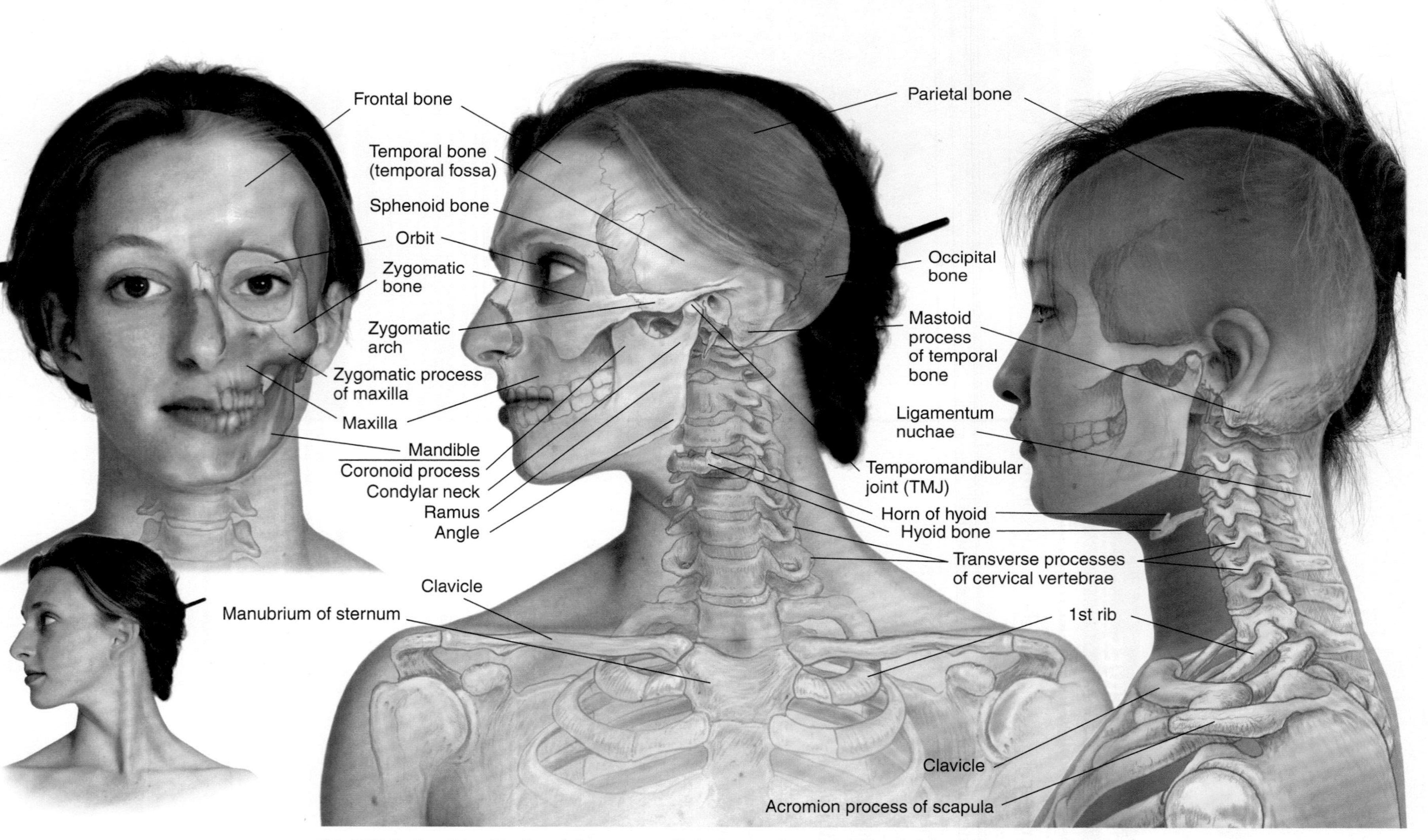

PLATE 3-1 ■ Skeletal features of the anterior and lateral head and neck

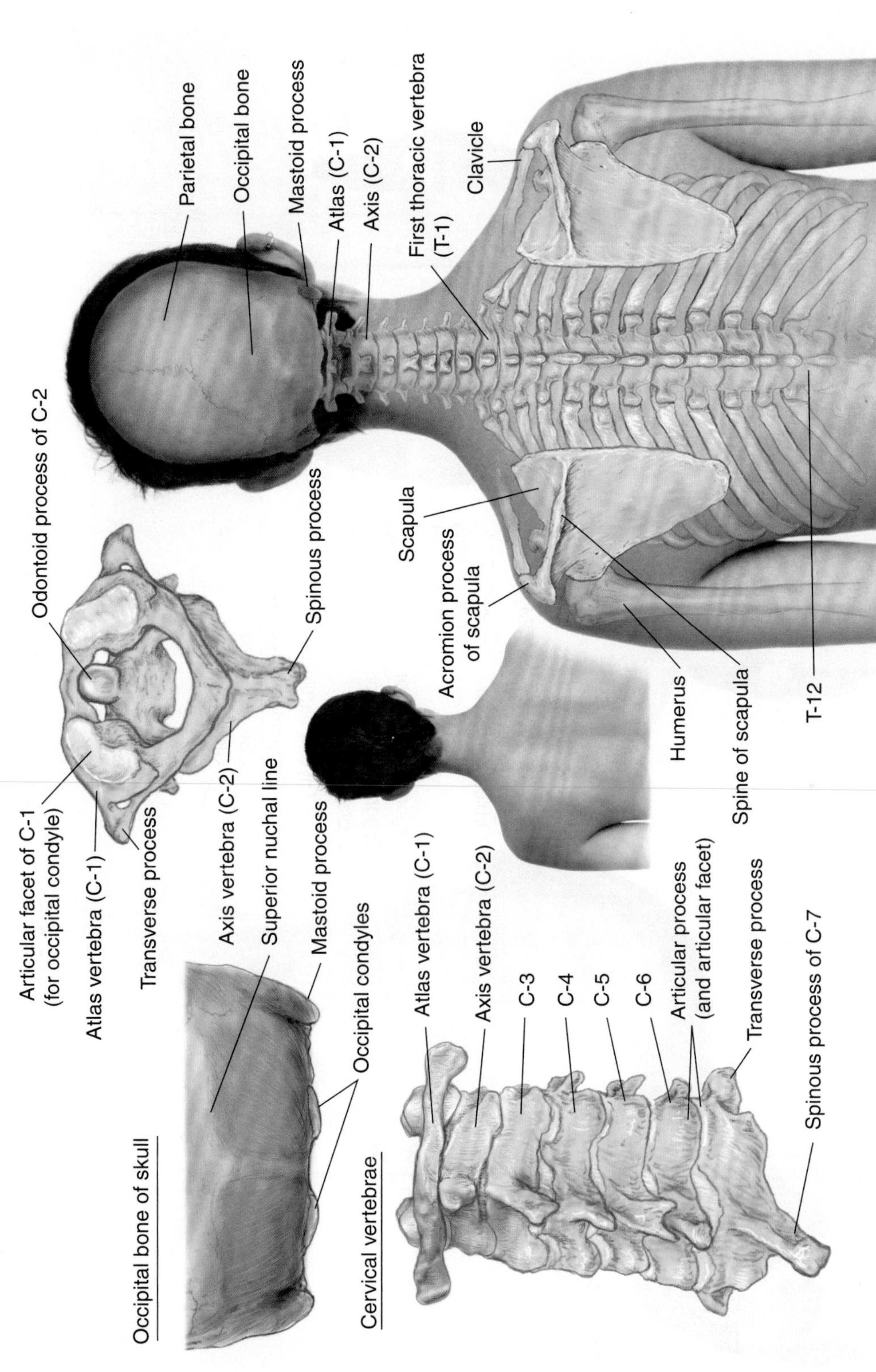

PLATE 3-2 ■ Skeletal features of the posterior head and neck

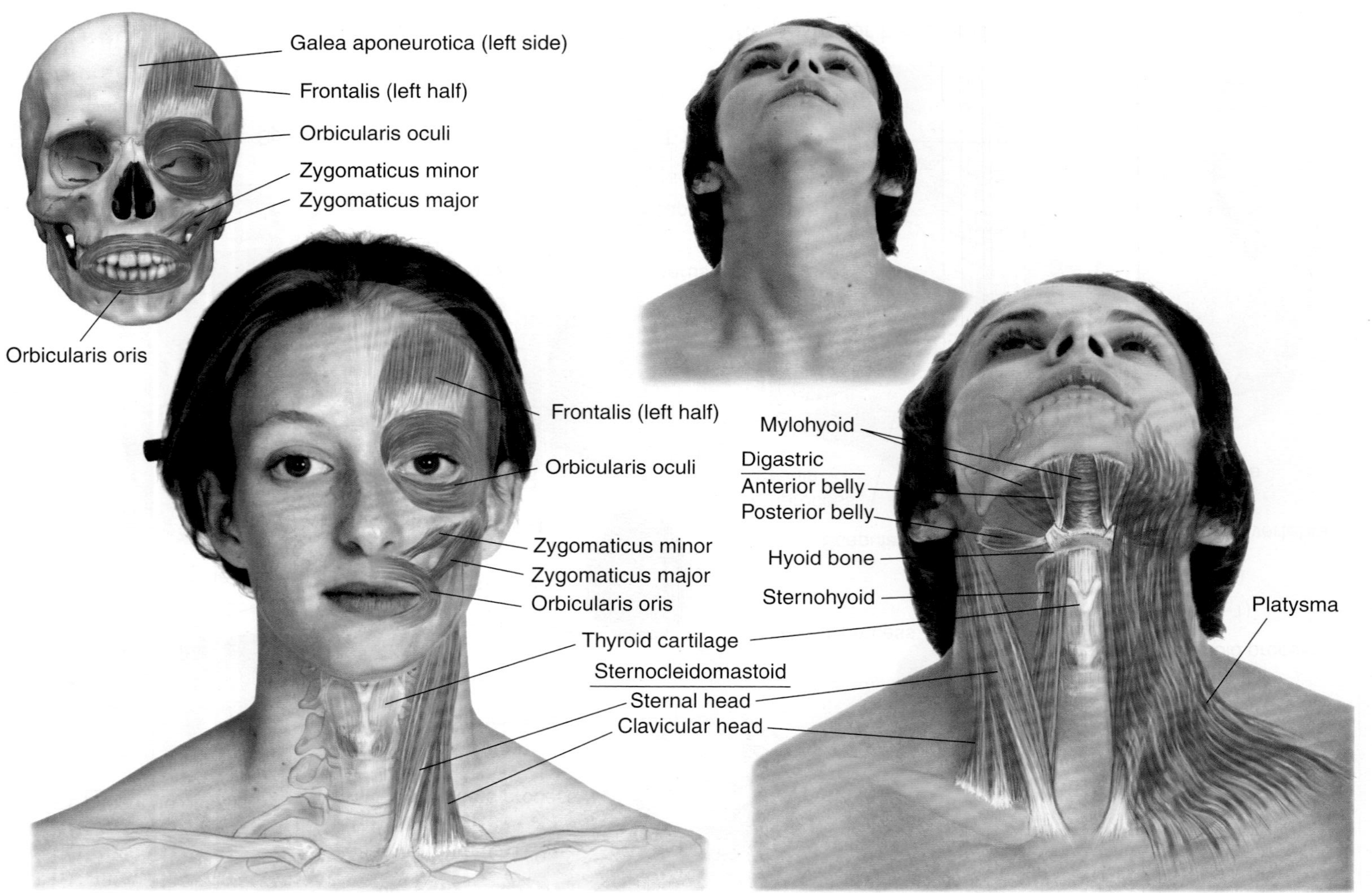

PLATE 3-3 ■ Muscles of the anterior head and neck

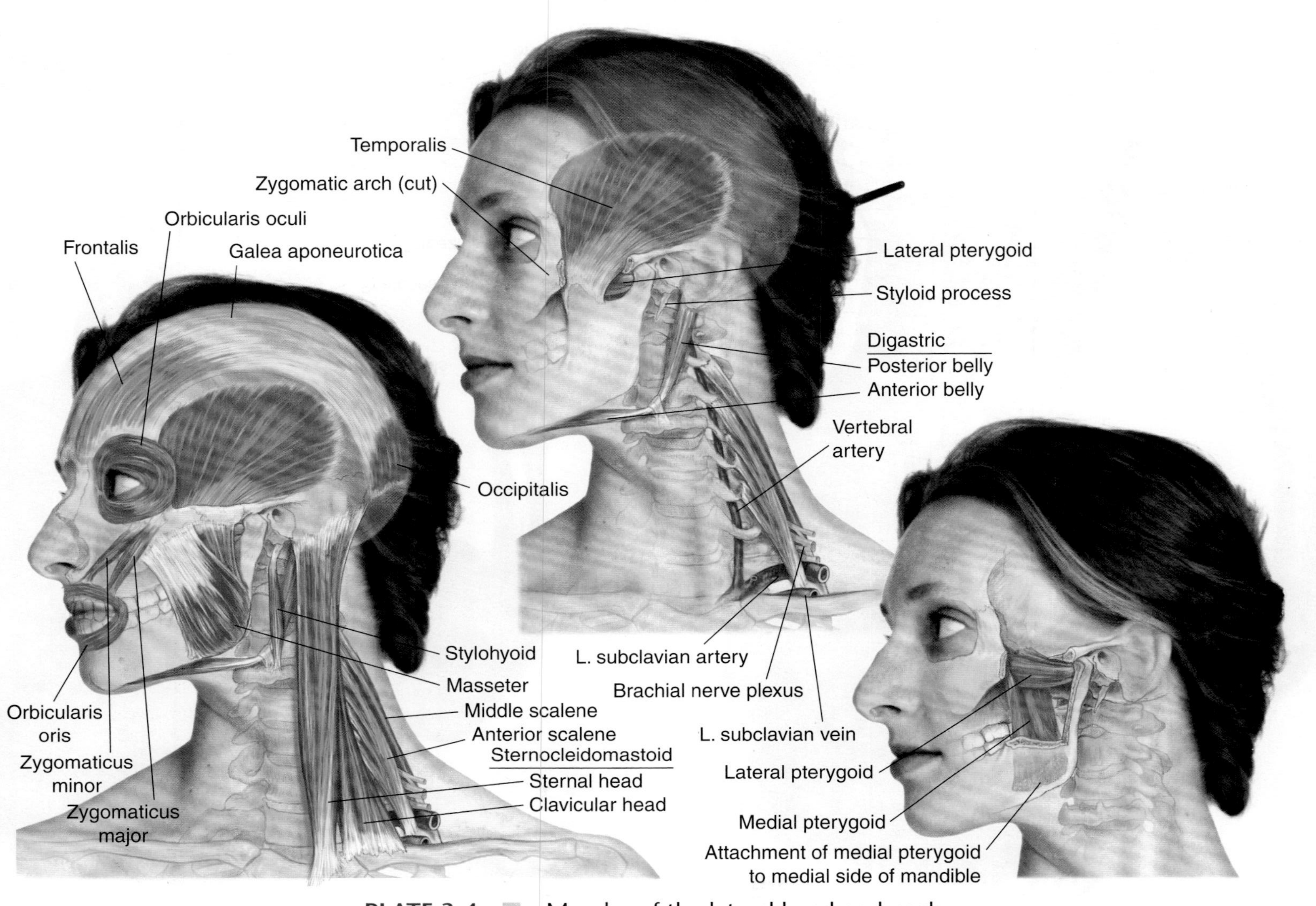

PLATE 3-4 ■ Muscles of the lateral head and neck

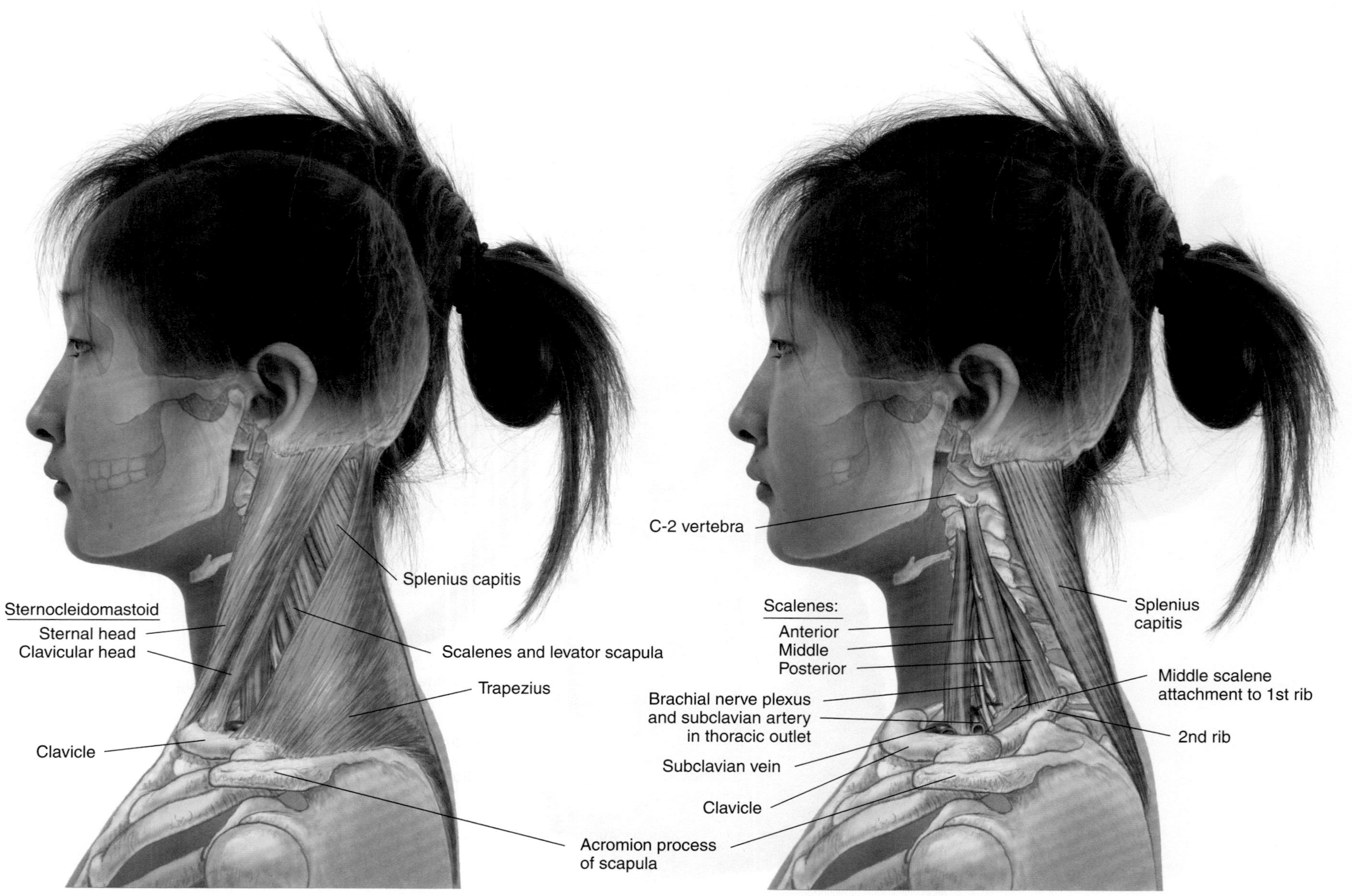

PLATE 3-5 ■ The scalene muscles and lateral neck anatomy

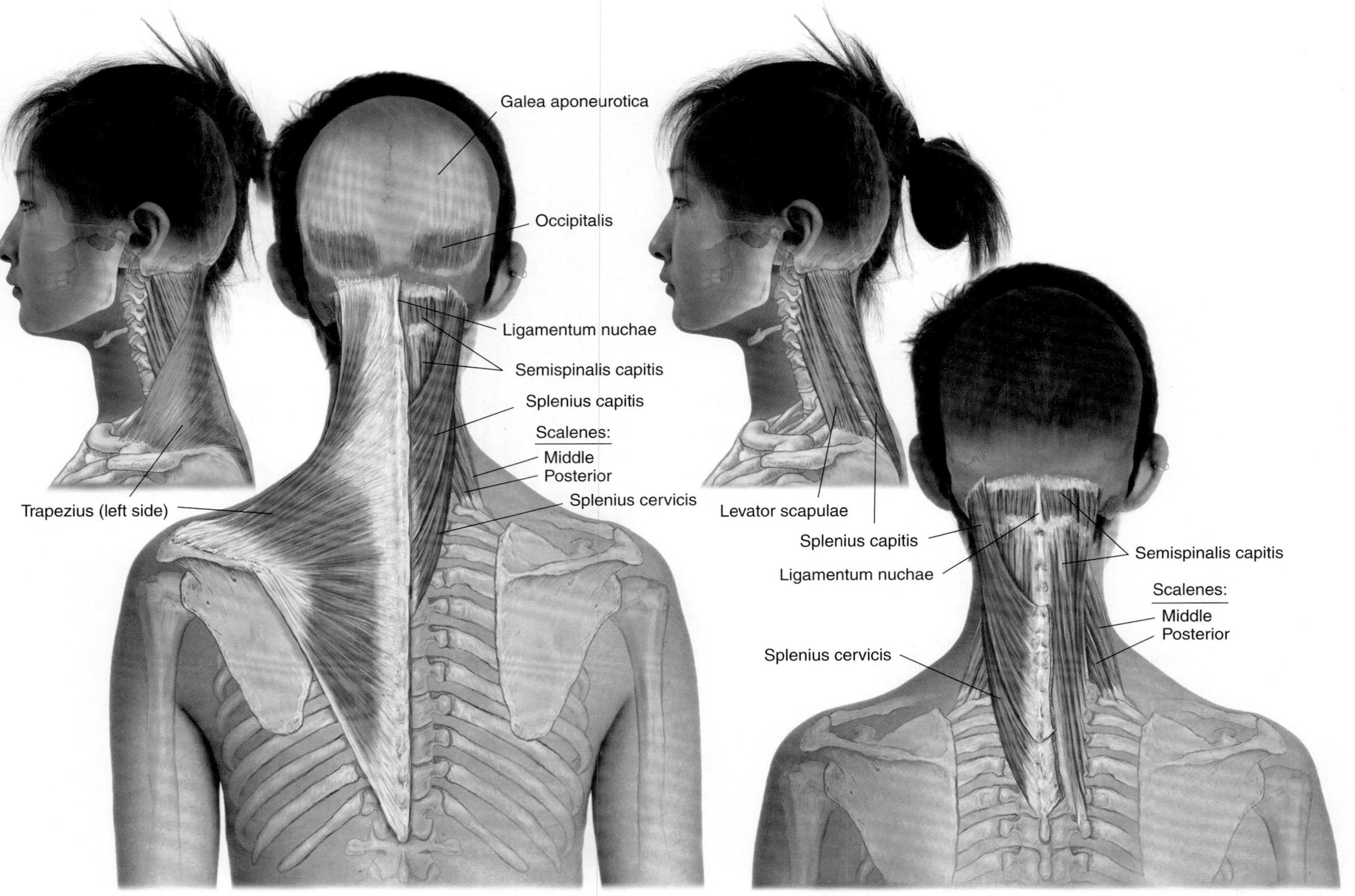

PLATE 3-6 ■ Superficial muscles of the posterior head and neck

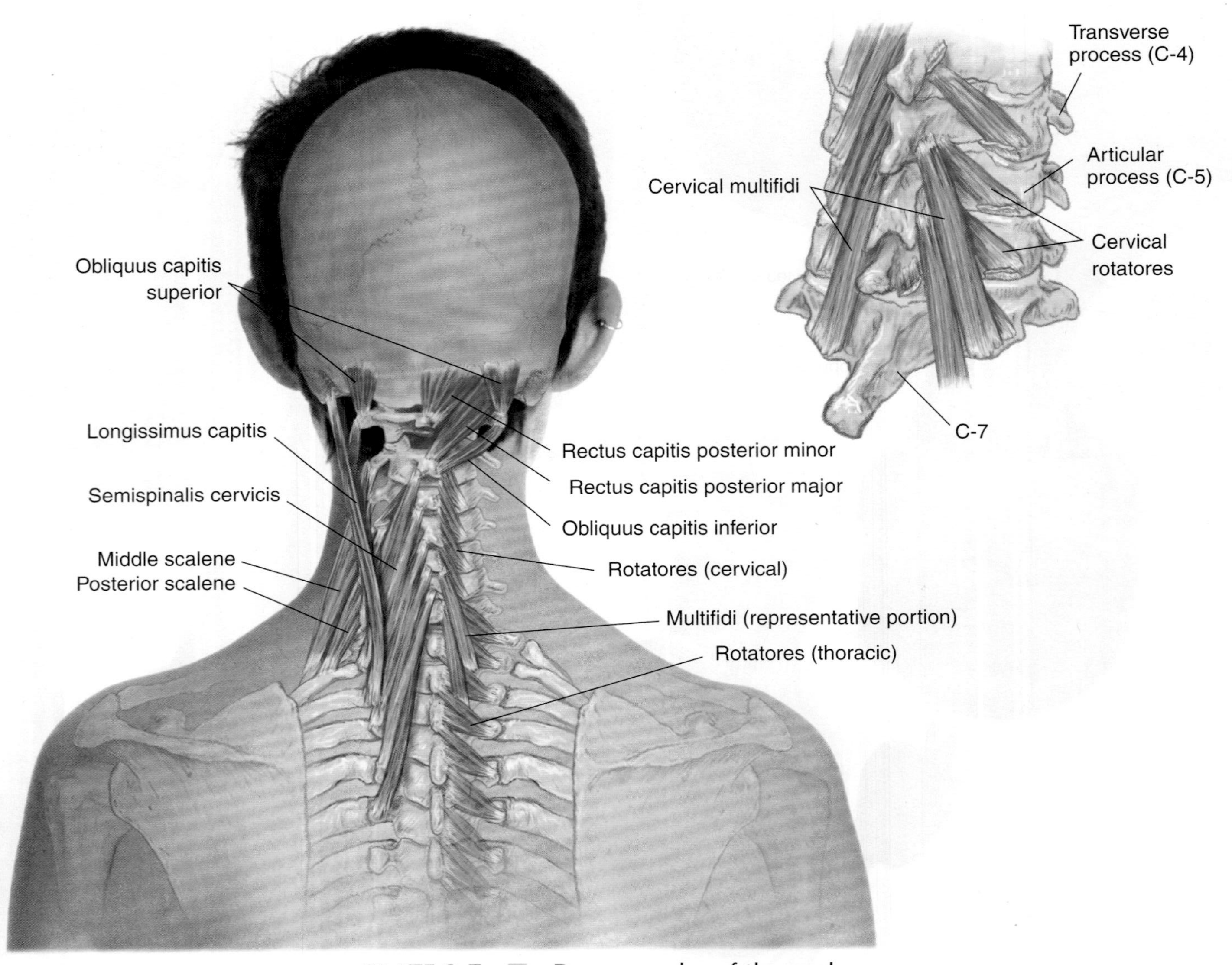

PLATE 3-7 ■ Deep muscles of the neck

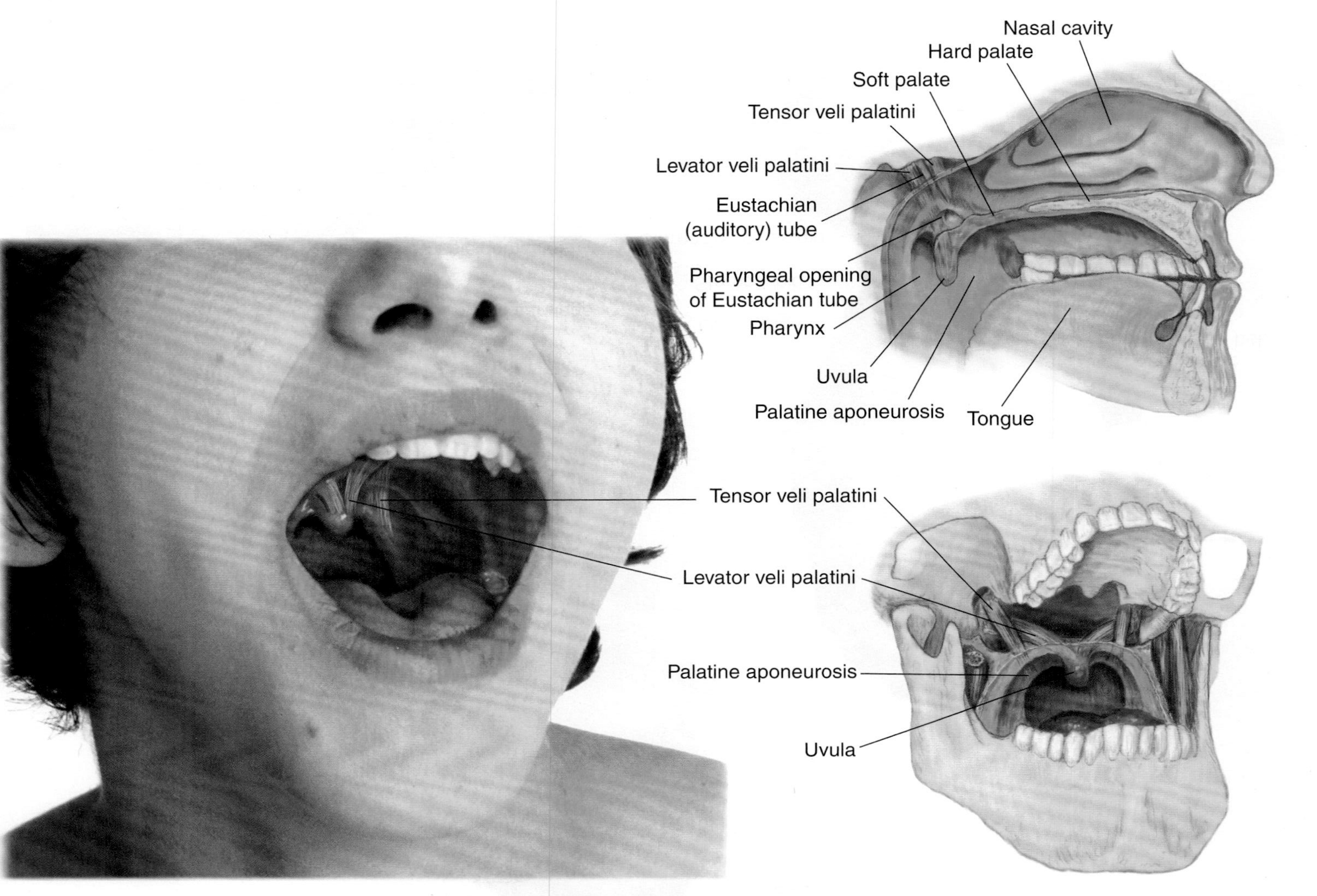

PLATE 3-8 ■ Intraoral anatomy

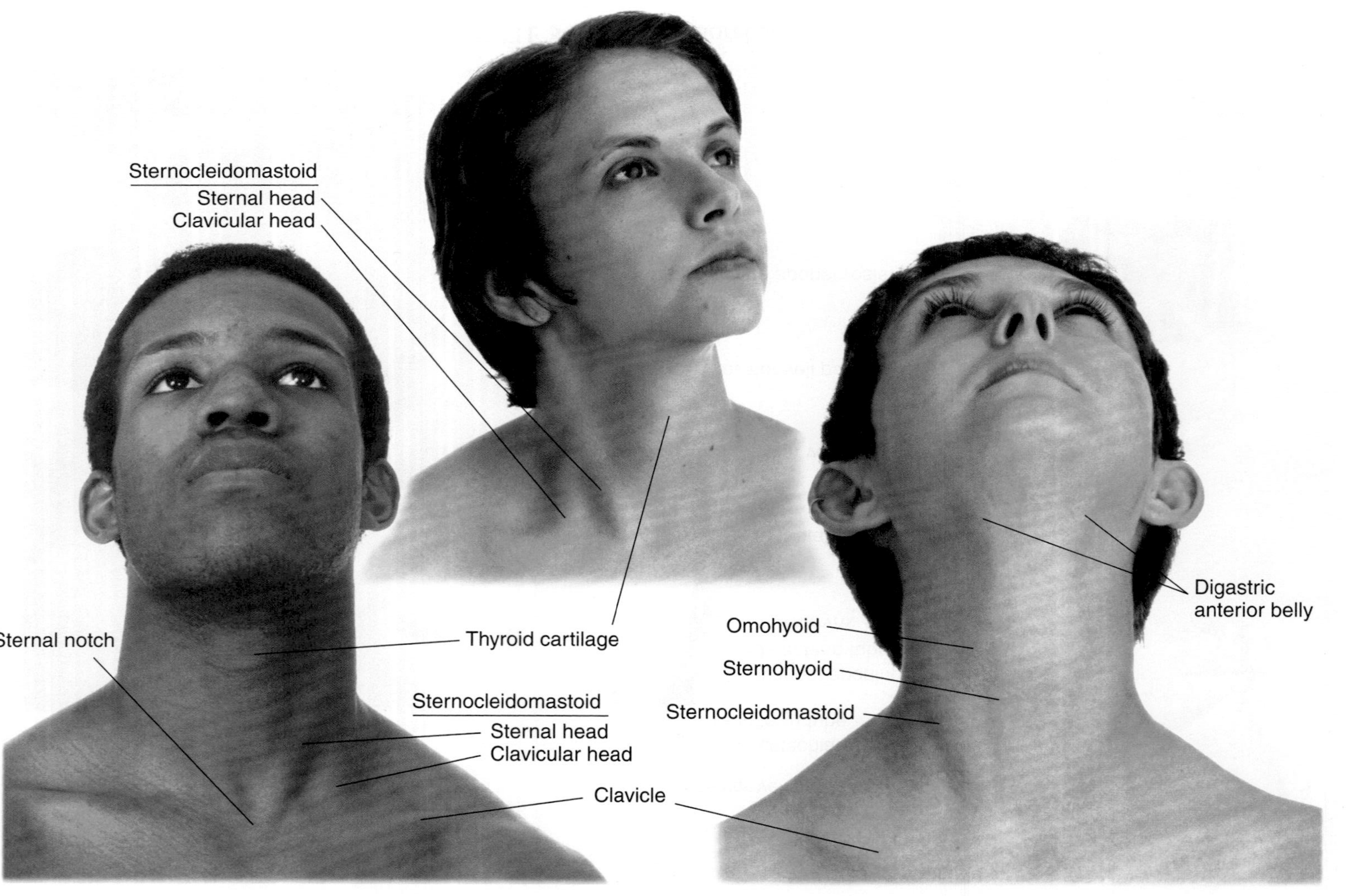

PLATE 3-9 ■ Surface anatomy of the anterior neck

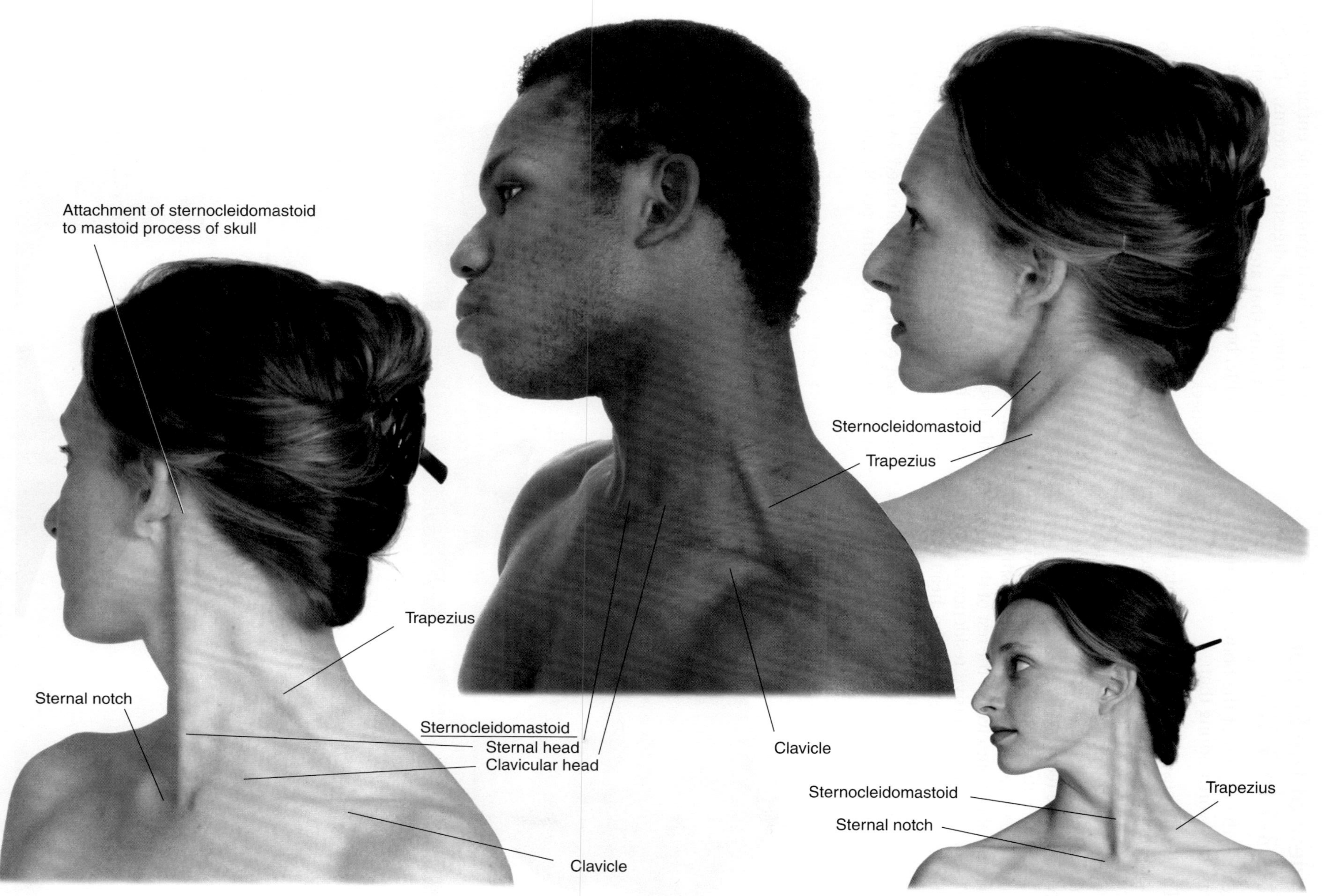

PLATE 3-10 ■ Surface anatomy of the lateral and posterior neck

Overview of the Region (Plates 3-1 to 3-10)

The head is the capital of the body. It is the headquarters. It is worth noting that:

- The head houses the brain—the control center of the body and, according to some, the seat of consciousness.
- The head is the home of the face. The face tells others who we are and, through expression, what we are feeling (Fig. 3-1).
- The head is the point from which the voice issues. The voice is how we verbally transmit information about ourselves to the rest of the world.
- The head is the exclusive residence of four of the five traditional senses. The head houses the organs of vision, hearing, taste, and smell. In addition, the head contains the primary organs of balance.
- Finally, the head contains the entrance to the respiratory and digestive systems. The two functions that are essential to the sustenance of life, breathing and eating, begin here.

The neck serves two essential functions:

- It connects the head and its functions to the rest of the body.
- It supports and moves the head.

The Centers for Disease Control and Prevention reports that headaches are the second most common cause of pain in adults over 18, behind back pain,[1] with neck pain coming in third place. Clinical observation confirms that many tension-type headaches are often triggered by stress, and many originate in trigger points in the neck muscles. Such headaches can be reduced in frequency and intensity, if not completely eliminated, by resolution of these trigger points. Many people carry their heads

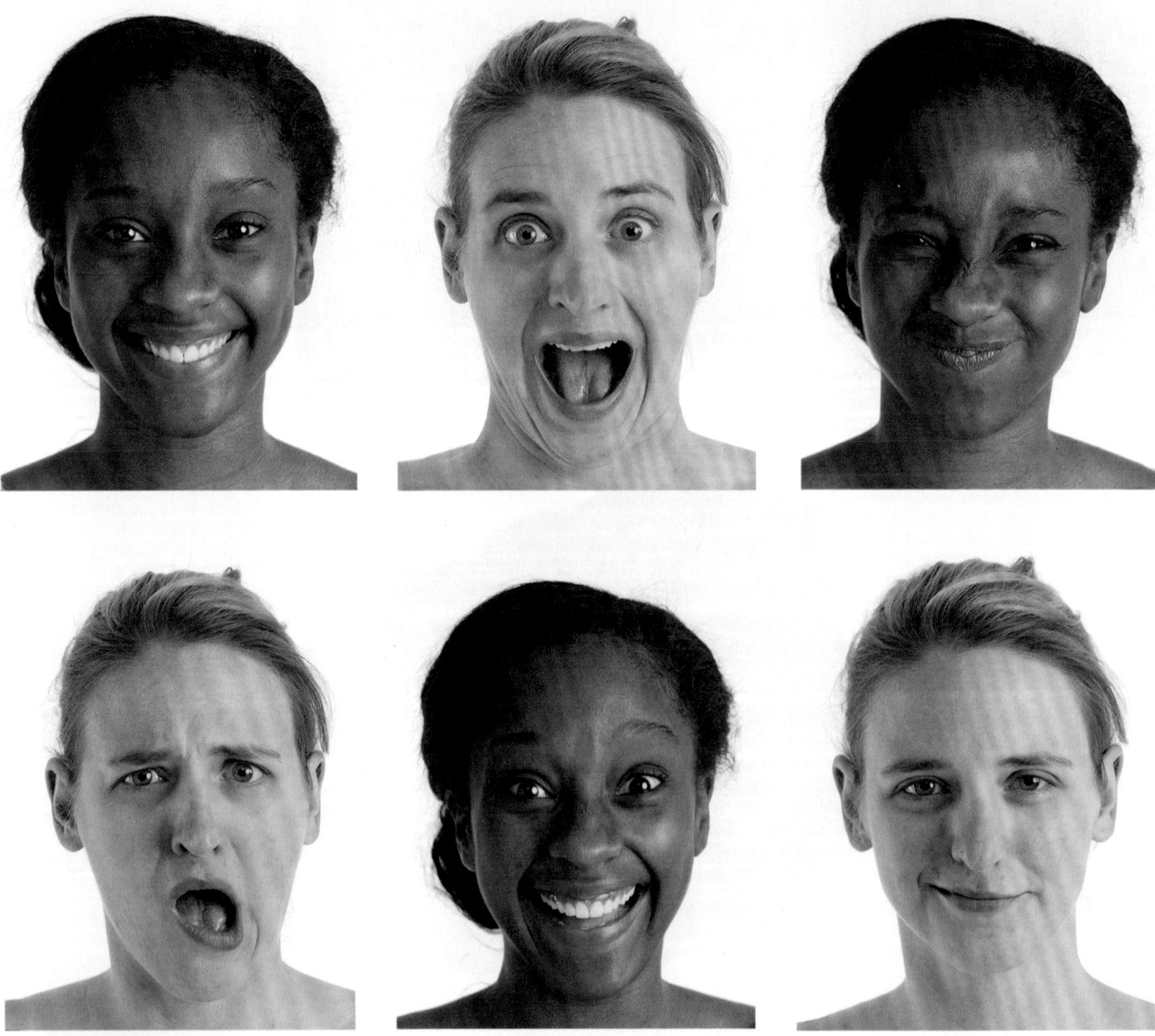

FIGURE 3-1 Muscles produce facial expressions

with the ears well forward of the sagittal midline (Fig. 3-2). This misalignment often results in the development of myofascial trigger points in the posterior neck. According to Simons, "The head-forward posture activates posterior neck MTrPs [myofascial trigger points] by overloading them, causing chronic contraction without relaxation periods" (David G. Simons, MD, private communication, September 23, 2001). Note, however, that the treatment of the posterior cervical trigger points alone will seldom solve the pain problem. If poor postural habits are the cause or a contributor to the pain, then overall correction of the causes of postural misalignment is required to achieve long-term relief. People who do office work, sitting at a computer all day and those who are constantly looking down at their phone (commonly known as "text neck"), are particularly vulnerable. Educating the clients about their posture and about using proper ergonomics in the workplace can help alleviate the problem.

Erik Dalton has popularized the theory of the "42-pound head," noting that for every inch the head is forward of the shoulders, weight is amplified by 10 lb. Dalton states that as a result, a 12-lb head held 3 inches forward causes the cervical extensors (semispinalis, splenii, longissimus, upper trapezius, etc.) to isometrically battle 42 lb against the relentless force of gravity.[2] That's why it's important to educate the client about poor postural habits; otherwise, we're just offering them a very temporary fix for a long-standing problem caused by their own tendencies and holding patterns.

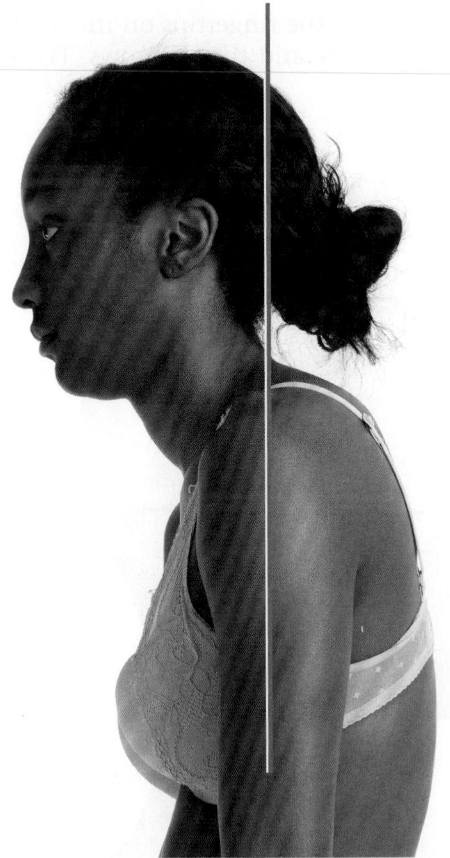

FIGURE 3-2 Posture with ear forward of sagittal midline

Other research has concluded that forward head posture and reduced cervical lordosis did not correlate with the location or the number of trigger points and myofascial pain syndrome in the neck and shoulders. Further studies are needed to delineate the mechanism of neck pain in patients with forward head posture.[3] We do have to remember that (a) not all pain is caused by poor posture, (b) not everyone who has poor posture has pain, and (c) plenty of people who have good posture have pain. While chronic poor posture patterns should certainly be brought to the client's attention, we cannot have the expectation that correcting that alone will entirely get rid of the issues. Stress and pain are very connected; so although correcting posture is good, the client's stress level is a separate factor.

The skull consists of 22 cranial bones, only one of which, the mandible, is generally considered movable. The cranial bones are connected by fibrous joints called sutures and are regarded by most anatomists as being fused. This fusion becomes literal as we age, to the extent that in the elderly, many of the suture "joints' have been converted to solid bone. Craniosacral therapists believe that the cranial bones are capable of small but significant movement, and their treatment approach attempts to influence the movement and positioning of these bones; most scientists scoff at the theory, and there is a lack of credible research to support it. The arguments for and against craniosacral theory are beyond the scope of this book.

The skull itself rests on the first cervical vertebra or atlas; the occipital condyles of the skull rest on two kidney-shaped facets on the superior surface of the atlas. The atlas vertebra is a bony ring with essentially no body or spinous process. In turn, the atlas rests on the second cervical vertebra, or axis, which has a toothlike projection, the odontoid process, projecting up into the ring of the atlas (see Plate 3-2). Turning the head consists partly of the rotation or pivoting of the atlas around the odontoid process.

Because of the significant weight of the head and the importance of its mobility in using the senses (particularly vision), the neck muscles are numerous, and many are thick and strong. They are all susceptible to pain and dysfunction.

The muscles of the head, face, and neck can be classified as follows:

- Scalp muscles, primarily occipitalis and frontalis (or occipitofrontalis, if viewed as one muscle). These muscles move the scalp and forehead.

- Face muscles, involved primarily in controlling facial expressions
- Jaw muscles, which open and close the jaw by moving the mandible
- Neck muscles, which support and balance the head on the spinal column and move it in all directions

Note: Some of the treatment techniques described in this chapter require work inside the mouth. Several principles should be observed:

- Working inside any body orifice may have emotional implications for the client. Always obtain permission first and discuss any hesitations the client may have.
- Examination gloves should always be worn when working inside any body orifice. Avoid latex and powdered gloves, to which many people are allergic.
- Remove your hand from the mouth frequently to give the client a chance to swallow and decrease any discomfort.

CAUTION Intraoral work is considered to be outside the scope of practice for massage therapists in many states in the USA. You should check with your state regulatory board before performing any intraoral work.

FRONTALIS

fron-TAL-is

ETYMOLOGY Latin, pertaining to the front

Overview

Frontalis (Fig. 3-3) is sometimes regarded as one belly of the muscle occipitofrontalis, since it is connected directly to the occipitalis by the galea aponeurotica, a tendinous sheet of connective tissue that lies over the skull from front to back. Taut bands of muscle in either the frontalis or occipitalis muscle (bellies) may produce an overall sense of tightness in the scalp. Note that the frontalis connects partially to the orbicularis oculi (see also Plates 3-3 and 3-4); both muscles are commonly involved in headaches.

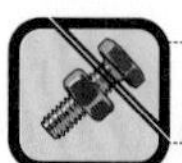

ATTACHMENTS

- Origin: the galea aponeurotica
- Insertion: the skin over the eyebrow, partially to the orbicularis oculi

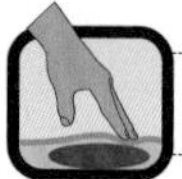

PALPATION

Press gently with the fingertips on the forehead between the hairline and the eyebrows. The muscle's

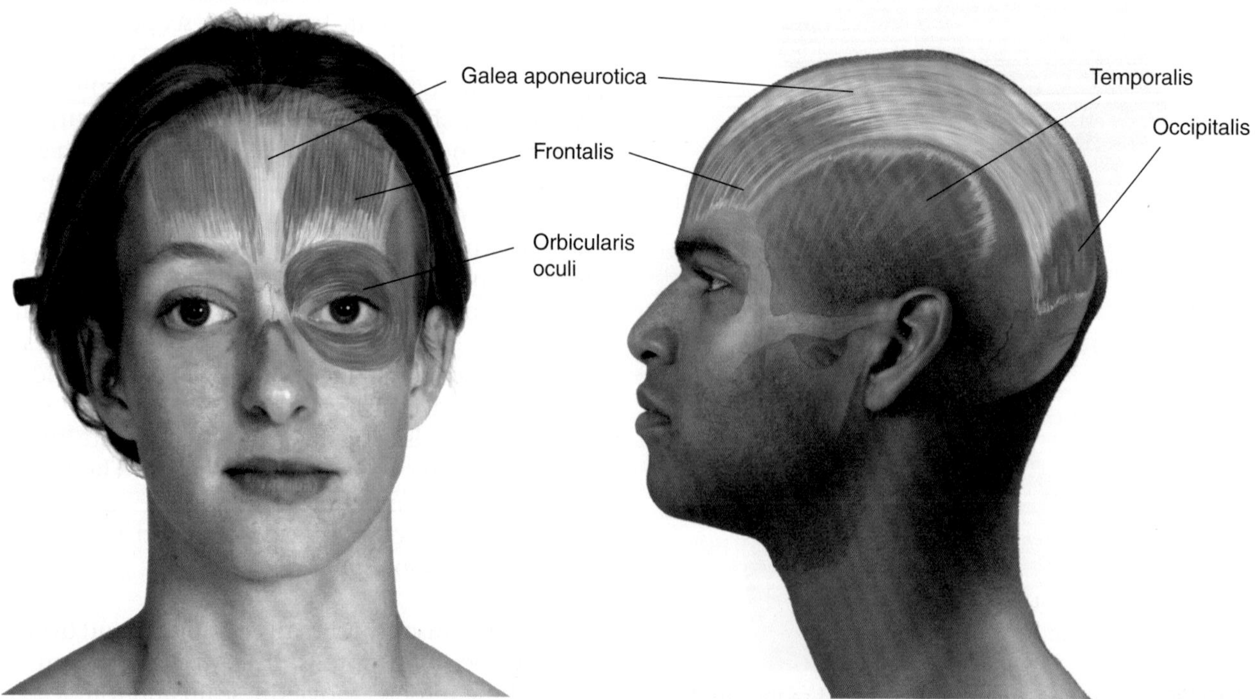

FIGURE 3-3 Anatomy of frontalis (occipitofrontalis), and galea aponeurotica

architecture is parallel, and the fiber direction is superior/inferior. The more taut the muscle, the more palpable it will be.

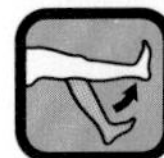

ACTIONS

- Raises the eyebrow and wrinkles the forehead
- Working with occipitalis, helps shift the scalp anteriorly and posteriorly

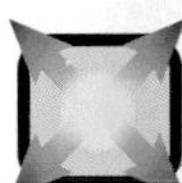

REFERRAL AREA

Local, with pain radiating over the forehead

OTHER MUSCLES TO EXAMINE

- Occipitalis
- Orbicularis oculi
- Temporalis
- Sternocleidomastoid
- Zygomaticus major
- Scalenes
- Posterior neck muscles

CAUTION Remember the general cautions for the head, face, and neck: Avoid dragging downward on the skin of the face. The skin around the eyes is very thin, so exercise extra caution. Having hands on the face and the front of the neck makes some people feel claustrophobic, so be attentive of the client's comfort.

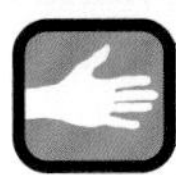

MANUAL THERAPY

Cross-fiber Stroking

- The client lies supine.
- With the fingers spread over the sides of the client's head, place the thumbs at the center of the forehead just over the eyebrows.
- Pressing firmly into the tissue, slowly spread the thumbs apart (Fig. 3-4) until they have covered the forehead to the lateral ridges of the frontal bone.
- Shifting your hands superiorly, repeat this process as far as the hairline.

Stripping

- The client lies supine.
- Place the tip or flat of the thumb on the forehead at the hairline just next to the central line of the forehead.

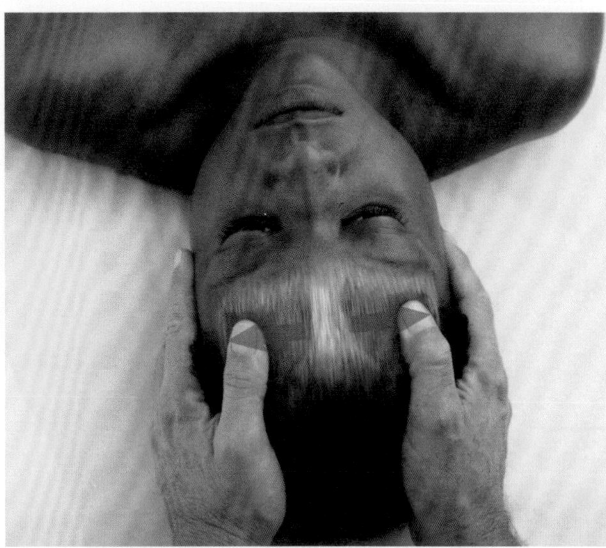

FIGURE 3-4 Cross-fiber stroking of frontalis

- Pressing firmly into the tissue, slide the thumb inferiorly to the medial end of the eyebrow.
- Shifting your hand laterally, repeat this process as far as the lateral end of the eyebrow.

CAUTION Remember, when performing *any* deep techniques, it's a good idea to warm the tissue first with strokes of Swedish massage, particularly effleurage, and to use it as a transitional stroke between cross-fiber work and stripping.

OCCIPITALIS

ock-sip-it-TAL-is

ETYMOLOGY Latin ***occiput***, back of the head

Overview

Occipitalis (Fig. 3-5) is also regarded as the posterior belly of the muscle occipitofrontalis, since it is connected directly to the frontalis by the galea aponeurotica, a tendinous sheet of connective tissue that lies over the skull from front to back. Taut bands of muscle in either the frontalis or occipitalis muscle (bellies) may produce an overall sense of tightness in the scalp.

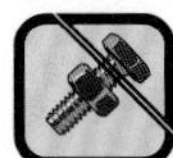

ATTACHMENTS

- Origin: the galea aponeurotica
- Insertion: the superior nuchal line of the occipital bone

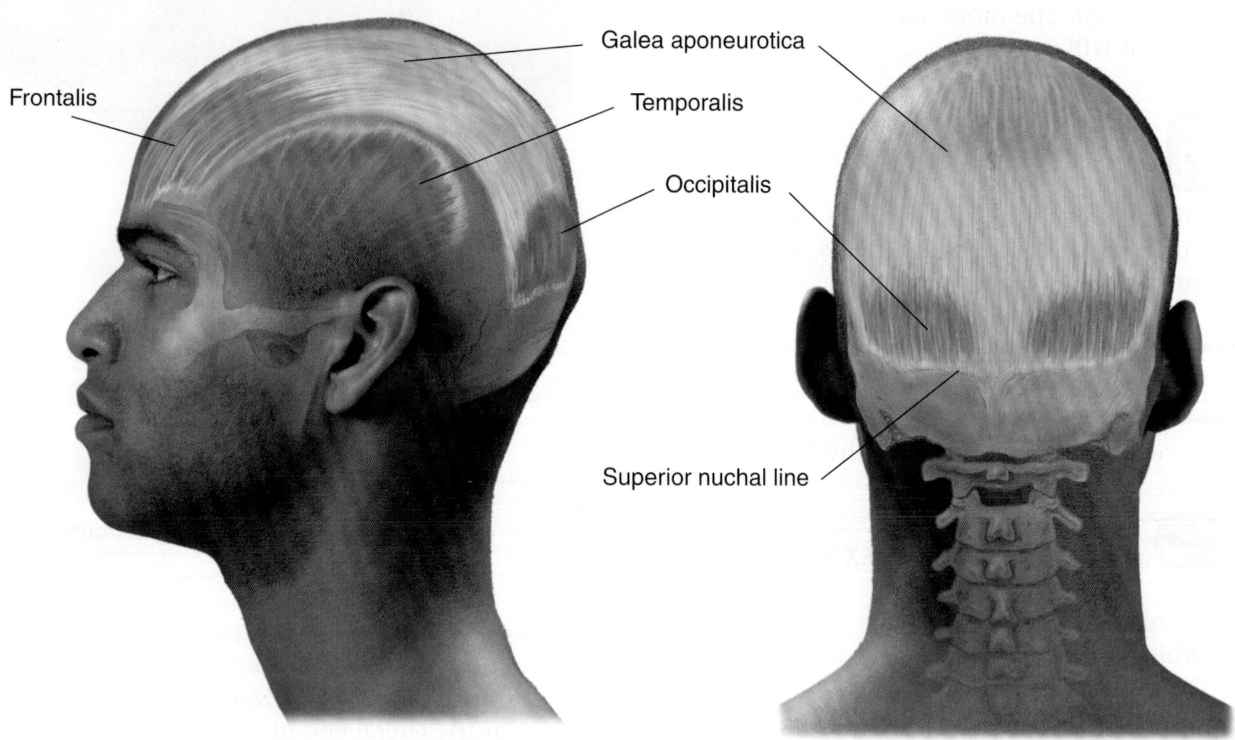

FIGURE 3-5 Anatomy of occipitalis

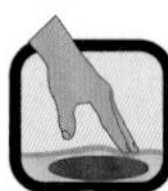

PALPATION

Place your fingertips under the head of the supine client directly under the two clearly defined protrusions of the skull. Occipitalis covers these protrusions. The muscle's architecture is parallel, and the fiber direction is superior/inferior.

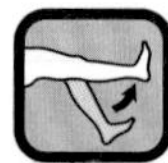

ACTION

Anchors and retracts the galea aponeurotica, thus pulling the scalp posteriorly. See Frontalis for further discussion.

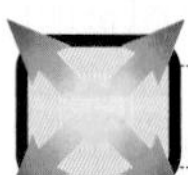

REFERRAL AREA

Radiates pain locally to the back and top of the head and can refer pain to the ipsilateral eye

OTHER MUSCLES TO EXAMINE

- Frontalis
- Temporalis
- Orbicularis oculi
- All lateral and posterior neck muscles

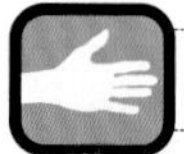

MANUAL THERAPY

Stripping (1)

- The client lies supine.
- Place the hands under the head, the fingers curled upward so that the fingertips touch the base of the skull.
- Pressing superiorly and using the weight of the client's head to generate pressure, draw the hands very slowly toward you, so that the fingertips treat the entire occipitalis belly (Fig. 3-6).
- Pause where the client reports tender points.

Stripping (2)

- The client lies either supine or prone with the head turned away from the therapist.
- Holding the head with one hand, place the other thumb at the central line of the occiput, on a line with the upper part of occipitalis.
- Pressing firmly into the tissue, draw the thumb laterally across occipitalis.
- Placing the thumb in a position closer to the neck, repeat the procedure until you have covered the entire muscle belly.

Stripping (3)

- The client lies either supine or prone with the head turned away from the therapist.

- Hold the client's head in both your hands, so that the thumbs rest on the upper part of occipitalis at its center.
- Pressing firmly into the tissue, spread the thumbs apart as far as the outer aspects of the muscle belly (Fig. 3-7).
- Shifting the thumbs to a position nearer the neck, repeat the procedure until the whole muscle belly has been treated.

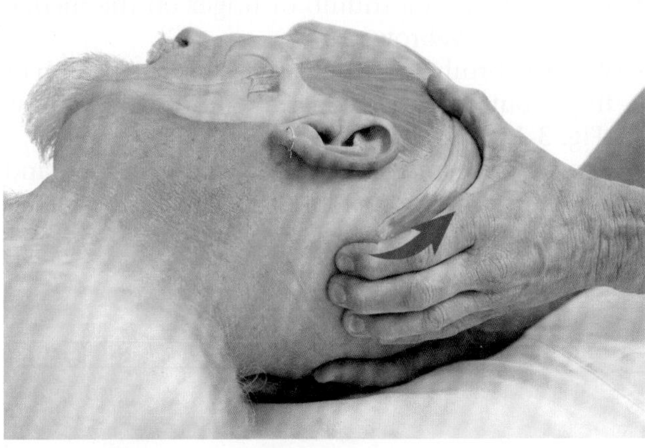

FIGURE 3-6 Stripping occipitalis with the fingertips

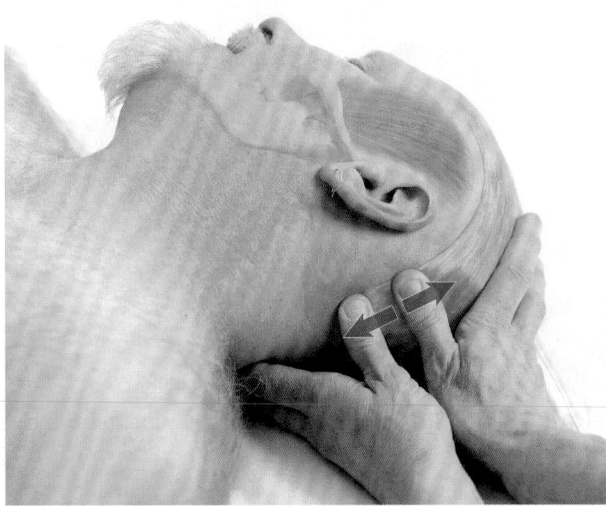

FIGURE 3-7 Stripping of occipitalis with thumbs

ORBICULARIS OCULI

or-bic-yu-LAR-is OCK-yu-lee (or OCK-yu-LYE)

ETYMOLOGY Latin: ***orbiculus,*** a small disk + ***oculi,*** of the eye

Overview

Orbicularis oculi (Fig. 3-8) encircles the eye and provides for voluntary closure of the eyelid. Its trigger points can be activated by frowning and squinting and by trigger points in sternocleidomastoid.

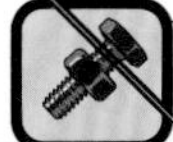

ATTACHMENTS

- Origin: the medial palpebral ligament, frontal and maxillary bones, and to the tissue of the eyelid
- Insertion: the orbit

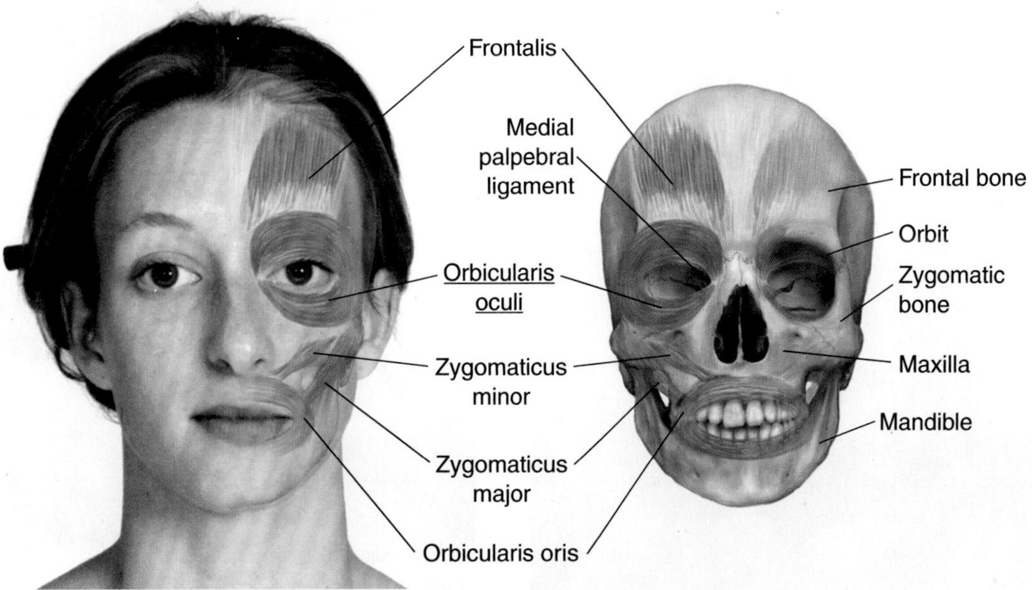

FIGURE 3-8 Anatomy of orbicularis oculi

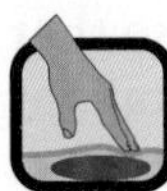

PALPATION

This muscle surrounds the eye. The muscle's architecture is parallel, and the fiber direction is roughly concentrical around the eye. Asking the client to intentionally forcefully close and open the eye will allow you to feel the muscle contractions.

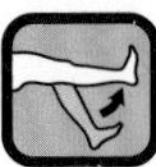

ACTIONS

- Intentional blinking and strong closure of the eyelid
- Squinting

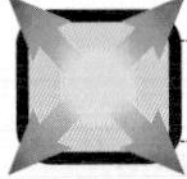

REFERRAL AREA

Superior to the eye and down the side of the nose

MANUAL THERAPY

Compression

- Using the thumb, seek a common tender or trigger point near the lateral end of the eyebrow.
- Compress and hold for release (Fig. 3-9).

CAUTION The thinnest skin on the body is around the eyes and is typically more delicate than elsewhere on the face. Use care and stroke only outwardly and upward; do not drag down.

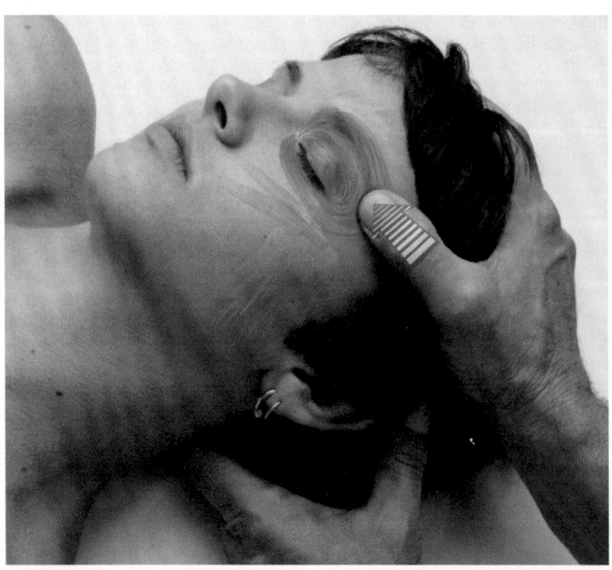

FIGURE 3-9 Trigger point compression of orbicularis oculi

Stripping

- Place the tip of a thumb or finger on the medial end of the eyebrow.
- Pressing firmly into the tissue, slide the thumb or finger outward to the lateral end of the eyebrow (Fig. 3-10).
- Repeat once just superior to the eyebrow, and again just inferior to it, pressing superiorly against the orbit (Fig. 3-11).

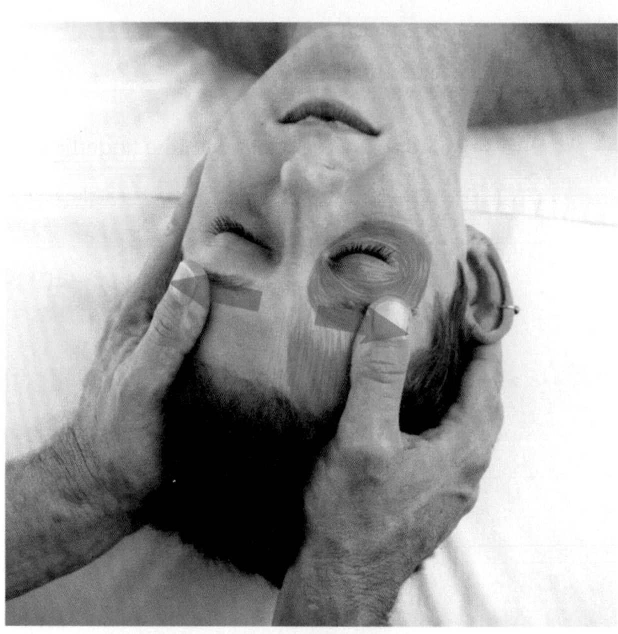

FIGURE 3-10 Stripping orbicularis oculi superior to the orbit

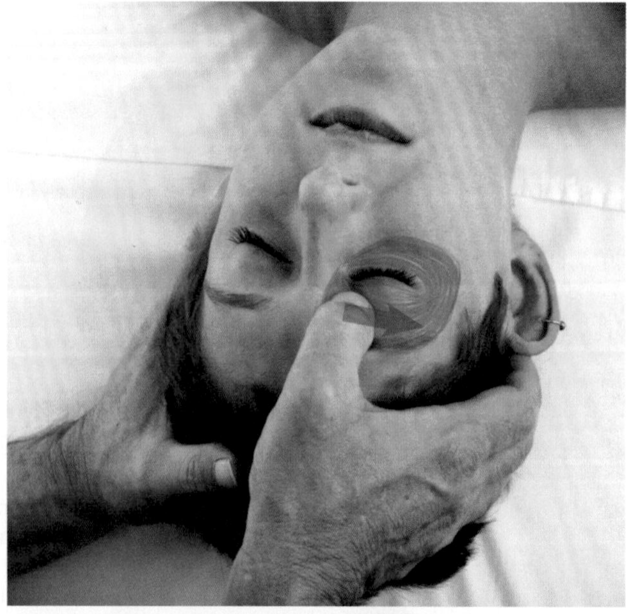

FIGURE 3-11 Stripping orbicularis oculi pressing upward against the orbit

ZYGOMATICUS MAJOR AND MINOR

zye-go-MAT-ik-us

ETYMOLOGY Greek *zygon*, yoke or joining

Overview

Zygomaticus major and **minor** (Fig. 3-12) are the principal smiling muscles; their trigger points arise from trigger point activity in the chewing muscles (masseter and the pterygoids) (see Plates 3-3 and 3-4). It is best examined by pincer palpation with the index finger in the mouth and the thumb outside the mouth, or vice versa; check your state law first to be sure any intraoral work is permitted.

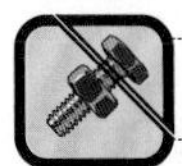

ATTACHMENTS

Zygomaticus major:
- Origin: anterior to zygomaticotemporal suture
- Insertion: the tissues at the corners of the mouth (modiolus), blending with fibers of orbicularis oris

Zygomaticus minor:
- Origin: zygomatic bone, posterior to zygomaticomaxillary suture
- Insertion: orbicularis oris of the upper lip

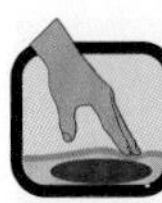

PALPATION

Place your index fingertip just under the zygomatic prominence with your fourth fingertip resting on the skin over the canine tooth. By moving your fingertips back and forth, you can feel the muscles clearly. The muscle's architecture is parallel, and the fiber direction is diagonal.

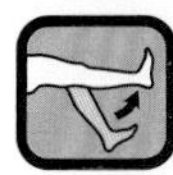

ACTION

- Zygomaticus major: pulls the corners of the mouth up and back, as in smiling
- Zygomaticus minor: elevates the upper lip

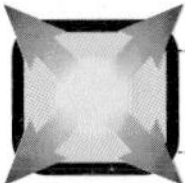

REFERRAL AREA

Up the cheek and along the side of the nose, past the medial corner of the eye and the eyebrow, and over the medial aspect of the forehead

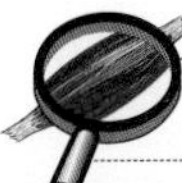

OTHER MUSCLES TO EXAMINE

- Masseter
- Pterygoids
- Orbicularis oculi

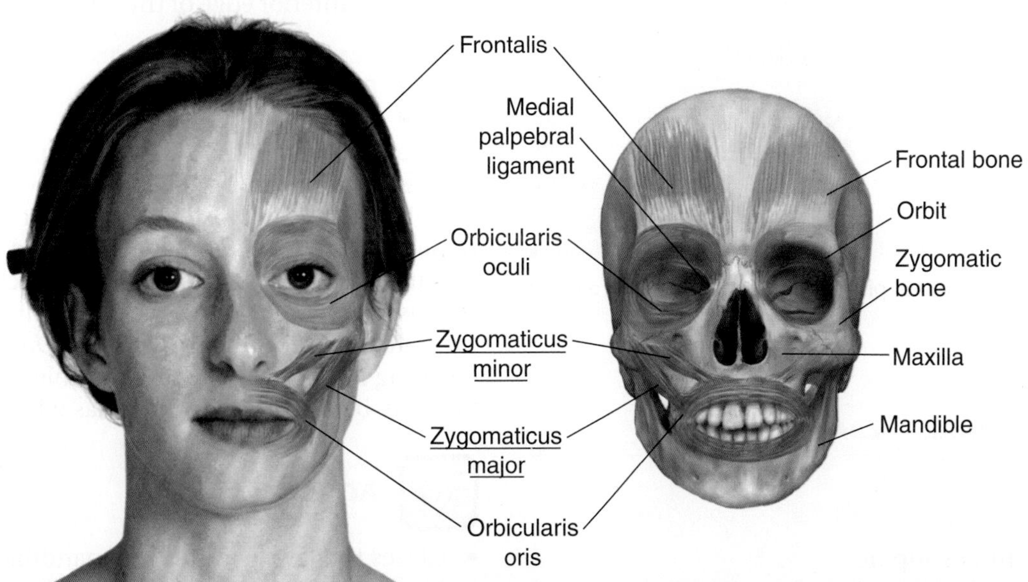

FIGURE 3-12 Anatomy of zygomaticus major and minor

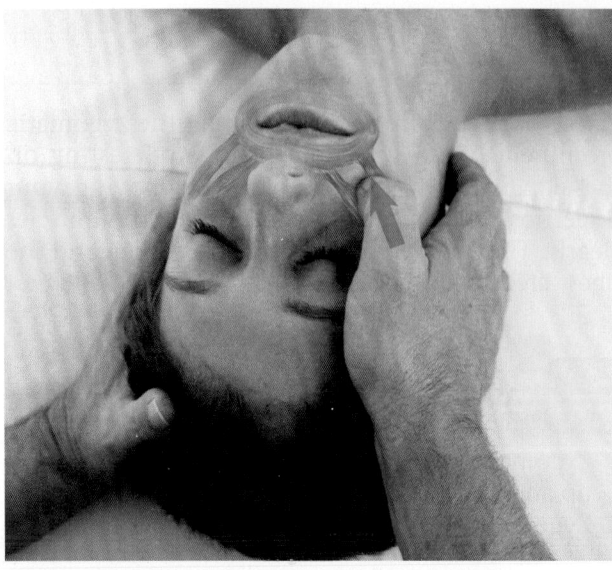

FIGURE 3-13 Stripping of zygomaticus

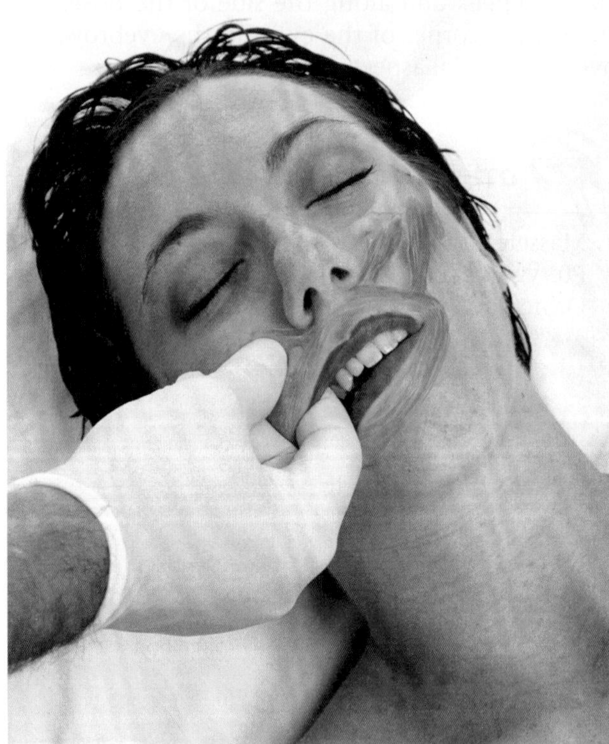

FIGURE 3-14 Intraoral pincer compression of zygomaticus

MANUAL THERAPY

Stripping

- The client lies supine.
- Place the edge of the thumb against the zygomatic bone (cheekbone).
- Pressing firmly into the tissue, slide the thumb slowly inferiorly to the corner of the mouth (Fig. 3-13).

Compression

- The client lies supine.
- Place the index finger inside the mouth in the pouch of the cheek.
- Place the tip of the thumb on the outside of the cheek.
- Using pincer palpation, explore the length of the muscle for trigger points or tender points. Compress and hold each point until it releases (Fig. 3-14).

TEMPORALIS

TEM-per-AL-is

ETYMOLOGY Latin, relating to the temple

Overview

Temporalis (Fig. 3-15) is a large, scallop-shaped muscle covering the side of the head in front of, superior to, and behind the ear. It is a muscle of the temporomandibular joint (TMJ). It should be examined and treated in all clients complaining of headaches or TMJ problems. Therapists usually pay a lot of attention to the anterior and middle portions, but the posterior section of the muscle should be addressed as well.

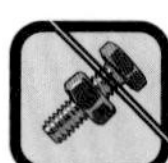

ATTACHMENTS

- Origin: the bone and fascia in the temporal fossa superior to the zygomatic arch
- Insertion: the coronoid process of the mandible and the anterior edge of the ramus of the mandible

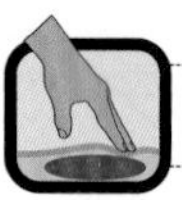

PALPATION

Although covered by a fairly tough layer of fascia, temporalis can be palpated between the sphenoid bone and the posterior aspect of the temporal bone down to the zygomatic arch, and a very small amount just below the arch. The muscle's architecture is convergent, and the fiber direction varies from diagonal to superior/inferior. Due to its fascial covering it is scarcely distinguishable when relaxed, but may be distinguished in areas where it is tight.

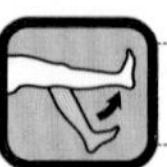

ACTIONS

- Closes the jaw (elevates the mandible)
- Moves the jaw posteriorly and laterally
- Maintains the resting position of the mandible

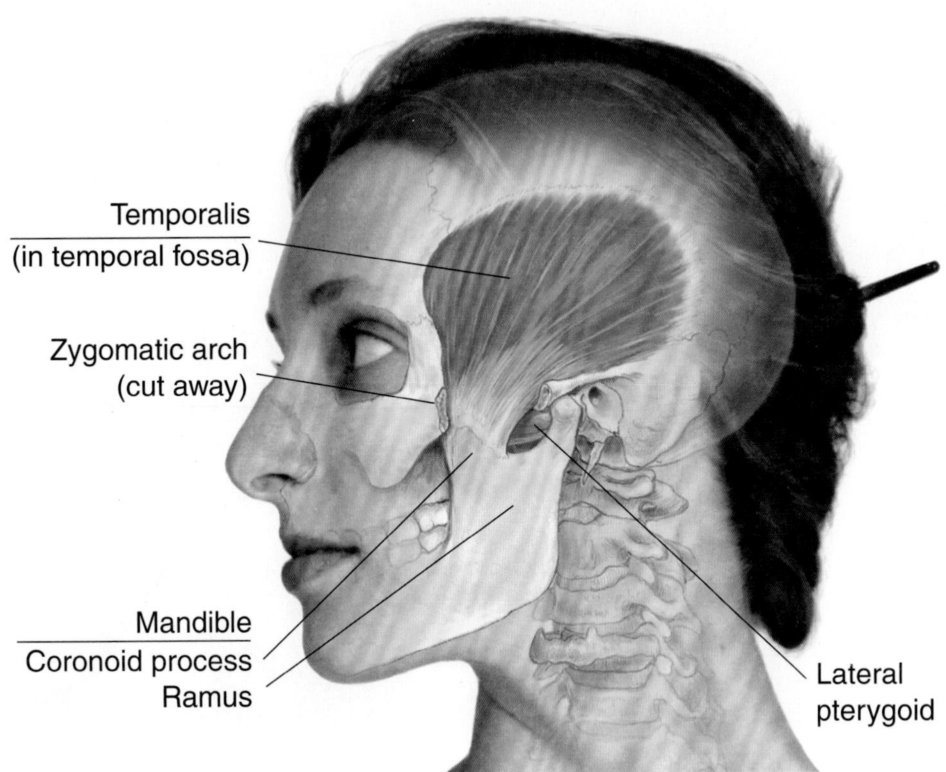

FIGURE 3-15 Anatomy of temporalis

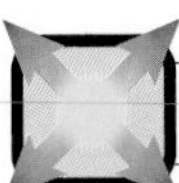

REFERRAL AREA

To all or part of temporal region, eyebrow region, cheek, and incisor and molar teeth

OTHER MUSCLES TO EXAMINE

- Masseter
- Pterygoids
- All facial muscles
- All anterior, lateral, and posterior neck muscles

MANUAL THERAPY

Stripping

- The client lies supine.
- Place fingertips at top of anterior part of muscle (superior and lateral to eyebrow).
- Pressing firmly medially, glide the fingertips inferiorly toward zygomatic arch.
- Place fingertips at the top of the muscle more posteriorly on head. (Note that the muscle is shaped like a scallop, so that it begins higher on the head toward its center, and then lower toward the back of the head.) Repeat movement toward zygomatic arch, pressing firmly.
- Continue until the entire muscle is covered.

Stroking Across the Fiber (1)

- The client lies supine.
- Place fingertips on sides of client's forehead at the anterior edge of temporal fossa (superior to lateral end of eyebrows).
- Pressing firmly, glide the fingertips across the muscle to its posterior edge behind the ear.
- Moving downward, repeat the procedure to cover the entire muscle.

Stroking Across the Fiber (2)

- The client lies supine.
- Hold the client's head in your spread hands, with your thumbs resting together on the anterior aspect of temporalis.
- Pressing firmly into the muscle with the edges of your thumbs, glide your thumbs apart, so that each thumb slides an inch or two (Fig. 3-16). Move the hands posteriorly, repeating the procedure until the entire temporalis muscle is covered.

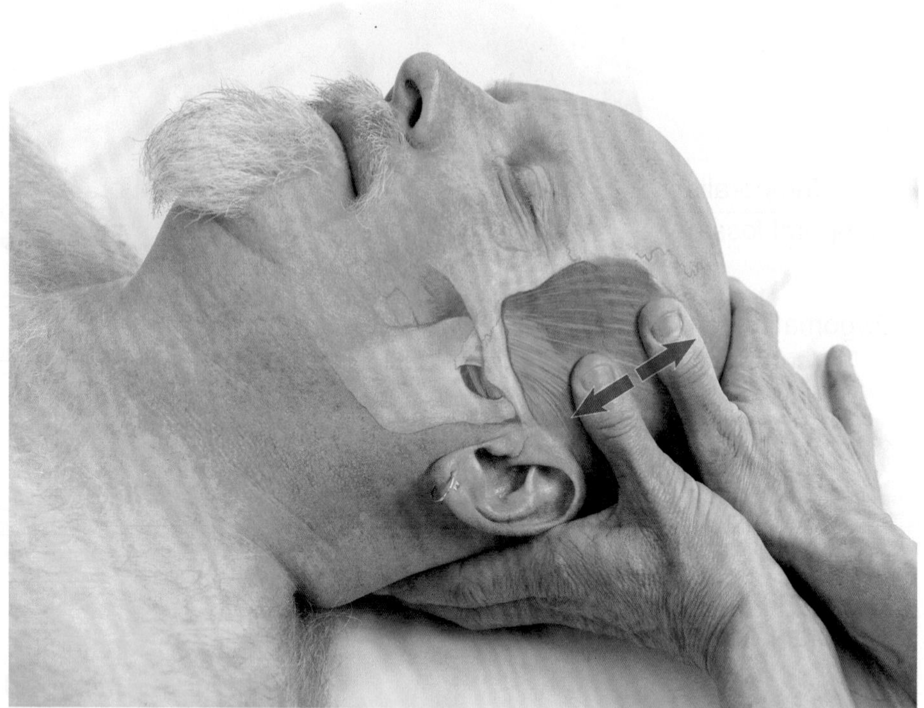

FIGURE 3-16 Cross-fiber stroking of temporalis with thumbs

MASSETER

MASS-e-ter

ETYMOLOGY Greek, masticator

Overview

Masseter (Fig. 3-17) is the most prominent chewing muscle. It should be treated first in TMJ problems, since it is in an easily accessible position.

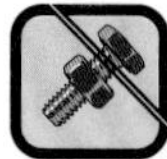

ATTACHMENTS

- Origin: zygomatic process of the maxilla and to the zygomatic arch
- Insertion: superficial layer of muscle to external surface of the mandible at its angle and to the inferior half of its ramus; deep layer of muscle to superior half of the ramus, possibly extending to the angle of the mandible

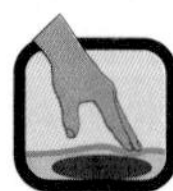

PALPATION

Masseter is distinctly palpable from just below the zygomatic arch to the mandible. It is internally palpable by placing the gloved finger in the mouth against the cheek and pressing posteriorly. The muscle's architecture is parallel, and the fiber direction is superior/inferior.

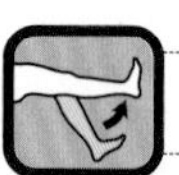

ACTION

- Elevates, protracts, and retracts the mandible at the TMJs (temporomandibular joints)

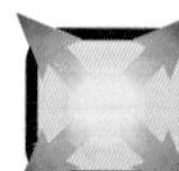

REFERRAL AREAS

- To upper and lower jaw, side of face, ear, and superior to eyebrow
- TMJ dysfunction may also cause tinnitus (ringing in the ears).

OTHER MUSCLES TO EXAMINE

- Temporalis
- Pterygoids
- All facial muscles
- All muscles of anterior, lateral, and posterior neck

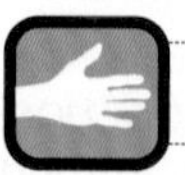

MANUAL THERAPY

Stripping

- The client lies supine.

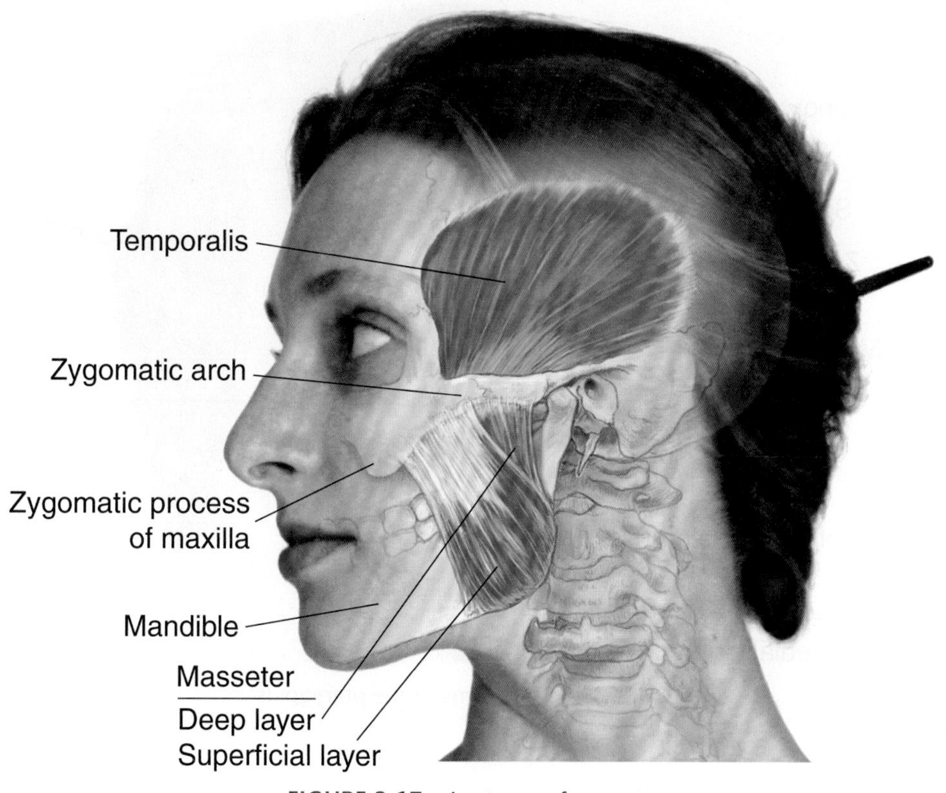

FIGURE 3-17 Anatomy of masseter

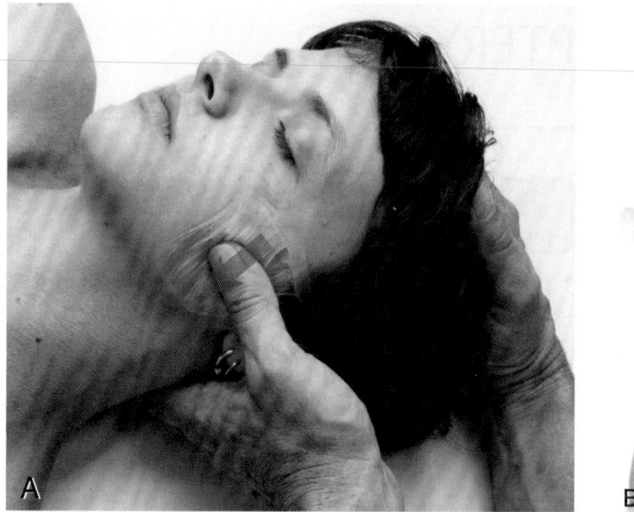

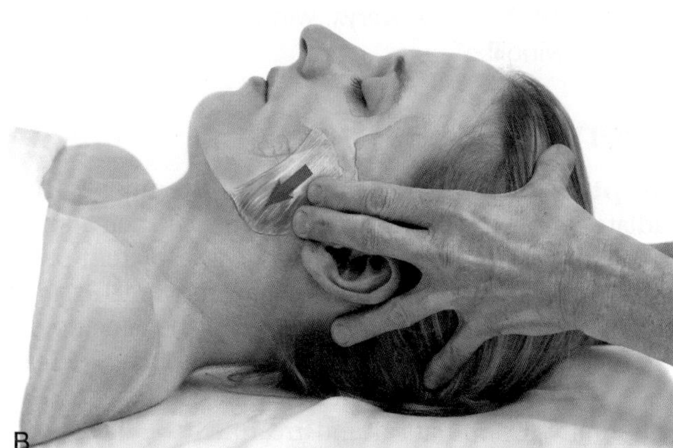

FIGURE 3-18 External stripping of masseter **(A)** with the thumb and **(B)** with the fingertips

- Place the thumb or fingertips at the upper aspect of the muscle, just anterior to the opening of the ear canal.
- Pressing firmly inward, glide the thumb (Fig. 3-18A) or fingertips (Fig. 3-18B) downward along the length of the muscle to the mandible.
- Pause at barriers or tender spots until release is felt.
- Make as many passes as necessary, starting nearest the ear and working forward, to cover the entire muscle (usually one or two passes will suffice).
- When a great deal of tenderness is present, repeat the above process, beginning lightly and pressing in more deeply each time.

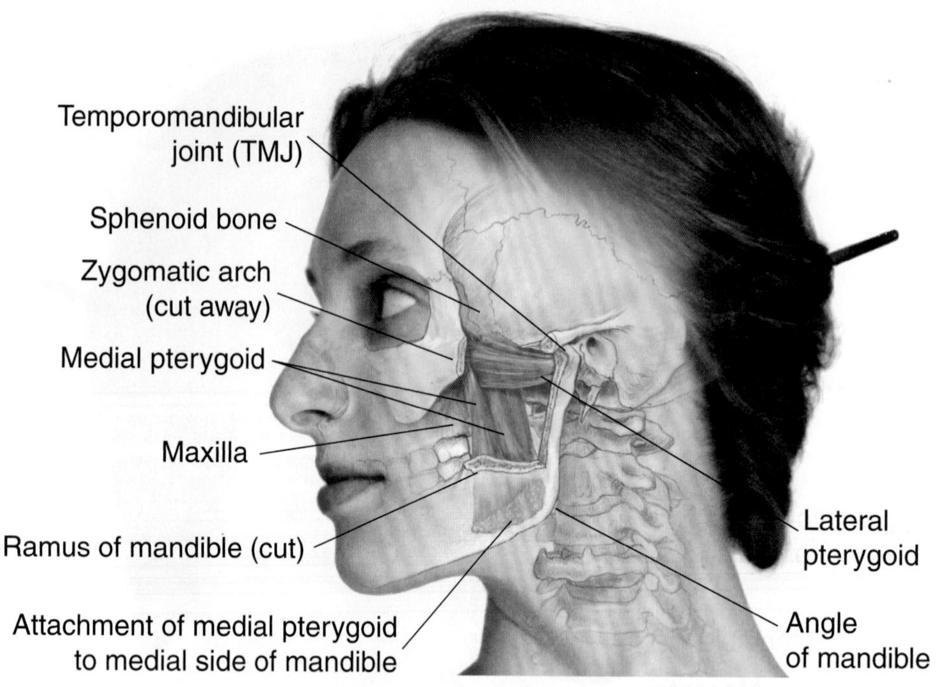

FIGURE 3-19 Anatomy of the pterygoids

PTERYGOIDS

TER-ri-goids

ETYMOLOGY Greek ***pteryx***, wing + ***eidos***, resemblance; "winglike"

Overview

The **pterygoids** (Fig. 3-19) are jaw (TMJ) muscles that radiate in a winglike pattern, and hence their name. They are a complex set of muscles, with different parts of the muscles participating in all jaw movements, and stabilization of the TMJ. A small part of the lateral pterygoid can be accessed from outside the mouth, whereas the medial pterygoids must be examined and treated intraorally. Examination and treatment of the pterygoid muscles can be somewhat awkward and uncomfortable, but they are often key factors in pain in the jaw, face, and ear. They are also major players in TMJD (temporomandibular joint dysfunction) syndrome.

Note: The head is anatomically complex, and the attachments of the pterygoids are particularly challenging to illustrate. For this reason, and because these attachments are not necessarily relevant to the massage therapist, not all of them can be seen in the anatomy plates. The student interested in more detail should consult an anatomy atlas.

MEDIAL OR INTERNAL PTERYGOID

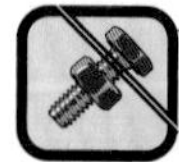

ATTACHMENTS

- Origin: the inner surface of the lateral pterygoid plate and the lateral surface of the palatine bone, and the pterygoid fossa
- Insertion: the lower, medial border of the ramus of the mandible, close to the angle of the mandible, and to the medial surface of the ramus of the mandible near the angle

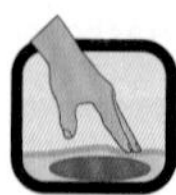

PALPATION

Pterygoids are palpable in three primary areas: (1) directly between the maxilla and mandible anterior to the joint, (2) along the medial surface of the mandible on the lateral aspect of the face, and (3) internally by pressing laterally at the joint of the maxilla and mandible. The muscles' architectures are parallel, and the fiber directions vary.

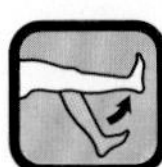

ACTIONS

- Participates in protruding the mandible, along with the lateral pterygoid
- Protracts the mandible
- Acting alternately, moves the mandible from side to side in grinding motion

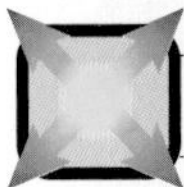

REFERRAL AREAS

- Jaw in front of ear
- Side of jaw (both outside and inside mouth)

LATERAL OR EXTERNAL PTERYGOID

This muscle has two divisions: superior and inferior. Note that the two divisions of the lateral pterygoid are antagonists. Although they have different origins, they share the same insertions.

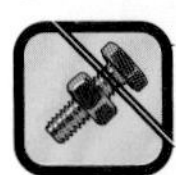

ATTACHMENTS

Superior lateral pterygoid:

- Origin: great wing of the sphenoid and pterygoid plate
- Insertion: neck of the mandibular condyle, articular disc of the TMJ

Inferior lateral pterygoid:

- Origin: lateral surface of the lateral pterygoid plate
- Insertion: neck of the mandibular condyle, articular disc of the TMJ

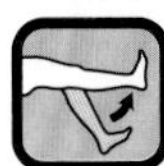

ACTIONS

- The two divisions of this muscle act together in raising and lowering the mandible, as well as moving the mandible posteriorly, anteriorly, and laterally.
- Depresses and protracts the mandible
- Acting alternately, produces side-to-side grinding
- The superior head closes the jaw (elevates the mandible).
- The inferior head opens the mouth by protruding the mandible.

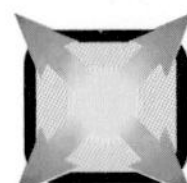

REFERRAL AREAS

- TMJ region
- Face around cheekbone

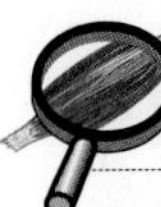

OTHER MUSCLES TO EXAMINE

- Masseter
- Temporalis
- All facial muscles
- Anterior, posterior, and lateral neck muscles

MANUAL THERAPY

All of the following are performed with the client supine.

External Compression (1)

- Use the thumb to find the space just anterior to the TMJ.
- Compress upward, downward, and forward, seeking tender points (Fig. 3-20). Hold each tender point until it releases.

External Compression (2)

- Place the thumb or two fingertips just under the angle of the mandible.
- Press superiorly and into the medial surface of the mandible, moving slowly and gently, seeking tender points.
- Compress any tender points against the medial surface of the mandible (Fig. 3-21).

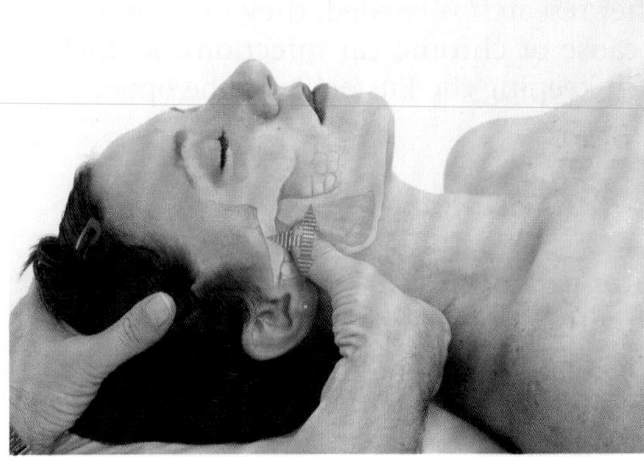

FIGURE 3-20 Compression of pterygoids (1)

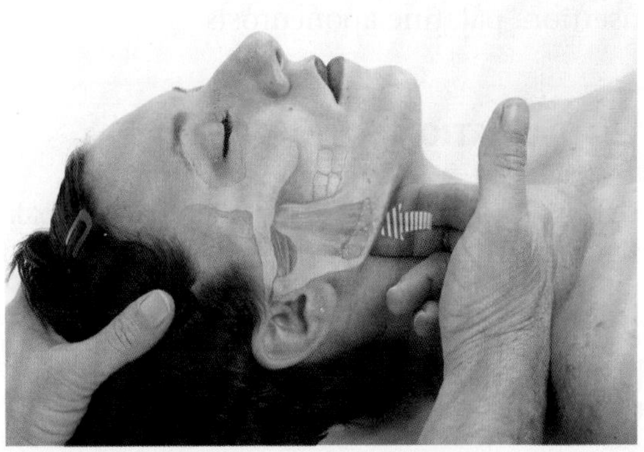

FIGURE 3-21 Compression of pterygoids (2)

LEVATOR VELI PALATINI, TENSOR VELI PALATINI, AND THE PALATINE APONEUROSIS

le-VAY-ter VEL-lee pa-LAT-in-ee

TEN-ser VEL-lee pa-LAT-in-ee

PAL-a-tine ap-o-new-RO-sis

ETYMOLOGY

Levator veli palatini: Latin ***levator***, raiser + ***velum***, veil or sail + ***palatini***, of the palate; "raiser of the veil of the palate"

Tensor veli palatini: Latin ***tensor***, tightener + ***velum***, veil or sail + ***palatini***, of the palate; "tightener of the veil of the palate"

Aponeurosis: Greek, the end of a muscle, where it becomes tendon, from ***apo*** + neuron, ***sinew***

Overview

Levator and **tensor palatini** (Fig. 3-22) both attach to the Eustachian (auditory) tube at one end and the palatine aponeurosis at the other. Although further research is needed, they may be involved in the cause of chronic ear infections, as they play a role in keeping the Eustachian tube open.

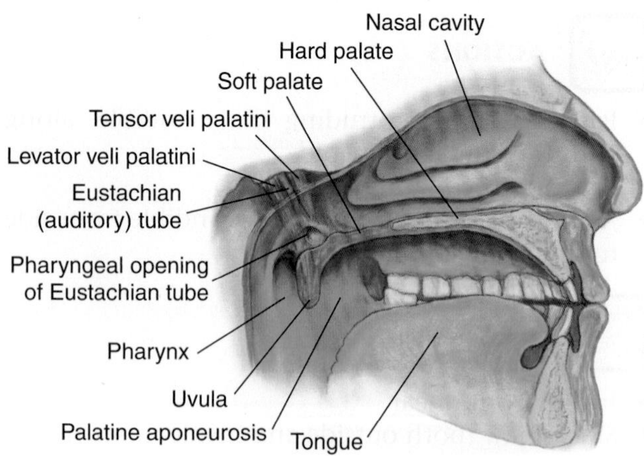

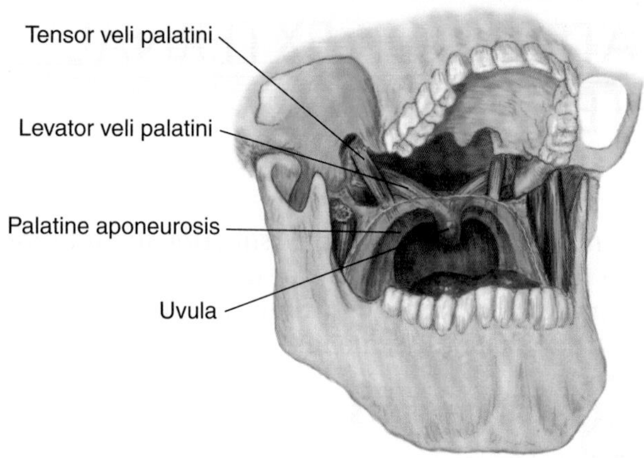

FIGURE 3-22 Anatomy of tensor and levator veli palatini

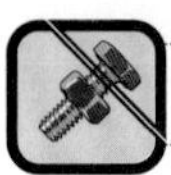

ATTACHMENTS

Levator palatini:
- Origin: cartilage of auditory tube and petrous part of temporal bone
- Insertion: palatine aponeurosis

Tensor palatini:
- Origin: cartilage of auditory tube, medial pterygoid plate, and spine of sphenoid bone
- Insertion: palatine aponeurosis

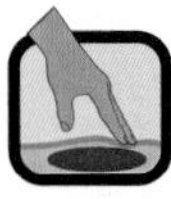

PALPATION

These muscles are not palpable, other than the palatine aponeurosis. Their architecture is parallel, and the fiber direction varies from superior/inferior to diagonal.

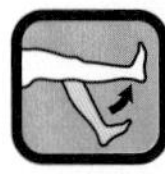

ACTIONS

As their names imply, the levator raises the soft palate, and the tensor tenses the soft palate. Both muscles also open the auditory tube to equalize air pressure between the middle ear and pharynx.

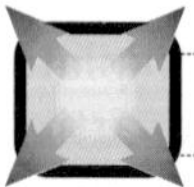

REFERRAL AREA

These muscles can be accessed only via the palatine aponeurosis; thus, we have no knowledge of trigger points or referral zones for them. They are highly suspect, however, in the presence of ear pain and infection.

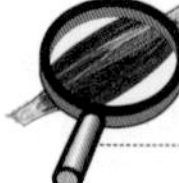

OTHER MUSCLES TO EXAMINE

- Temporalis
- Masseter
- Pterygoids
- All anterior, lateral, and posterior neck muscles

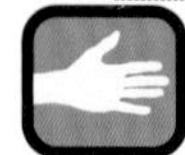

MANUAL THERAPY FOR THE JAW MUSCLES: INTRAORAL WORK

All of the following are performed with the client supine. Have the client open the mouth as wide as is comfortable.

CAUTION Intraoral work is considered to be outside the scope of practice for massage therapists in many states in the USA. You should check with your state regulatory board before performing any intraoral work.

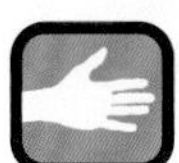

MANUAL THERAPY FOR THE PALATINE APONEUROSIS (LEVATOR VELI PALATINI, TENSOR VELI PALATINI)

- Place the gloved fingertip on the roof of the mouth just medial to the upper molars.
- Pressing firmly (but gently) superiorly, glide the fingertip back toward the pharynx.
- Maintaining pressure, carefully glide the fingertip along the soft palate toward the center (medially).

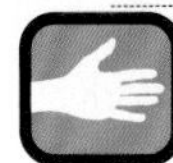

MANUAL THERAPY FOR THE INNER ASPECT

- Beginning just posterior to the last upper molar on the medial side, press the tissue against the bone firmly, gliding in a deep (posterior) direction. The movement should form a "U" shape (Figs. 3-23 and 3-24) as it passes over the inner

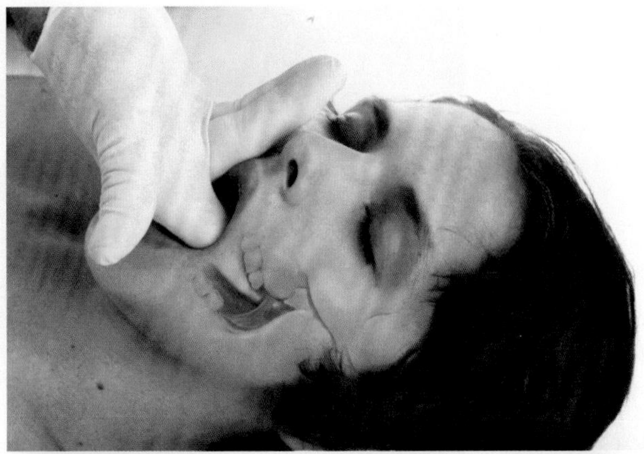

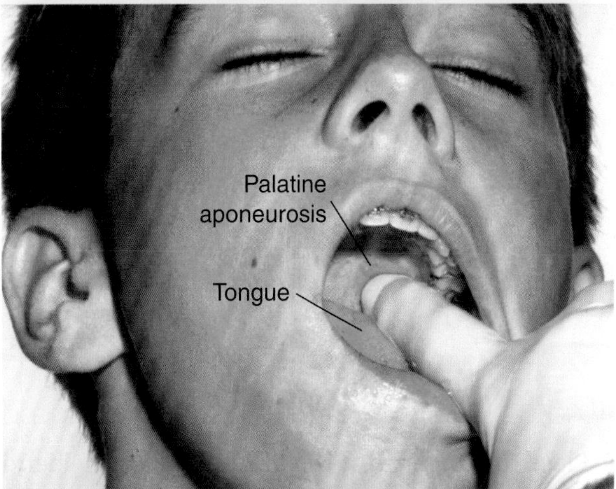

FIGURE 3-23 Release of palatine aponeurosis (1)

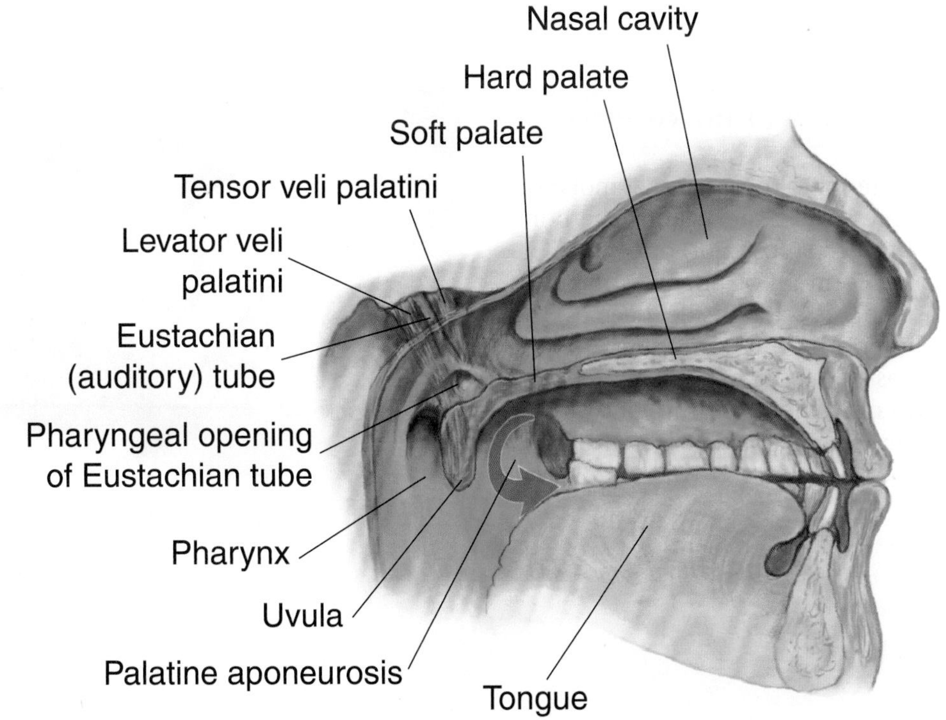

FIGURE 3-24 Release of palatine aponeurosis (2)

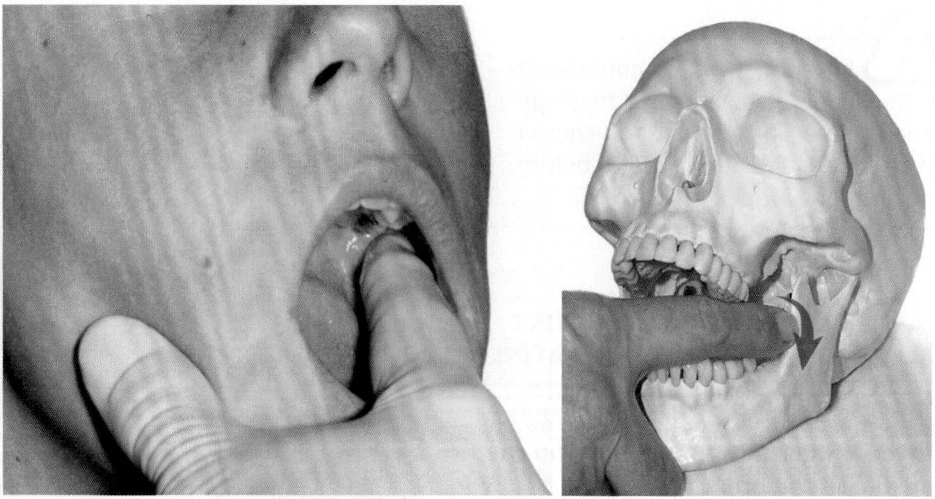

FIGURE 3-25 Stroking between the maxilla and mandible

aspect of the maxilla and mandible just posterior to the teeth, first inferiorly, then anteriorly just posterior to the last upper molar.

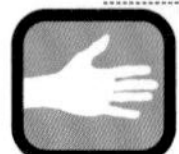

MANUAL THERAPY BETWEEN THE MAXILLA AND MANDIBLE

- Place the fingertip at the deepest point (the bend) of the "U" movement just made, that is, on the medial aspect of the mandible.
- Pressing the tissue firmly against the bone, move the finger laterally between the teeth (Fig. 3-25).

MANUAL THERAPY OF OUTER ASPECT

- Beginning just posterior to the last upper molar on the lateral side, press the tissue against the bone firmly, moving in a deep (posterior) direction. The movement should form a "U" shape as it passes over the coronoid process and inside (deep to) the masseter, first inferiorly, then anteriorly to just posterior to the last lower molar (Fig. 3-26).
- Repeat the above movement pressing outward to work the masseter from inside. You can also work the front border of the masseter with the fingertip (Fig. 3-27).

CAUTION 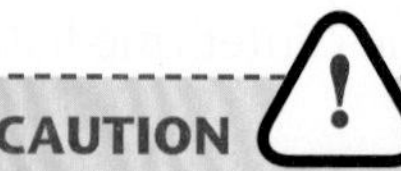

- If you are worried about being bitten, use a finger of the nontreating hand to press the cheek between the client's teeth.
- To suppress the gag reflex while working medially, have the client curl the tongue backward into the pharynx.
- Remove your hand from the mouth frequently for the client's comfort.

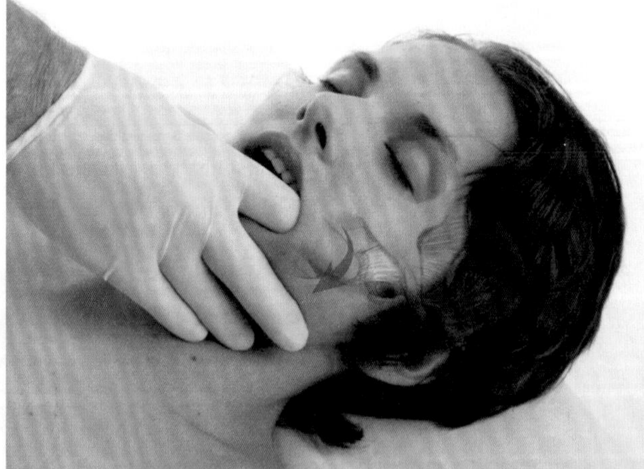

FIGURE 3-26 Intraoral stroke over the coronoid process

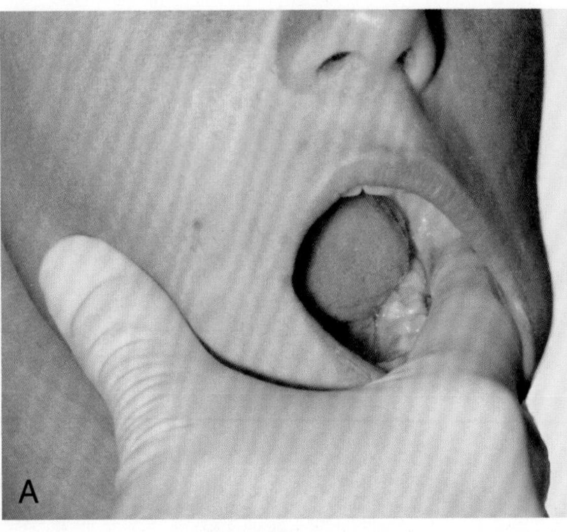

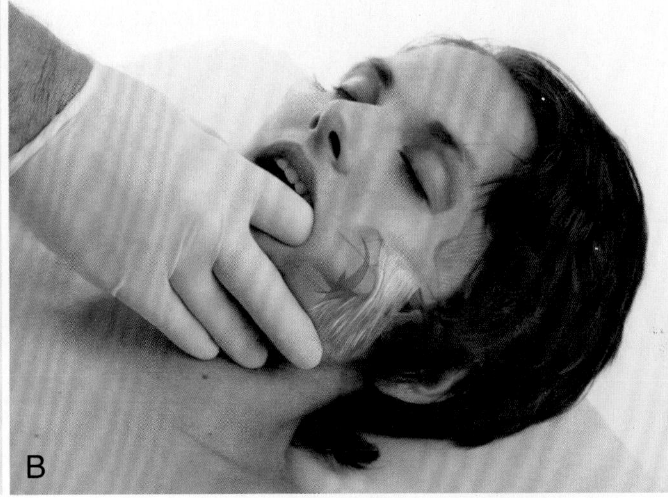

FIGURE 3-27 Intraoral moving compression of masseter: **(A)** intraoral view, **(B)** lateral view

PLATYSMA

pla-TIZ-ma

ETYMOLOGY Greek, a flat plate

Overview

Platysma (Fig. 3-28) is a thin, flat, subcutaneous muscle. It lies parallel to sternocleidomastoid, and its trigger points tend to occur in conjunction with that muscle.

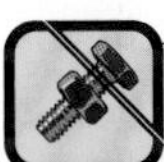

ATTACHMENTS

- Origin: the corner of the mouth and the other facial muscles in that region, and to the lower aspect of the mandible
- Insertion: the superficial fascia of the upper anterior chest

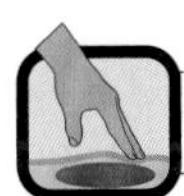

PALPATION

Asking the client to grimace or make the sound "eeeeee" will allow you to feel the edges of it on the neck just under the midpoint of the mandible.

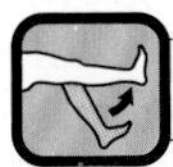

ACTIONS

- Pulls the corner of the mouth downward and the skin of the chest upward
- Tenses the skin of the neck (as in horror)

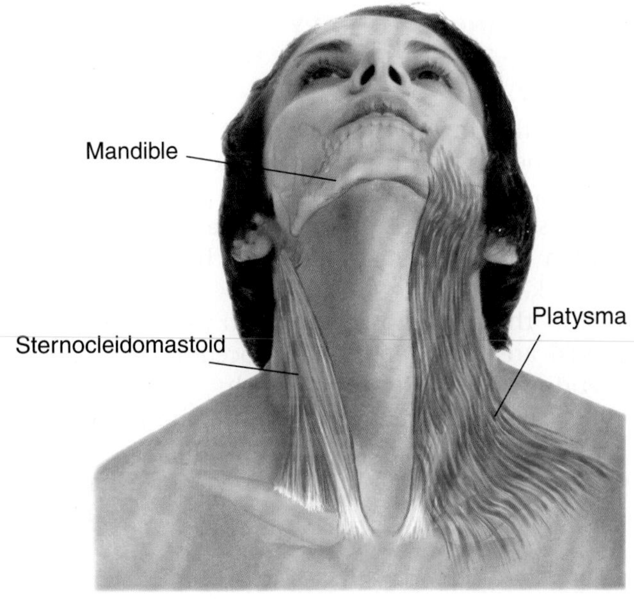

FIGURE 3-28 Anatomy of platysma

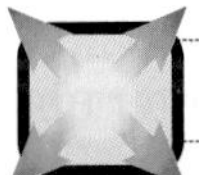

REFERRAL AREA

Over the anterior neck in the area of the sternocleidomastoid; may also be a hot, prickly sensation to the upper chest

OTHER MUSCLES TO EXAMINE

Sternocleidomastoid

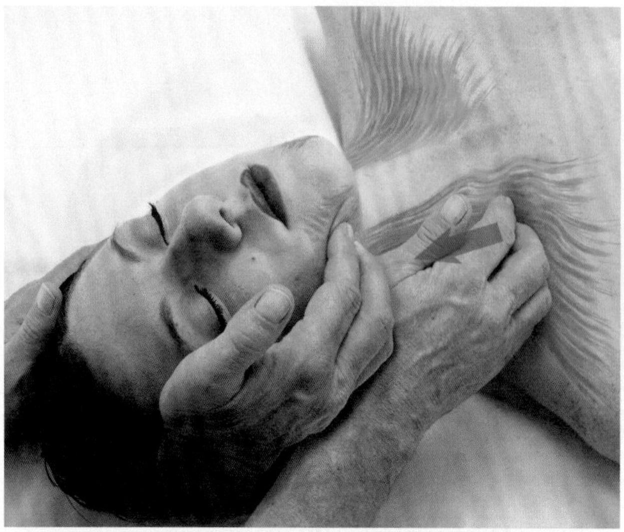

FIGURE 3-29 Stripping platysma with fingertips

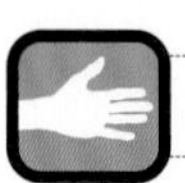

MANUAL THERAPY

Stripping

- Place the fingertips on the chest 2 or 3 inches below the clavicle, just medial to the anterior deltoid.
- Pressing firmly into the tissue, glide the fingertips superiorly over the clavicle and up the neck, then over the mandible and halfway up the cheek.
- Shift the fingertips medially to the next uncovered area and repeat the procedure (Fig. 3-29), ending the stroke at the mouth.
- Repeat the procedure across the chest, with the last stroke beginning at the sternum.
- The same procedure may be performed from superior to inferior using the edge of the thumb.

MUSCLES ATTACHED TO THE HYOID BONE

Etymology Greek, *hyoeides,* shaped like the letter upsilon (u- or v-shaped)

Overview

The **hyoid bone** lies just superior to the thyroid cartilage where the angle below the jaw meets the angle of the neck, approximately at the level of the body of the third cervical vertebra. It is the first resistant structure below the chin. To find it, place your thumb and index finger on either side of the anterior neck below the chin about 3 or 4 inches apart. Squeeze gently. If you don't feel resistance, shift your fingers a little farther down and squeeze again. Repeat until you feel a resistant structure (Fig. 3-30). It may also help to ask the client to swallow, which will cause a palpable movement of the hyoid bone.

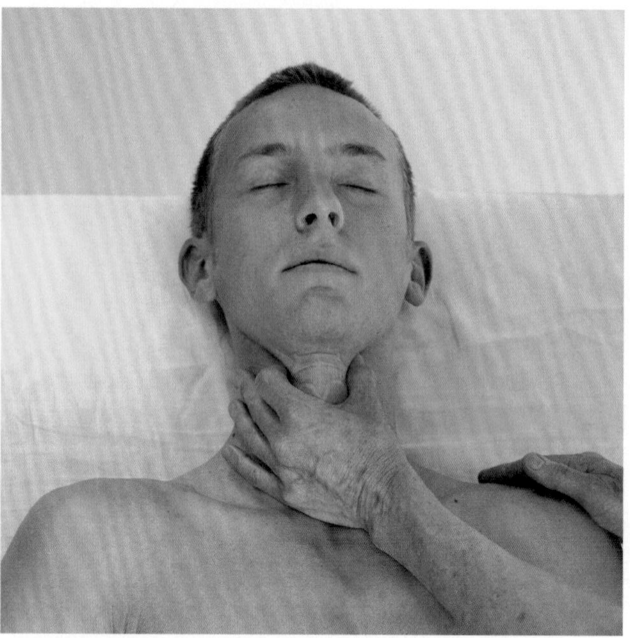

FIGURE 3-30 Locating the hyoid bone by palpation

CAUTION Working near the hyoid and other locations on the anterior neck sometimes makes clients feel claustrophobic—your hands are on their throat. Be conscious of that and remain in communication with the client about whether or not they are comfortable.

The hyoid is the only bone in the body that does not articulate with another bone, but many muscles are attached to the hyoid bone (Fig. 3-31). Those muscles superior to the hyoid bone are called **suprahyoid** muscles; those inferior, **infrahyoid** muscles. They fan out from the hyoid bone both above and below. It is not necessary in basic clinical massage therapy, and therefore in this book, to distinguish them all; they can be worked as a group above and below. The principal muscle involved in pain referral and clinical treatment is the digastric muscle, which is discussed separately. Geniohyoid and sternothyroid are not illustrated because they lie deep to mylohyoid and sternohyoid; their anatomical details are not essential to the purposes of this book.

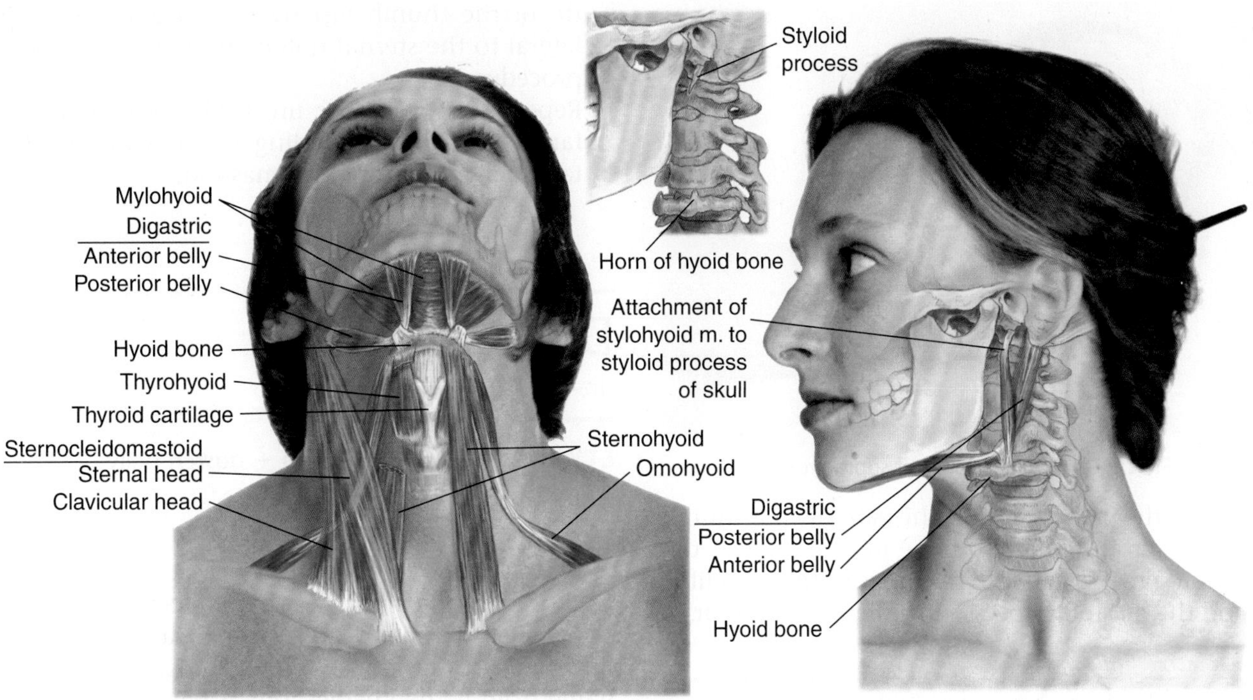

FIGURE 3-31 Anatomy of the hyoid bone and attached muscles

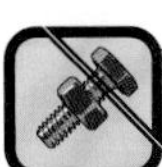

ATTACHMENTS

Suprahyoid muscles:

- Digastric (treated separately; see later listing)
- Stylohyoid
  - Origin: styloid process of temporal bone
  - Insertion: lateral margin of hyoid
- Mylohyoid
  - Origin: inner surface of mandible off the mylohyoid line
  - Insertion: along the midline of the body of the hyoid
- Geniohyoid: lies deep to the anterior belly of the digastric (not illustrated)

Infrahyoid muscles:

- Sternohyoid
  - Origin: posterior aspect of the manubrium, sternal end of the clavicle
  - Insertion: body of the hyoid
- Thyrohyoid
  - Origin: oblique line of thyroid cartilage
  - Insertion: lateral side of hyoid
- Omohyoid
  - Superior belly attaches to the hyoid, lateral to the sternohyoid.
  - Inferior belly attaches to the superior scapular border, medial to the suprascapular notch.
  - Both bellies meet at the clavicle and are attached to the clavicle by a pulley tendon.
- Sternothyroid: connects the manubrium of the sternum to the thyroid cartilage (not illustrated)

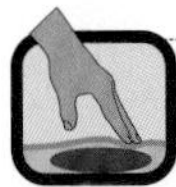

PALPATION

Place your thumb and index finger on either side of the anterior neck below the chin about 3 or 4 inches apart. Squeeze gently. If you don't feel resistance, shift your fingers a little farther down and squeeze again. Repeat until you feel a resistant structure (Fig. 3-30).

It may also help to ask the client to swallow, which will cause a palpable movement of the hyoid bone. The attached muscles are palpable, but not really discernible.

MANUAL THERAPY OF THE SUPRAHYOID MUSCLES

Stripping

- Locate the hyoid bone with your thumb and index finger.
- Place your thumb just superior to the hyoid bone medial to its horn (end) (Fig. 3-32).
- Pressing gently into the tissue, glide the tip of your thumb slowly superiorly to the inner surface of the mandible at the center.
- Starting again superior to the hyoid bone, place your thumb slightly lateral to the previous starting point.
- Slide the thumb slowly superiorly to the inner surface of the mandible, parallel to the first pass.

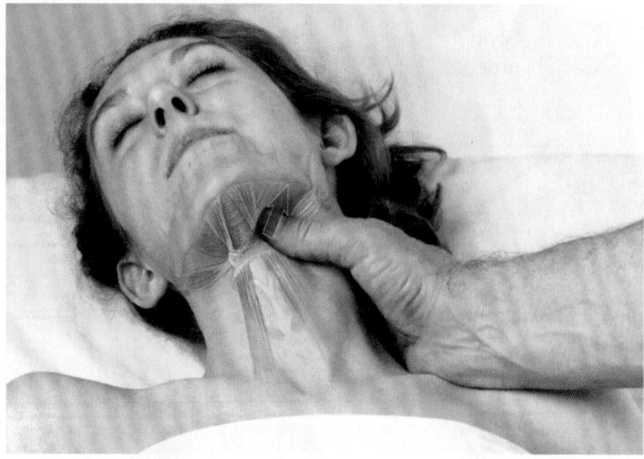
FIGURE 3-32 Stripping of suprahyoids

- Repeat the process, letting the path of your thumb fan out from the hyoid bone until it ends at the styloid process between the angle of the mandible and the mastoid process, just inferior to the ear.

CAUTION Do not exert excessive pressure on the styloid process, as it can be broken. All "stripping" of muscles in the hyoid area should be gentler than stripping the thicker, more prominent muscles of the neck.

MANUAL THERAPY OF THE INFRAHYOID MUSCLES

Stripping

- With the side of one thumb or finger, gently press the thyroid cartilage laterally away from you.
- Place the thumb or fingertips of the other hand just superior to the manubrium next to the trachea.
- Pressing gently, glide the thumb or fingertips slowly up to the hyoid bone (Fig. 3-33). Place the tip of the thumb just over the clavicle slightly lateral to the sternal notch and repeat the above procedure.
- Repeat this procedure until you have covered a fan-shaped area extending to the clavicular attachment of sternocleidomastoid.

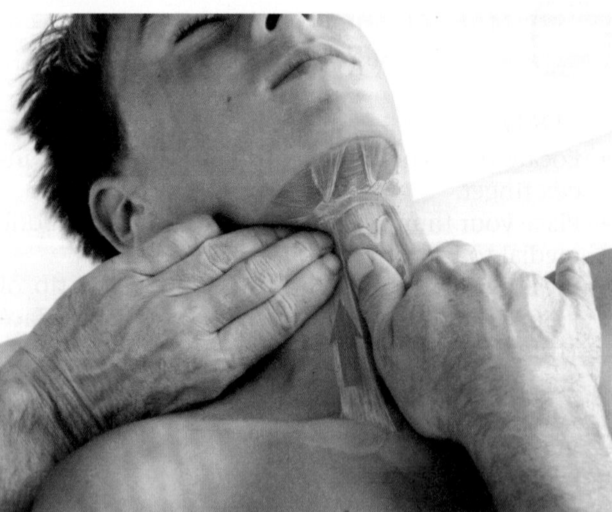
FIGURE 3-33 Stripping of infrahyoids

DIGASTRIC

die-GAS-trick

ETYMOLOGY Greek ***di***, two + ***gaster***, belly

Overview

One of a group of muscles that attach to the hyoid bone, digastric (Fig. 3-34) is close to, and difficult to distinguish from, the stylohyoid. Digastric takes its name from its two bellies: one is between the mastoid process and the hyoid bone, the other between the hyoid bone and the mandible.

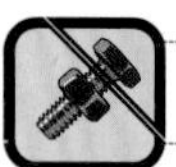

ATTACHMENTS

- Posterior belly attaches at the mastoid process of the temporal bone, deep to the longissimus capitis, splenius capitis, and sternocleidomastoid.
- Anterior belly attaches at the digastric fossa of the internal mandible.
- Both bellies meet and attach at the lateral aspect of the body of the hyoid by a pulley tendon.

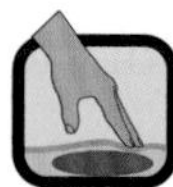

PALPATION

Digastric is palpable under the ear and under the mandible, but not truly discernable. As with many muscles that are not easily discernable in a state of rest, placing your hand on the muscle while asking the client to perform the action(s) of the muscle will often allow you to palpate with more accuracy.

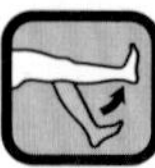

ACTIONS

- Lowers the mandible (opening the jaw)
- Raises the hyoid bone
- Retracts the mandible
- Participates in swallowing and coughing
- Steadies the hyoid in coughing, swallowing, and sneezing

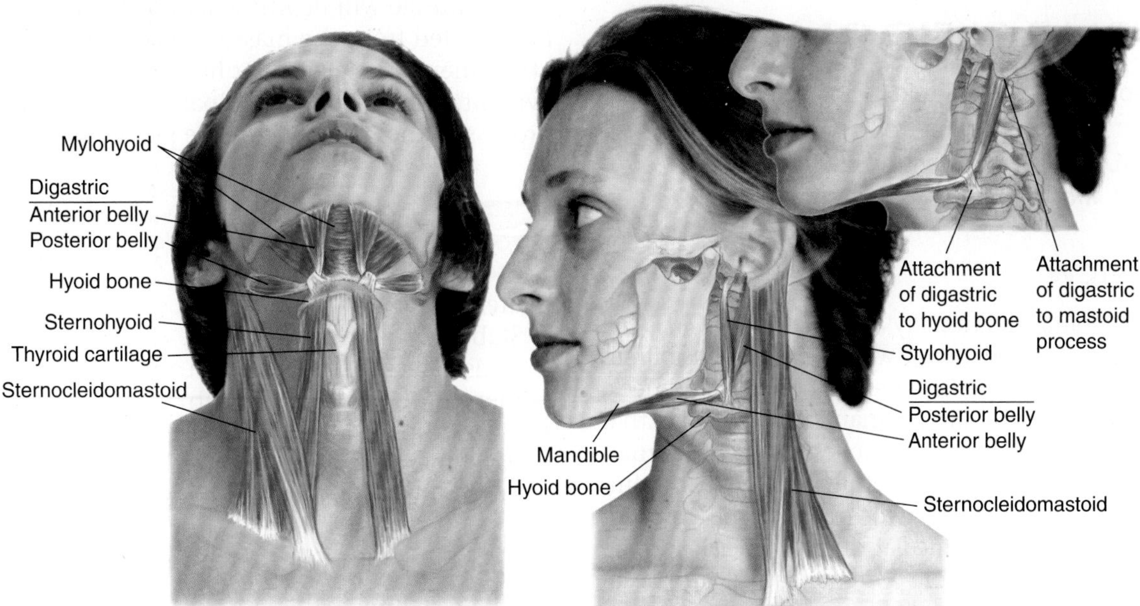

FIGURE 3-34 Anatomy of digastric and stylohyoid

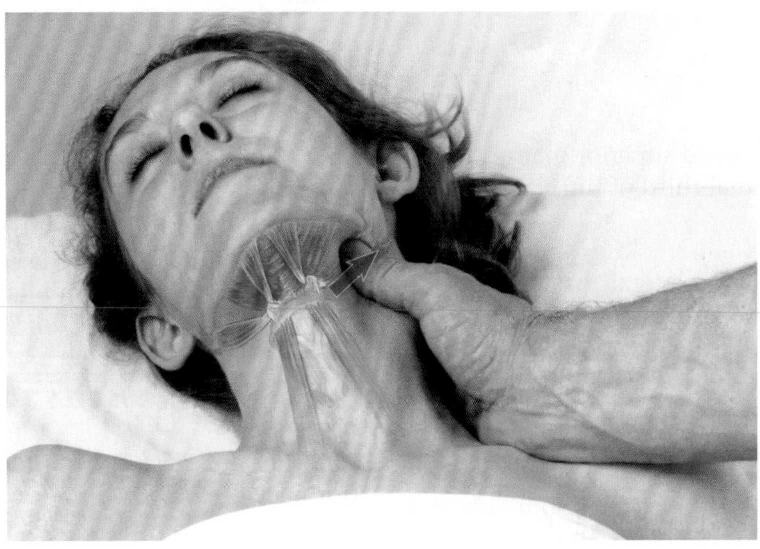

FIGURE 3-35 Stripping of posterior belly of digastric

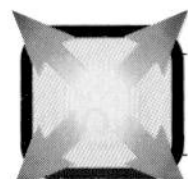

REFERRAL AREAS

- Posterior belly: inferior to, over, and behind the angle of the mandible; over the mastoid process; into the occipital region
- Anterior belly: to the four lower incisors and directly inferior to them

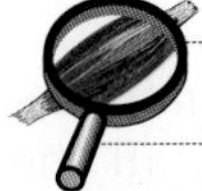

OTHER MUSCLES TO EXAMINE

- Other muscles of the anterior and lateral neck
- Occipitalis

MANUAL THERAPY

Stripping

- Gently locate the hyoid bone using the tips of your thumb and index finger.
- Place the tip of the thumb or a finger just superior to one side of the hyoid bone.
- Pressing gently, follow the posterior belly to the mastoid process (Fig. 3-35).
- Starting at the same position, follow the anterior belly toward the chin to a point just to one side of the center of the underside of the mandible.
- Pause where tenderness is found and wait for release.
- Repeat on the opposite side.

STERNOCLEIDOMASTOID

STERN-o-KLIDE-o-MASS-toid

ETYMOLOGY Greek: ***sternon,*** chest + ***kleis,*** clavicle + ***mastos,*** breast + ***eidos,*** resemblance

Overview

Sternocleidomastoid (usually abbreviated as **SCM**) (Fig. 3-36) is a two-headed muscle with major responsibilities for stabilizing, turning, and flexing the head and neck. It is also a common site for many trigger points that cause a wide variety of headaches. Sternocleidomastoid should be examined carefully in all clients complaining of headaches. Its two heads are the **sternal**, which is more anterior, medial, and superficial; and the **clavicular**, which is more posterior, lateral, and deep. The sternocleidomastoid helps maintain posture by stabilizing the head when the body is in movement.

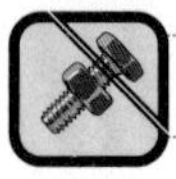

ATTACHMENTS

Origin

- Sternal head: anterior and superior manubrium
- Clavicular head: medial third of the clavicle

Insertion

- Both heads insert at the lateral mastoid process of the temporal bone and the lateral half of the superior nuchal line of the occipital bone.

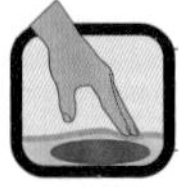

PALPATION

Have the supine client turn the head to one side and raise it off the table. In most clients, the sternal head of the muscle will be immediately evident, and can be palpated from the mastoid process to the sternal attachment. The clavicular head is much less visibly evident, but can also be palpated from the mastoid process to the insertion on the posterior clavicle.

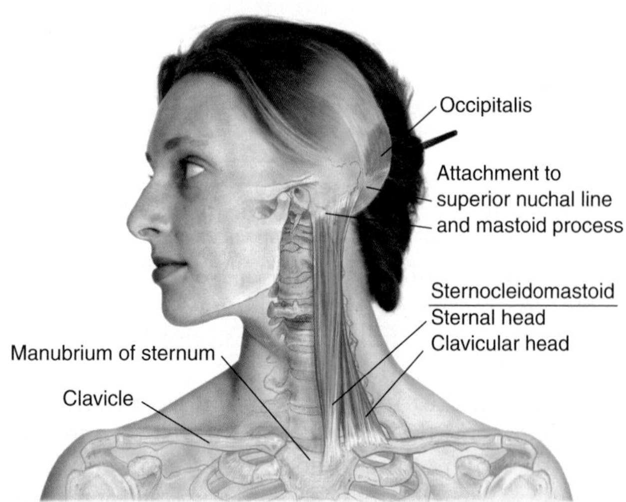

FIGURE 3-36 Anatomy of SCM

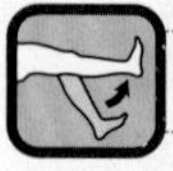

ACTIONS

Bilateral:

- Stabilizes the head and neck
- Resists neck hyperextension and backward movement of the head (whiplash)
- Flexes the neck
- Participates to some degree in swallowing and breathing by raising the rib cage

Unilateral:

- Rotates face to the opposite side
- Tilts face upward
- With trapezius, bends the head and neck to the side

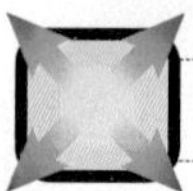

REFERRAL AREAS

- Sternal head: into the occipital region, in an arc over the eye, the top of the head, the cheek, and areas on and inferior to the chin
- Clavicular head: into the ear, behind the ear, and into the frontal region bilaterally

OTHER MUSCLES TO EXAMINE

All other muscles of the anterior, lateral, and posterior neck

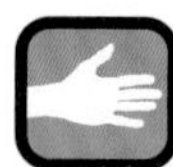

MANUAL THERAPY

Stripping

- The client is supine. Hold the client's head in one hand and turn it slightly to the side opposite to the muscle you intend to work on.
- Place the thumb or fingertips of the other hand on the attachment of the muscle at the mastoid process.
- Pressing firmly into the tissue, slide the thumb or fingertips slowly down the sternal head all the way to the attachment at the manubrium, pausing at tender spots until they release (Fig. 3-37).
- Beginning at the superior attachment again, repeat the process on the clavicular head, all the way to the attachment on the clavicle (Fig. 3-38).
- Repeat the above process on the other side.

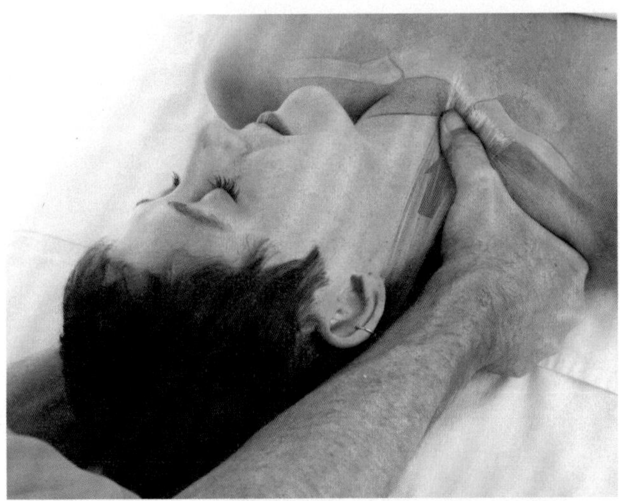

FIGURE 3-37 Stripping of sternal head of SCM

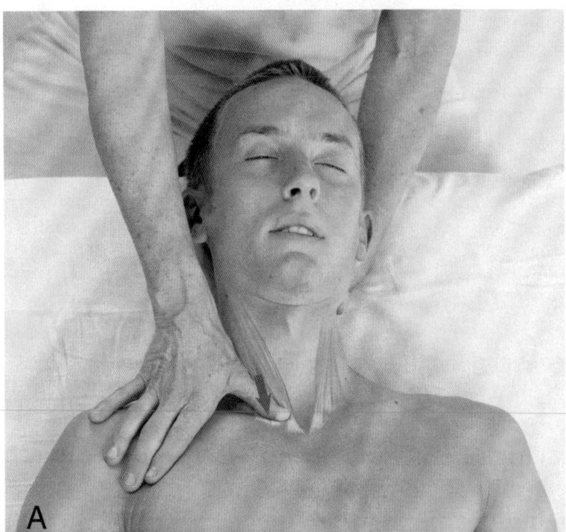

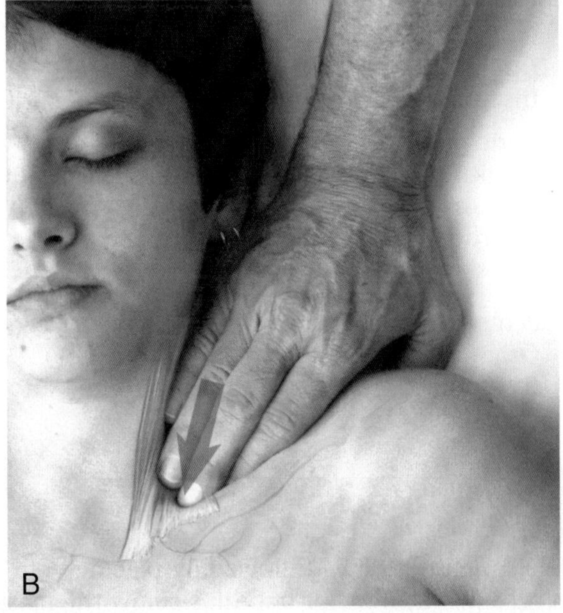

FIGURE 3-38 Stripping of clavicular head of SCM with thumb **(A)** and fingertips **(B)**

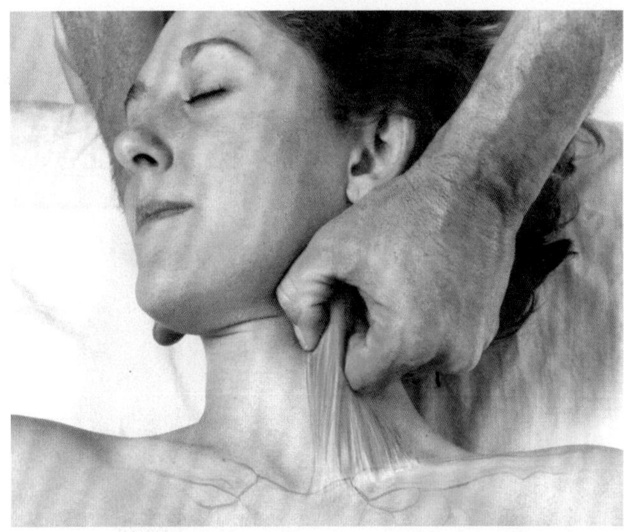

FIGURE 3-39 Pincer compression of SCM

Pincer Compression

- Hold the client's head in one hand, firmly supporting the back of the head and the base of the skull.
- Lift the head a few inches to induce sternocleidomastoid to stand out; turn the head slightly away from the side on which you intend to work.
- Starting as close as possible to the mastoid attachment, grasp the sternal head between your thumb and either the side of your index finger or the tips of your index and middle fingers (Fig. 3-39).
- Compress firmly but gently, asking the client for feedback about tenderness and/or pain referral. If tightness or tenderness is present, hold until release.
- Shift your fingers down slightly, repeating until you get as close to the manubrium as possible.
- Turn the client's head a little farther from the side you are working on, and repeat the above process with the clavicular head. Note that this head is more difficult to grasp, as it lies deeper than the sternal head.
- Repeat the entire process on the other side.

SCALENI (SCALENES)

ska-LEN-ee

ETYMOLOGY Greek, ***skalenos***, uneven

Overview

The **scalenes** (Fig. 3-40) are known for their propensity to refer pain. Although they have the fairly simple function of tilting the head to either side, we also tend to use them to hold up the rib cage and

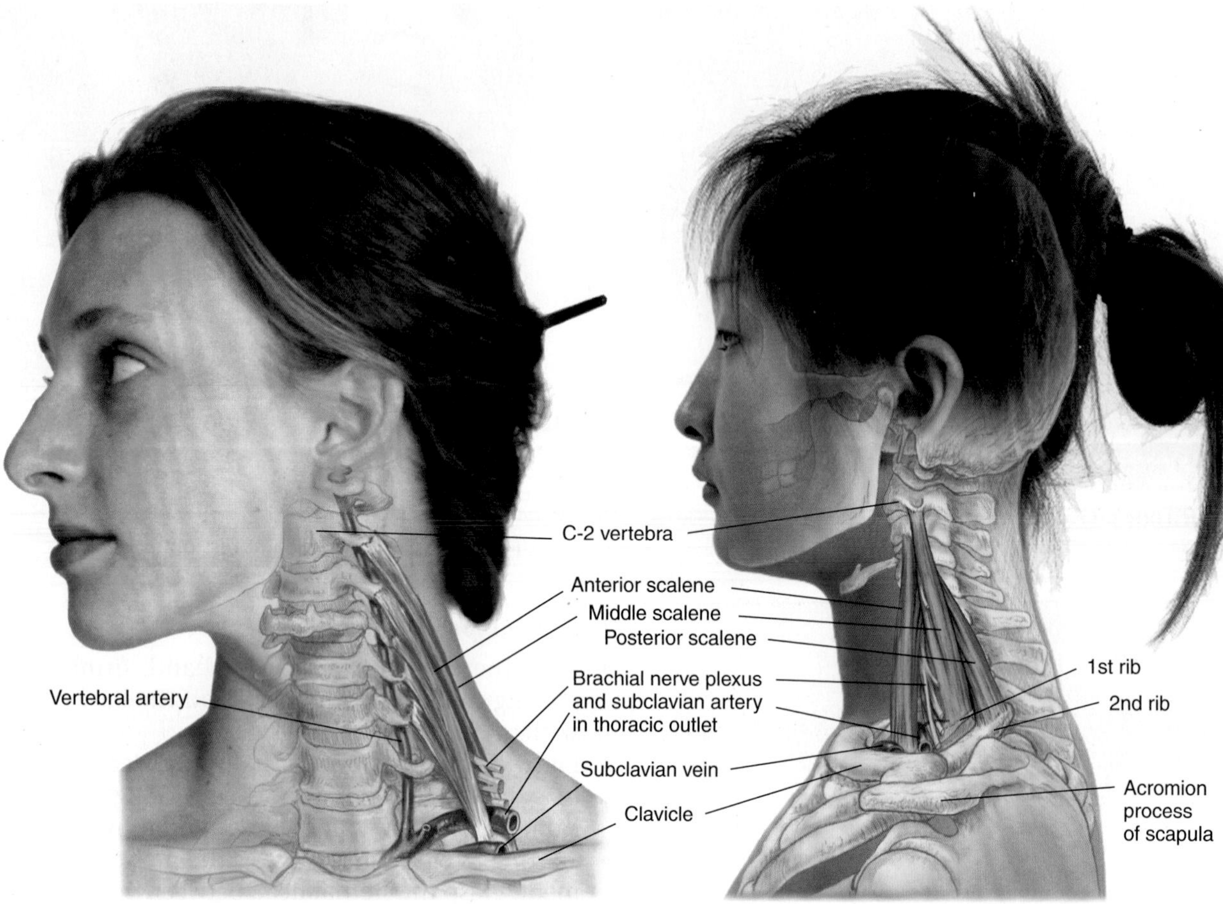

FIGURE 3-40 Anatomy of the scalenes and the thoracic outlet

as inappropriate accessory muscles in paradoxical breathing (see Muscles of Breathing in Chapter 4). As a result, we subject the scalenes to substantial tension. Few people escape problems with these muscles.

The term **thoracic outlet** is used to refer to the entire area defined by scalenes and the first rib, or to the passage between the anterior and middle scalenes. On their way to the arm, the axillary (subclavian) artery and brachial plexus pass between these two muscles, then between the first rib and the clavicle. They can become entrapped at some point in this area by tightness in the anterior and middle scalenes. It is sometimes difficult to distinguish pain referred by the scalenes from pain resulting from entrapment of the brachial plexus.

Note: Scalenus minimus (not illustrated) is not found in everyone, and often occurs on only one side. Individuals with this muscle may be at greater risk of entrapment symptoms. Although it can have a trigger point, it is difficult to isolate manually, and may be treated as an aspect of the anterior scalene.

ATTACHMENTS

Anterior scalene (scalenus anterior):

- Origin: anterior tubercules of the transverse processes of C3 through C6
- Insertion: the inner upper edge of the first rib

Middle scalene (scalenus medius):

- Origin: the posterior transverse processes of C2 through C7
- Insertion: the outer upper edge of the first rib

Posterior scalene (scalenus posterior):

- Origin: the posterior transverse processes of C5 or C6 and C7
- Insertion: the lateral surface of the second rib, and sometimes also the third

Scalenus minimus (found in some, but not all, people):

- Origin: the anterior transverse process of C7
- Insertion: the top of the pleural dome and the inner edge of the first rib

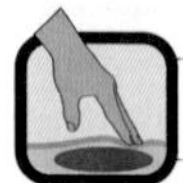

PALPATION

The scalenes may be followed by placing your fingertips just in front of trapezius below the mastoid process (they do not attach there, but are first discernible there) and tracing them downward to their respective attachments on the ribs and the pleural dome. Posterior scalene may be traced by following the anterior edge of trapezius. Anterior scalene may be followed from just below the mastoid process down to the first rib. Middle scalene may be followed from the same location down to the first rib. Their architecture is largely convergent.

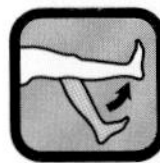

ACTIONS

- Primary lateral flexors of the cervical spine
- Anterior scalenes: bilaterally, assist in flexion and rotation of the neck
- Posterior scalenes: stabilizers of the neck, participate in inspiration, also tend to be involved in raising the rib cage in lifting and carrying

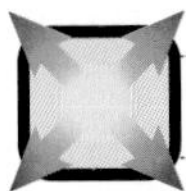

REFERRAL AREAS

- Over the shoulder and down the medial side of the shoulder blade
- Over the upper anterior chest
- Down the front of the upper arm
- Down the radial half of the forearm and into the thumb and fingers, especially the index finger
- Scalenus minimus: dorsum of the forearm and hand

OTHER MUSCLES TO EXAMINE

All muscles of the rotator cuff, anterior chest, and arm

MANUAL THERAPY

Stripping (1)

- The client lies supine.
- Stand at the client's head. Hold the head underneath with one hand.
- Place the fingers of the other hand under the client's neck, and with the thumb find the upper part of the anterior scalene (Fig. 3-41).
- Pressing firmly into the tissue, slide the thumb slowly along the muscle as far as you can reach, into the space behind the clavicle.
- Repeat the process, this time finding the middle scalene.
- Repeat the process, this time finding the posterior scalene and following it as far as you can into the space just anterior to the edge of trapezius (Fig. 3-42).
- Repeat the entire process on the other side.

As an alternative to this procedure, you can use the fingertips rather than the thumb (Fig. 3-43).

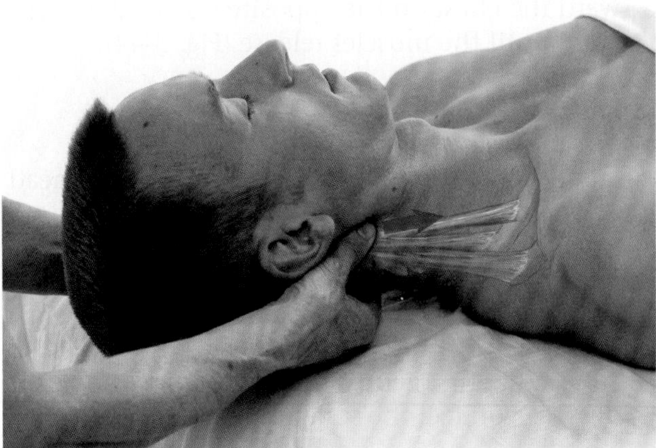

FIGURE 3-41 Stripping of anterior scalene

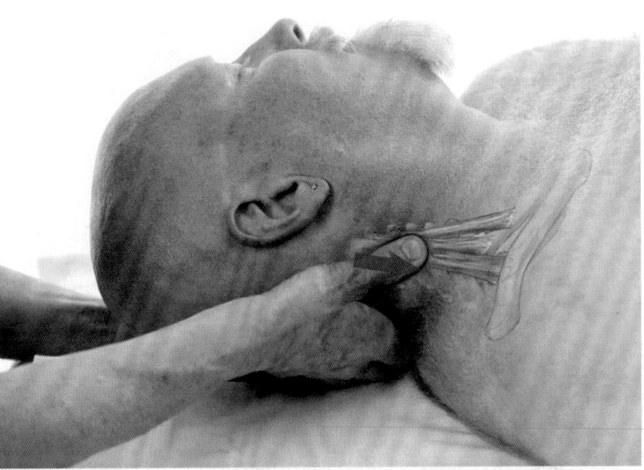

FIGURE 3-42 Stripping of posterior scalene with thumb

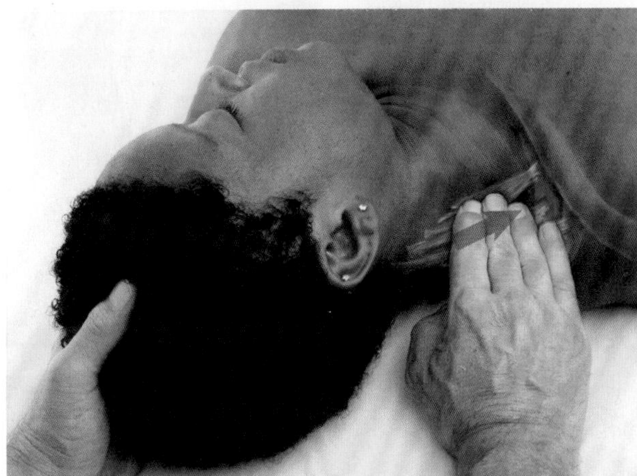

FIGURE 3-43 Stripping of scalenes with fingertips

Deep Compression

- The client lies supine.
- Stand or sit at the client's head. Place the fingertips on the scalenes at the base of the neck. Press

deeply into the tissues in a diagonal direction toward the chest on the opposite side of the client. Hold until the muscles release (Fig. 3-44).

Compression

- The client lies prone.
- Stand beside the client, facing the client's head. Place your hand at the base of the client's neck, with the heel of the hand resting over trapezius and levator scapulae.
- Curl the fingers over trapezius so that they grasp the scalenes at the base of the neck.
- Squeeze, at first gently, then with increasing firmness, as you feel the scalenes release.

Stripping (2)

- The client lies prone.
- Stand at the client's head, facing the client.
- Holding the head steady with one hand, find the superior portion of the middle scalene with the other thumb.
- Pressing firmly into the tissue just anterior to the edge of trapezius (Fig. 3-45), slide the thumb along the anterior scalene as far as it will go.
- Repeat for posterior scalene.
- The previous procedure may also be performed using the knuckles (Fig. 3-46).

Stripping (3)

- The client is seated.
- Stand behind the seated client.
- Place the thumb on the middle scalene at its superior attachment (Fig. 3-47).
- Pressing deeply into the tissue, glide the thumb along the muscle to its inferior attachment.
- Repeat this procedure for anterior and posterior scalenes.

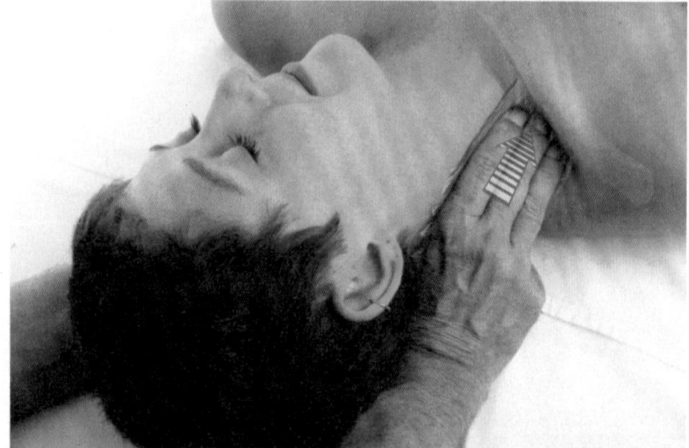

FIGURE 3-44 Deep compression of scalenes

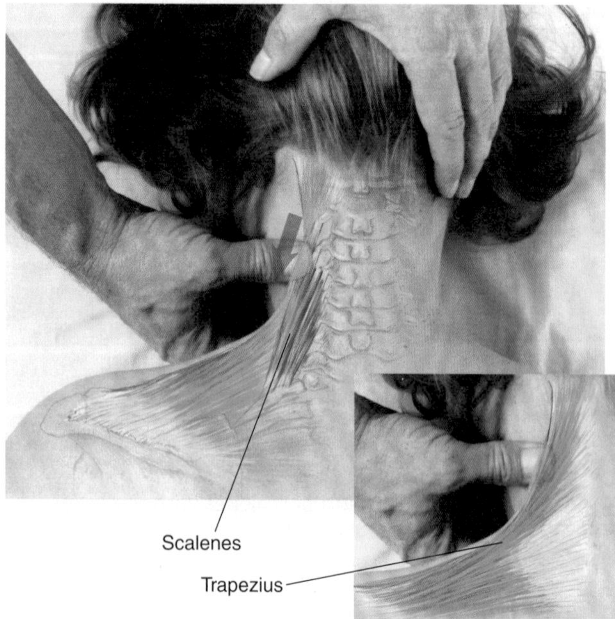

FIGURE 3-45 Stripping of scalenes with client prone: thumb is on the scalenes (inset shows thumb under the edge of trapezius)

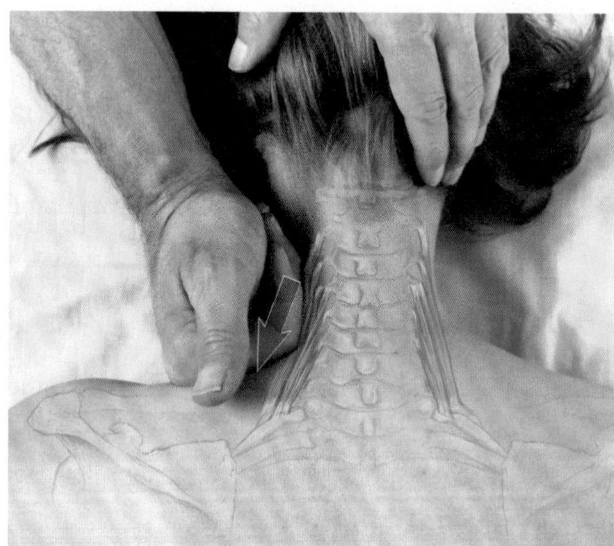

FIGURE 3-46 Stripping of the scalenes with the knuckles

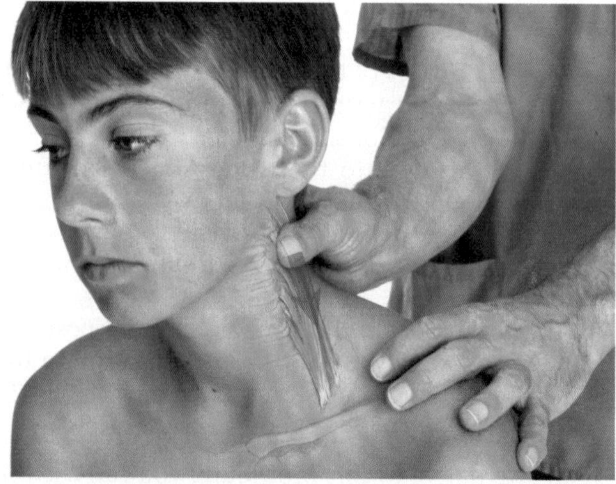

FIGURE 3-47 Stripping of scalenes with client seated

Overview of the Posterior Neck Muscles

The large number of overlapping muscles in the posterior neck makes it difficult to isolate them and their tender points manually. When you find a tender point by pressing deeply a little inferior to the skull, for example, is the tender point located in trapezius, splenius capitis, or semispinalis capitis? Often, you can only make an educated guess, usually based on the referral area.

Fortunately, for the purposes of this book, it is not necessary to isolate the location of a trigger point in a particular muscle of the posterior neck with absolute precision. Because all of these muscles are frequently in a state of strain due to reading, desk work, or poor posture, and because they are all commonly responsible for headaches, they should be treated together. It is important, however, to become familiar with their individual attachments and actions, since more advanced approaches require precise isolation.

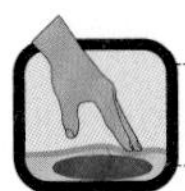

PALPATION

Although easily palpable as a group, most of these muscles are difficult to discern individually. Semispinalis and longissimus capitis are parallel and their fibers are superior/inferior; splenius capitis and cervicis are convergent and their fibers are diagonal. The suboccipital muscles are also palpable but not individually discernible, and their fibers are convergent and diagonal.

TRAPEZIUS

tra-PEEZ-ee-us

ETYMOLOGY Greek, ***trapezium***, a table, from tetra, four + ***pous***, foot

Overview

Trapezius (Fig. 3-48) covers a vast territory and performs a wide variety of functions. Although it is an important posterior neck muscle, it is also a shoulder and back muscle producing several movements of the scapula. Problems in trapezius may cause a great deal of pain and discomfort. It is the muscle most commonly addressed in informal back rubs between friends, because it is so accessible and because manual therapy of trapezius gives tremendous relief. For most people, it is the chief repository of day-to-day tension.

Trapezius lies superficial to all other muscles of the posterior neck, shoulders, and upper back; therefore, examination and treatment of the other muscles of this region inherently involve examination and treatment

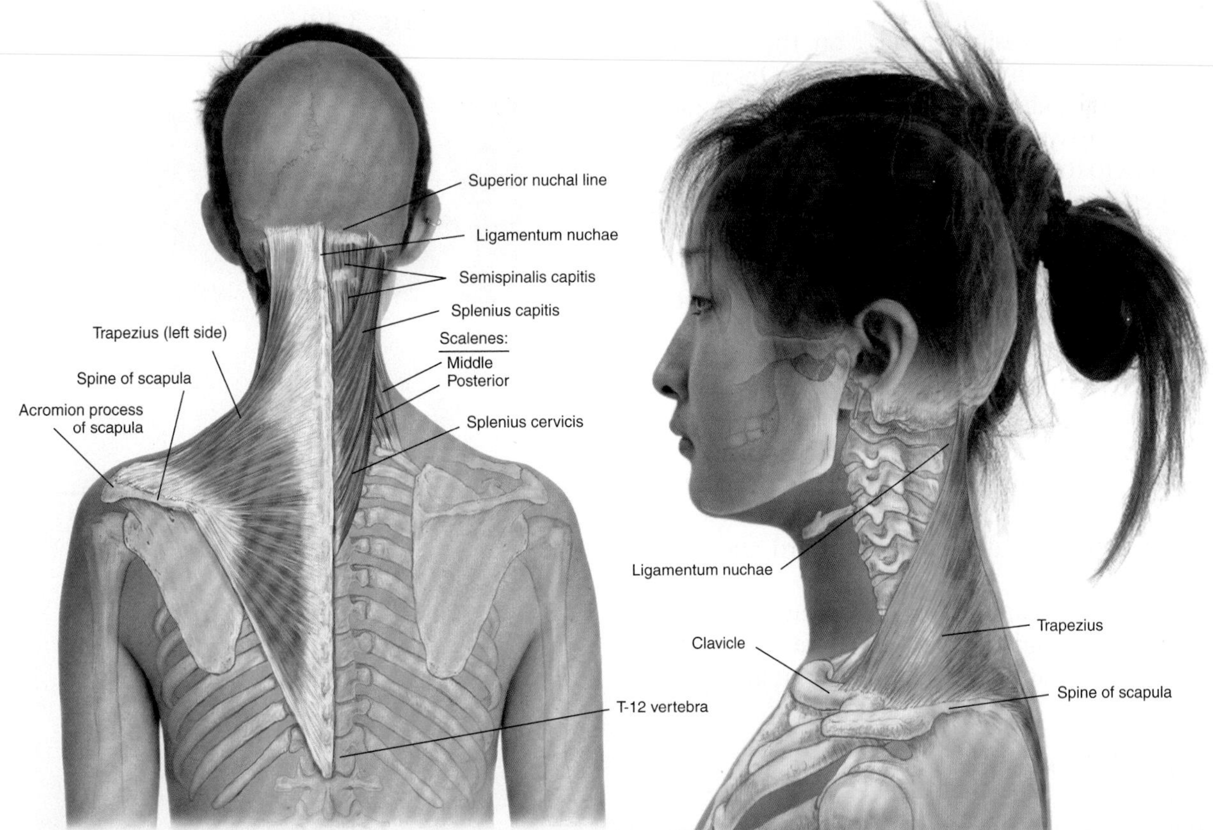

FIGURE 3-48 Anatomy of trapezius

of trapezius. It is important to be aware of its attachments, actions, and referral patterns because of the major role it plays in upper body pain and dysfunction.

In general, examination and treatment of the cervical portion of trapezius are accomplished through examination and treatment of the other muscles of the posterior neck. The same is true for the portions of middle trapezius over and around the scapula.

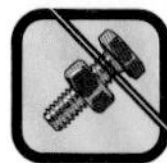

ATTACHMENTS

Upper trapezius:

- Origin: the superior nuchal line, the ligamentum nuchae, and the spinous processes of C1 through C5
- Insertion: the outer third of the clavicle

Middle trapezius:

- Origin: the spinous processes and ligaments of C6 through T3
- Insertion: the acromion and upper aspect of the spine of the scapula

Lower trapezius:

- Origin: the spinous processes and ligaments of T4 through T12
- Insertion: the medial end of the spine of the scapula, next to the lower attachment of levator scapulae

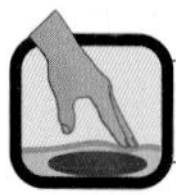

PALPATION

Trapezius is most easily palpated on the shoulders, where it is almost invariably taut, simply by grasping it in the hand. Asking the client to shrug his shoulders makes it very easy to grasp the tissue. One can follow it up the neck to the superior nuchal line from that point. It is not easily discernible on the upper back except at the borders, and even that discernment depends on positioning and individual muscle development. Architecture is highly variable, but largely convergent.

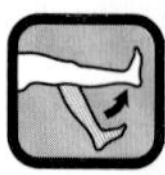

ACTIONS

- Elevates the scapula (with levator scapulae)
- Rotates the scapula upward (moves the glenoid fossa upward)
- Retracts the scapula (pulling toward the spinal column)
- Depresses the scapula (lower trapezius)
- Extends the head and neck (bilateral action)
- Rotates the head and neck (unilateral action)

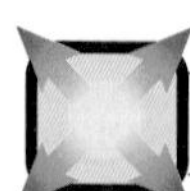

REFERRAL AREAS

- Trigger points in the part of upper trapezius overlying the shoulder refer pain up the neck to the mastoid process and over the ear to the temporal region; also to the angle of the mandible.
- Trigger points in middle and lower trapezius refer pain into the posterior neck at the base of the skull, across the posterior shoulders, and between the shoulder blades.
- Trigger points in middle trapezius, particularly toward the lateral end near the acromion, refer pain to the outer surface of the arm proximal to the elbow.

OTHER MUSCLES TO EXAMINE

All muscles of the posterior and lateral neck, the upper back, and around the scapula

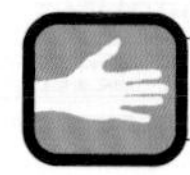

MANUAL THERAPY

Stripping

- The client lies prone.
- Stand at the client's head and place one hand flat on the client's shoulder at the base of the neck, the fingers pointing inferiorly.
- Using your body weight and pressing firmly into the tissue, slide the hand inferiorly between the vertebral column and the scapula all the way to the end of the thoracic spine, transmitting your weight primarily to the client through the heel of your hand (Fig. 3-49).

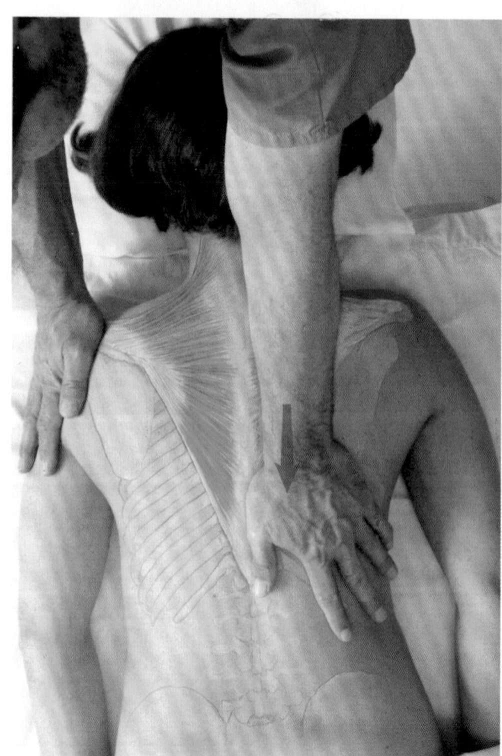

FIGURE 3-49 Deep stripping of trapezius

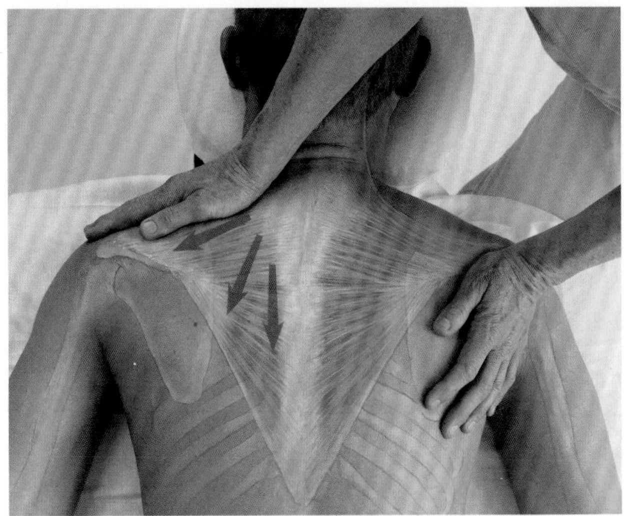

FIGURE 3-50 Deep stripping of superolateral trapezius

- Place the same or opposite hand—whichever is most comfortable for you—at the same starting point.
- Using the same weight and motion, and shifting the position of your feet so that your weight is behind the movement of your hand, slide your hand diagonally along the back just inside the medial edge of the scapula, past the inferior angle of the scapula.
- Place the heel of your opposite hand just lateral to the lower cervical vertebrae.
- Pressing firmly, slide your hand over the upper aspect of the scapula, continuing to the acromion (Fig. 3-50).
- Repeat this procedure on the other side.

Pétrissage

- Stand at the side of the prone client at the elbow, facing the client's head.
- Place both hands on the client's near shoulder on the upper trapezius.
- Squeeze and pull the tissue, first with one hand, then with the other, beginning gently and allowing your grasp to become firmer as the tissue relaxes.
- To finish, grasp the muscle with one hand and shake it several times.
- Move to the other side of the client and repeat the procedure.

Pincer Compression

- Stand at the side of the prone client at the elbow, facing the client's head.
- Place the hand that is closest to the client's head on the client's upper trapezius.
- Grasp it firmly between your fingers and thumb, and hold it. Begin with a gentle grasp, assessing the tissue, and allow your grasp to become firmer as the tissue releases (Fig. 3-51).

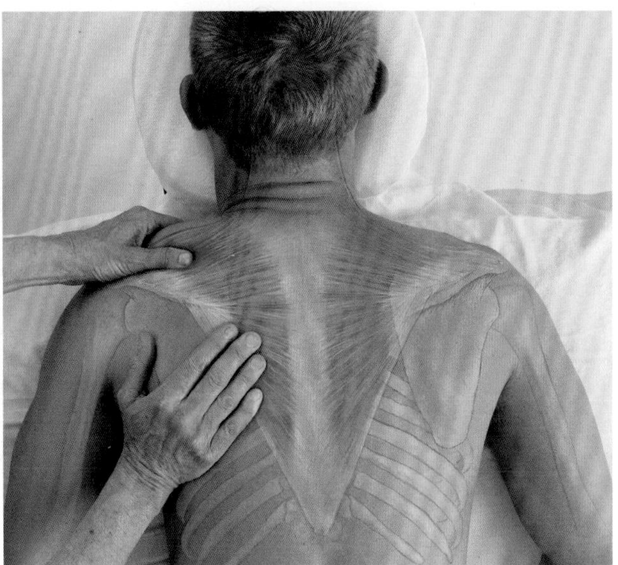

FIGURE 3-51 Pincer compression of trapezius

- Alternate holding the tissue with a back and forth movement of your thumb and fingers.

SEMISPINALIS CAPITIS AND CERVICIS, LONGISSIMUS CAPITIS

SEM-ee-spin-AL-iss CAP-it-iss
SERV-iss-iss
long-GISS-im-us

ETYMOLOGY Latin ***semi***, half + ***spinalis***, of the spine + ***capitis***, of the head; ***semi***, half + ***spinalis***, of the spine + ***cervicis***, of the neck; ***longissimus***, longest + ***capitis***, of the head

Overview

Semispinalis capitis and **cervicis and longissimus capitis** (Fig. 3-52) are involved in support of the head when carried or tilted forward. As a result, they are commonly overused and in a state of strain and are among the chief culprits in headache pain.

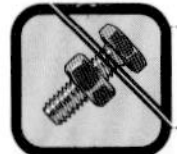

ATTACHMENTS

Semispinalis cervicis:

- Origin: the transverse processes of T1 through T6
- Insertion: spinous processes of C2 through C5

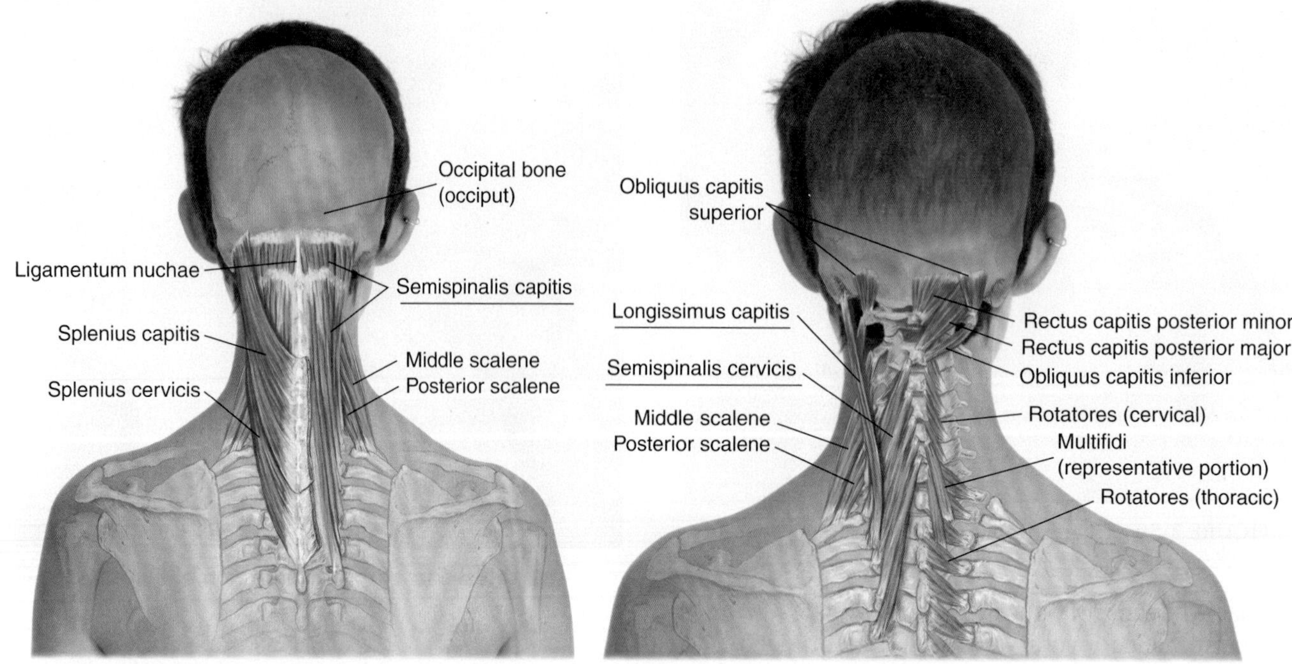

FIGURE 3-52 Anatomy of posterior neck muscles

Semispinalis capitis:

- Origin: the transverse processes of C7 through T6, also articular processes of C4 through C7
- Insertion: between the superior and inferior nuchal lines of the occipital bone

Longissimus capitis:

- Origin: transverse processes of T1 through T5 and articular processes of C4 through C7
- Insertion: posterior margin of the mastoid process, between the splenius capitis and the sternocleidomastoid

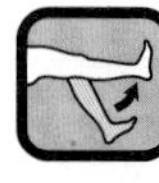

ACTIONS

Semispinalis capitis and longissimus capitis:

- Extends neck and bends it laterally to the same side (lateral flexion)
- Rotates the head to same side
- Supports the head when tilted forward

Semispinalis cervicis:

- Extends neck and bends it laterally to the same side (lateral flexion)
- Rotates the head to opposite side

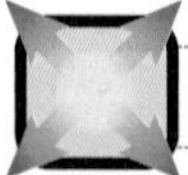

REFERRAL AREAS

- Semispinalis and longissimus capitis: a band across the side of the head, especially in the anterior part of the temporal region
- Semispinalis cervicis: back of the head (the classic tension headache)

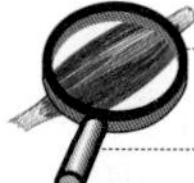

OTHER MUSCLES TO EXAMINE

- All other posterior, lateral, and anterior neck and head muscles
- Levator scapulae

SPLENIUS CAPITIS, SPLENIUS CERVICIS

SPLEN-ee-us CAP-it-iss
SER-viss-is

ETYMOLOGY Latin ***splenius***, bandage (from Greek, ***splenion***, bandage) + ***capitis***, of the head; ***splenius***, bandage (from Greek, ***splenion***, bandage) + ***cervicis***, of the neck

Overview

Splenius capitis and splenius cervicis (Fig. 3-53) are head-turners and neck extenders, and are involved in much headache pain.

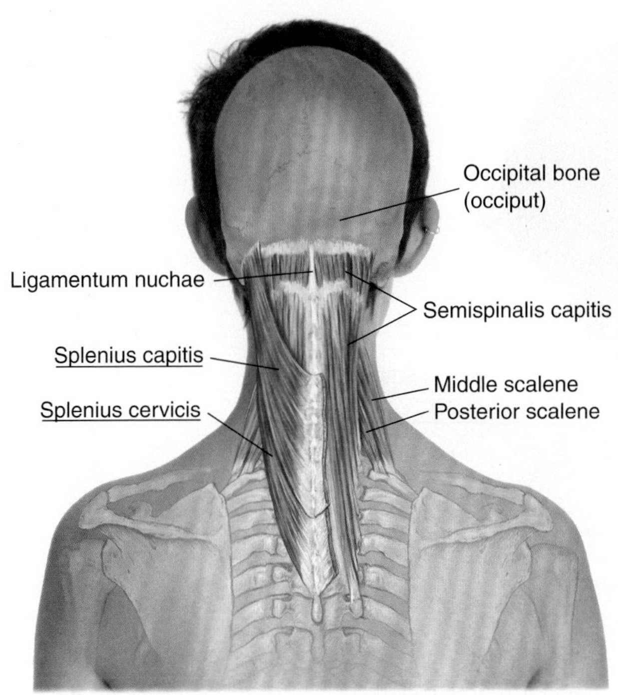

FIGURE 3-53 Anatomy of splenius capitis and splenius cervicis

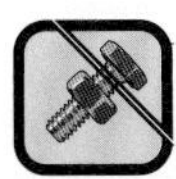

ATTACHMENTS

Splenius capitis:

- Origin: inferior half of the ligamentum nuchae, spinous process of C7, spinous processes of T1 through T3 or possibly T4
- Insertion: mastoid process of the temporal bone, and on the occipital bone inferior to the lateral third of the superior nuchal line

Splenius cervicis:

- Origin: spinous processes of T3 through T6
- Insertion: posterior tubercles of the transverse processes of C1 through C3

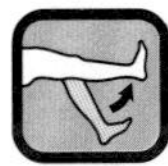

ACTIONS

These muscles extend the neck and rotate the head to the same side.

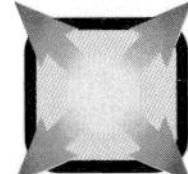

REFERRAL AREAS

Splenius capitis:

- To the top of the head

Splenius cervicis:

- To the eye
- Over the temporal region and the ear to the occipital region
- To the angle of the neck

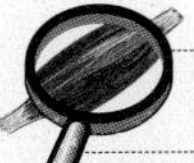

OTHER MUSCLES TO EXAMINE

- All posterior neck muscles
- Levator scapulae
- Trapezius
- Sternocleidomastoid

MULTIFIDI AND ROTATORES

mul-TIFF-id-ee
ro-ta-TORE-ace

ETYMOLOGY Latin, ***multus***, much + ***findus***, divided; Latin, ***rotatores***, rotators

Overview

Multifidi and **rotatores** (Fig. 3-54) are small, deep intervertebral muscles that occur over the entire length of the spine. They function less as movers than as restrainers; they keep the individual vertebrae from bending or rotating too far out of position when the spine is bent by larger muscles.

Rotatores lie deep to the multifidi. The rotatores in the cervical region are poorly defined and not present in everyone. The multifidi are identified as four separate regions, due to their origin, and cross two to four vertebral joints, while rotatores cross only one or two (Fig. 3-55).

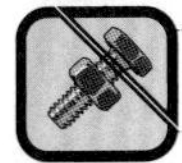

ATTACHMENTS

Origin

- Cervical multifidi: the articular processes of the four lower vertebrae
- Thoracic multifidi: all the transverse processes
- Lumbar multifidi: all the mamillary processes
- Sacral multifidi: from the back of the sacrum, as low as the fourth sacral foramen, from the aponeurosis of origin of the sacrospinalis, from the medial surface of the posterior superior iliac spine, and from the posterior sacroiliac ligaments

Insertion

- All multifidi cross superiorly 2 to 4 vertebrae to the spinous processes.

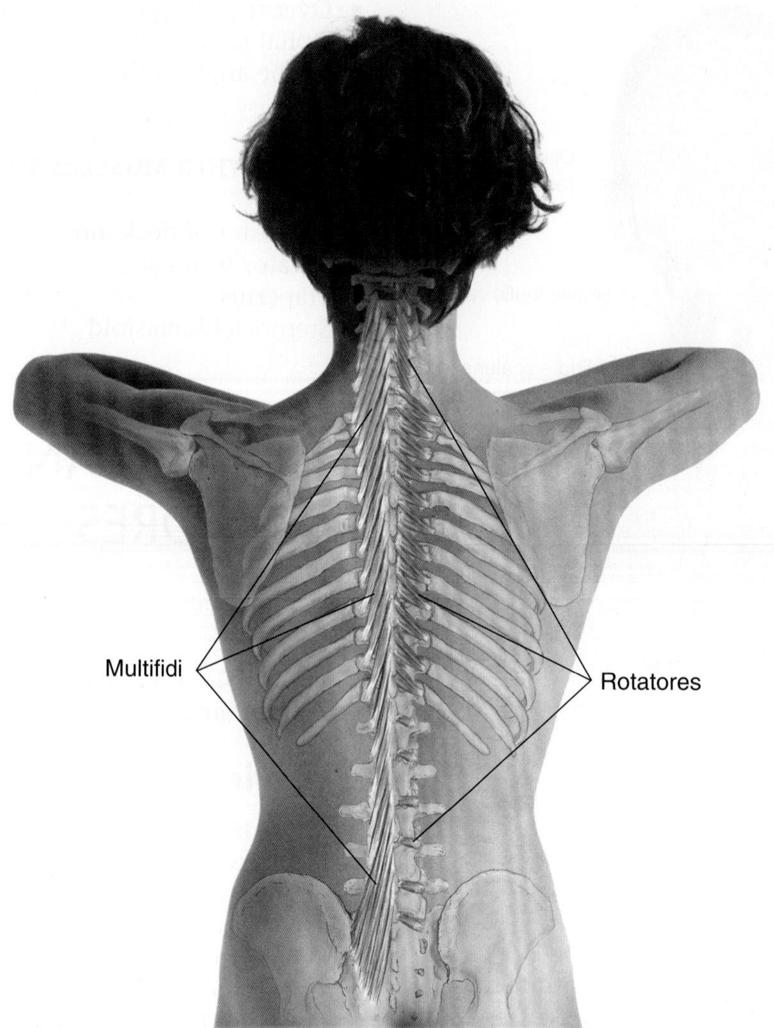

FIGURE 3-54 Attachment patterns of multifidi and rotatores of entire spine

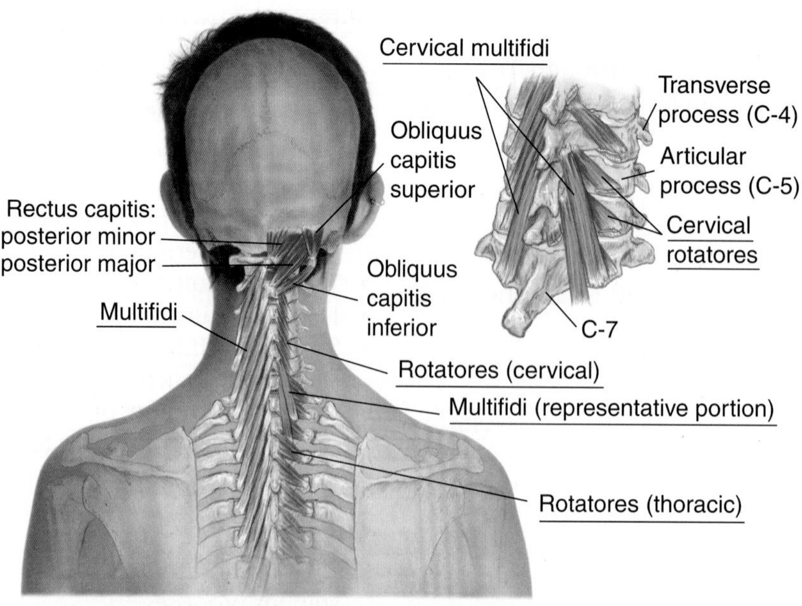

FIGURE 3-55 Anatomy of cervical multifidi and rotatores

ROTATORES

Origin: superior and posterior aspect of the transverse process
Insertion: inferior border and lateral surface of the lamina of the vertebra above

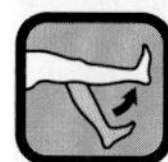

ACTIONS

Although technically considered extensors, lateral flexors, and rotators of the spine, these functions are actually carried out primarily by larger muscles. These small muscles seem to be chiefly involved in small positional adjustments of individual vertebrae and providing sensory feedback on spinal movement (proprioception).

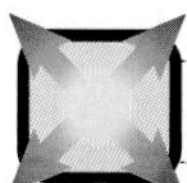

REFERRAL AREAS

- To an area just inferior to the base of the skull and another just medial to the root of the spine of the scapula
- To a band between those areas extending slightly over the shoulder

OTHER MUSCLES TO EXAMINE

- Other posterior neck muscles
- Levator scapulae
- Serratus posterior superior

SUBOCCIPITAL MUSCLES

Obliquus capitis superior, obliquus capitis inferior, rectus capitis posterior major, rectus capitis posterior minor

ETYMOLOGY

Latin ***sub***, under + ***occiput***, back of head
Latin ***obliquus***, oblique + ***capitis***, of the head + ***superior***, higher
Latin ***obliquus***, oblique + ***capitis***, of the head + ***inferior***, lower
Latin ***rectus***, straight + ***capitis***, of the head + ***posterior***, toward the back + ***major***, larger
Latin ***rectus***, straight + ***capitis***, of the head + ***posterior***, toward the back + ***minor***, smaller

Overview

The triangle formed by the suboccipital muscles (Fig. 3-56) (except rectus capitis posterior minor) is called the **suboccipital triangle**; it surrounds the vertebral artery. The suboccipital triangle muscles, which are often involved with other posterior neck muscles in general headache pain, are treated along with these other muscles. Their trigger points are virtually impossible to differentiate from those of the overlying muscles. They are best treated with compression and stretching.

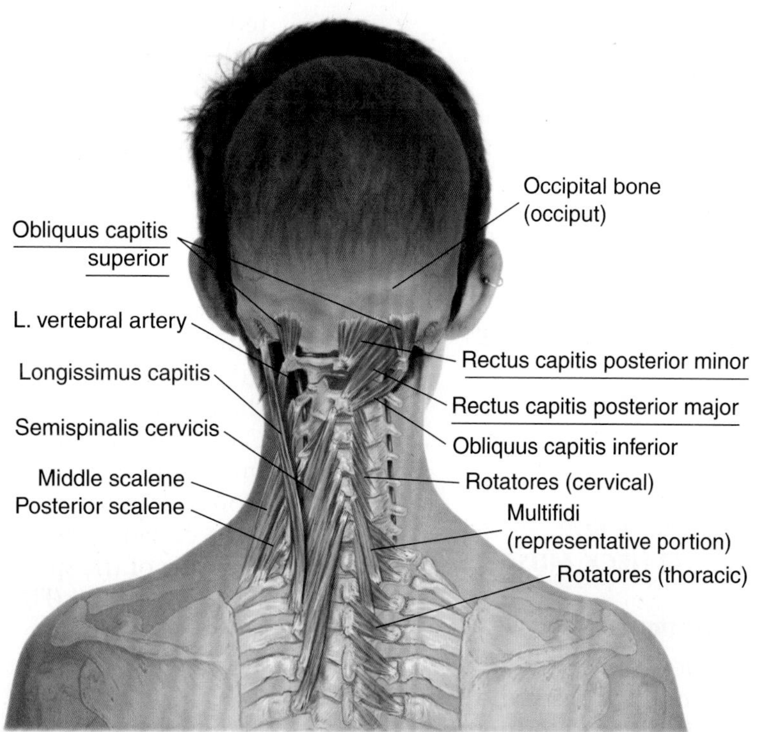

FIGURE 3-56 Anatomy of suboccipital muscles

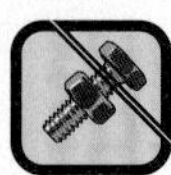

ATTACHMENTS

Obliquus capitis superior:
- Origin: transverse process of atlas (C1)
- Insertion: between the superior and inferior nuchal line of occiput

Obliquus capitis inferior:
- Origin: spinous process of axis (C2)
- Insertion: transverse process of atlas (C1)

Rectus capitis posterior major:
- Origin: spinous process of axis (C2)
- Insertion: inferior nuchal line of the occipital bone

Rectus capitis posterior minor:
- Origin: tubercle on the posterior arch of the atlas (C1)
- Insertion: medial aspect of the inferior nuchal line of the occipital bone and the surface between it and the foramen magnum

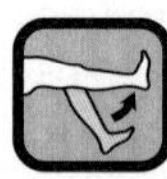

ACTIONS

Obliquus capitis superior:
- Bilaterally extends the head
- Laterally flexes the head to the contracted side

Obliquus capitis inferior:
- Rotates the head to the contracted side

Rectus capitis posterior major:
- Bilaterally extends the head
- Rotates the head to the contracted side

Rectus capitis posterior minor:
- Bilaterally extends the head

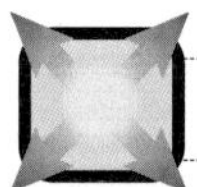

REFERRAL AREAS

- Over the back of the head
- In a band over the side of the head to the eye

OTHER MUSCLES TO EXAMINE

- All other posterior neck muscles
- Sternocleidomastoid

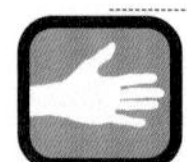

MANUAL THERAPY FOR ALL POSTERIOR NECK MUSCLES

Stripping and Compression

- The client lies supine.
- Seated beside the client's head and using the hand nearest the client's head to support it from underneath, place the other hand under the client's neck with the fingers on the far side and the thumb on the near side.

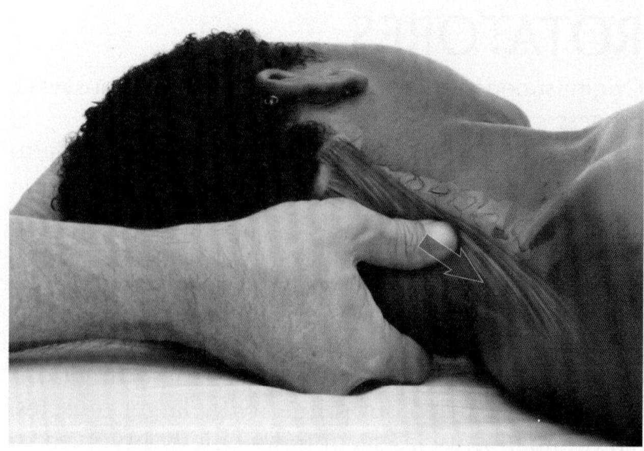

FIGURE 3-57 Stripping of posterior neck muscles with thumb

- Press the thumb into the posterior muscles of the neck at the base of the skull just lateral to the spinous processes of the upper cervical vertebrae.
- Pressing firmly into the tissue, glide the thumb toward the torso, pausing at tight or tender spots and waiting for them to release (Fig. 3-57). Take the thumb as far as it will comfortably go along the base of the neck.
- Slide the thumb back along the same path to the base of the skull, again stopping at tender or tight spots to release them (Fig. 3-58A).
- Shift the thumb laterally toward yourself and repeat the process until you have covered the posterior neck as far as the posterior aspect of the scalenes. This may be done with the fingertips as well (Fig. 3-58B)
- At the base of the skull, press the fingertips upward and deep into the suboccipital muscles.
- Hold for release (Fig. 3-59).

Moving Compression with Fingertips

- The client lies supine.
- Seated centrally at the client's head, push both hands flat under the client's shoulders on both sides until your fingertips rest on either side of the thoracic spine.
- Curl your fingers so that their tips press into the muscles on either side of the spine.
- Slowly draw your hands toward yourself, gliding your curled fingertips along the muscles on either side of the spine until your fingers reach the base of the skull (Fig. 3-60).

Cross-fiber Stroking

- The client lies supine.
- Standing at the client's head and facing the client, place one hand under the client's neck at the base

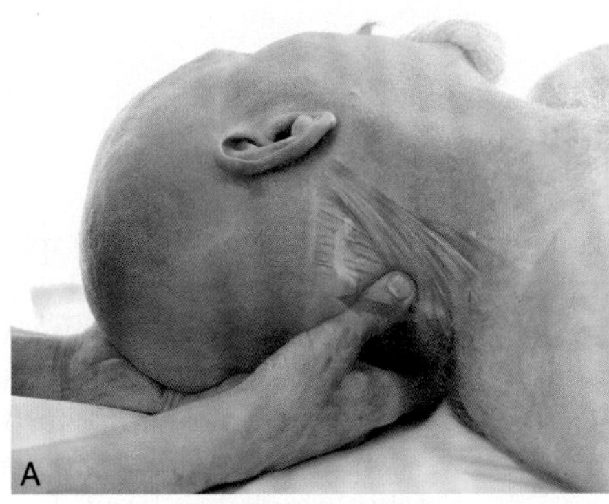

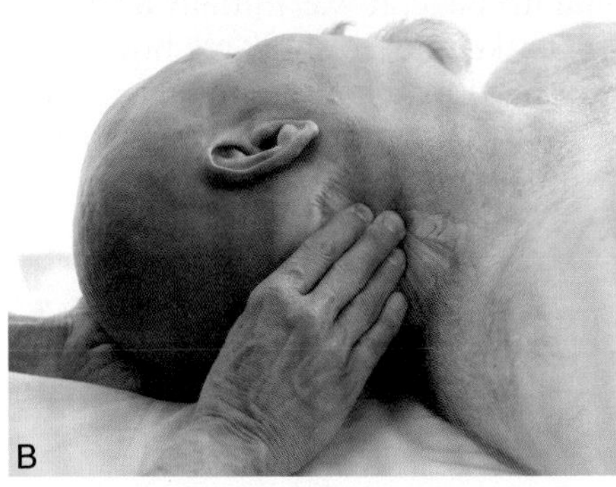

FIGURE 3-58 Bidirectional stripping of posterior neck muscles with thumb (A) or fingers (B)

of the occiput and curl the fingertips into the lateral aspect of the posterior neck muscles (Fig. 3-61).

- Pressing firmly up into the tissue, continue to curl the fingers, drawing the tips toward you until they reach the spine.
- Move the hand downward toward the base of the neck and repeat.
- Repeat on the other side.

Cross-fiber Stroking with the Thumb

- The client lies prone.
- Standing at the client's head and facing the neck, hold the head steady with the far hand.
- Place your fingertips on the far side of the client's neck and the tip of your thumb on the cervical spine at the base of the skull.
- Pressing firmly into the tissue, slide your thumb across the neck muscles toward your fingers (Fig. 3-62). (Note: At the base of the skull, direct your pressure partially against the occipital bone.)
- Shift your hand down the neck an inch or two and repeat the process; repeat until you reach the base of the neck.
- Move to the opposite side of the client and repeat the procedure on the other side.

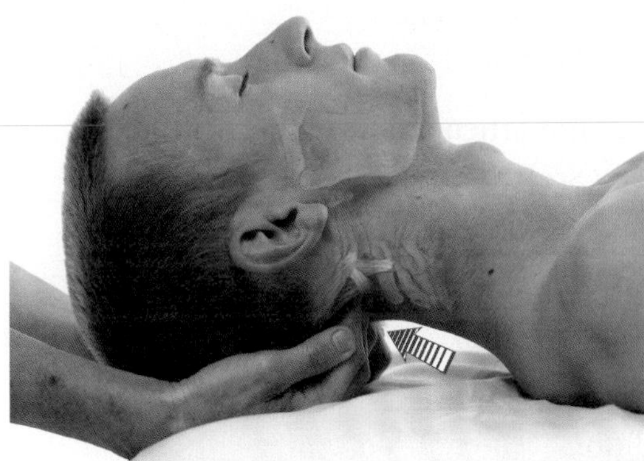

FIGURE 3-59 Compression of suboccipital muscles

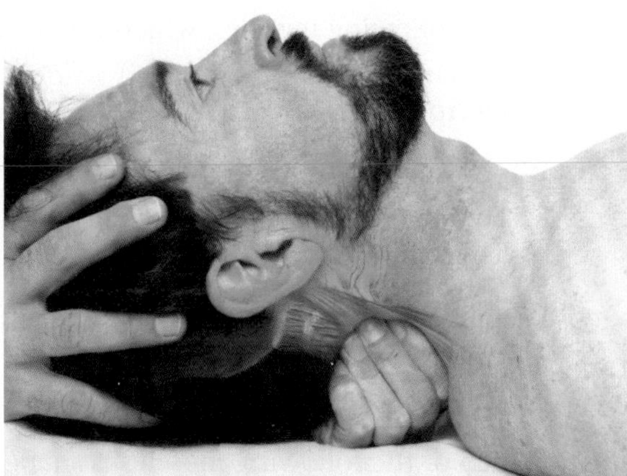

FIGURE 3-61 Cross-fiber stroking of posterior neck muscles with fingertips

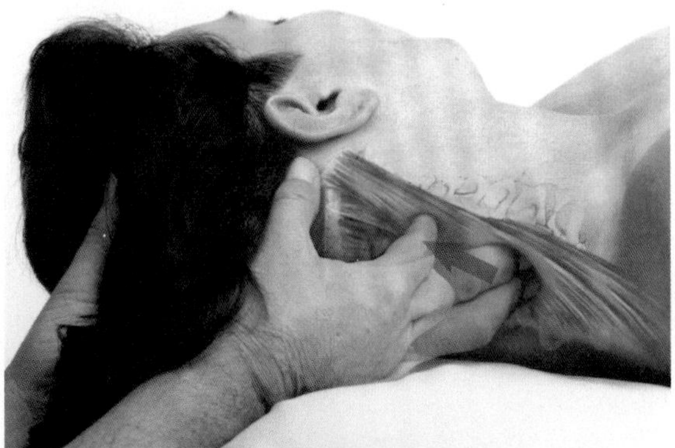

FIGURE 3-60 Moving compression of posterior neck muscles with fingertips

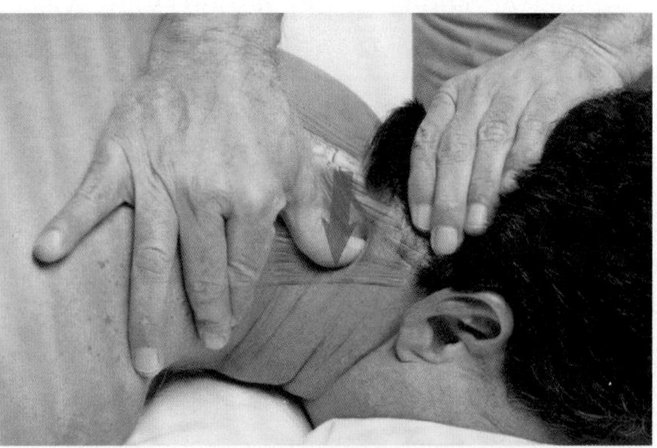

FIGURE 3-62 Cross-fiber stroking on posterior neck muscles with the thumb

CHAPTER REVIEW

CASE STUDY

I treated Mrs. Owens about 10 years ago for TMJD, and to this day it remains one of the most special sessions of my career. Mrs. Owens was 85 years old at the time of her visit. Her granddaughter had been seeing me for TMJD work and asked me if Mrs. Owens was too old to receive treatment. I assured her she was not. When Mrs. Owens arrived here, she was basically talking through clinched teeth. She stated that she had been suffering for several years and that she only ate soft foods like soup, oatmeal, mashed potatoes, and other things that she did not have to chew. I started the session with Swedish massage strokes to warm her tissues. After approximately 40 minutes of myofascial work and deep stripping on her head, face, neck, and shoulders, all of which were very taut, I performed intraoral massage. It was initially a struggle just to get a finger into her mouth. After 10 minutes of intraoral work, I asked her to show me how far she could open her mouth. She slowly opened her mouth to full range of motion, a smile came over her face, and she exclaimed, "I'm going to go get a hot dog!" I laughed and cried at the same time. She had a follow-up session a few weeks later and was just thrilled at being able to eat her favorite foods again. She died not too long after I started seeing her, but I'm glad that her last year was more pleasant for her.

L.A., LMBT

REVIEW QUESTIONS

1. What is another term for the first cervical vertebra?
   a. Atlantic joint
   b. Axis
   c. Cranium
   d. Atlas

2. Of the following muscles, which one would move the scalp?
   a. Buccinator
   b. Occipitalis
   c. Zygomaticus
   d. Pterygoid

3. Which bone has a lot of muscle attachments, but does not articulate with another bone?
   a. Hyoid
   b. Thyroid
   c. Scalenes
   d. Scapula

4. Which "neck" muscles also cover the entire length of the spine?
   a. Splenius capitis
   b. Levator scapulae
   c. Multifidi
   d. Trapezius

5. Which of the following muscles is shaped like a scallop?
   a. Frontalis
   b. Temporalis
   c. Masseter
   d. Levator palatini

thePoint Additional helpful resources are available at http://thePoint.lww.com.

CHAPTER 4

The Shoulder Region and Upper Thorax

LEARNING OBJECTIVES

At the end of this chapter, the learner will be able to:

- State the correct terminology of the muscles of the shoulders and upper thorax.
- Palpate the muscles of the shoulders and upper thorax.
- Identify their attachments at the origins and insertions.
- Explain the actions of the muscles.
- Describe their pain referral areas.
- Recall related muscles.
- Recognize any endangerment sites and ethical cautions for massage therapy.
- Demonstrate proficiency in manual therapy techniques for muscles of the shoulders and upper thorax.

The Overview of the Region begins on page 107, after the anatomy plates.

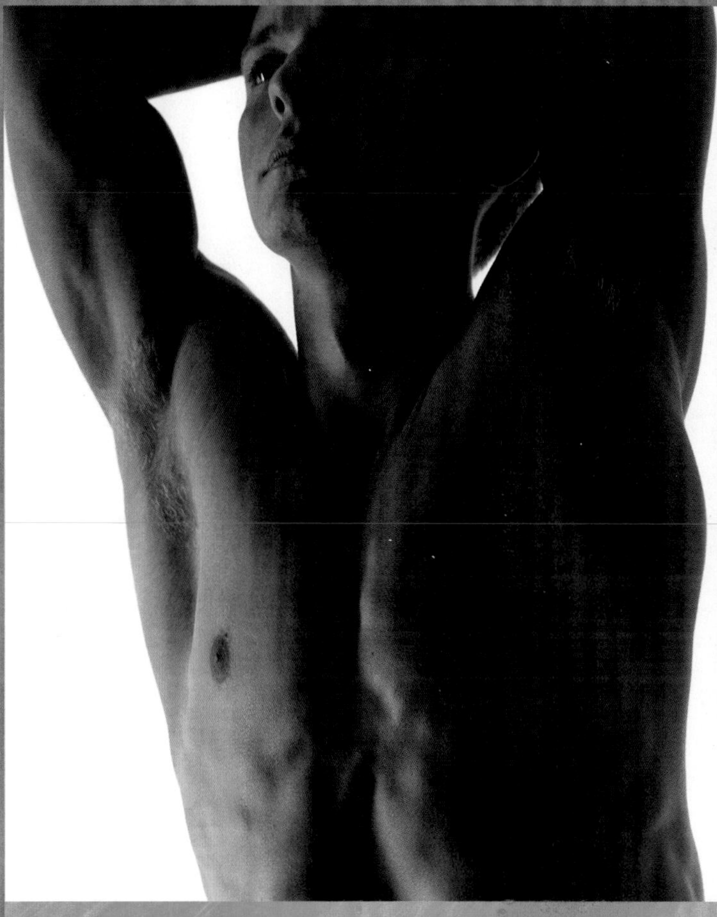

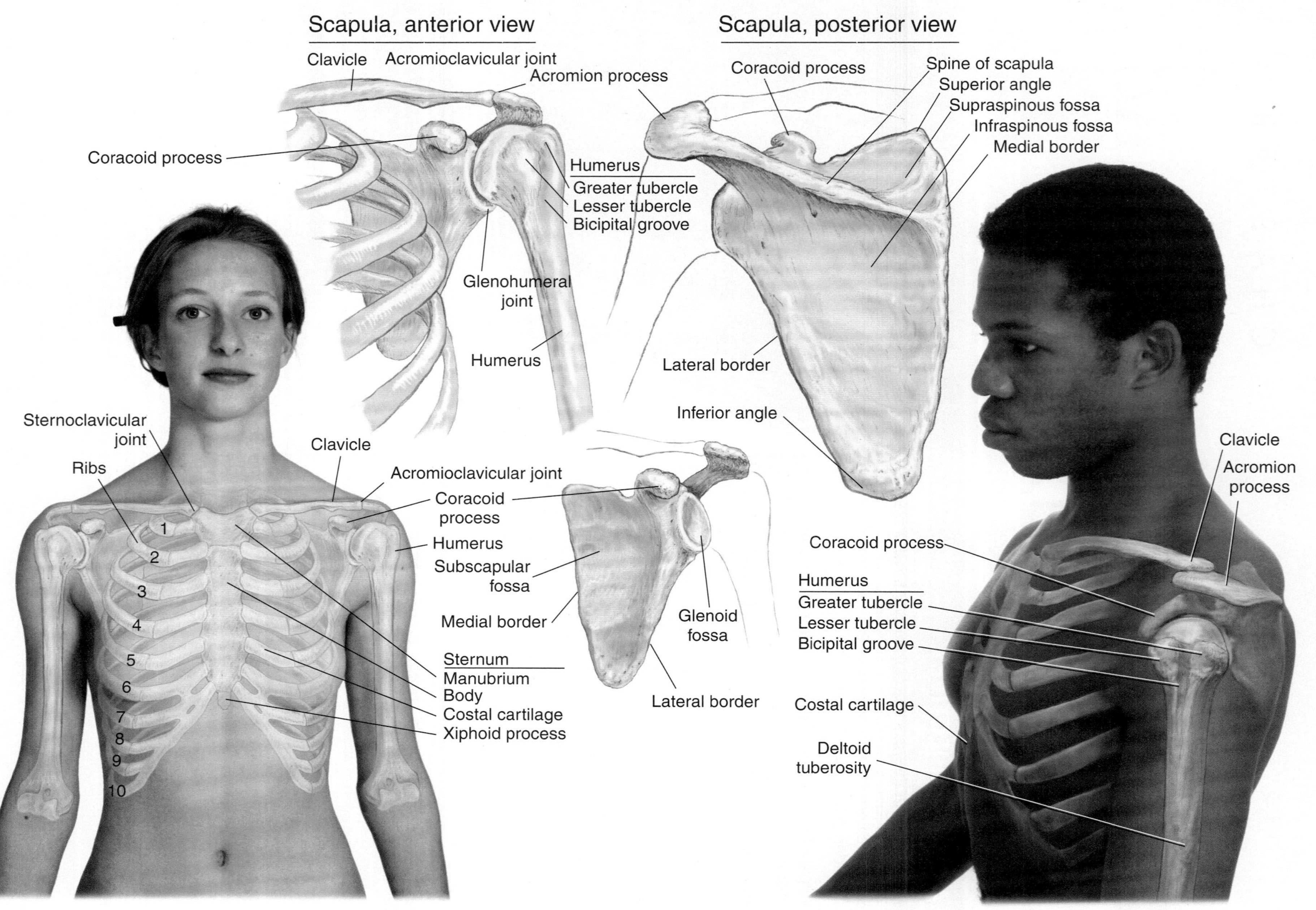

PLATE 4-1 ■ Skeletal features of the scapula, chest, and shoulder

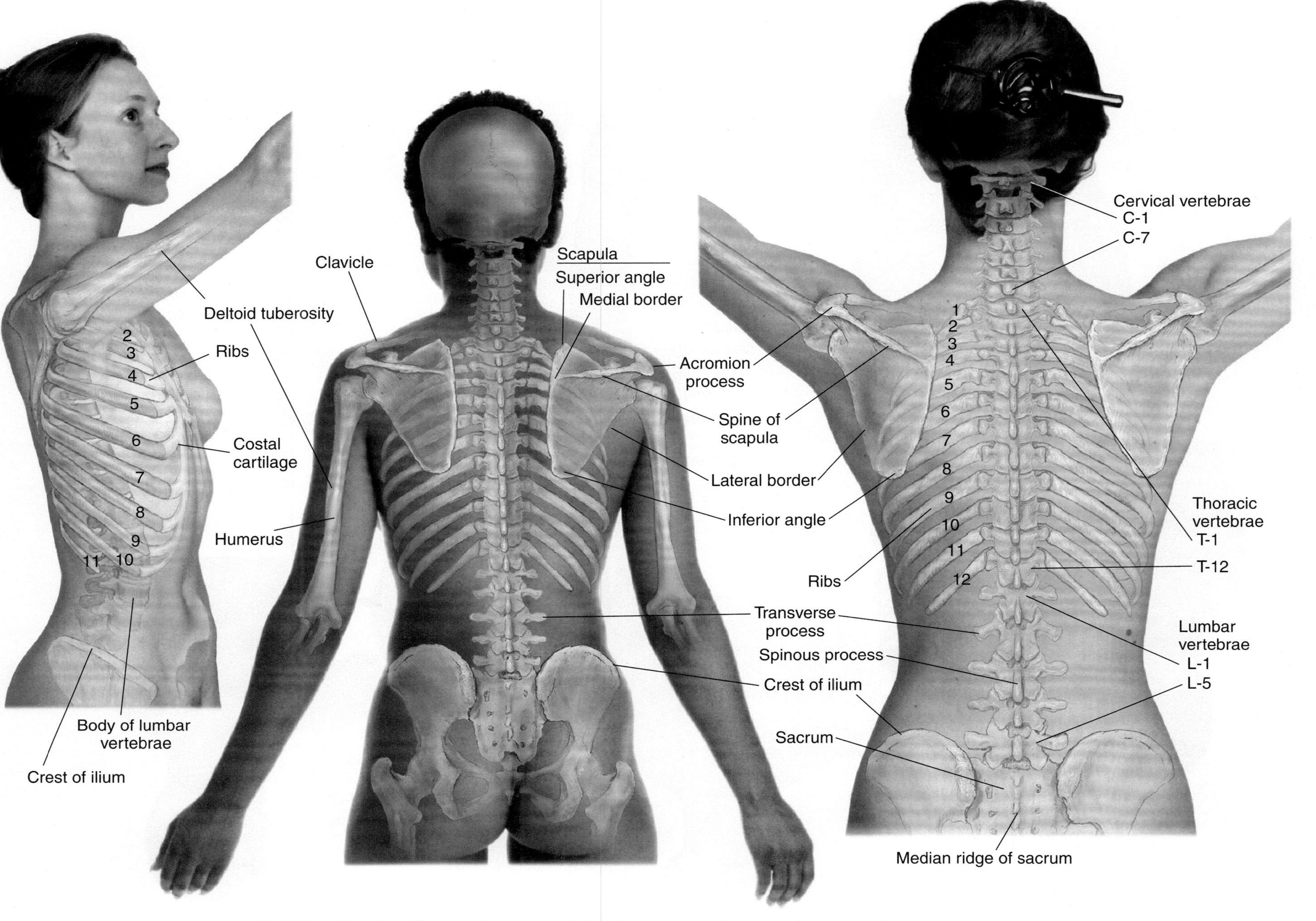

PLATE 4-2 ■ Skeletal features of the lateral chest, posterior shoulder, and upper back

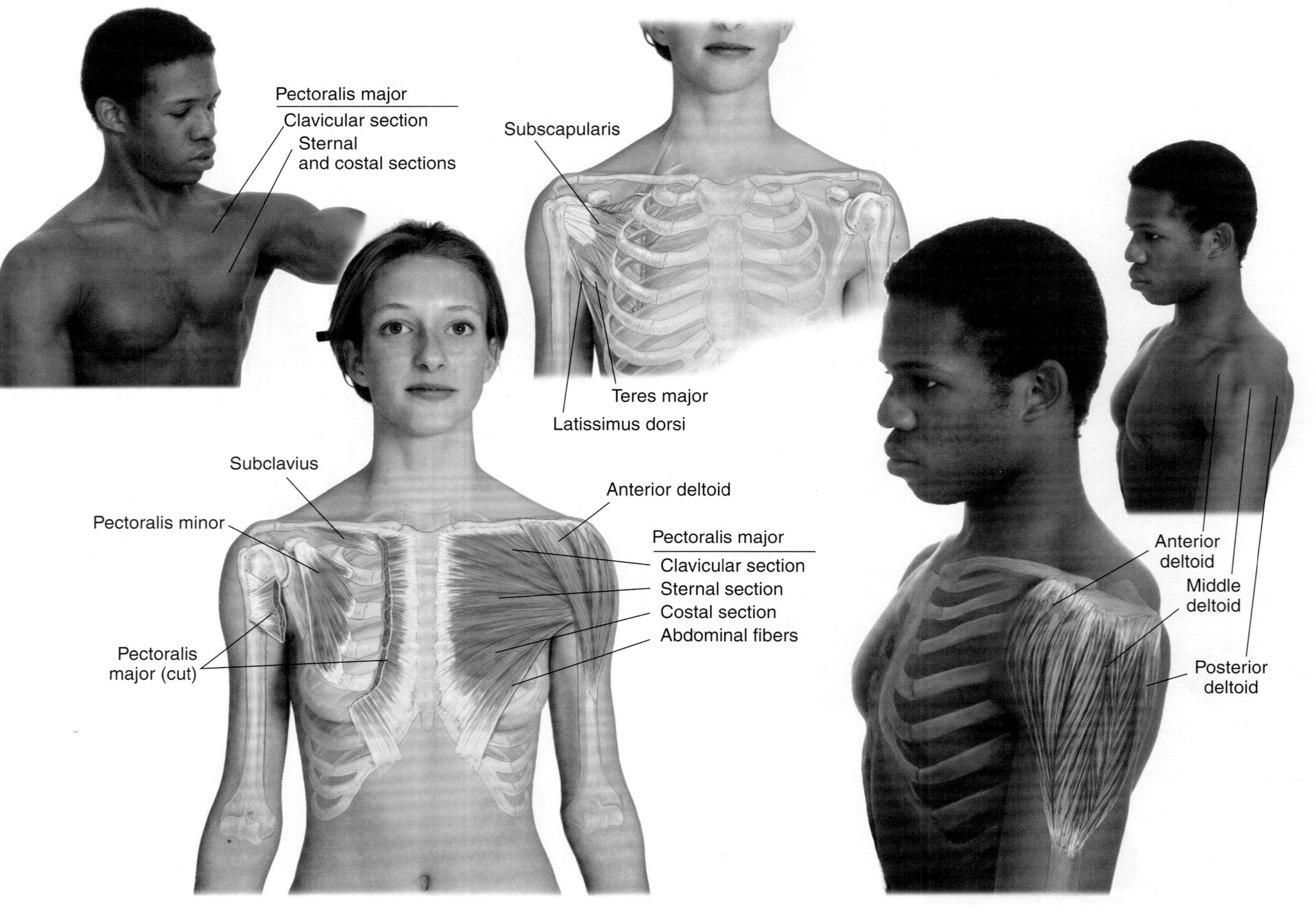

PLATE 4-3 ■ Muscles of the chest and shoulder

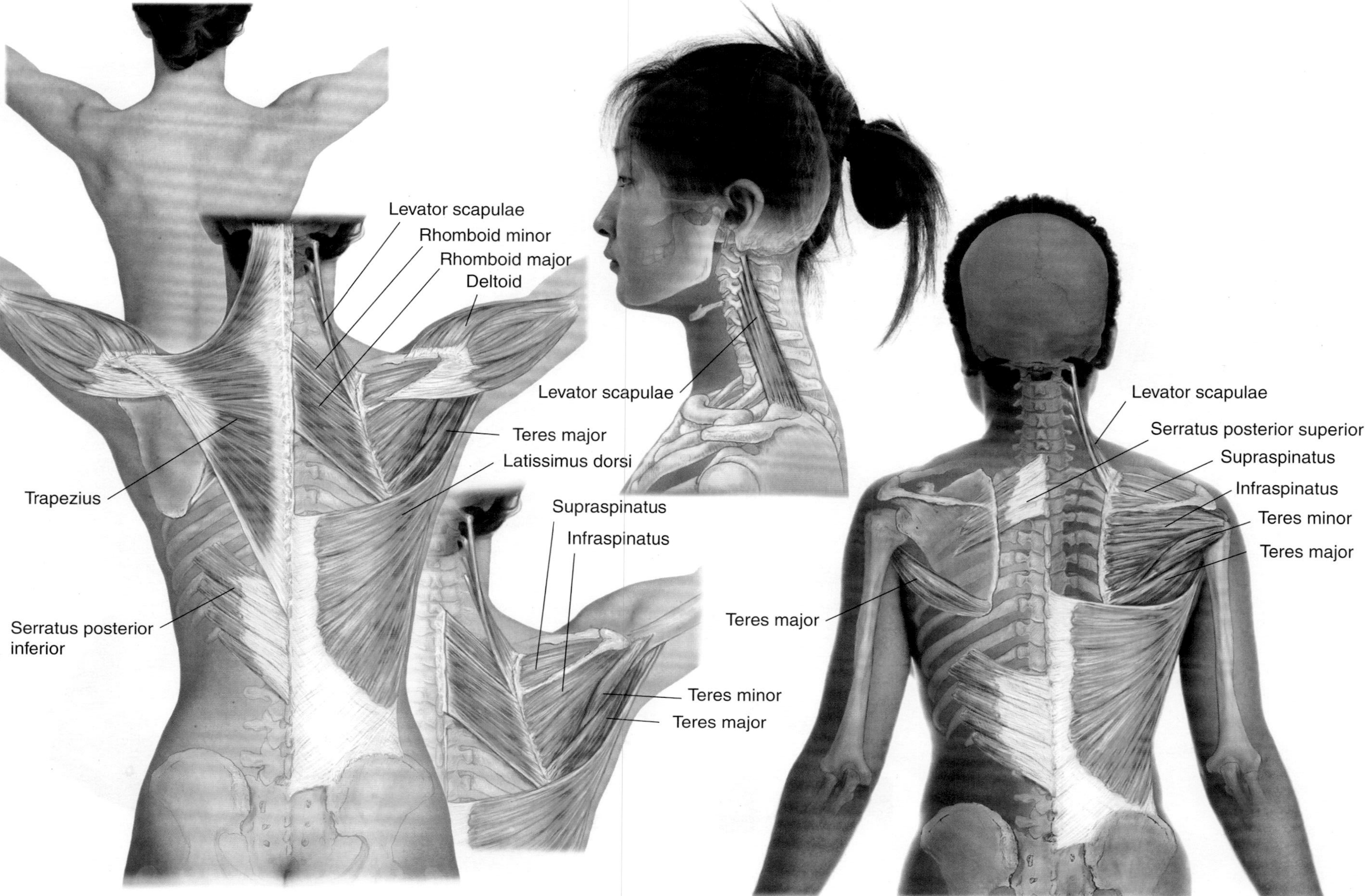

PLATE 4-4 ■ Muscles of the shoulder and upper back

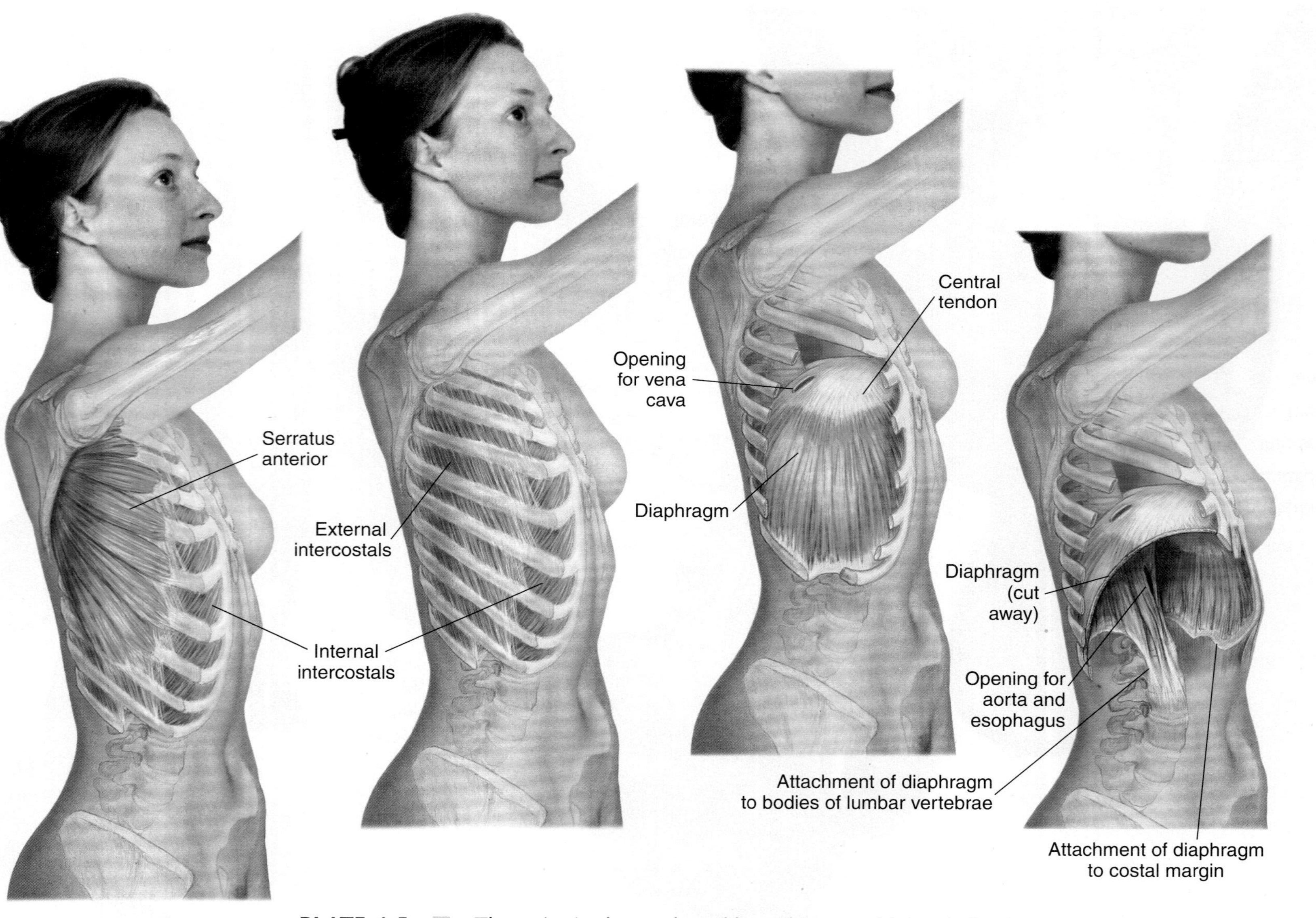

PLATE 4-5 ■ The principal muscles of breathing and lateral chest

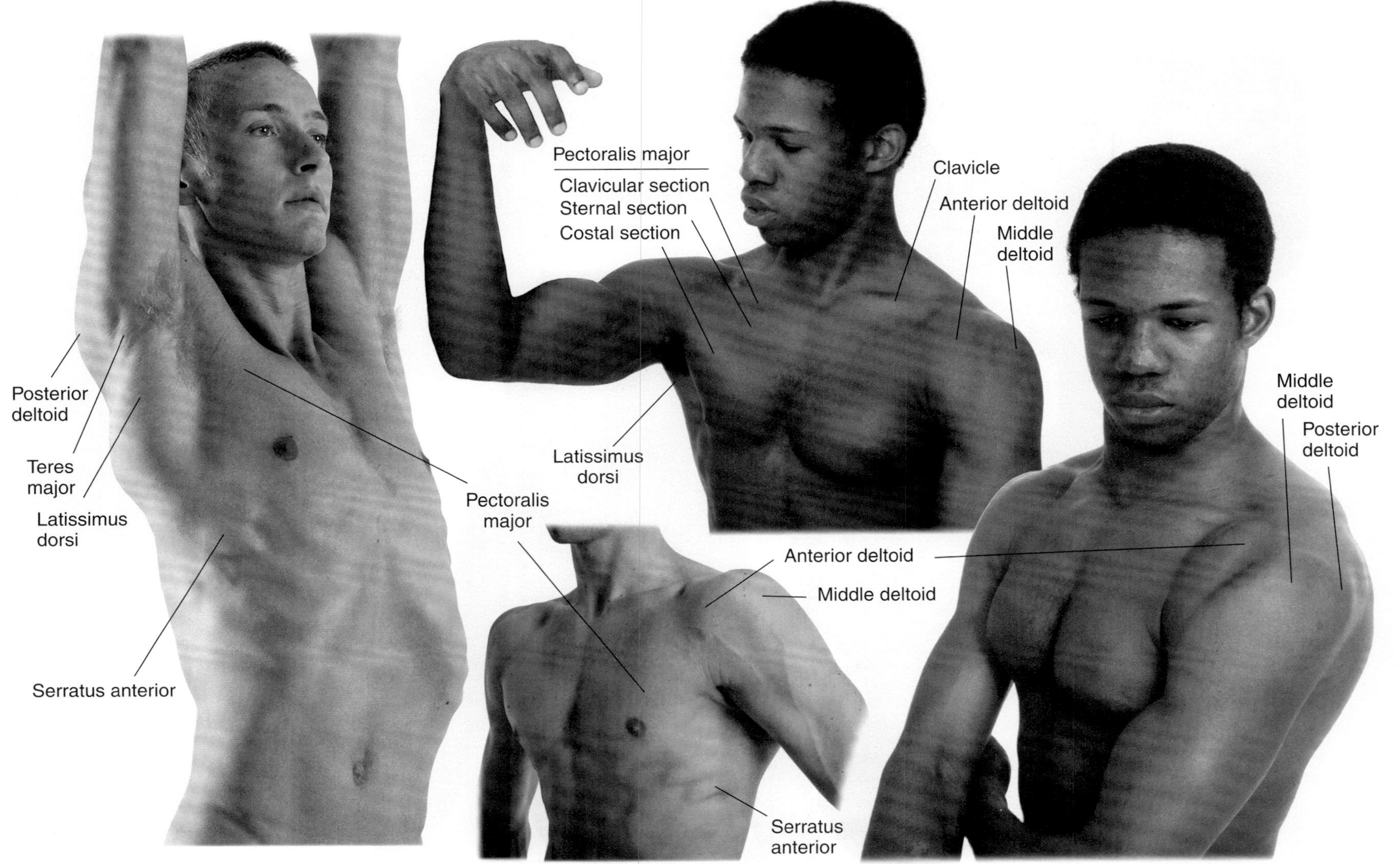

PLATE 4-6 ■ Surface anatomy of the chest and shoulder

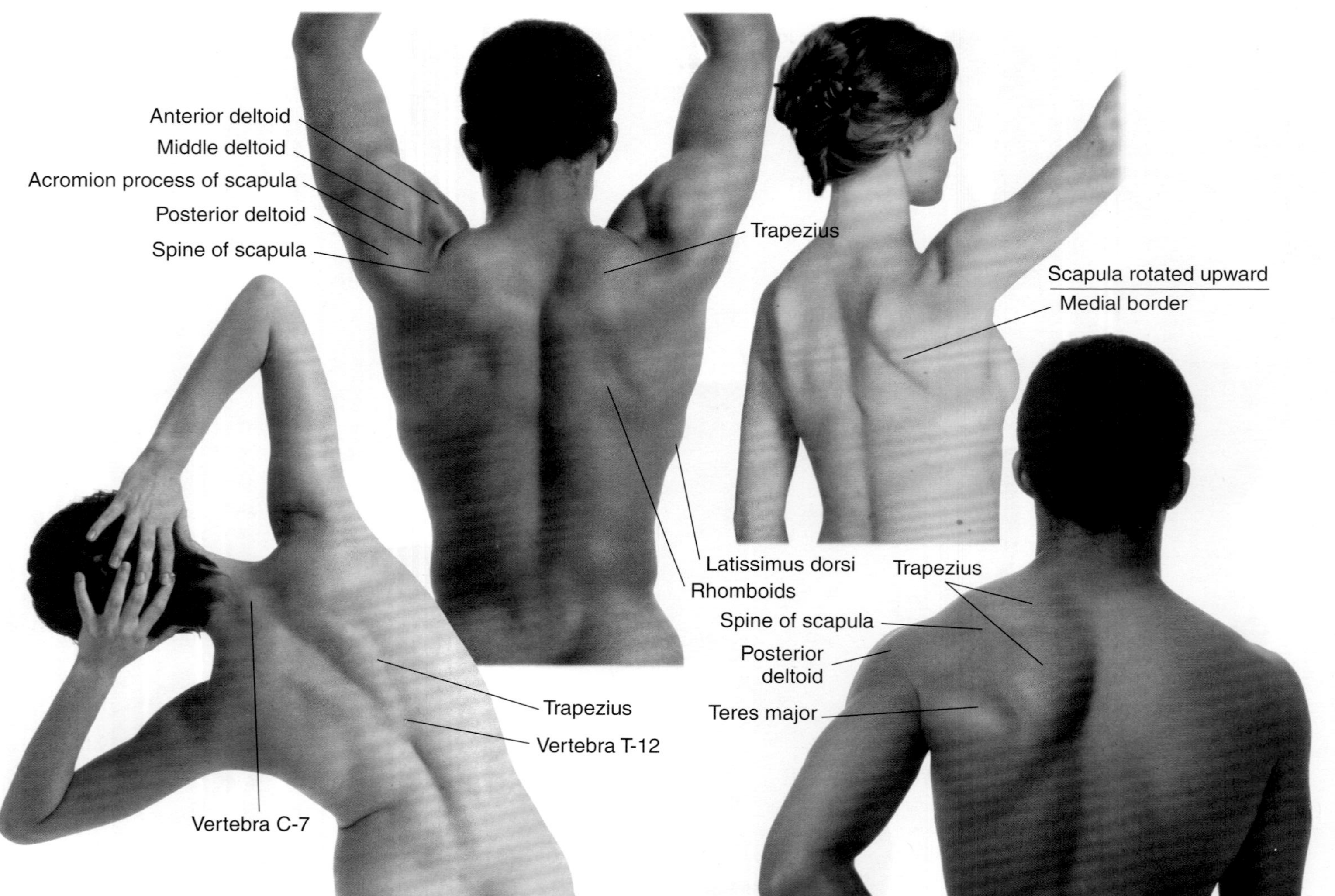

PLATE 4-7 ■ Surface anatomy of the shoulder and upper back

Overview of the Region (Plates 4-1 to 4-7)

The shoulder region and upper thorax includes the clavicle, scapula and proximal humerus. Movement in this region includes the glenohumeral joint (the shoulder joint, itself) and the scapula. Although the movement terminology describes changes to the position of the scapula, the joints involved in its movement are the sternoclavicular and acromioclavicular joints. The muscles of the shoulder region and upper thorax are grouped because of their physical proximity, and because the majority of the chest and upper back muscles are either directly involved in the control of the shoulder or strongly influence it. Although we may be in the habit of thinking of the pectoralis as a chest muscle and the latissimus as a back muscle, the only muscles in this area that are not actually shoulder muscles are those of the ribs and respiration.

Although we have already seen trapezius in Chapter 3, we need to remember that its territory is vast, covering the posterior shoulders and upper back. It plays a major role in moving and stabilizing the shoulders and is usually involved in problems of the upper back and shoulders.

The Shoulder Region

Perhaps the most important thing to understand about the shoulder region is that it and the entire upper extremity are connected to the rest of the skeletal structure by only one joint, the sternoclavicular joint. Aside from this one rather tenuous connection, the entire shoulder structure, including the scapula, clavicle and humerus, is supported by soft tissues. Although this arrangement allows considerable freedom of movement for the arm, it also renders the shoulder highly vulnerable to soft tissue injury.[1,2]

The shoulder girdle is a bony ring comprising the manubrium of the sternum, the clavicles, and the two scapulae. It is an incomplete ring, since the scapulae are not joined in the back. Each side of the shoulder girdle might be compared to the boom on a sailboat (the clavicle) swinging freely from the mast (the sternum). Its considerable range of motion is limited only by the soft tissues.

Thus, the shoulder combines great flexibility with great vulnerability:

- Great flexibility, because the soft tissues (muscles, tendons, and fascia) that connect the arm and shoulder to the back, chest, and neck are soft and stretchable, allowing for movement in many directions.
- Great vulnerability, because movement too far in any direction can result in dislocation or separation of shoulder joints or injury to the soft tissues.

Shoulder Region Components

Two bones make up the shoulder region (not counting the glenohumeral joint with the humerus) (see Plate 4-1):

- Anteriorly, the clavicle, or collarbone, which joins the arm and shoulder to the rest of the skeleton at the manubrium of the sternum, by means of the sternoclavicular joints
- Posteriorly, the scapula or shoulder blade

The clavicle is actually one of the most frequently broken bones in the body. Interestingly, it is the first bone to ossify in a human fetus, and the last one to finish development—usually around age 25. The clavicle has its own muscle, the subclavius, which attaches it inferiorly to the top rib. It is a fairly simple bone, but the scapula is intricate and complex. It is rather like the famous Swiss Army knife, in that it includes several extensions that serve a variety of purposes.

THE SCAPULA

Most of the bones in the body serve as rigid spacers, similar to tent poles. A few, however, act as anchors for soft tissues and other bones. The scapula, or shoulder blade, is one of the most important of these "anchors."

We usually think of the shoulder blade as the essentially flat, triangular bone that we can see on the surface at the back of each shoulder. This part of the scapula serves mainly as an anchor for several muscles, four of which make up the rotator cuff of sports injury notoriety—four muscles that help rotate the arm (supraspinatus, infraspinatus, teres minor, and subscapularis). According to the American Academy of Orthopedic Surgeons, more than 2 million people per year seek help for rotator cuff injuries.

The posterior section of the scapula is divided into two areas by a bony ridge running across it at a slightly upward angle from the horizontal. This ridge is called the spine of the scapula. Muscles are attached to the two fossas superior and inferior to the spine of the scapula, and to the spine itself.

The spine of the scapula extends beyond the flat, triangular portion to form the acromion process (a process is an extension of a bone.) The function of the acromion process is to join with the clavicle at the acromioclavicular joint. It also forms a hood or roof over the glenohumeral joint inferior to it, the head of the humerus, and the tendons that pass just under it, giving them some protection.

Just inferior to the acromion process and the acromioclavicular joint, the upper outer corner of the triangular bone forms a socket for the arm. The socket is called the glenoid fossa (a fossa is a cavity or hollow), and the ball-and-socket joint where the arm bone, or humerus, fits into the glenoid fossa is called the glenohumeral joint. Compared to the hip joint, the glenohumeral joint is a very shallow and open ball-and-socket joint. It functions well only because of the additional protection of the acromion process and attached tendons and ligaments. Even so, dislocations of the shoulder are much more common than those of the hip—another way in which flexibility is gained at the price of vulnerability.

Finally, another process extends from the front of the superolateral corner of the scapula. This process, the coracoid process, serves as an anchor for muscles such as pectoralis minor, coracobrachialis, and the short head of the biceps. (These last two muscles will be presented in Chapter 5.)

Since the scapula provides the socket for the arm, it must be able to move freely in all directions. It can move up or down, it can move somewhat forward and closer to the ribs, and, most importantly, it can rotate both upward and downward (clockwise and counterclockwise).

Six muscles hold the scapula in position and move it in these various directions:

- Pectoralis minor
- Rhomboid major
- Rhomboid minor
- Levator scapulae
- Trapezius
- Serratus anterior

Three other powerful muscles move the humerus and can move the scapula when the humerus (glenohumeral joint) is stabilized:

- The deltoid muscle, or deltoideus, which covers the superior, anterior, posterior, and lateral aspects of the shoulder joint structure, with attachments to the spine of the scapula, the acromion process, the clavicle, and the humerus. It is often referred to as three muscles: anterior deltoid, lateral deltoid, and posterior deltoid.
- Pectoralis major covers the anterior chest and attaches to the humerus.
- Latissimus dorsi is a shoulder muscle extending from the iliac crest over much of the back and attaching to the humerus.

Muscles of the Ribs and Respiration

The muscles of the ribs are the internal and external intercostals, serratus anterior, and serratus posterior superior and inferior.

The mechanical and physiological aspects of the breathing process are key factors in neuromuscular integrity. Therefore, the muscles of breathing are an essential consideration in bodywork. Although other muscles assist, the primary muscle of respiration is the diaphragm.

Anterior Shoulder

SUBCLAVIUS

sub-CLAY-vee-us

ETYMOLOGY Latin ***sub***, under + ***clavis***, key (***claviculus***, little key)

Overview

For such a small muscle, the subclavius (Fig. 4-1) can refer pain over a broad expanse. It should always be treated along with the other anterior chest muscles.

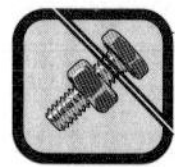

ATTACHMENTS

- Origin: first rib and cartilage
- Insertion: subclavian groove on the inferior surface of the medial one-third of the clavicle

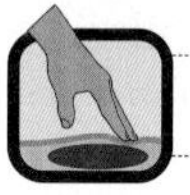

PALPATION

Place four fingertips just under the clavicle with the little finger just medial to the acromion process. The fibers are parallel and slightly diagonal.

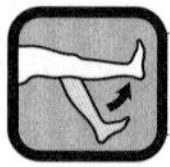

ACTIONS

- Fixes the clavicle or elevates the first rib
- Helps protract (abduct) the scapula, drawing the shoulder down and forward
- Helps stabilize the sternoclavicular joint

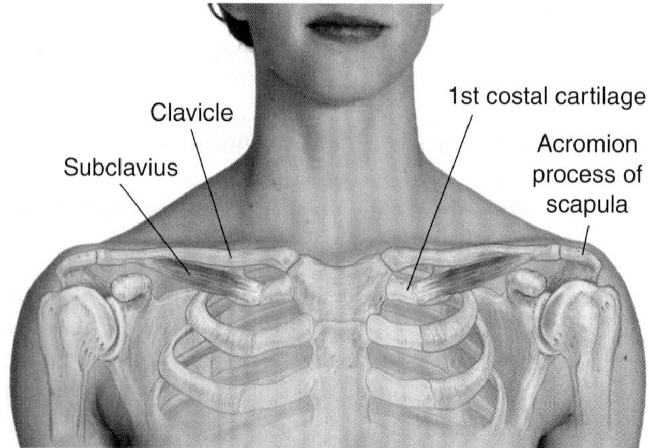

FIGURE 4-1 Skeletal features of the scapula, chest, and shoulder

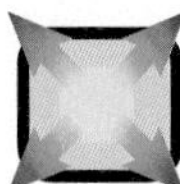

REFERRAL AREA

Laterally along the clavicle, over the front of the shoulder and upper arm, along the radial side of the forearm and into the thumb and first two fingers

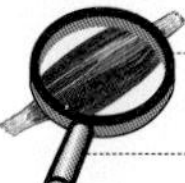

OTHER MUSCLES TO EXAMINE

- Pectoralis major and minor
- Scalenes

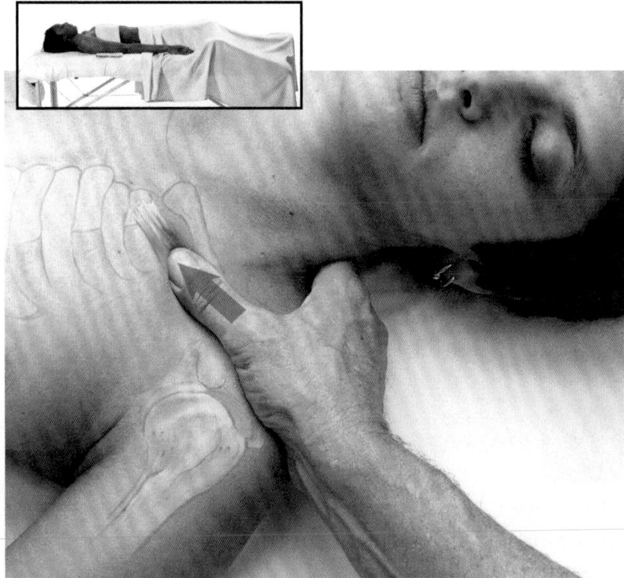

FIGURE 4-2 Stripping massage of subclavius

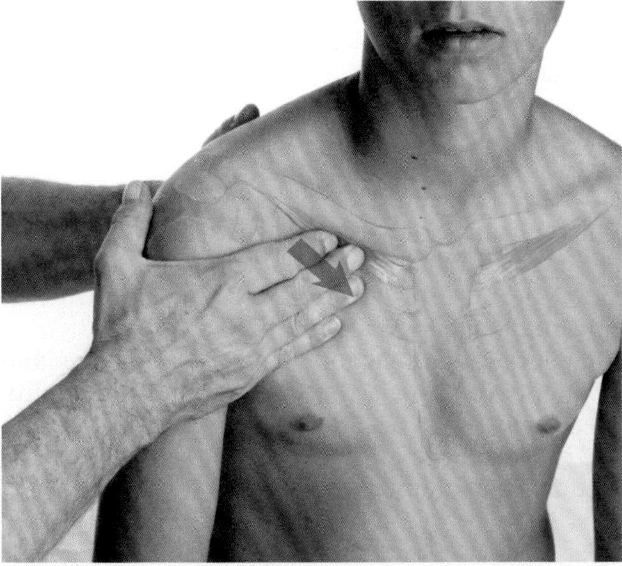

FIGURE 4-3 Stripping of subclavius in sitting position

MANUAL THERAPY

Stripping

- The client lies supine.
- Place the thumb or fingertips on the subclavius just medial to the head of the humerus and just inferior to the clavicle.
- Pressing firmly, glide your thumb or fingertips along the muscle as far as the medial end of the clavicle (Fig. 4-2).
- This technique may also be performed with the client seated (Fig. 4-3).

PECTORALIS MAJOR

PECK-tor-AL-is MAY-jer

ETYMOLOGY Latin ***pectus, pectoris***, breast (chest) + ***major***, larger; "the larger muscle of the breast"

Overview

Pectoralis major (Fig. 4-4) has three sections named for their attachments: clavicular, sternal, and costal, with additional fibers to the abdominal aponeurosis. The fibers of each of these sections run in different directions. The muscle crosses three joints: sternoclavicular, acromioclavicular, and glenohumeral. Each section performs or assists in different actions.

Pectoralis major plays an important role in postural alignment, particularly with regard to the "head-forward" posture discussed in Chapter 3. David G. Simons, MD, writes that "the [head-forward] posture is often caused by pectoralis major MTrPs [myofascial trigger points] that pull the shoulder blades forward, creating a round-shouldered posture that includes a forward positioning of the head. Correction of that posture is rarely successful for any length of time unless you correct the Pec[toralis] Major problem" (David G. Simons, MD, private communication, September 23, 2001).

We do need to always be conscious that the entire body is connected and that it is difficult to attribute postural faults on just one part of the body. Any dysfunction in one area is likely to have effects somewhere else. Any postural correction made by the therapist will also rarely be successful for any length of time, unless the client makes a concerted effort to change their own bad postural habits. You may want to demonstrate some useful stretches to

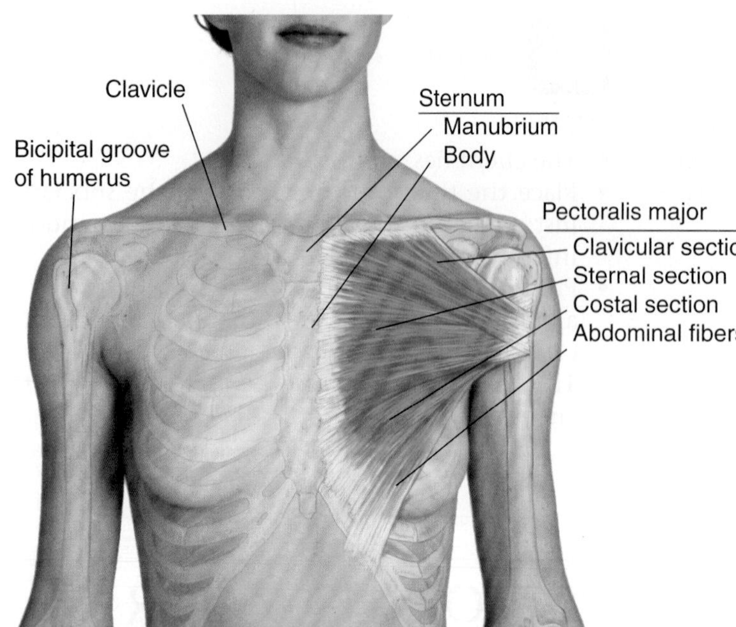

FIGURE 4-4 Pectoralis major

be done at home or offer suggestions or educational articles on how the client could improve the ergonomics of their workspace. The therapist should always remember that a postural fault may not be causing any pain at all, while someone with good posture may have pain.

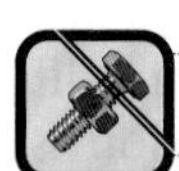

ATTACHMENTS

- Origin: clavicular part, to the medial half of the clavicle; sternal and costal parts, to the anterior surface of the manubrium and the body of the sternum and cartilages of the first to the sixth ribs; abdominal part, to the aponeurosis of the external oblique
- Insertion: lateral lip of the bicipital groove of the humerus

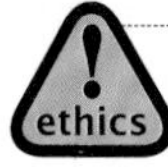

ETHICAL CAUTION

Anytime you are working around breast tissue, informed consent and clear and direct client communication are of vital importance. Keeping the client draped in the most secure manner possible while still allowing you to reach the tissue will reinforce their feelings of comfort and safety. Be especially tuned in to body language and nonverbal cues—clients sometimes hesitate to state that they feel threatened or uncomfortable; so it is crucial to have a professional and reassuring demeanor. Also bear in mind that the client has the right of refusal at any time, even if they have already given informed consent. Be careful never to touch the nipple.

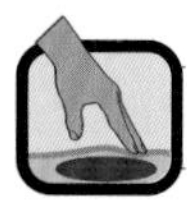

PALPATION

The upper attachment is palpable just under the lesser tubercle of the humerus and at the bicipital groove. The upper medial aspect is easily palpable by pincer palpation just medial to the armpit. The superior aspect is palpable under the clavicle and subclavius to the sternum. The medial aspect is palpable along the sternum. The lateral aspect is easily palpable with the fingertips along the rib cage, continuing diagonally to the lower rib cage. The clavicular, sternal, and costal sections are convergent.

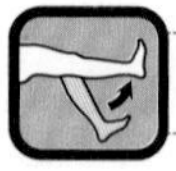

ACTION

The clavicular, sternal, and costal sections all adduct and medially rotate the shoulder; they also assist in elevating the ribs during forced inhalation (when the arm is stabilized and supported).

The clavicular section flexes the shoulder and horizontally adducts the shoulder at the glenohumeral joint.

The costal section extends the shoulder at the glenohumeral joint.

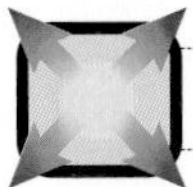

REFERRAL AREA

In the ipsilateral (on the same side) breast and anterior chest, over the anterior shoulder, down the volar (referring to the palm of the hand) surface of the upper arm, over the volar surface of the forearm just below the elbow, and into the middle and ring fingers

OTHER MUSCLES TO EXAMINE

- Pectoralis minor
- Scalenes
- Sternocleidomastoid
- Sternalis
- Subclavius
- Deltoid
- Biceps brachii
- Coracobrachialis

MANUAL THERAPY

Pincer Compression

- The client lies supine.
- The therapist stands at the client's shoulder beside the head.
- Grasp the pectoralis major just medial to the humerus between the thumb and the first three fingers. Squeeze the muscle firmly and wait for release (Fig. 4-5).
- Move the thumb and fingers to a position farther away from the shoulder as the muscle widens; squeeze and wait for release.
- Continue this process, moving farther along the muscle as it widens, until you have worked as much of the muscle as you can reasonably grasp.

Stripping

- The client lies supine.
- The therapist stands beside the client's shoulder, facing the client.
- Place the fingertips on the muscle just medial to the humerus.
- Pressing firmly into the tissue, glide the fingertips medially across the muscle to its attachments on the sternum.
- Beginning at the same spot, repeat this procedure, sliding diagonally along the muscle just inferior to the path you traced in the last movement.
- Repeat the same procedure, beginning each time at the same point, with the paths of your movement forming a fan shape, ending with a path along the lateral edge of the muscle (Fig. 4-6).
- With a female client with developed breasts, each path should end when you reach the bulk of the breast tissue ahead of your fingers (Fig. 4-7).

Compression

- The client lies supine.
- The therapist stands beside the client facing the client's head.
- Place the hand nearest the client flat on the client's rib cage with the fingertips resting on the inferior aspect of the pectoralis major.

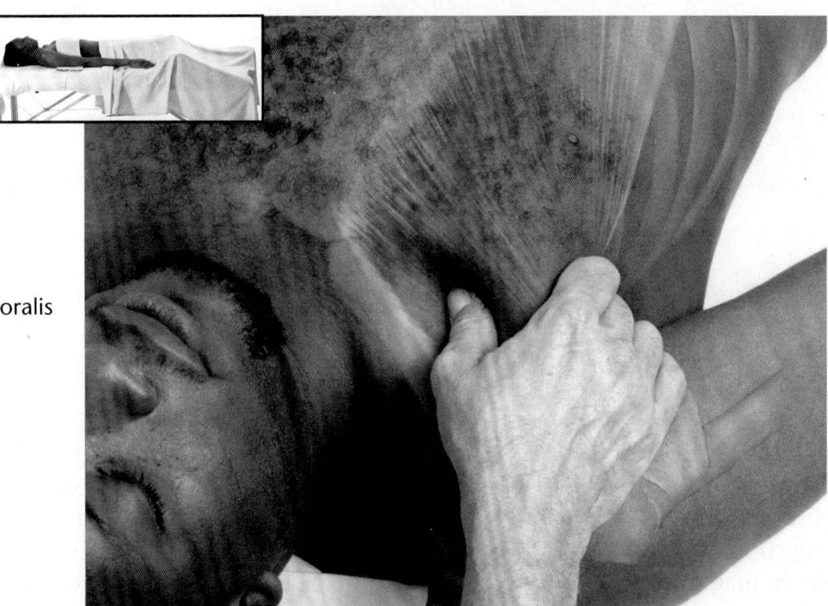

FIGURE 4-5 Pincer compression of pectoralis major

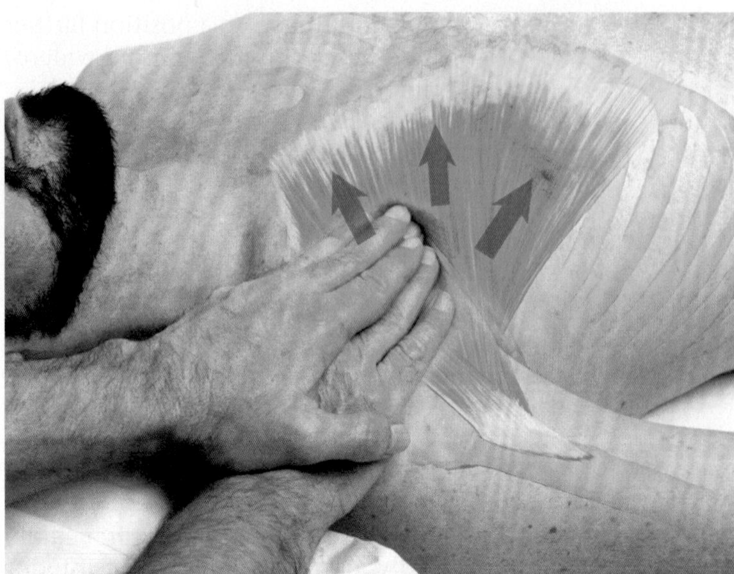

FIGURE 4-6 Stripping massage of pectoralis major

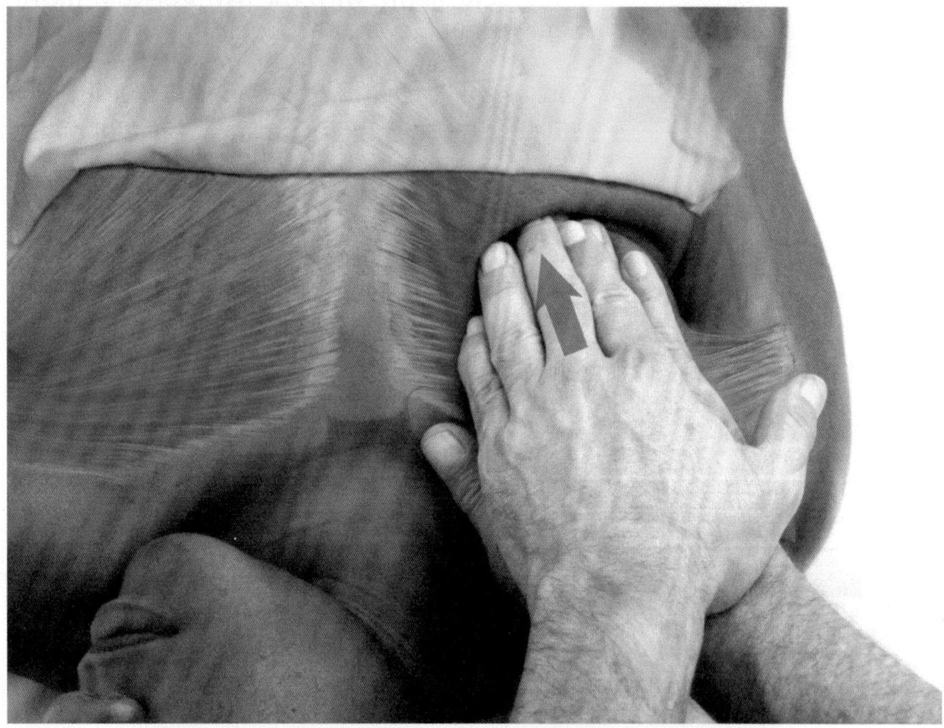

FIGURE 4-7 Treatment of pectoralis major in a female client

- Press firmly into the tissue, searching for tender spots. Hold for release.
- Move the hand upward so that the fingertips are just superior to the previous spot.
- Repeat this procedure until you reach the upper aspect of the muscle.
- Start again at the lower rib cage, with your hand just medial to the original starting point. Keep moving superiorly to new positions on the muscle on a slight diagonal until you reach the superior aspect.
- Continue this procedure, moving up the medial aspect of the muscle along the sternum, until you have covered the entire muscle in a fan-shaped pattern.
- With a female client with developed breasts, continue each path as far as the breast tissue allows you to remain in contact with the muscle (Fig. 4-8A). When you have worked as much of the muscle as you can from this position, move to the client's shoulder and repeat the process,

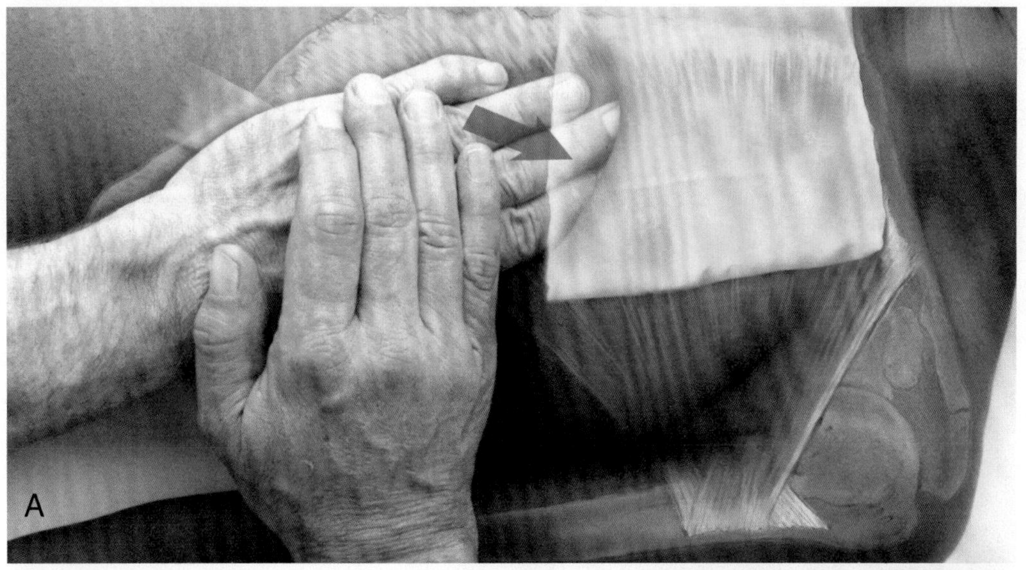

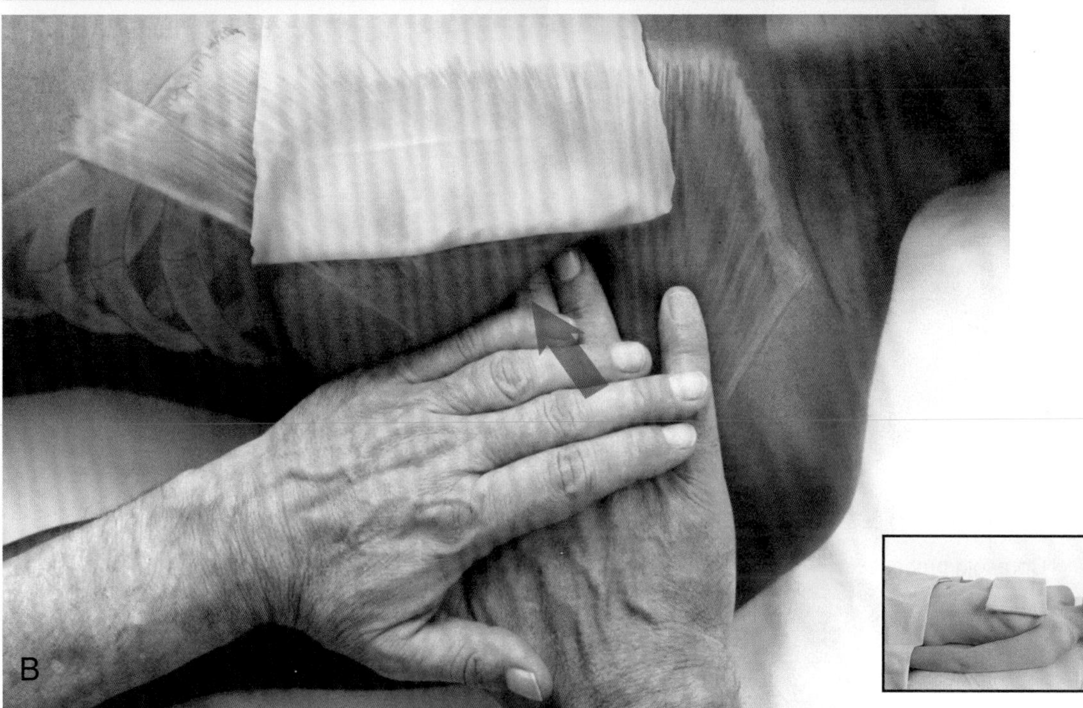

FIGURE 4-8 Compression of pectoralis major in a female client: medial inferior portion **(A)**, lateral portion **(B)**

working inferiorly (Fig. 4-8B). You should be able to cover all the muscle tissue underlying the breast in this way without being invasive.

PECTORALIS MINOR

PECK-ter-AL-is MY-ner

ETYMOLOGY Latin ***pectus***, pectoris, breast (chest) + ***minor***, smaller; "the smaller muscle of the breast"

Overview

Pectoralis minor (Fig. 4-9) anchors the scapula to the chest. It is therefore susceptible to injury from inferior motions of the arm and commonly refers pain to the arm as far as the fingertips. Pain in pectoralis minor is often accompanied by pain in the upper back muscles such as the rhomboids. Because the brachial plexus (the bundle of nerves leading to the arm) passes directly underneath the attachment to the coracoid process, tautness in pectoralis minor can entrap the nerve, causing numbness in the arm (Fig. 4-10), especially when the arm is raised.

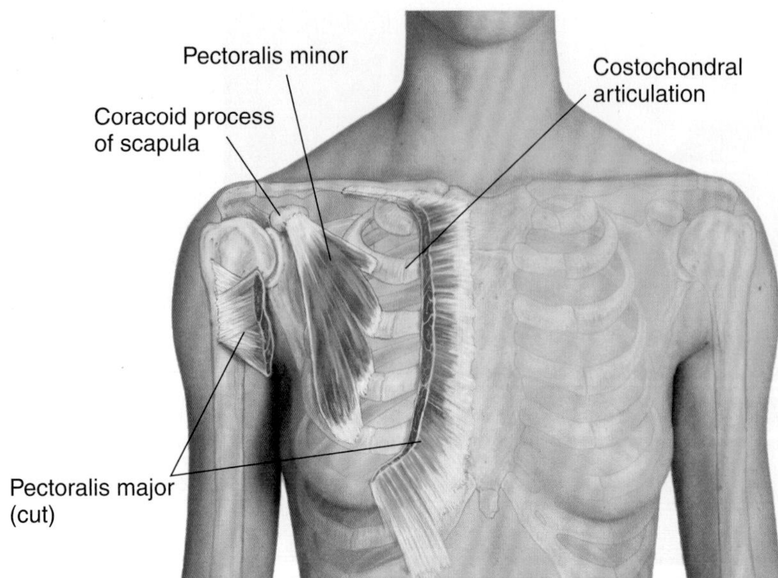

FIGURE 4-9 Pectoralis minor

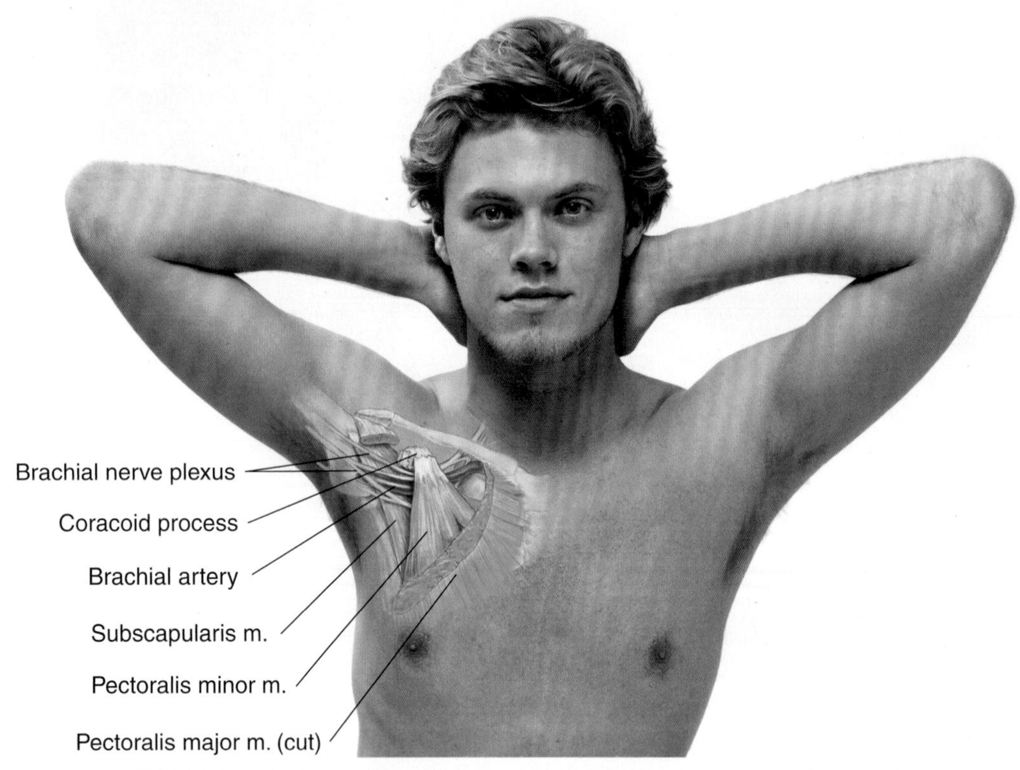

FIGURE 4-10 Position of brachial nerves and vessels relative to pectoralis minor

CAUTION The axilla, or armpit, is the area directly inferior to the glenohumeral joint, and lies within a cavity formed posteriorly by a bundle of muscles made up of teres major and minor and latissimus dorsi, and anteriorly by pectoralis major. Caution must be taken when working in the axilla, on account of the major brachial nerves, lymph nodes, and blood vessels that pass through the area. To avoid them, move into the axilla slowly while maintaining constant contact with the muscle itself.

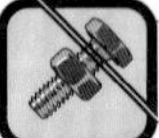

ATTACHMENTS

- Origin: third, fourth, and fifth rib at the costochondral articulations
- Insertion: tip of the coracoid process of the scapula

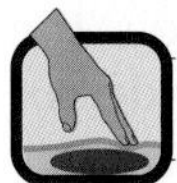

PALPATION

Place your fingertips on the rib cage at the edge of pectoralis major at the level of the nipple. Press medially under pectoralis major. Pectoralis minor is generally palpable here. Moving superiorly, continue to press against the ribs under pectoralis major, further under the muscle as your hand moves superiorly to find the more medial aspects of the muscle. When you reach the armpit, you should be able to follow pectoralis minor all the way to its attachment to the coracoid process. Its inferior attachments may be palpated on the second or third rib to the fifth rib. Its architecture is convergent.

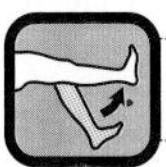

ACTION

Rotates scapula downward or draws it inferiorly (depression), and, with scapula fixed, assists in elevating ribs

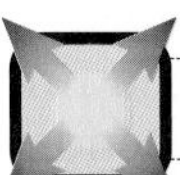

REFERRAL AREA

Over the anterior shoulder, into the anterior chest and along the volar surface of the arm into the last three fingers

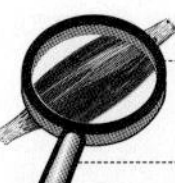

OTHER MUSCLES TO EXAMINE

- Pectoralis major
- Scalenes
- Sternocleidomastoid
- Rotator cuff

MANUAL THERAPY

Stripping

- The client lies supine, with the arm nearest the therapist slightly abducted and bent at the elbow.
- The therapist stands beside the client's shoulder.
- Place the fingertips on the rib cage just lateral to the pectoralis major slightly superior to the nipple, with your fingers pointing diagonally across the chest below the nipple. Push the fingers under the pectoralis major along the rib cage until they encounter the attachment of pectoralis minor to the fifth rib.
- Pressing your fingertips against the muscle, turn your arm and hand so that the fingertips glide along the muscle from an inferior to superior position (Fig. 4-11).

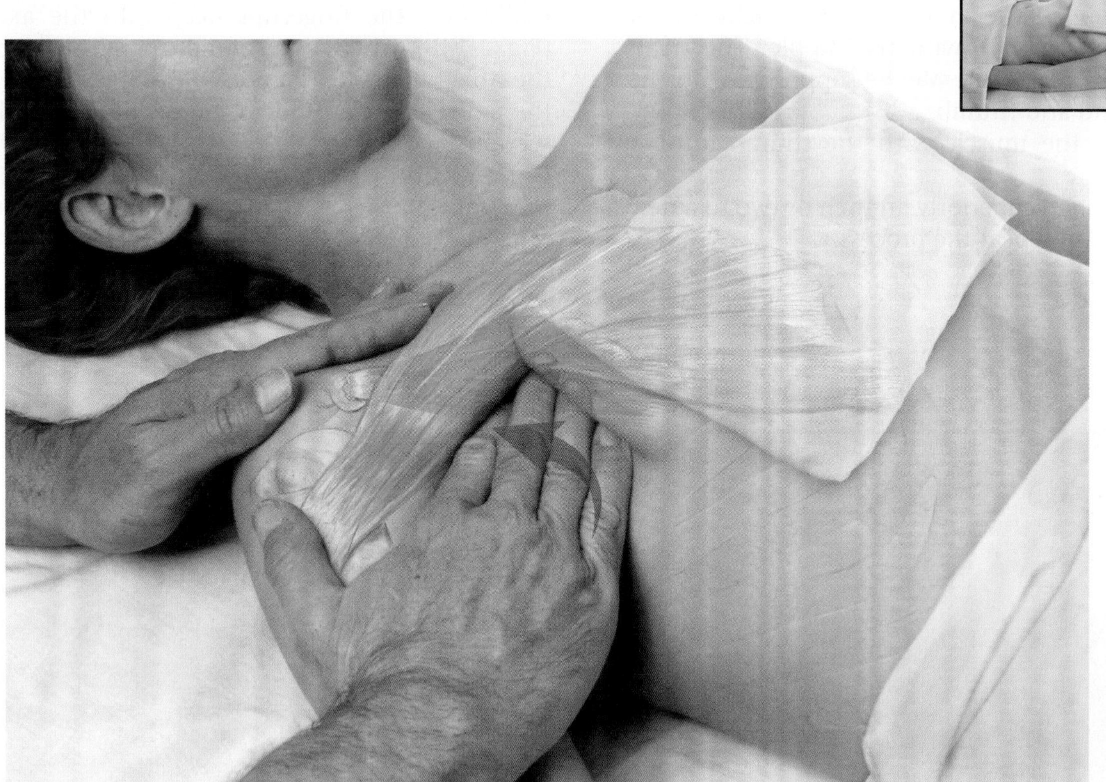

FIGURE 4-11 Treatment of pectoralis minor in supine position

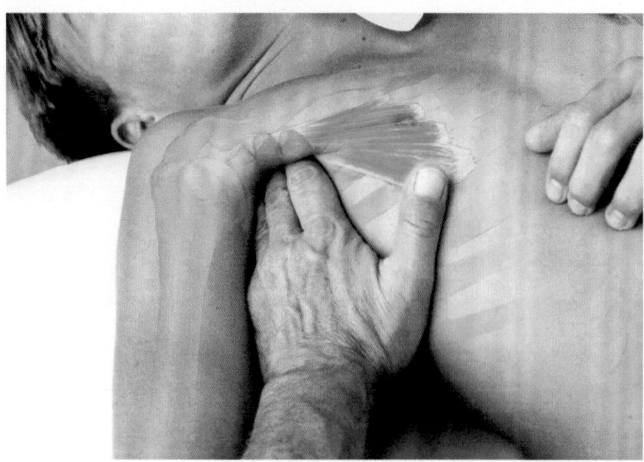

FIGURE 4-12 Compression of pectoralis minor attachment to coracoid process

- Move your hand up to a point just below the axilla and repeat the procedure, with the fingertips finally pressing deeply into the axilla under the pectoralis major, contacting the attachment of pectoralis minor to the coracoid process (Fig. 4-12).

Compression (1)

- The client lies on the side opposite to that to be treated, with the arms raised diagonally upward. The therapist stands in front of the client at the chest.
- Place the treating hand on the rib cage with the thumb on the most inferior attachment of the muscle, in line with the nipple. The treating hand and thumb may be supported with the other hand and thumb.
- Compress the muscle with the thumb until it releases.
- Shift the hand superiorly an inch or two to a new position and repeat the process.
- As you move superiorly, begin to glide the thumb laterally at each level to find tender or trigger points in all the branches of the muscle (Fig. 4-13).
- Continue this process so that the thumb gradually moves diagonally toward the coracoid process of the scapula. This movement will eventually take the thumb deep into the axilla, where you should carefully seek out the attachment to the coracoid process deep in the axilla (see Caution at the beginning of this section).

Compression (2)

- The client lies on the side opposite to that to be treated, with the arms raised diagonally upward. The therapist stands behind the client at the chest.
- Place the treating hand on the rib cage.
- Pressing pectoralis major medially with the fingertips, contact the inferior attachments of pectoralis minor at the level of the nipple and compress the muscle until it releases (Fig. 4-14A).
- Shift the hand superiorly an inch or two to a new position and repeat the process.
- As you move superiorly, begin to glide the fingertips laterally at each level to find tender or trigger points in all the branches of the muscle.
- Continue this process so that the fingertips gradually move diagonally toward the coracoid process of the scapula. This movement will eventually take the fingertips deep into the axilla (Fig. 4-14B), where you should carefully seek out the attachment to the coracoid process deep in the axilla (see Caution at the beginning of this section).
- Compression may also be performed with the thumb on a client in supine position (Fig. 4-15).

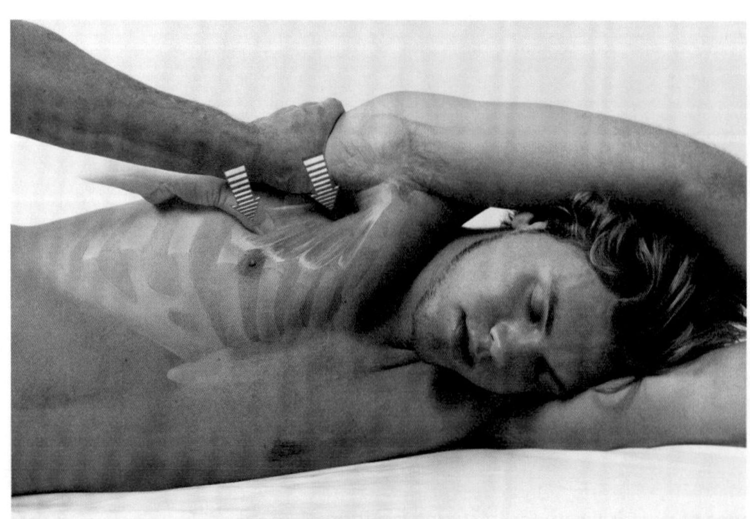

FIGURE 4-13 Treating pectoralis minor in side-lying position

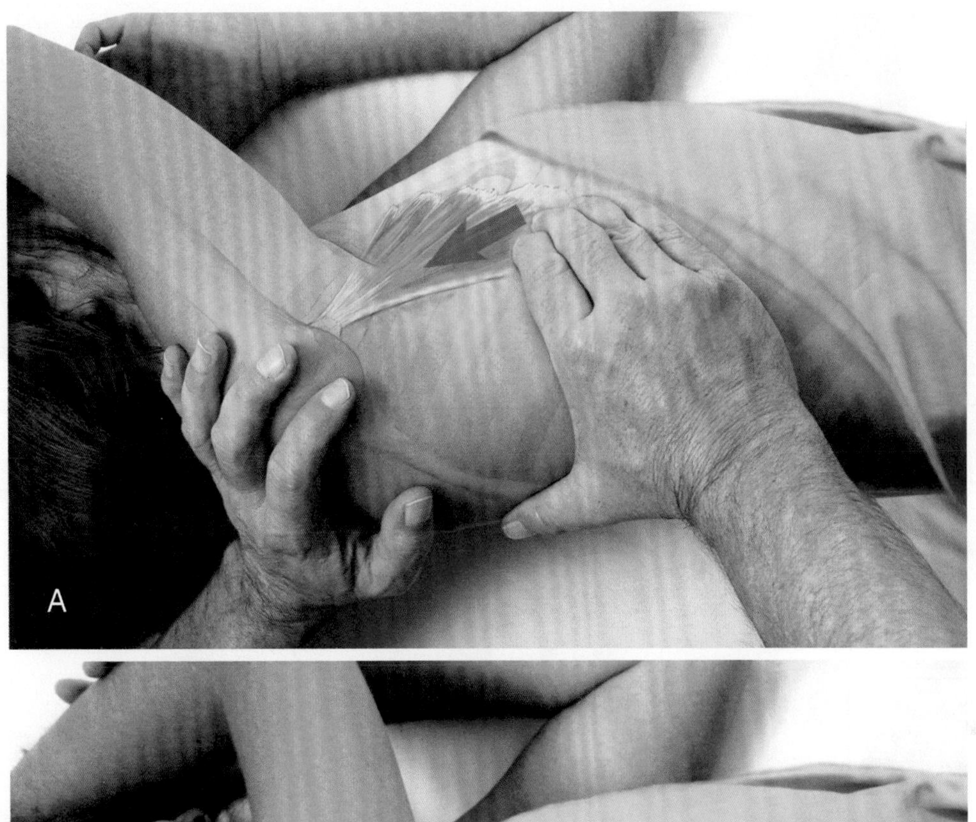

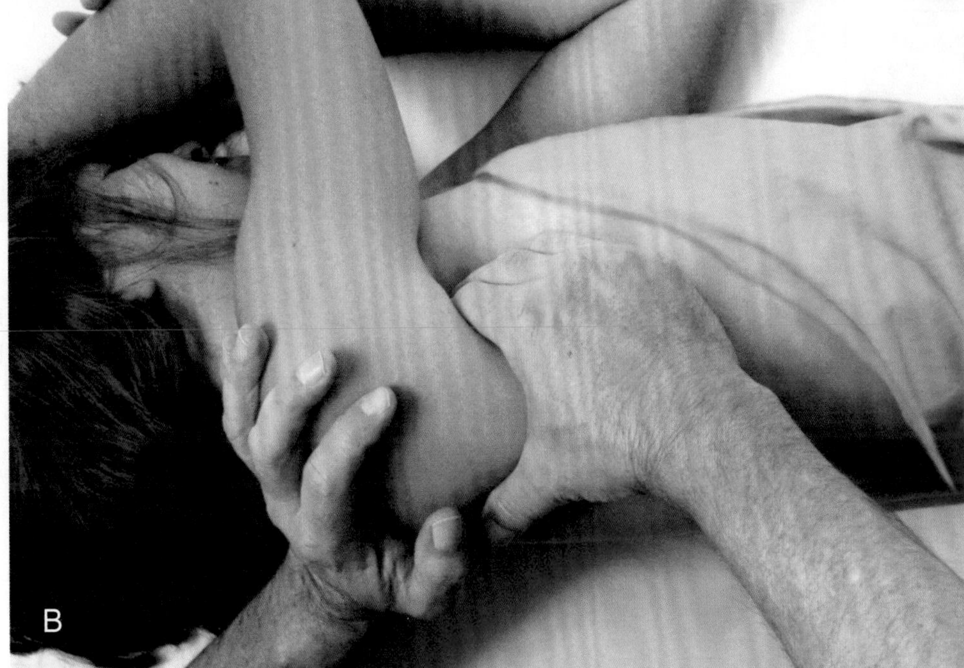

FIGURE 4-14 Side-lying treatment of pectoralis minor from behind the client from starting position **(A)** to final position **(B)**

Fingertip Compfression, Client Seated

- The client sits upright and the therapist stands behind the client. The client's forearm on the side to be treated rests at the side, with the arm slightly abducted and rotated medially to slacken the pectoralis major.
- Place the nontreating hand on the client's shoulder contralateral (on the opposite side) to the side to be treated.
- Place the treating hand on the client's rib cage, sliding the fingertips under pectoralis major at the level of the nipple.
- Compress the muscle at that level, holding until release (Fig. 4-16).
- Move the treating hand to a position just superior to the last, repeating the aforementioned procedure.
- At each level, glide the fingertips outward to contact all the branches of the muscle.

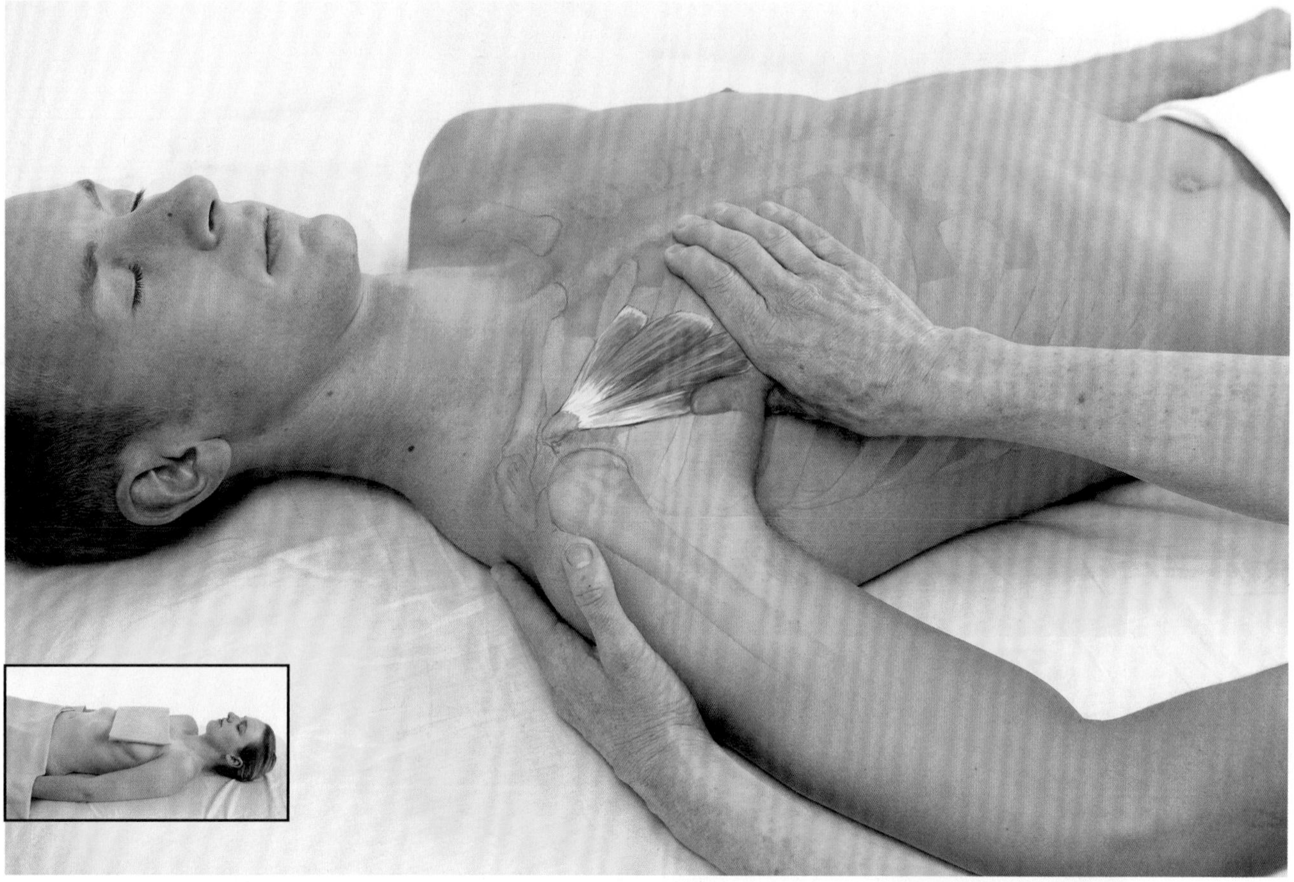

FIGURE 4-15 Compression of pectoralis minor with thumb

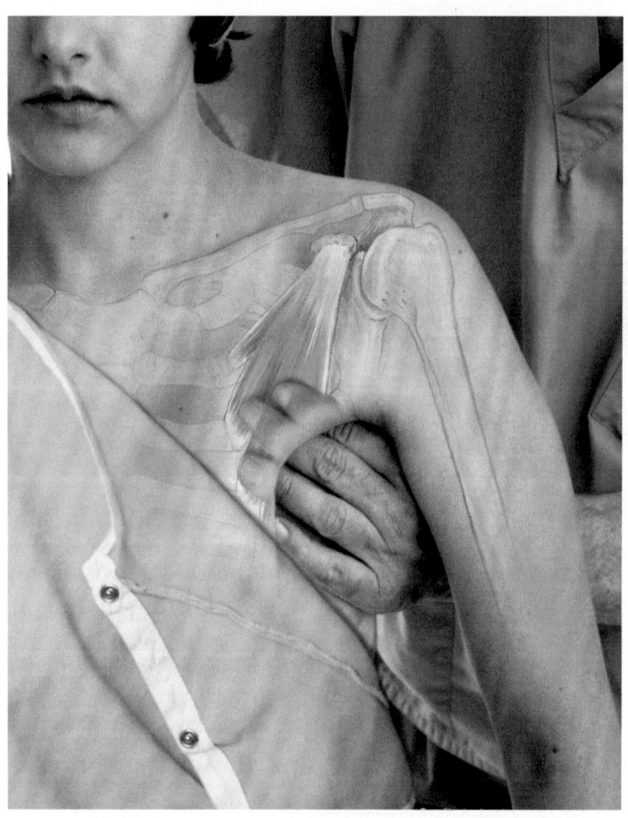

FIGURE 4-16 Compression of pectoralis minor on seated client

- As the fingertips move into the axilla, turn the hand gradually so that the fingertips are pointing superiorly into the axilla, finally encountering the attachment of the muscle to the coracoid process of the scapula.

Upper Thorax

There is a lot of overlap in the muscles of the shoulder and upper thorax. Some muscles act to stabilize the scapulae and clavicle, while others move the actual shoulder joint. The complexity of the region makes it difficult to put these muscles in nice, clean categories. Pain and dysfunction in one often means pain and dysfunction in other related muscles.

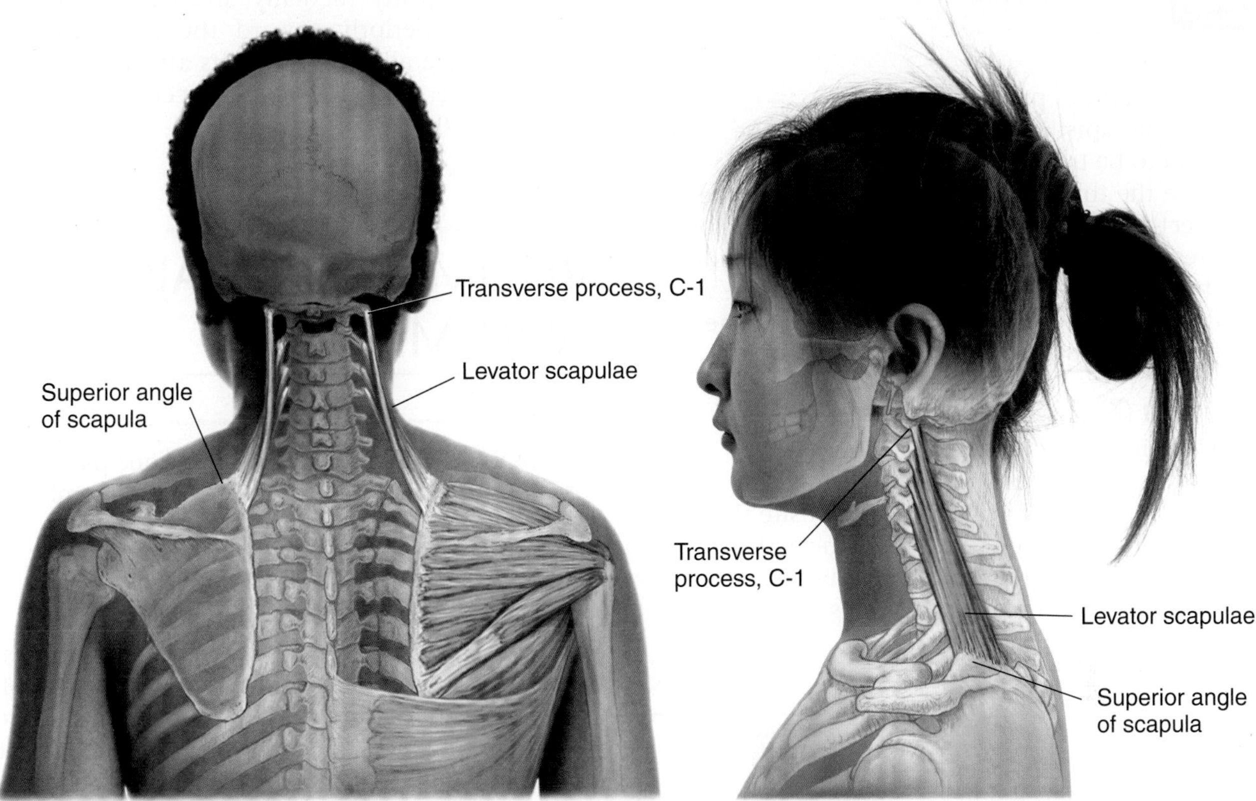

FIGURE 4-17 Levator scapulae

LEVATOR SCAPULAE

le-VAY-ter SKAP-you-lay

ETYMOLOGY Latin ***levator***, raiser + ***scapulae***, of the shoulder blade

Overview

After trapezius, levator scapulae (Fig. 4-17) is probably the most common site of pain and tension in the neck and shoulders. It is one of the muscles most abused by the carrying of heavy backpacks and shoulder bags. It assists trapezius in raising the scapula and the rhomboids in rotating the glenoid fossa downward.

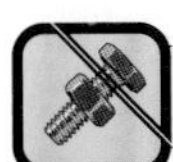

ATTACHMENTS

- Origin: posterior tubercles of transverse processes of four upper cervical vertebrae
- Insertion: medial border of scapula between the superior angle and the superior portion of the spine of the scapula

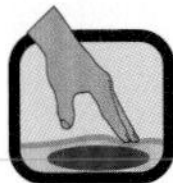

PALPATION

Find the superior angle of the scapula by pressing along the superior edge and the medial edge. You should be able to palpate levator scapulae easily at this point. Follow it up to the transverse processes of the upper four cervical vertebrae. Its architecture is parallel, and its fibers are diagonal.

ACTION

Raises (elevates) the scapula

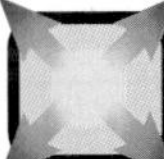

REFERRAL AREA

Locally over the muscle, along the medial border of the scapula, across the upper scapula to the back of the upper arm

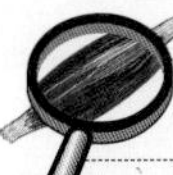

OTHER MUSCLES TO EXAMINE

- Rhomboids
- Trapezius
- Supraspinatus
- Posterior neck muscles

MANUAL THERAPY

Stripping (1)

- The client lies prone.
- The therapist stands at the side of the client's head to be treated, facing the shoulder.
- Place the thumb of the treating hand on the neck over the transverse processes of the cervical vertebrae.
- Pressing firmly medially and deeply, glide the thumb inferiorly along the muscle all the way to its attachment on the superior angle of the scapula (Fig. 4-18).

Stripping (2)

- The client lies prone.
- The therapist stands at the client's side, facing diagonally toward the client's opposite shoulder.
- Place the treating hand on the near shoulder of the client, with the thumb resting on the attachment of levator scapulae at the superior angle of the scapula.
- Pressing firmly medially and deeply, glide the thumb superiorly toward the neck, following the muscle all the way to its attachment to the transverse processes of the cervical vertebrae (Fig. 4-19).

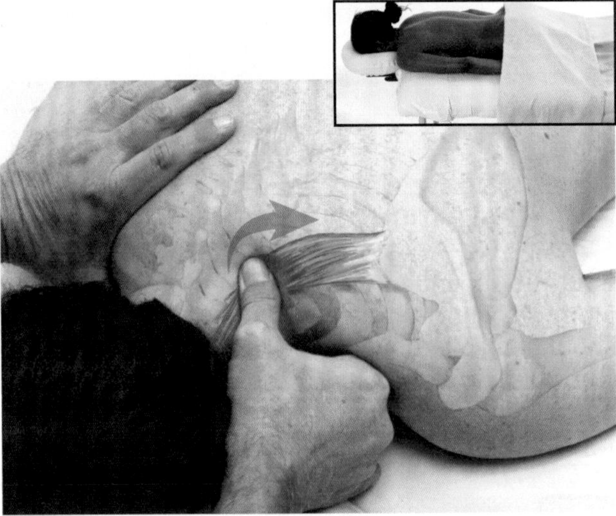

FIGURE 4-18 Stripping massage of levator scapulae (1)

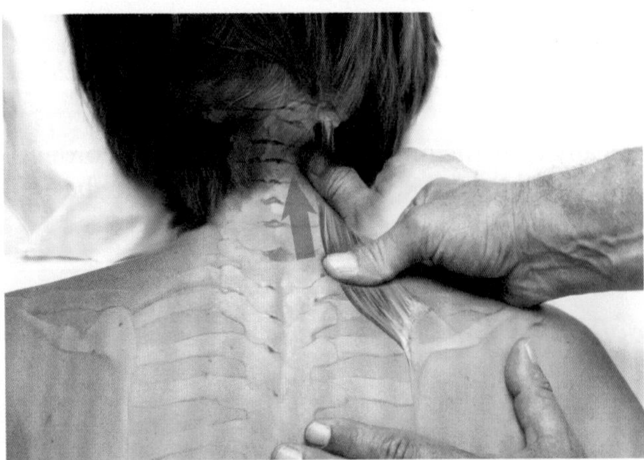

FIGURE 4-19 Stripping massage of levator scapulae (2)

RHOMBOIDS MAJOR AND MINOR

ROM-boydz

ETYMOLOGY Greek ***rhombo***, an oblique parallelogram, but having unequal sides + ***eidos***, resembling

Overview

The rhomboids (Fig. 4-20) are a major source of upper back pain. They rotate the scapula downward to lower the glenohumeral joint, and they retract the scapula. Keep in mind that they are in constant tension with the forces of the chest muscles and serratus anterior, which pull the scapula forward. Therefore, tautness of the rhomboids is almost always associated with tautness in the pectoral muscles.

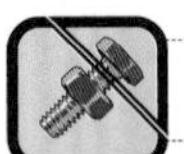

ATTACHMENTS

Rhomboid major

- Origin: spinous processes and corresponding supraspinous ligaments of the T2-T5
- Insertion: medial border of scapula from the scapular spine to the inferior angle.

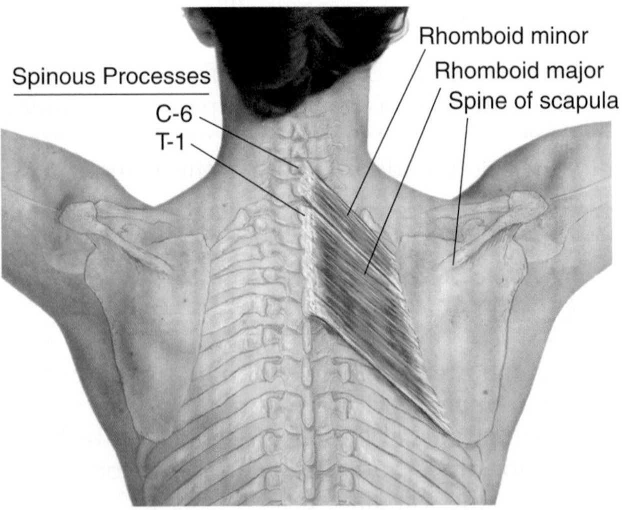

FIGURE 4-20 Rhomboids major and minor

Rhomboid minor

- Origin: spinous processes of the C7 and T1 vertebrae, and corresponding ligamentum nuchae and supraspinous ligaments
- Insertion: medial margin of the scapula above the spine

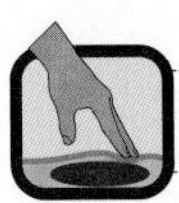

PALPATION

The rhomboids are palpable but not easily discernible except along the medial border of the scapula, although their position is clear. Their fibers are diagonal and parallel, resembling an upside-down Christmas tree, when the therapist is standing at the client's head, looking toward the foot of the table.

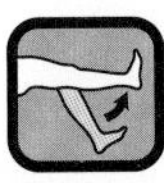

ACTION

Draws the scapula toward the vertebral column (adduction); both also draw it slightly upward (elevate)

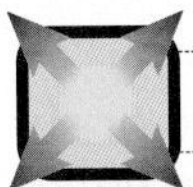

REFERRAL AREA

Along the medial border of the scapula and over the superior angle of the scapula

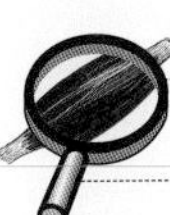

OTHER MUSCLES TO EXAMINE

- Serratus posterior superior
- Levator scapulae
- Thoracic paraspinal muscles
- Serratus anterior
- Pectoralis major

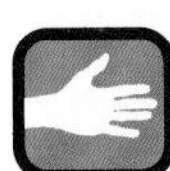

MANUAL THERAPY

Stripping

- The client lies prone. The therapist stands beside the client's head, facing the client's back.
- Place the supported fingertips (or the supported thumb) just lateral to the spinous process of the sixth cervical vertebra.
- Pressing deeply, glide the fingertips (or thumb) slowly diagonally until you encounter the medial border of the scapula (Fig. 4-21).
- Place the fingertips (or thumb) at a point just below the previous starting point and repeat the process.
- Repeat the process until you have reached the inferior angle of the scapula.

Compression/Stretch

- The client lies prone. The therapist stands beside the client's head, facing the client's back.

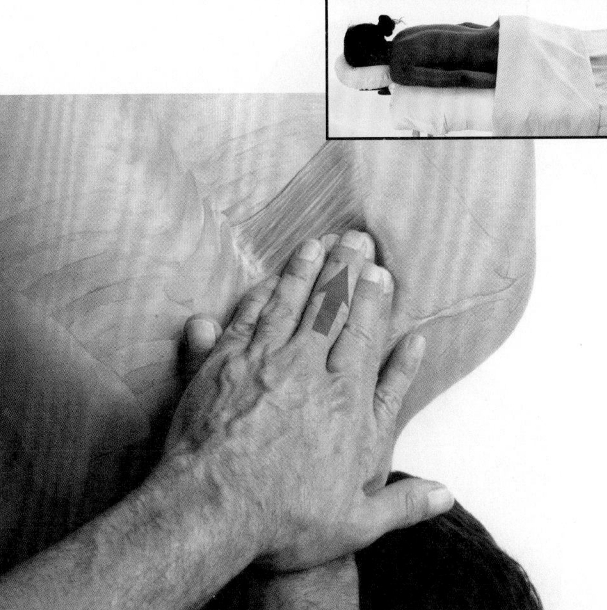

FIGURE 4-21 Stripping massage of the rhomboids

- Place the fingertips at the medial border of the scapula, pointing laterally.
- With the other hand, lift the client's shoulder at the glenohumeral joint while inserting the fingertips under the scapula (Fig. 4-22).

Compression/Stretch

- The client is seated, and the therapist sits next to the client.
- Place the hand flat on the back, the index finger aligned with the medial border of the scapula.
- With the other hand, press back on the client's shoulder at the glenohumeral joint while pressing the index finger under the medial border of the scapula (Fig. 4-23).

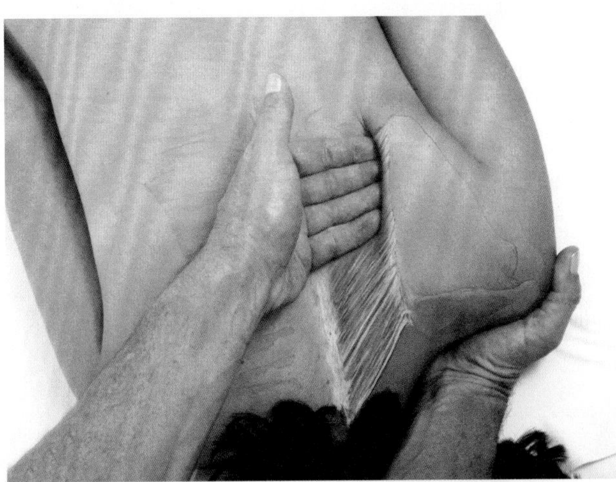

FIGURE 4-22 Rhomboid stretch, prone

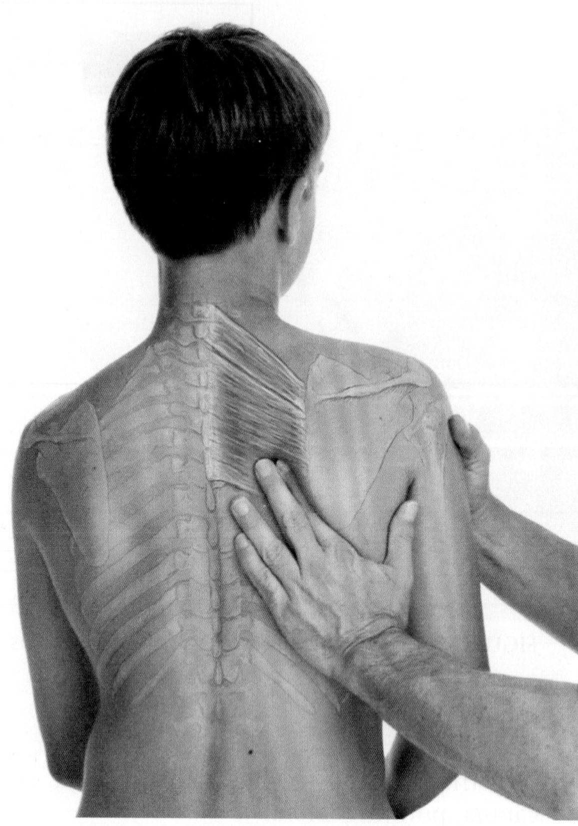

FIGURE 4-23 Stretch of rhomboids, client seated

LATISSIMUS DORSI

La-TISS-imus DOR-see

ETYMOLOGY Latin ***latissimus***, widest (from latus, wide) + ***dorsi***, of the back (from ***dorsum***, back)

Overview

A large and powerful muscle, latissimus dorsi (Fig. 4-24) allows us to pull ourselves up by the arms (or pull things down and back with the arms, e.g., paddling a canoe). It covers the lower posterior torso as trapezius covers the upper posterior torso: It extends up the back and side, and attaches to the anterior aspect of the upper humerus thus anchoring the arm to the lower back and pelvis. With teres major, it forms the muscle bundle that defines the posterior border of the axilla.

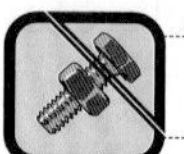

ATTACHMENTS

- Origin: spinous processes of the lower five or six thoracic and the lumbar vertebrae, to the median ridge of sacrum, and to the outer lip of the iliac crest

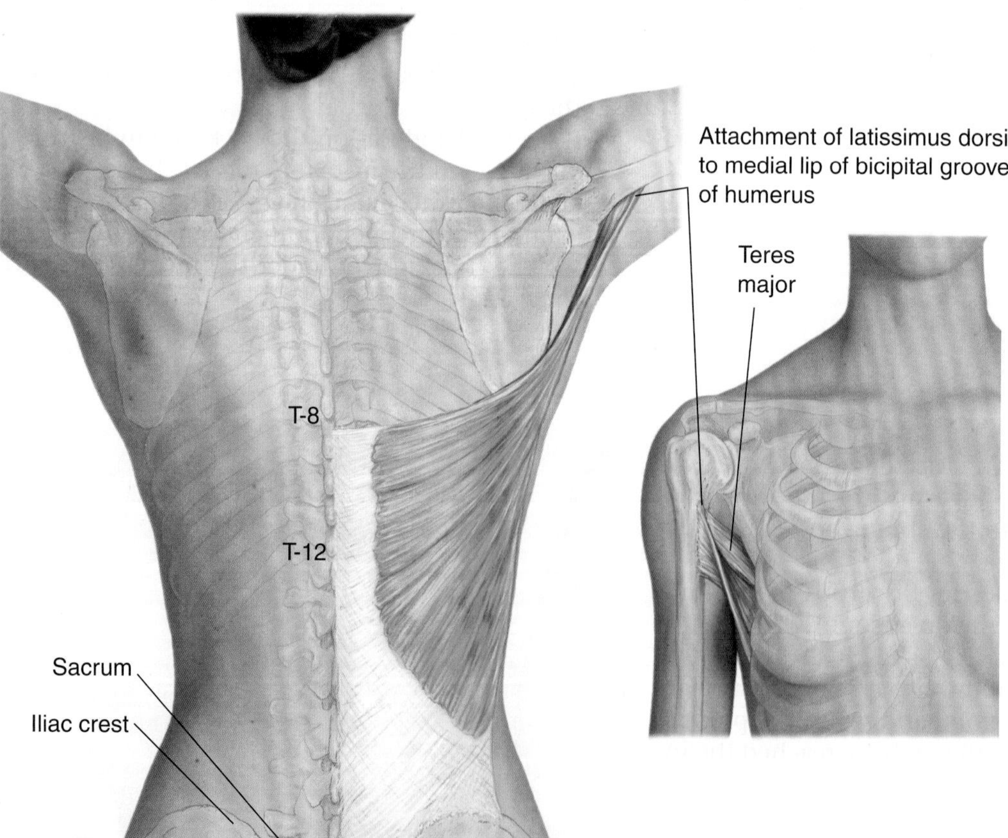

FIGURE 4-24 Latissimus dorsi

- Insertion: with teres major into the medial lip of the bicipital groove of the humerus

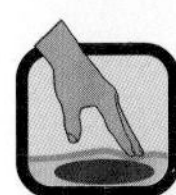

PALPATION

Find the inferior edge of the scapula and, moving laterally a couple of inches, follow it to its attachment on the bicipital groove.

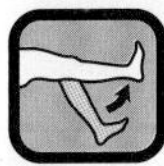

ACTION

Adducts, medially rotates, and extends the shoulder joint (glenohumeral)

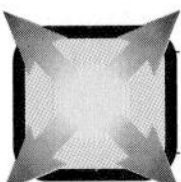

REFERRAL AREAS

- Around the inferior angle of the scapula, across the scapula to the axilla, and down the back of the arm to the last two fingers
- Over the anterior deltoid
- On the side at the waist

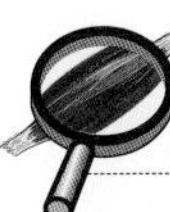

OTHER MUSCLES TO EXAMINE

- Serratus posterior inferior
- Teres major
- Teres minor
- Pectoralis minor
- Serratus anterior
- Internal and external obliques

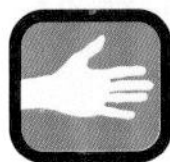

MANUAL THERAPY

Stripping

- The client lies prone.
- The therapist stands at the client's head on the side to be treated.
- Place the heel of the hand (or the knuckles or supported fingertips) lateral to the lateral border of the scapula just below the axilla.
- Pressing deeply, glide the hand inferiorly all the way to the iliac crest (Fig. 4-25). Repeat the aforementioned process, placing your hand on a more medial position on the iliac crest each time, then diagonally across to the spine, ending about a third of the way up the spine.

Pincer Compression

- The client may be prone or seated. The therapist stands beside the client if prone, or behind the client if seated, facing the axilla on the side to be treated.

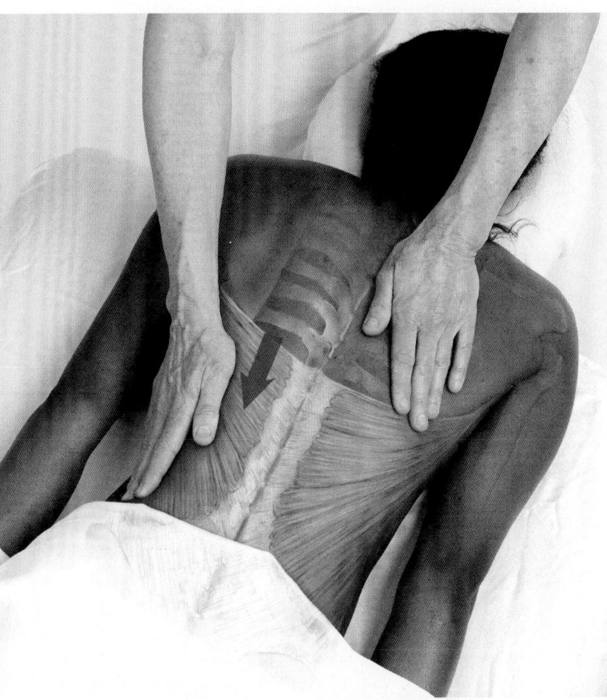

FIGURE 4-25 Stripping massage of latissimus dorsi

- Grasp the bundle of muscles that form the rear border of the axilla (latissimus dorsi and teres major).
- Squeeze firmly. Explore the posterior aspect of the bundle with your thumb, compressing as needed and holding for release (Fig. 4-26). Explore the anterior aspect of the bundle with your fingertips, compressing and holding for release as needed.
- Note that a trigger point is frequently found in the muscle near the bottom of the bundle; examine, in particular, for this trigger point and compress as needed (Fig. 4-27).

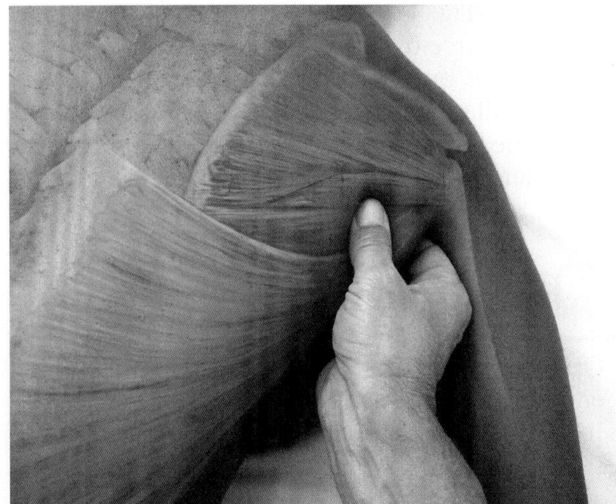

FIGURE 4-26 Pincer compression of latissimus dorsi

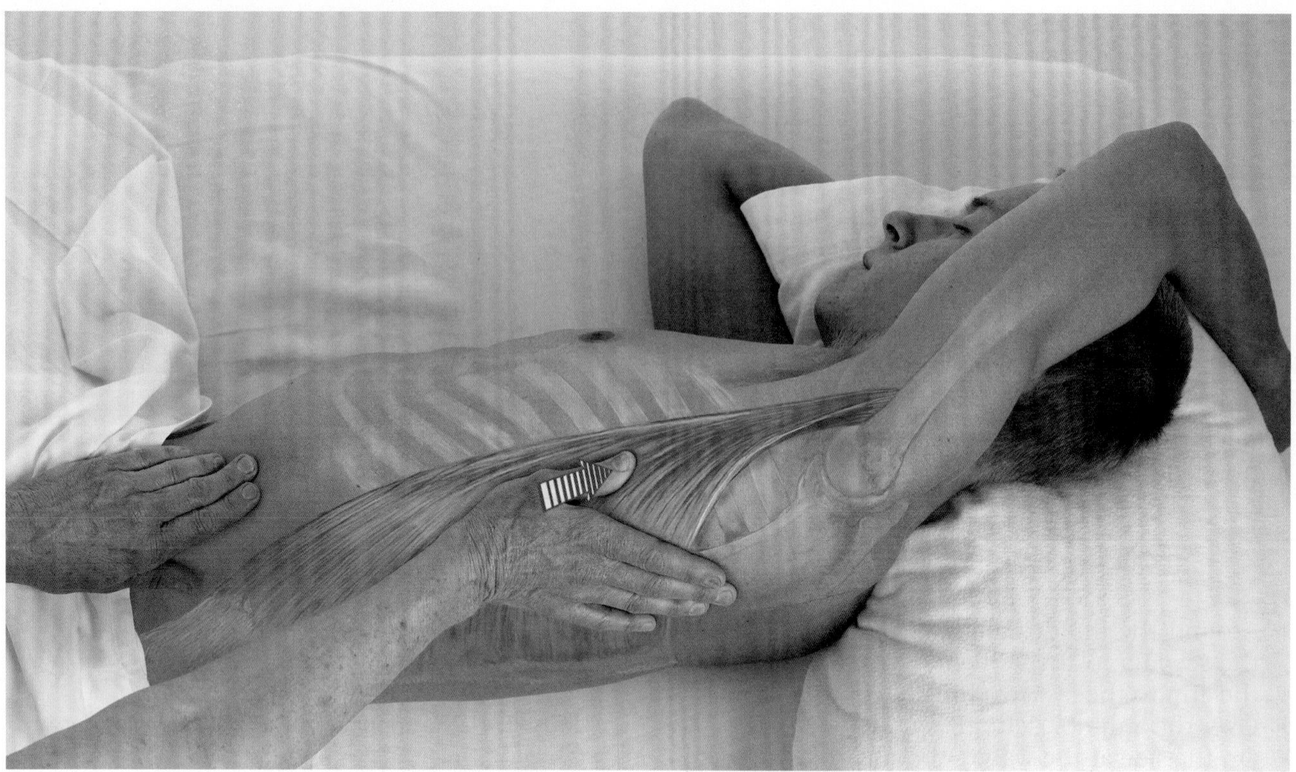

FIGURE 4-27 Trigger point compression in latissimus dorsi

TERES MAJOR

TERR-ease MAY-jer

ETYMOLOGY Latin ***teres***, round and long + ***major***, greater

Overview

Teres major (Fig. 4-28) works with latissimus dorsi, exerting its force from the scapula. These two muscles form the bundle of muscle tissue that passes into the axilla from the scapula and attaches to the front of the upper humerus. This bundle forms the rear border of the axilla.

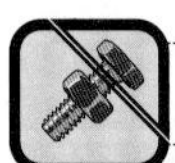

ATTACHMENTS

- Origin: inferior angle and lower third of the lateral border of the scapula
- Insertion: medial border of the bicipital groove of the humerus.

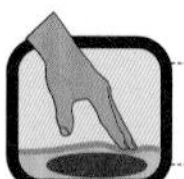

PALPATION

Press along the lower lateral border of the scapula. Follow the muscle along the posterior bundle forming the axilla to the bicipital groove. The fibers are parallel and diagonal.

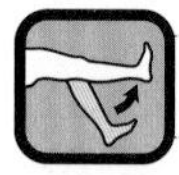

ACTION

Adducts, medially rotates, and extends the shoulder joint (glenohumeral)

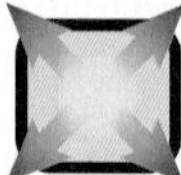

REFERRAL AREA

Over the middle deltoid area and the dorsal forearm

OTHER MUSCLES TO EXAMINE

- Teres minor
- Middle deltoid
- Infraspinatus
- Latissimus dorsi

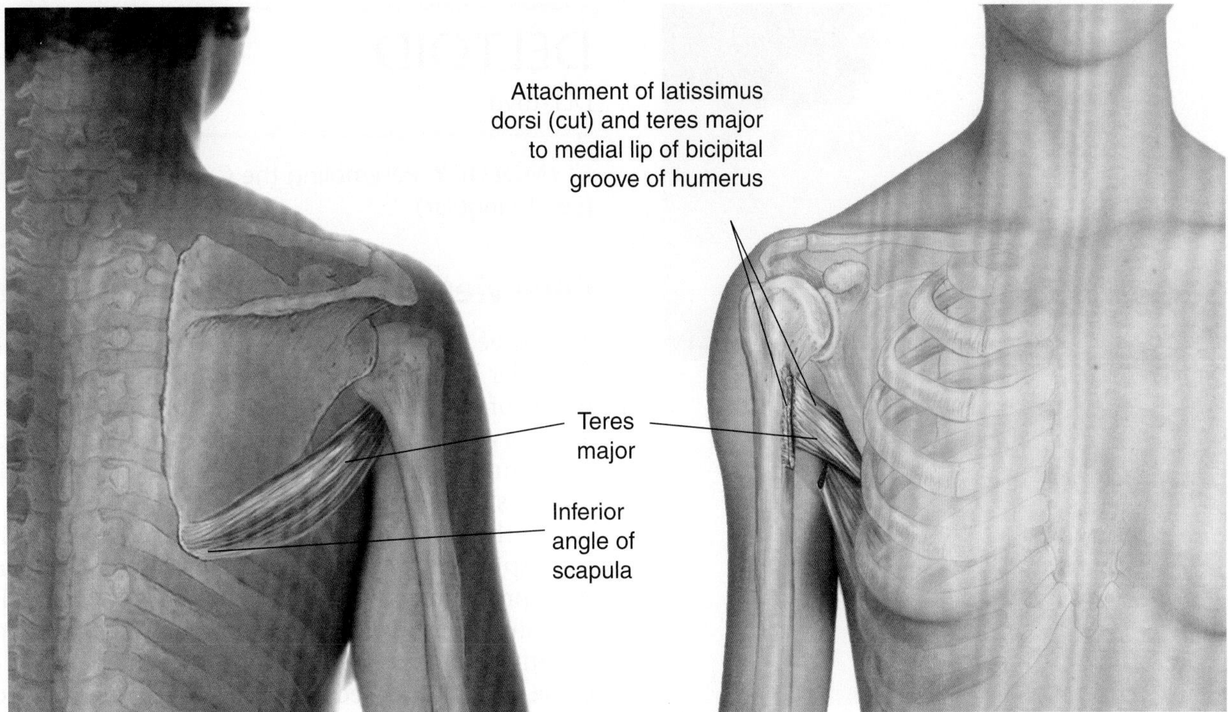

FIGURE 4-28 Teres major

MANUAL THERAPY

Pincer Compression

- The client may be prone or seated. The therapist stands beside the client if prone, or behind the client if seated, facing the axilla on the side to be treated.
- Grasp the bundle of muscles that form the rear border of the axilla (latissimus dorsi and teres major).
- Find teres major along the lateral border of the scapula just superior to latissimus dorsi.
- Squeeze firmly. Explore the posterior aspect of the bundle with your thumb, compressing as needed and holding for release (Fig. 4-29). Explore the anterior aspect of the bundle with your fingertips, compressing and holding for release as needed.
- Work the bundle with a kneading motion between your thumb and fingertips.

Stripping

- The client lies prone. The therapist stands beside the client, facing the shoulder to be treated.
- Place the thumb of the treating hand against the lateral border of the scapula near the inferior angle (Fig. 4-30).

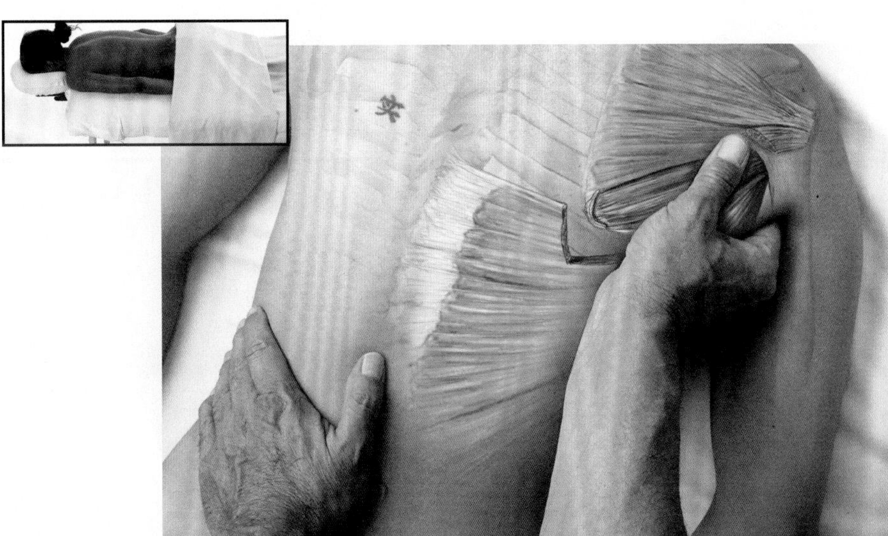

FIGURE 4-29 Pincer compression of teres major

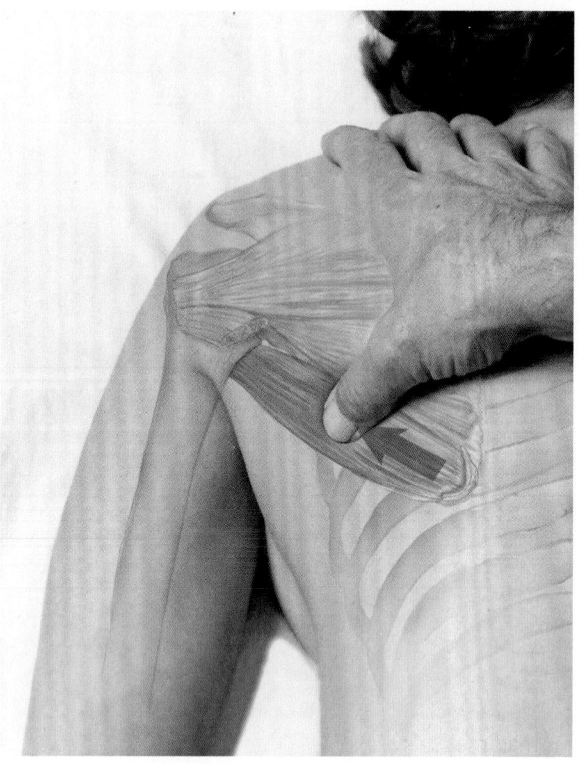

FIGURE 4-30 Stripping massage in teres major

- Pressing deeply and medially, glide the thumb superiorly toward the axilla. Continue until your thumb reaches the humerus.

DELTOID

DEL-toyd

ETYMOLOGY Resembling the Greek letter ***delta*** (i.e., triangular)

Overview

The three aspects of the deltoid (Fig. 4-31) cap the shoulder over the head of the humerus and provide much of the force that initiates movement of the arm forward, backward, and away from the body. This three-sided arrangement makes the anterior and posterior aspects of the deltoid antagonists to each other. The middle deltoid works closely with supraspinatus in abduction. The deltoids are common problem spots, but they are easy to treat with stripping massage. Deltoid trigger points are often interpreted as bursitis (an inflammation of the bursa, the fluid-filled sac that serves as a cushion underneath the muscle).

Note: The three aspects of the deltoid are often referred to as if they were three distinct muscles.

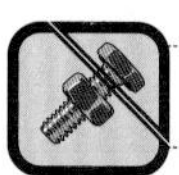

ATTACHMENTS

- Origin: lateral third of the clavicle, the lateral border of the acromion process, the lower border of the spine of the scapula
- Insertion: deltoid tuberosity of the humerus

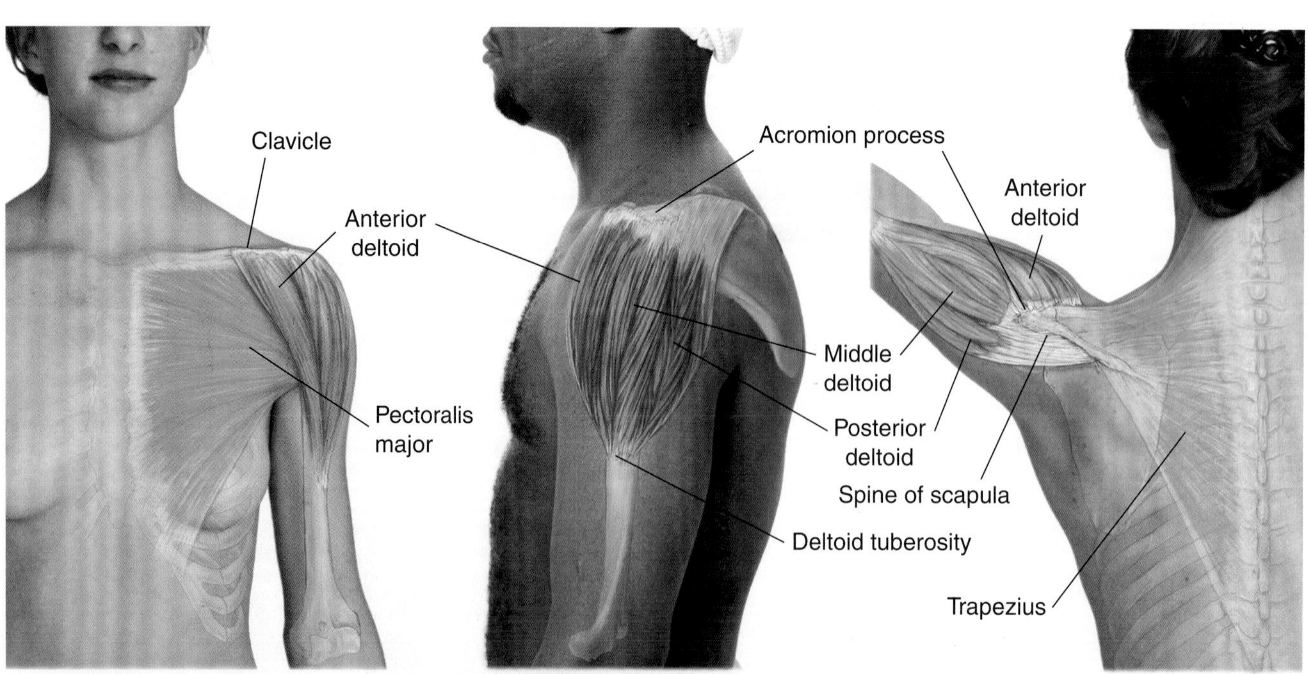

FIGURE 4-31 Deltoid anatomy

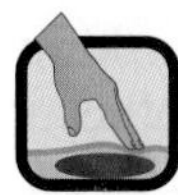

PALPATION

The deltoids are easily palpable and discernible over the front, side, and back of the shoulder. The fibers are multipennate and primarily diagonal.

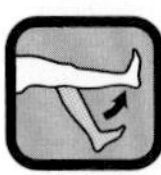

ACTION

All parts abduct the glenohumeral joint. The anterior portion flexes and medially rotates; the posterior portion extends and laterally rotates the glenohumeral joint.

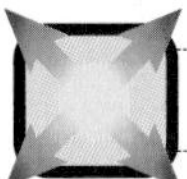

REFERRAL AREA

Radiating locally over the area of the muscle

OTHER MUSCLES TO EXAMINE

- Rotator cuff muscles, especially infraspinatus
- Teres major
- Pectoralis major

MANUAL THERAPY

Stripping (Fig. 4-32)

- The client lies supine. The therapist stands beside the client's head, facing the shoulder to be treated.
- Place the knuckles, fingertips, or thumb on the most superior aspect of the anterior deltoid at its medial border.
- Pressing deeply, glide inferiorly over the muscle to its attachment on the humerus.
- Reposition the hand laterally and repeat this procedure, moving on to the lateral deltoid and turning the hand as necessary.
- Continue repeating this procedure with the hand moving underneath the shoulder onto the posterior deltoid andwpressing upward, until the entire deltoid has been treated.

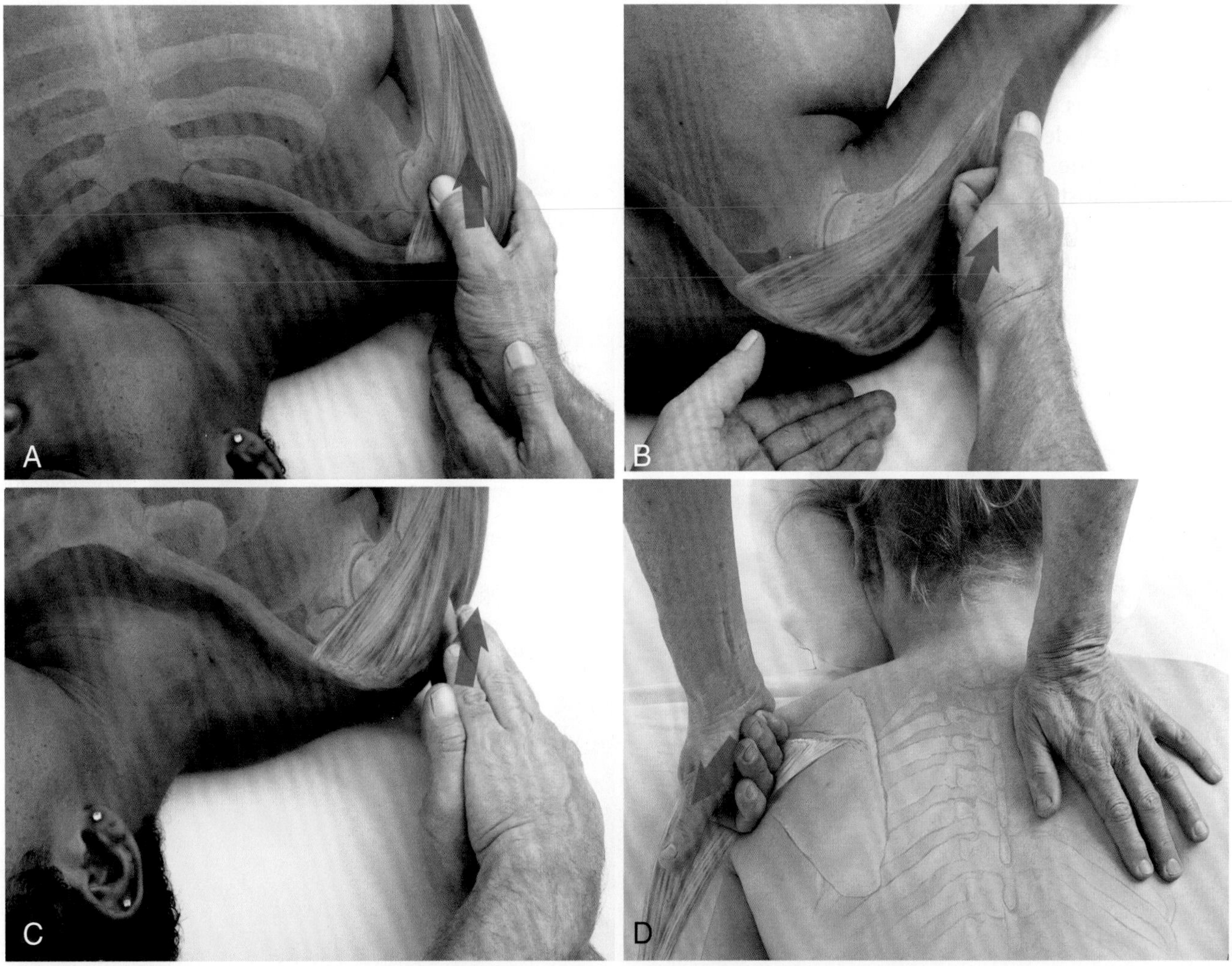

FIGURE 4-32 Stripping massage of all aspects of the deltoid: (from left) anterior **(A)**, middle (knuckles) **(B)**, middle (fingertips) **(C)**, and posterior **(D)**

- You may treat the posterior deltoid when the client is lying prone.

The Rotator Cuff

The rotator cuff is probably best known for its frequent injury in athletes, particularly baseball pitchers and football quarterbacks, because of the demands made on it by forceful throwing. The rotator cuff takes its name from the "cuff" of tendons of these four muscles that attach side by side at the head of the humerus. The traditional acronym for remembering the rotator cuff muscle is SITS: supraspinatus, infraspinatus, teres minor, and subscapularis.

SUPRASPINATUS

SOUP-ra-spin-ATE-us

ETYMOLOGY Latin ***supra***, above + ***spina***, spine; "above the spine (of the scapula)"

Overview

Supraspinatus (Fig. 4-33) is a surprisingly small muscle given the demands that are made on it. It functions with the middle deltoid in abduction of the arm, but most of its problems arise from its job as stabilizer of the glenohumeral joint. It is active in this capacity during all rotator cuff activities, such as holding a heavy weight in the hand or working with the arms raised. People who carry heavy objects such as suitcases or even heavy briefcases are likely to have problems with supraspinatus. Repetitive motions, such as using a computer mouse for long periods of time, also cause rotator cuff problems.

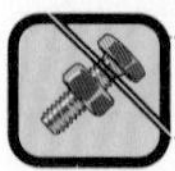

ATTACHMENTS

- Origin: supraspinous fossa of scapula
- Insertion: greater tubercle of the humerus

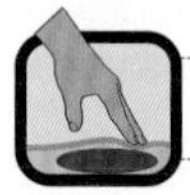

PALPATION

Find the upper angle of the scapula and the spine. Supraspinatus is quite palpable above the spine, and can be palpated all the way out to the acromion process. The attachment can be palpated just lateral to the acromion. The fibers are convergent and horizontal.

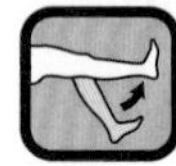

ACTION

Initiates abduction and stabilizes the glenohumeral joint

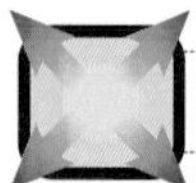

REFERRAL AREA

Over the shoulder, over the middle deltoid area, and down the radial aspect of the arm

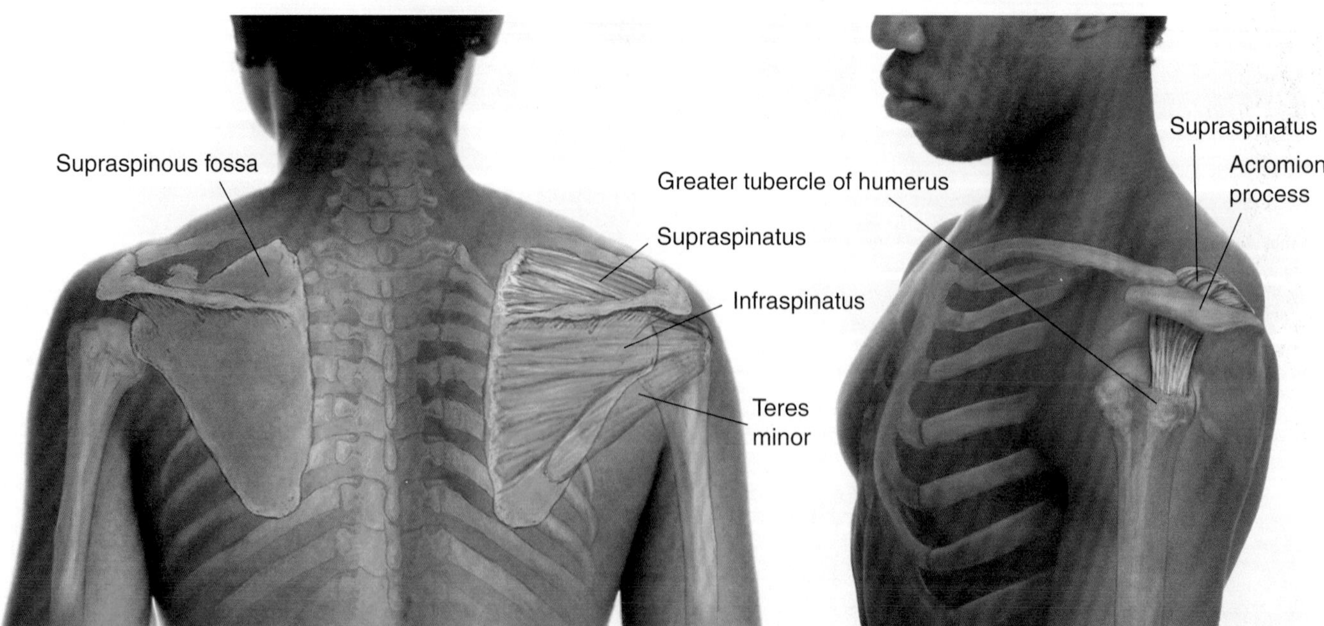

FIGURE 4-33 Supraspinatus

OTHER MUSCLES TO EXAMINE

- Middle deltoid
- Other rotator cuff muscles, especially infraspinatus

MANUAL THERAPY

Stripping

- The client lies prone. The therapist stands beside the client's head on the side to be treated.
- Place the thumb of the treating hand on the medial end of the muscle at the superior angle of the scapula (Fig. 4-34).
- Pressing deeply and inferiorly, move the thumb laterally along the muscle, pressing it into the trough formed by the spine of the scapula, until your thumb is stopped by the acromion process.
- This procedure may also be done with the fingertips or elbow (Fig. 4-35).
- The client may be prone or seated. The therapist stands beside the client.
- The client's hand on the side to be treated is placed behind the client's back at the waist to internally rotate the shoulder (Fig. 4-36A).
- Press the thumb deeply through the middle deltoid just under the acromion process until you encounter the attachment of the supraspinatus tendon to the greater tubercle of the humerus. Hold for release (Fig. 4-36B).

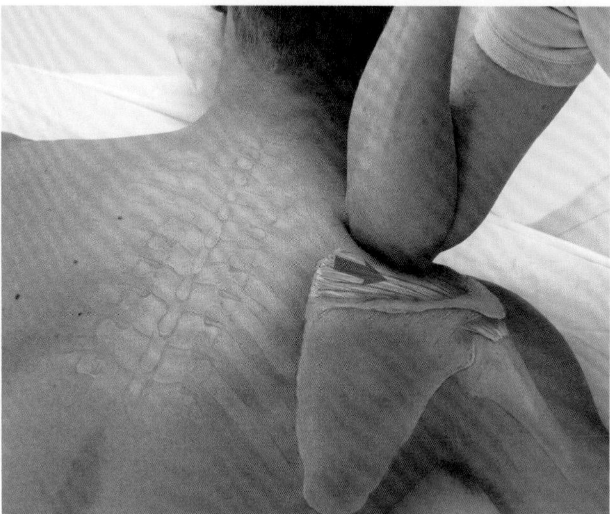

FIGURE 4-35 Stripping of supraspinatus with elbow

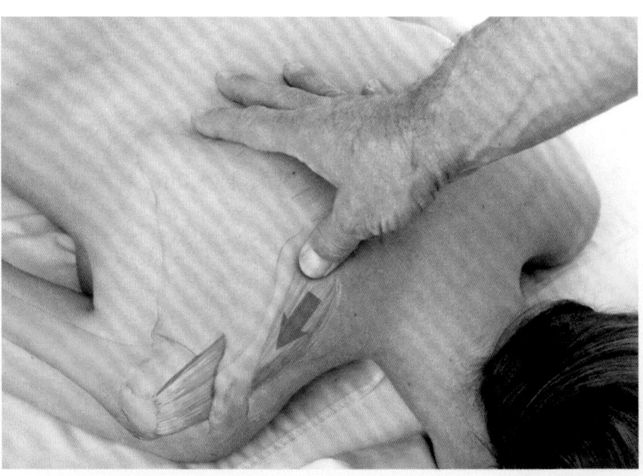

FIGURE 4-34 Stripping massage of supraspinatus

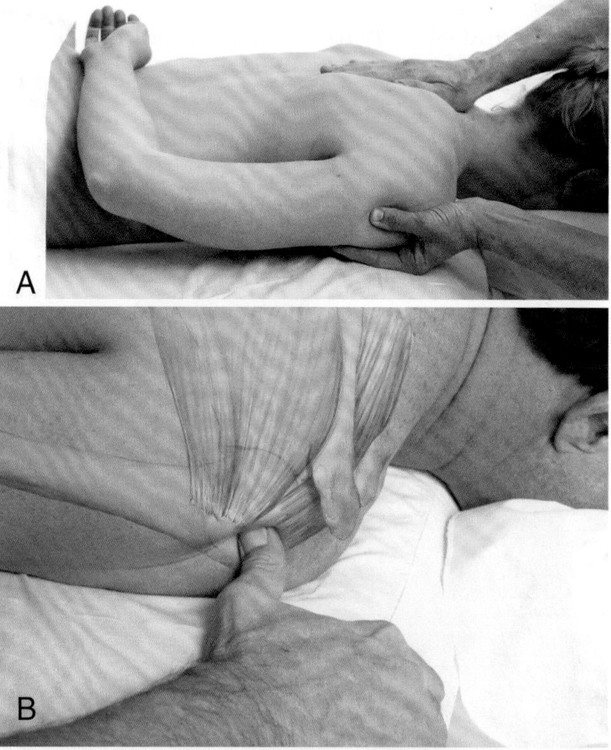

FIGURE 4-36 Compression of supraspinatus attachment

INFRASPINATUS

IN-fra-spin-ATE-us

ETYMOLOGY Latin *infra*, below + *spina*, spine, hence "below the spine (of the scapula)"

Overview

Infraspinatus (Fig. 4-37) is a lateral rotator and a stabilizer of the glenohumeral joint during arm movements. It is a common trouble spot, most often referring pain to the outer aspect of the upper arm from trigger points along the scapular spine and the medial border of the scapula.

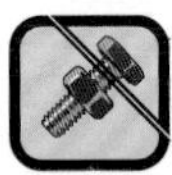

ATTACHMENTS

- Origin: infraspinous fossa of the scapula
- Insertion: greater tubercle of humerus

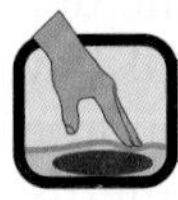

PALPATION

Palpation of the scapula below the spine is effectively palpation of infraspinatus. Fibers are convergent and diagonal.

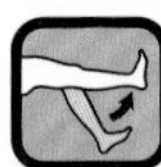

ACTION

Extends and laterally rotates the glenohumeral joint

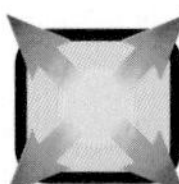

REFERRAL AREA

Along the medial border of the scapula, over the middle and/or anterior deltoid area, and down the radial aspect of the arm into the first two or three fingers

OTHER MUSCLES TO EXAMINE

- Deltoids
- Other rotator cuff muscles
- Biceps brachii
- Coracobrachialis

MANUAL THERAPY

Stripping (1)

- The client lies prone. The therapist stands at the client's shoulder opposite the side to be treated, facing the shoulder to be treated.
- Place the fingertips (Fig. 4-38A), knuckles (Fig. 4-38B), or supported thumb on the muscle at the medial border of the scapula just below the root of the scapular spine.
- Pressing deeply, glide laterally along the muscle just inferior to the spine of the scapula all the way to the attachment on the posterior aspect of the head of the humerus.
- Place the hand just inferior to the prior starting point and repeat the aforementioned procedure. Continue along the scapula inferiorly, shifting the angle as necessary, until the entire muscle has been treated.

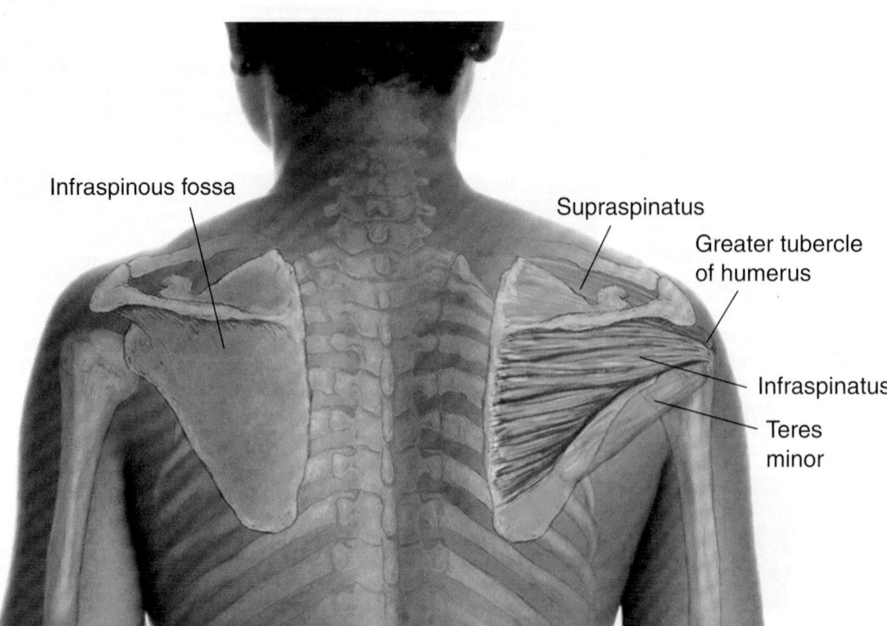

FIGURE 4-37 Infraspinatus

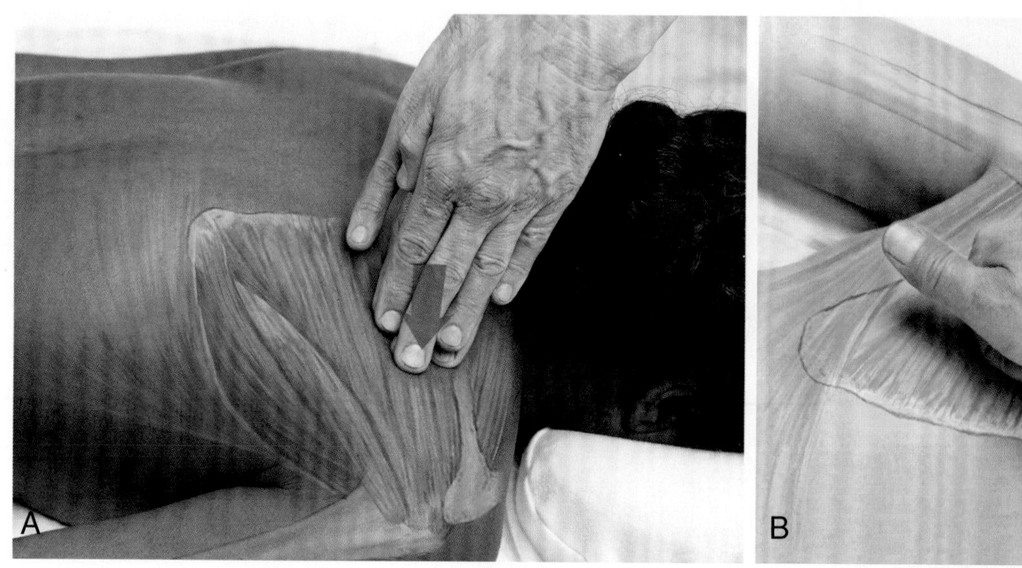

FIGURE 4-38 Stripping massage of infraspinatus with fingertips **(A)** and knuckles **(B)**

Stripping (2)

- The client lies prone. The therapist stands at the client's side, facing the scapula.
- Place the thumb on the scapula at the inferior angle.
- Pressing firmly into the muscle, glide the thumb up the lateral border of the scapula (Fig. 4-39) to the spine, then follow the muscle to the humerus.
- Either of the two aforementioned procedures may also be performed with the elbow (Fig. 4-40).

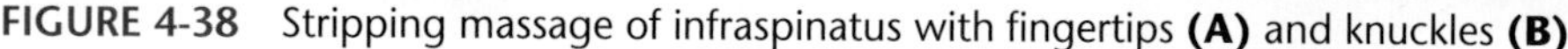

Compression

- The client lies prone. The therapist stands by the client's shoulder to be treated, facing the shoulder.
- Place the thumb on the muscle at its medial edge just inferior to the root of the spine of the scapula and press deeply.
- Repeat the procedure shifting the position of your thumb laterally, holding for release as necessary.
- When you have reached the lateral edge of the scapula, begin shifting the position of your thumb inferiorly along the lateral border of the scapula in the same way until you reach the inferior angle of the scapula (Fig. 4-41).

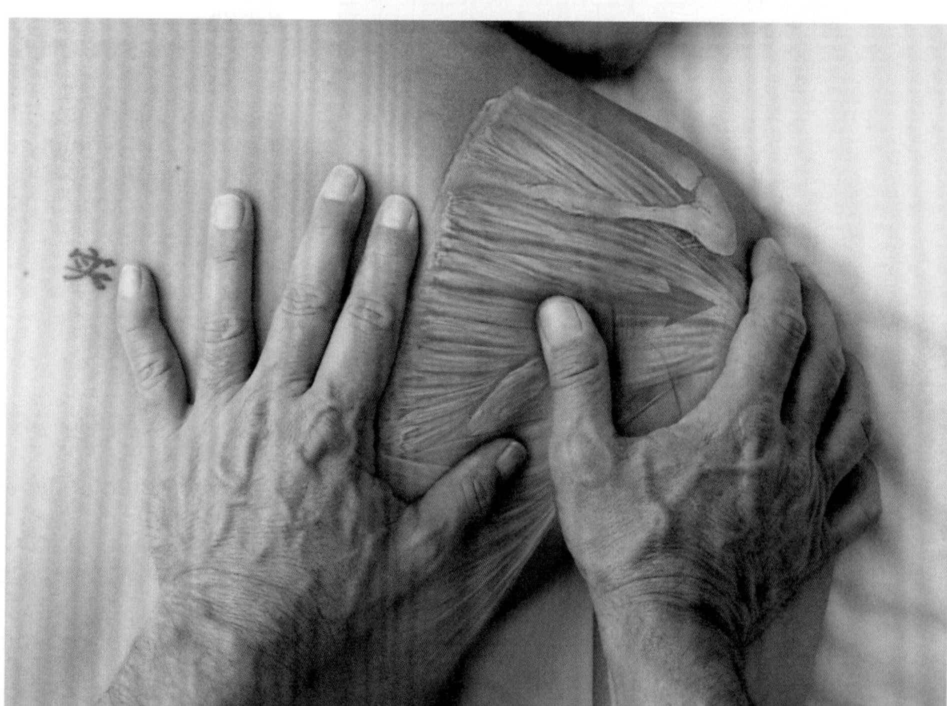

FIGURE 4-39 Stripping massage of infraspinatus from inferior angle

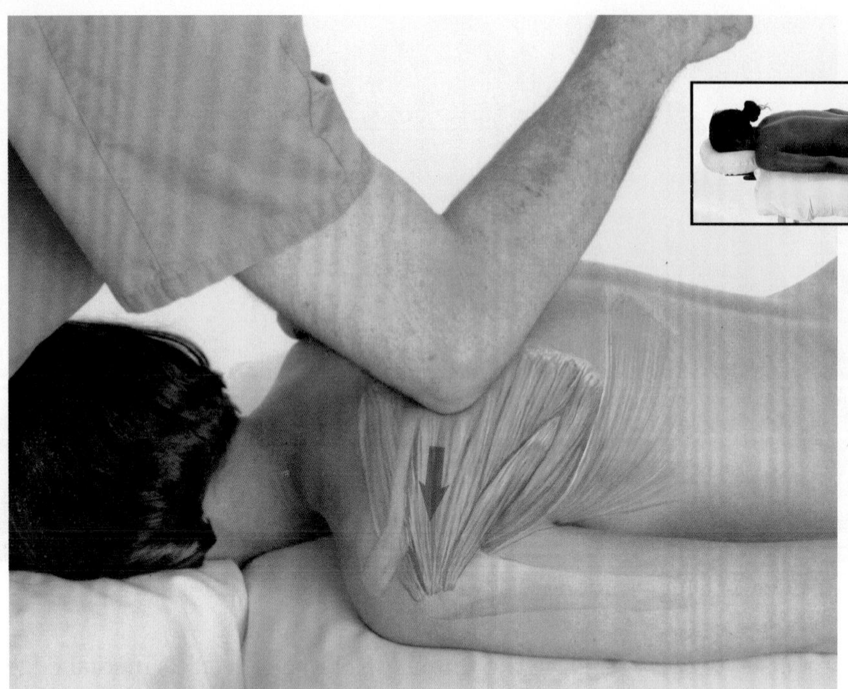

FIGURE 4-40 Stripping of infraspinatus with the elbow

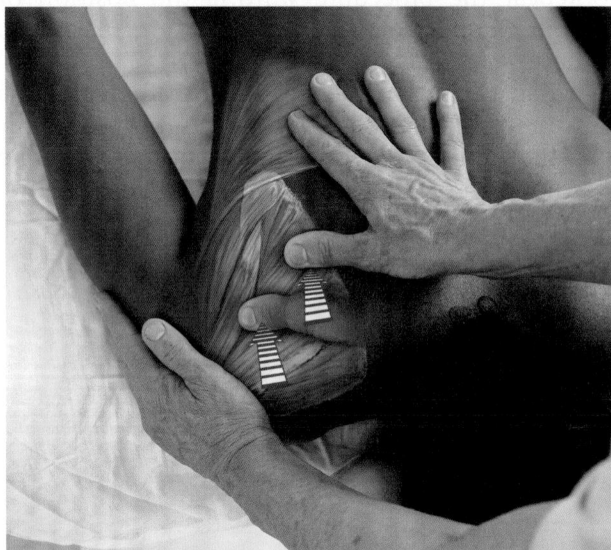

FIGURE 4-41 Compression of infraspinatus

TERES MINOR

TERR-ease MY-ner

ETYMOLOGY Latin *teres*, round and smooth

Overview

Teres minor (Fig. 4-42) is essentially an adjunct muscle to infraspinatus. It has the same function and, when it has trigger points, refers to the same area (outer aspect of the upper arm).

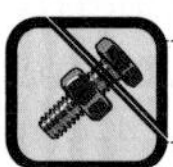

ATTACHMENTS

- Origin: upper two-thirds of the lateral border of the scapula
- Insertion: greater tubercle of the humerus just below infraspinatus

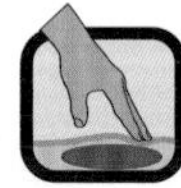

PALPATION

Find the upper lateral border of the scapula. Follow the muscle diagonally upward to the greater tubercle of the humerus. Its fibers are parallel and diagonal.

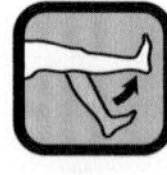

ACTION

Extends and laterally rotates the glenohumeral joint

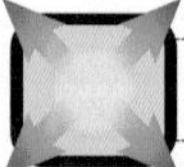

REFERRAL AREA

Over the outer, upper arm

OTHER MUSCLES TO EXAMINE

- Other rotator cuff muscles, especially infraspinatus
- Teres major
- Middle deltoid

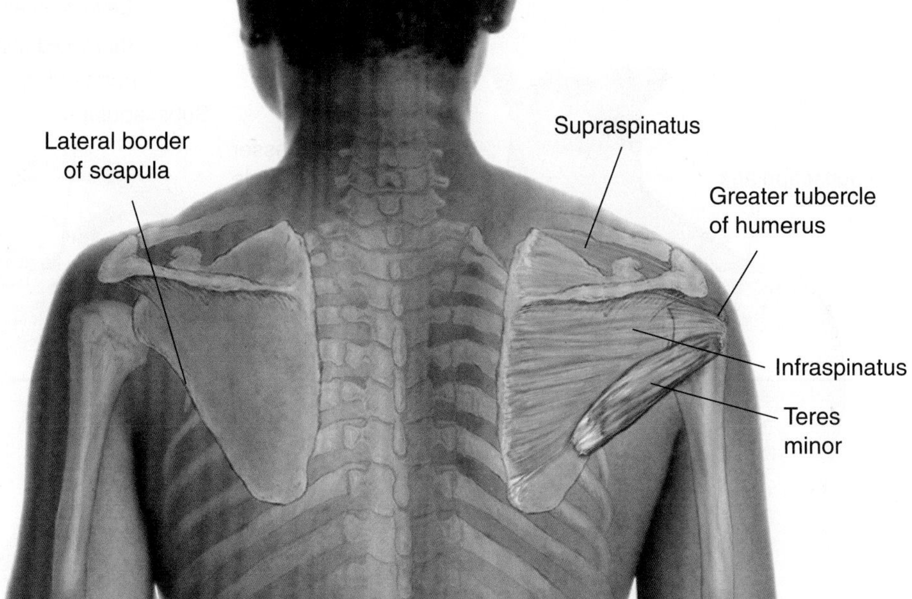

FIGURE 4-42 Teres minor

MANUAL THERAPY

Stripping

- The client lies prone. The therapist stands at the client's side to be treated, facing the client's shoulder.
- Use the thumb to find the muscle around the midpoint of the lateral edge of the scapula, between teres major and infraspinatus (Fig. 4-43).
- Pressing deeply with the supported thumb, glide along the muscle all the way to its attachment on the posterior aspect of the humerus.

FIGURE 4-43 Stripping massage of teres minor

SUBSCAPULARIS

SUB-SCAP-you-LAIR-iss

ETYMOLOGY Latin ***sub***, under + ***scapula***, shoulder blade

Overview

Subscapularis (Fig. 4-44) is a medial rotator and a stabilizer of the glenohumeral joint. It is stressed in heavy or repetitive lifting. An inability to raise the arm fully overhead can be a sign of a tight subscapularis.

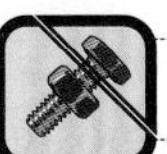

ATTACHMENTS

- Origin: subscapular fossa
- Insertion: lesser tubercle of humerus.

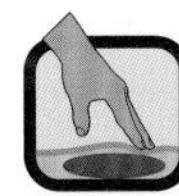

PALPATION

The lateral aspect of subscapularis is palpable by placing the fingertips under the muscle bundle consisting of latissimus dorsi and the teres muscles, directly into the axilla, and pressing posteriorly. From there, it can be followed to the lesser tubercle of the humerus. A small portion of the muscle may be palpable medially in relatively slender clients with fairly relaxed musculature by putting the hand behind the back, lifting the shoulder, and pressing under the medial border of the scapula.

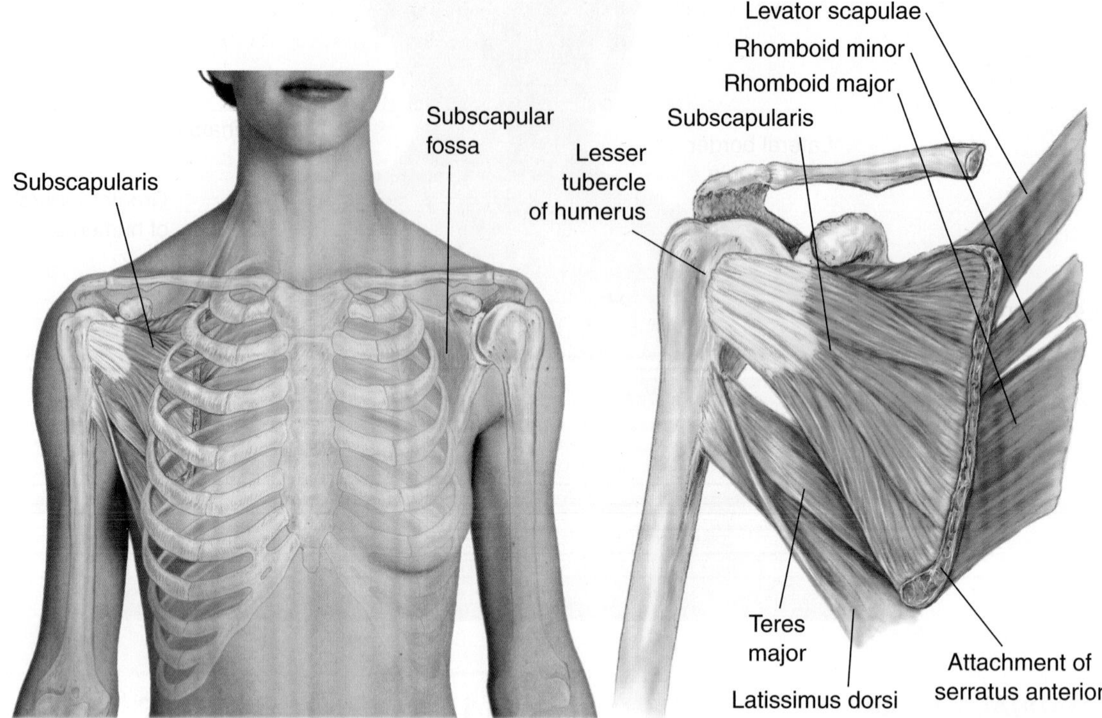

FIGURE 4-44 Subscapularis

Architecture is multipennate, and fiber direction is diagonal.

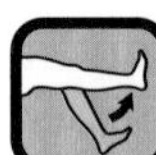

ACTION

Rotates the glenohumeral joint medially

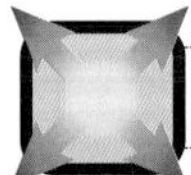

REFERRAL AREA

Over the scapula, behind the axilla, along the posterior arm, and into the wrist

OTHER MUSCLES TO EXAMINE

- Other rotator cuff muscles
- Teres major

MANUAL THERAPY

Stripping (1)

- The client lies prone. The therapist stands at the client's side, facing the shoulder to be treated.
- Abduct the client's arm, bending it at the elbow, and internally rotating it (palm up), to about 45°.
- Place the nontreating hand on the medial border of the scapula, pressing the scapula laterally and superiorly.
- Place the fingertips of the treating hand under the muscle bundle forming the rear boundary of the axilla, pressing lateral to the bundle into subscapularis (Fig. 4-45).
- Pressing firmly into the muscle, glide the fingertips from the superior to the inferior aspect of the muscle (or vice versa, according to what works best for you), covering as much of the muscle as possible.

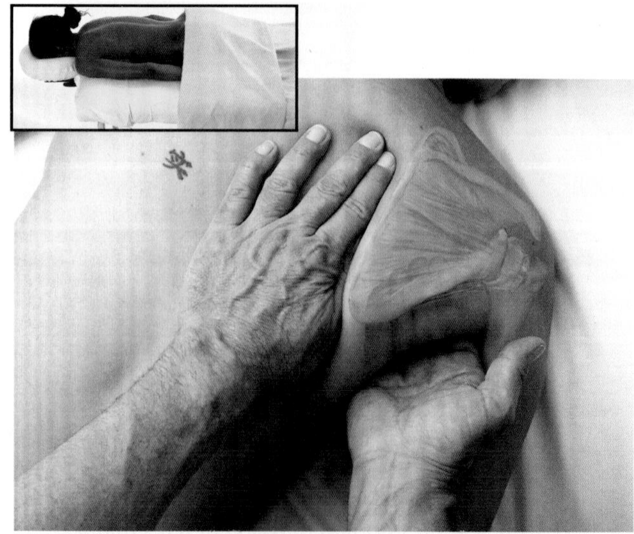

FIGURE 4-45 Stripping massage of subscapularis (1)

This technique may also be performed with the client sitting on the side of the table, using the thumb (Fig. 4-46A) or the fingertips (Fig. 4-46B), or with legs drawn up and arms wrapped around legs (Fig. 4-46C).

Compression

- To reach the inferior portion of the muscle, bend the client's arm at the elbow 45° behind the back.
- Lift the shoulder with your far hand.
- Insert the fingertips of your near hand underneath the inferior angle of the scapula and press upward (Fig. 4-47).

Stripping (2)

- The client lies supine with the arm abducted. The therapist stands at the client's side, facing the shoulder.

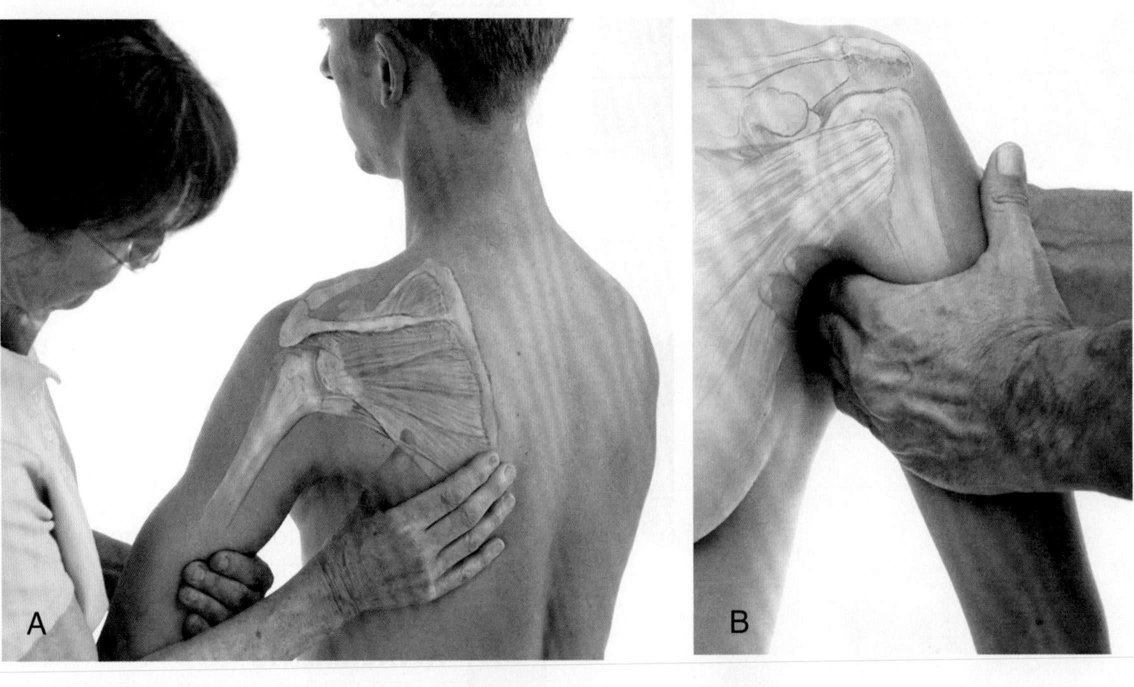

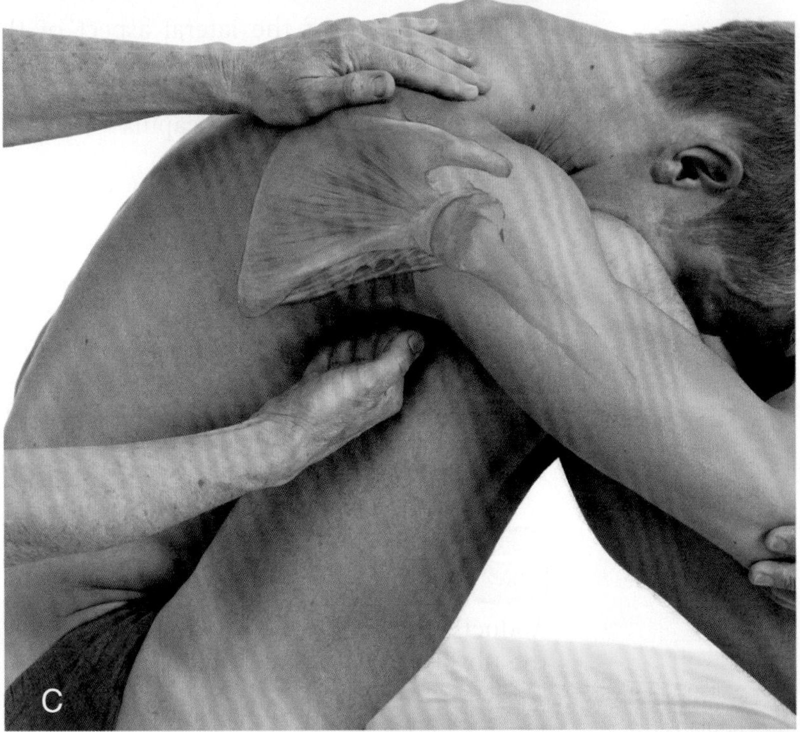

FIGURE 4-46 Accessing subscapularis with the client seated: with thumb **(A)**, with fingertips **(B)**, and with the client's hips and knees flexed and arms wrapped around knees **(C)**

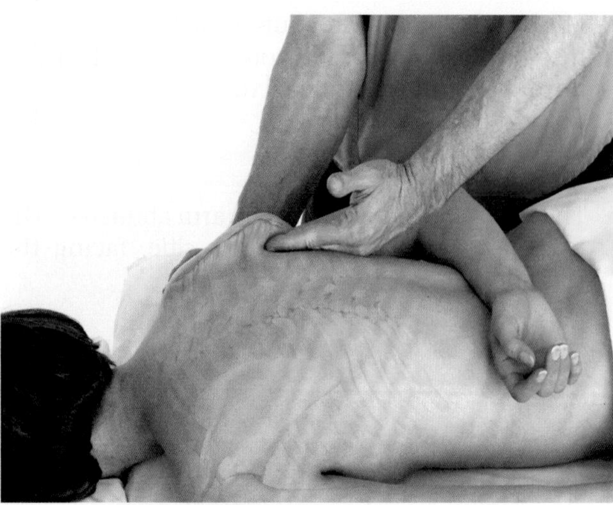

FIGURE 4-47 Compression of the inferior aspect of subscapularis

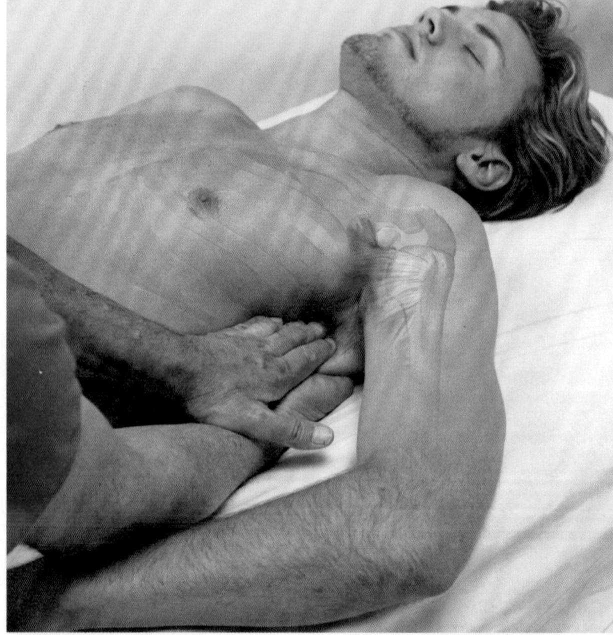

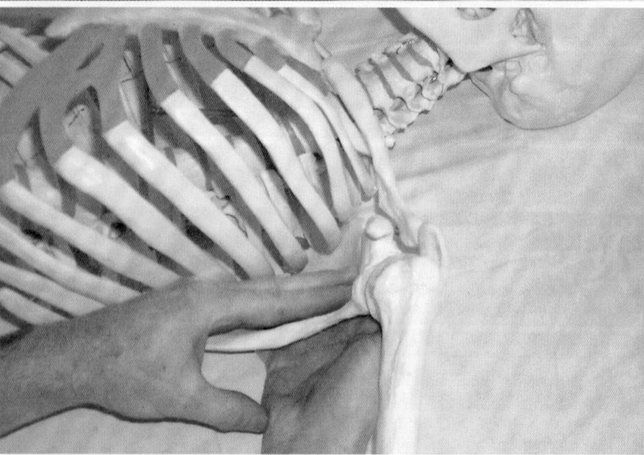

FIGURE 4-48 Stripping massage of subscapularis (2)

- Place the far hand under the client's scapula, with the fingertips hooked over the medial border, pulling the scapula laterally.
- With the fingertips of the near hand, press firmly just under the axilla into the underside of the scapula (Fig. 4-48).
- Glide the fingertips slowly inferiorly or superiorly along the muscle.

Muscles of the Ribs

SERRATUS ANTERIOR

serr-RATE-us an-TIER-ee-yore

ETYMOLOGY Latin ***serra***, saw + ***anterior***, more toward the front

Overview

Serratus anterior (Fig. 4-49) works with the pectoral muscles and opposes the rhomboids. It plays an important role in stabilizing the scapula to prevent adduction (retraction) during lifting or pushing with the arms. It can produce pain in the side of the chest and down the arm in a pattern similar to that of pectoralis minor, and it is most easily treated along with that muscle.

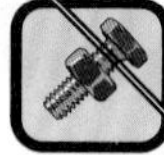

ATTACHMENTS

- Origin: center of the lateral aspect of the first eight to nine ribs
- Insertion: superior and inferior angles and intervening medial margin of scapula

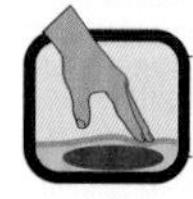

PALPATION

Serratus anterior can be palpated by placing the fingers flat against the rib cage just lateral to the scapula and moving them up and down in a superior/inferior direction, then moving them around toward the front of the chest, stopping before one reaches the pectoral muscles. Architecture is convergent, and fibers are diagonal.

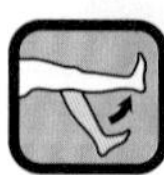

ACTION

Abducts the scapula and rotates it upward; elevates the ribs if scapula is stabilized

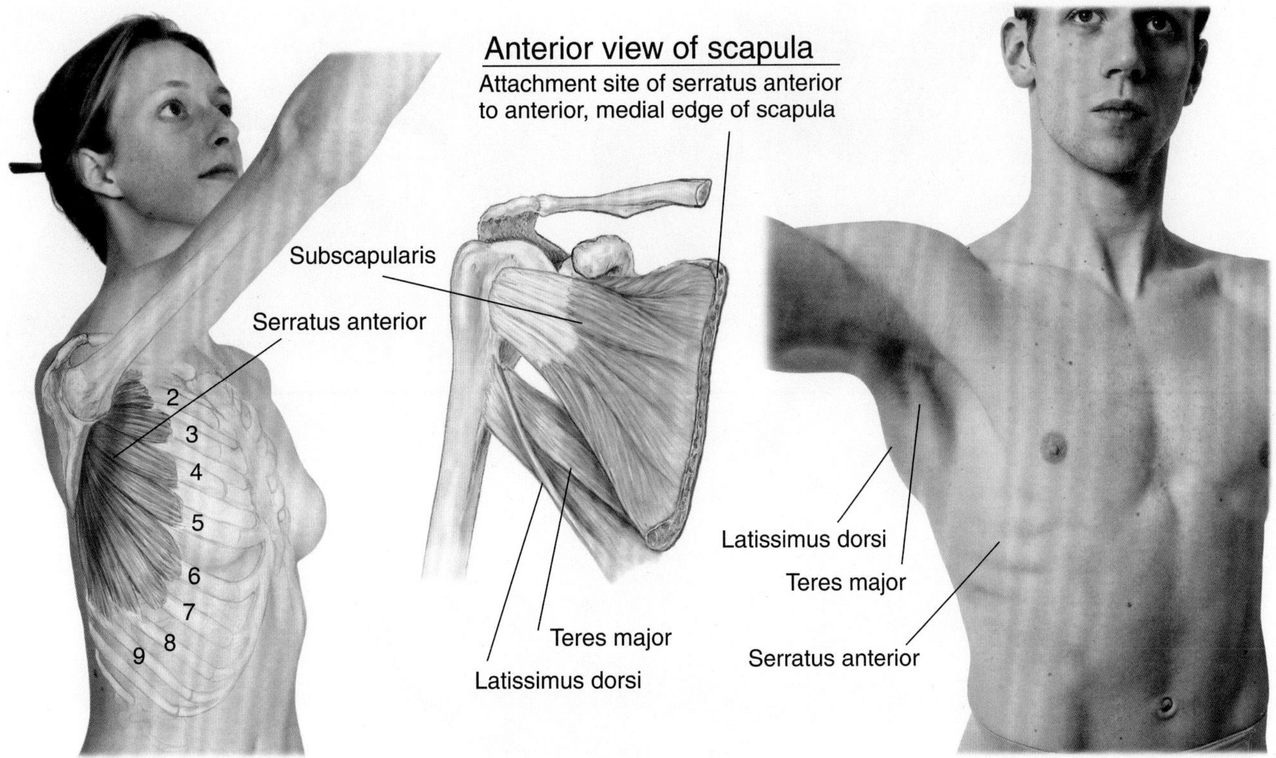

FIGURE 4-49 Serratus anterior

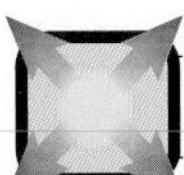

REFERRAL AREA

To the side of the chest at the middle of the rib cage, down the ulnar aspect of the arm to the last two fingers, and just medial to the inferior angle of the scapula

OTHER MUSCLES TO EXAMINE

- Latissimus dorsi
- Teres major
- Pectoralis minor
- Rhomboids

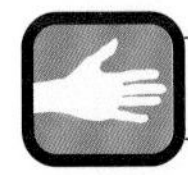

MANUAL THERAPY

Stripping

- The client lies on the side contralateral to that to be treated. The therapist stands in front of the client's chest.
- Place one hand on the side of the client's rib cage, with the fingers lying over the scapula and the thumb resting on the ninth rib.
- Pressing deeply, glide the thumb in an arc toward the scapula until it reaches the inferior angle.
- Shift the thumb one rib superiorly and repeat the process (Fig. 4-50) on the next page, each time ending slightly more superiorly on the lateral border of the scapula. As you encounter the bundle of muscles that forms the posterior boundary of the axilla, let your thumbs slip under the bundle to the scapula.

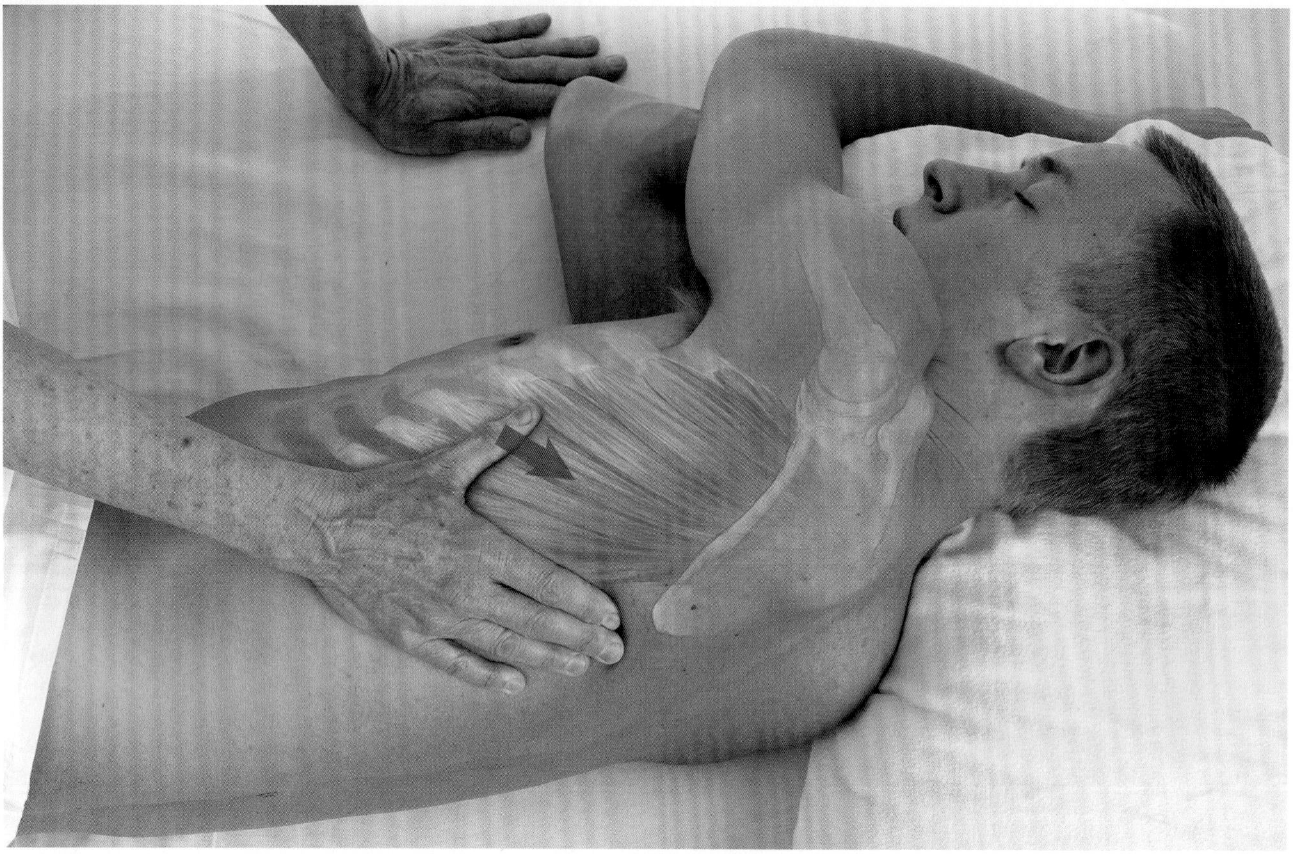

FIGURE 4-50 Stripping massage of serratus anterior in side-lying position

SERRATUS POSTERIOR INFERIOR

serr-RATE-us poss-TIER-ee-yore in-FEAR-ee-yore

ETYMOLOGY Latin *serra*, saw + *posterior*, toward the back + *inferior*, lower

Overview

Serratus posterior inferior (Fig. 4-51) assists in rotation and extension of the trunk, and assists in respiration. Its most common trigger point radiates locally.

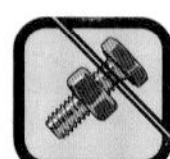

ATTACHMENTS

- Origin: with latissimus dorsi, from the spinous processes and supraspinous ligaments of T11 through L2
- Insertion: posterior aspect of ribs 9 to 12

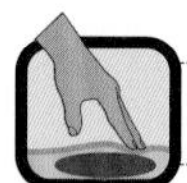

PALPATION

Unless it harbors the trigger point mentioned, this muscle is palpable but not discernible. Architecture is parallel and fibers are diagonal.

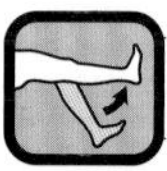

ACTION

Draws lower ribs backward and downward to assist forced expiration

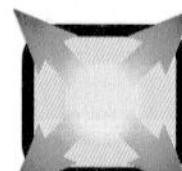

REFERRAL AREA

Radiating locally over the muscle

OTHER MUSCLES TO EXAMINE

- Quadratus lumborum
- Iliocostalis thoracis
- Psoas major
- Rectus abdominis
- Pyramidalis
- Diaphragm

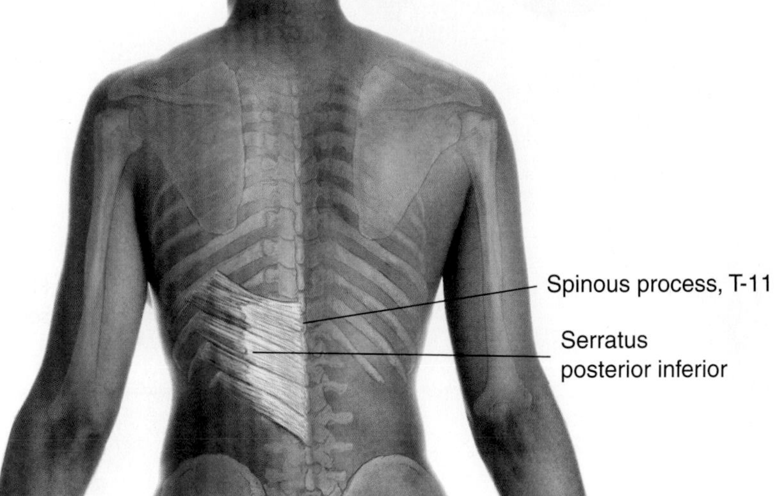

FIGURE 4-51 Serratus posterior inferior

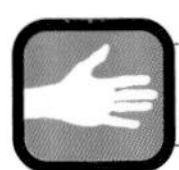

MANUAL THERAPY

Stripping

- Client lies prone; the therapist stands at the client's hips on the side contralateral to that to be treated.
- Place your supported fingertips at the upper lumbar vertebrae.
- Press deeply into muscle, moving the fingertips diagonally (inferiorly and laterally) over the lower two ribs.
- Move the fingertips up to the lowest two thoracic vertebrae and repeat (Fig. 4-52).
- In place of the fingertips, the thumb, elbow, or knuckles may be used.

Compression

- Palpate the area over the muscle with the thumb or supported fingertip until the client reports a sharp, radiating pain.
- Compress that point with the thumb or elbow until the pain eases (Fig. 4-53).

Muscles of Breathing

The proper way to breathe primarily involves the diaphragm. This dome-like muscle marks the boundary between the thoracic and abdominal cavities and pulls downward during inhalation, expanding the thoracic cavity to allow air to fill the lungs. The abdomen will expand as it does this. Upon exhaling quietly, the diaphragm relaxes as the abdominal tissues compressed by its contraction recoil elastically upward, moving air out of the lungs.

Breathing more rapidly, deeply and forcefully, during exercise for instance, will recruit the complex involvement of rib-moving and abdominal muscles. Using these muscles in normal circumstances, however, leads to inefficient breathing. Many people do not breathe properly, due to stress and anxiety, respiratory issues, sinus problems, or plain poor habits, such as shallow breathing in through the mouth.

Although many theories address why people learn improper breathing skills, they are beyond the scope of this book. Nevertheless, the clinical

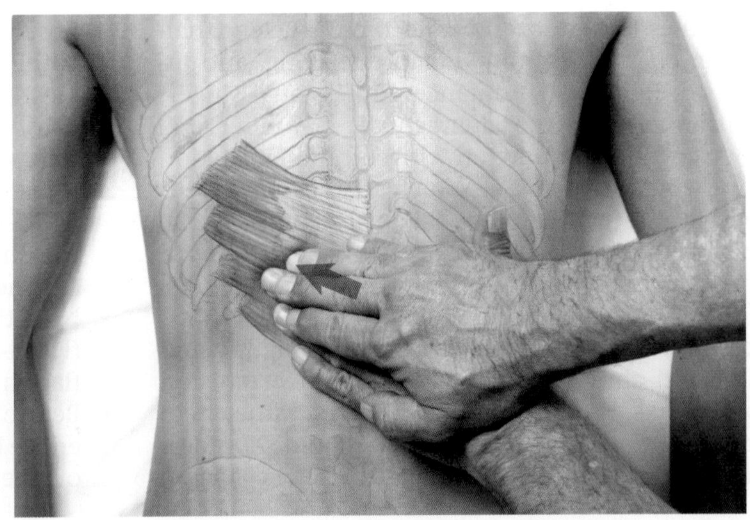

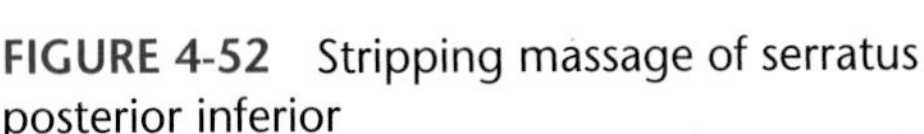

FIGURE 4-52 Stripping massage of serratus posterior inferior

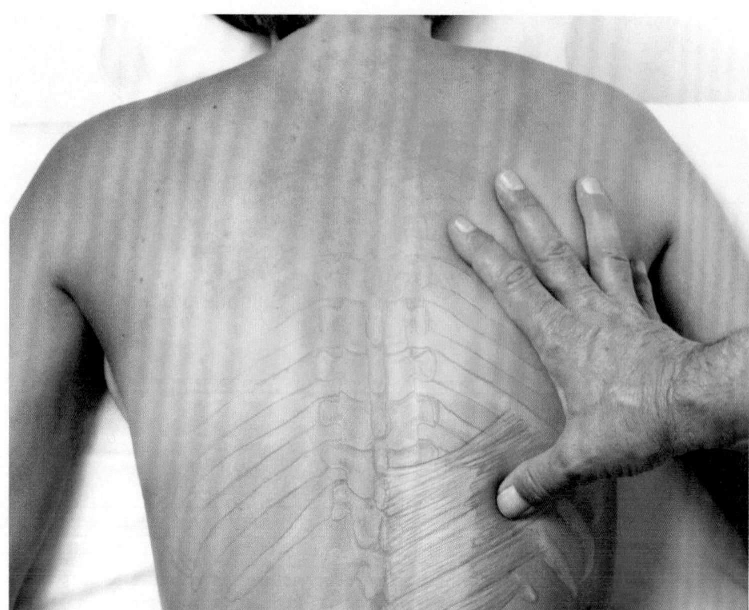

FIGURE 4-53 Compression of trigger point in serratus posterior inferior with the thumb

massage therapist is in an excellent position to enable clients to relearn breathing skills.

Two things are necessary: first, the therapist should work on the muscles of respiration so that they are free of constrictions and trigger points, have good muscle tone, and can move freely. Second, the therapist should teach the client good breathing skills and urge the client to practice them outside of therapy.

Many people tend to breathe from the neck, shoulders, and upper chest, allowing the upper rib cage to expand while tightening the abdominal muscles. This habit is called "paradoxical breathing," because the abdomen is contracted rather than expanded. In proper breathing, the lower rib cage and abdomen expand. This skill is called "diaphragmatic breathing."

Diaphragmatic breathing draws air more deeply into the lungs and increases breathing efficiency. It requires less effort and is far more efficient than "upper chest" breathing, is more relaxing, and increases respiratory endurance. Professional singers and musicians learn diaphragmatic breathing, and when used in conjunction with forceful exhalation using abdominal muscles such as the transversus abdominis, it will improve the quality of the voice. The latter advantage can be observed not only in opera singers but in the lusty cry of a baby!

Begin by evaluating the client's breathing practices. Although the shoulders may rise slightly and the upper chest expand somewhat, the expansion should take place from the bottom up, rather than from the top down. The upper chest and shoulders should be pushed slightly upward by the expansion of the inferior rib cage, rather than pulled upward by the scalenes. If the breathing motion expands the abdomen and lower rib cage, followed by a moderate expansion of the upper chest and a slight rise in the shoulders, the client is breathing properly, and you need only to work the respiratory muscles to loosen and relax them. If, however, the abdomen contracts, the shoulders rise significantly, and the upper chest expands pronouncedly, you'll need to teach proper breathing mechanics to the client.

MANUAL THERAPY

Initial Assessment

- The client may stand (Fig. 4-54), sit, or lie supine (Fig. 4-55).
- Ask the client to take a deep breath while you observe the shoulders, chest, and abdomen.
- If the client is breathing paradoxically, you will see the shoulders rise pronouncedly, the upper chest expand markedly, and the abdomen contract (Figs. 4-54A and 4-55A).
- If the client is breathing diaphragmatically, you will see the abdomen and lower rib cage expand, the shoulders rise slightly, and the upper chest expand moderately (Figs. 4-54B and 4-55B).
- Note the clearer delineation of the inguinal folds (Fig. 4-54B) when the abdomen expands, and the flattening of the inguinal folds on contraction.
- Before proceeding to teach breathing, release the entire breathing apparatus with myofascial work on the chest and manual therapy of the muscles

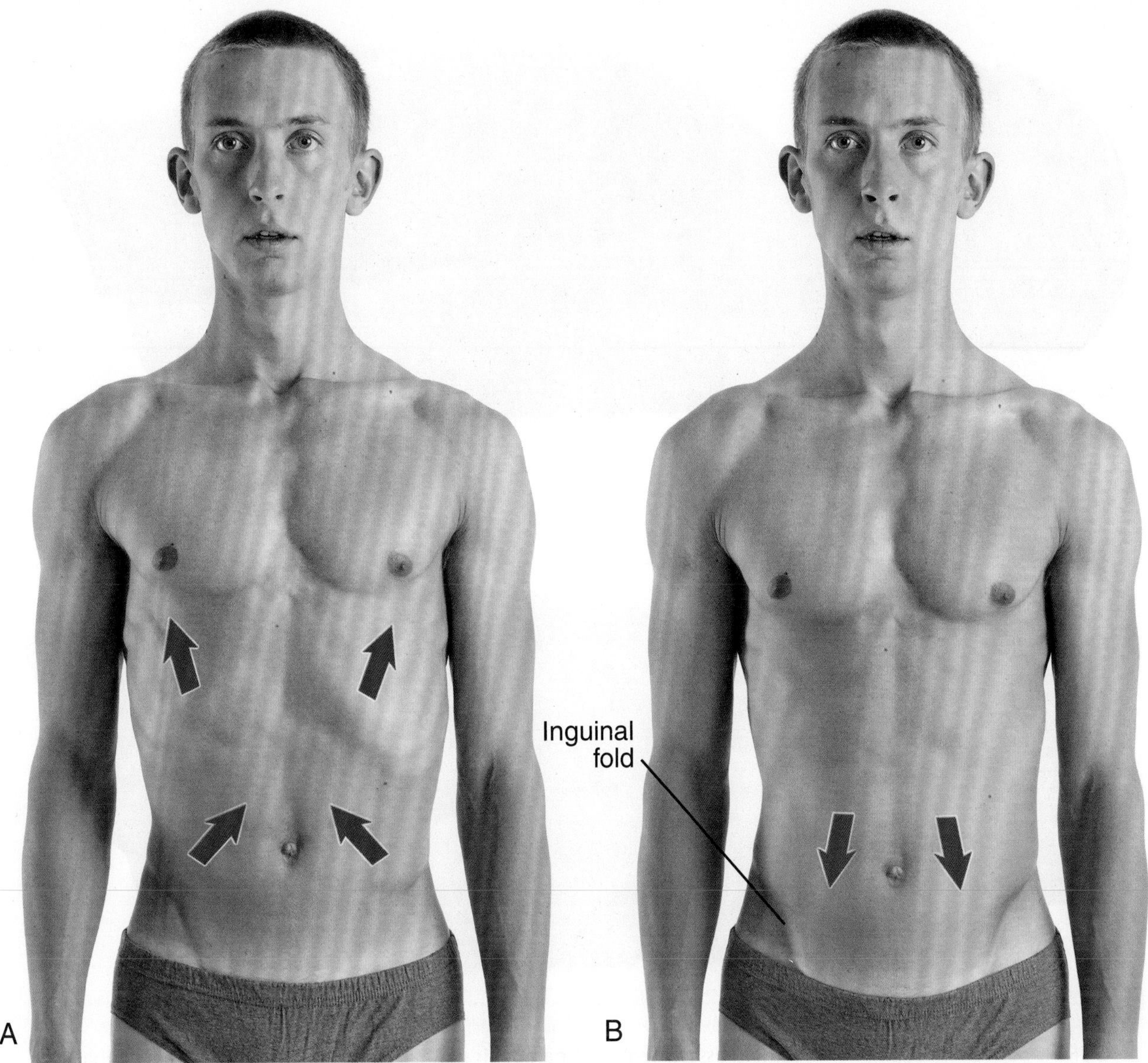

FIGURE 4-54 Client standing for breathing assessment: **(A)** paradoxical inhalation and **(B)** diaphragmatic inhalation

of breathing. First, examine the diaphragm. Place your hand on the abdomen with the fingers pointing superiorly just at the edge of the first rib. As the client exhales, press your fingers under the costal arch in a superior direction (Fig. 4-56). Repeat on the opposite side. Tautness or pain indicates constriction and probable trigger point activity in the breathing mechanism that can cause pain and prevent comfortable respiration.

Myofascial Release of the Chest (1)

- Have the supine client raise her or his arms overhead.
- Place one hand flat on the client's chest just medial to the axilla, with your fingers pointing superiorly. Cross the other hand over the first hand and place it flat on the chest just inferior to the first hand, the fingers pointing inferiorly (Fig. 4-57).
- Let your hands sink gently into the tissue until you feel the underlying superficial fascia. Press the two hands gently away from each other, stretching the myofascial tissue. Hold until you feel that the soft tissue has softened.
- Shift your hands medially by a hand's width and repeat the process.
- Repeat the procedure as far as the sternum, then move to the other side of the client and repeat.
- On female clients with developed breasts, discontinue this procedure at the breasts and continue on the medial side.

Myofascial Release of the Chest (2)

- Stand at the client's head.

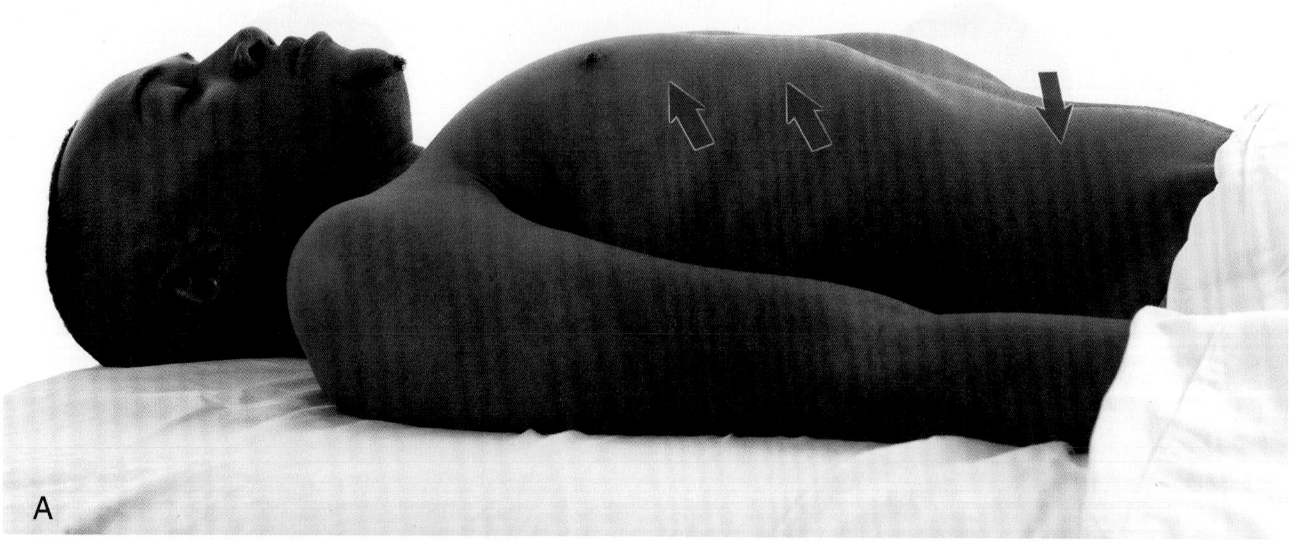

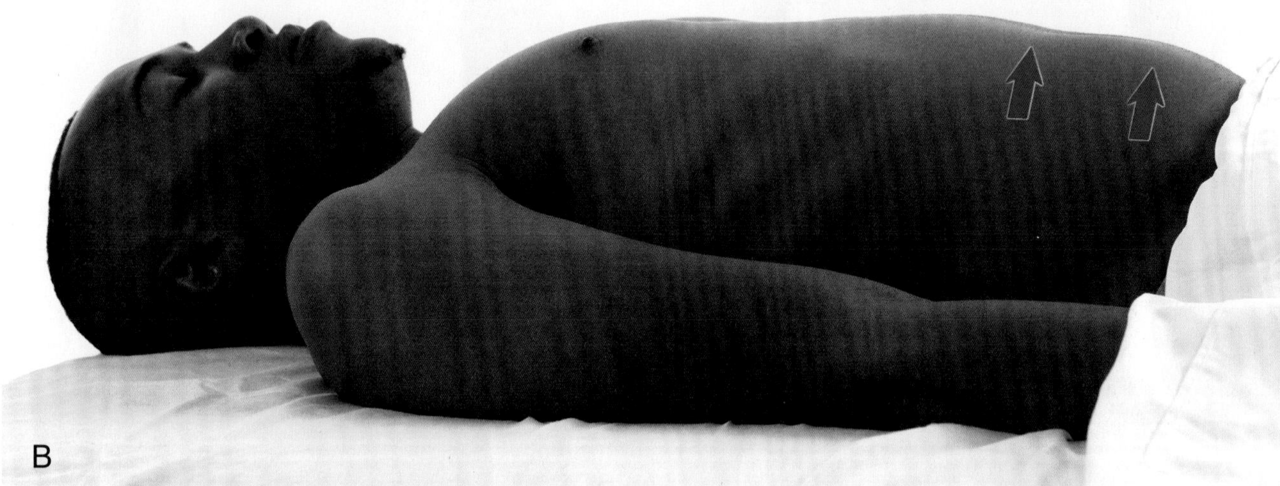

FIGURE 4-55 Client supine for breathing assessment: **(A)** paradoxical inhalation and **(B)** diaphragmatic inhalation

- Place one hand flat on the client's chest, with the heel of the hand resting on the sternum just below the manubrium, the fingers pointing laterally.
- Cross the other hand over and place it next to the first, the fingers pointing laterally in the other direction (Fig. 4-58).
- Let your hands sink gently into the tissue until you feel the underlying superficial fascia. Press the two hands gently away from each other, holding until you feel that the tissue has softened.
- Shift your hands inferiorly by a hand's width and repeat the process.
- Place one hand flat on the client's sternum just inferior to the manubrium, with your fingers pointing inferiorly (Fig. 4-59).
- Pressing gently into the tissue, glide your hand slowly down the sternum until the heel of your hand reaches the inferior end of the sternum.
- After warming the sternum with the heel of the hand, gently use your thumb to repeat the gliding motion down and around the sternum (Fig. 4-60).

CAUTION Be gentle and do not press too firmly on the xiphoid process. It can be broken with pressure, or may be tender.

Myofascial Work on the Chest (3)

- Standing beside the supine client at chest level, place your whole hand flat on the upper chest on the contralateral side of the client's body, the

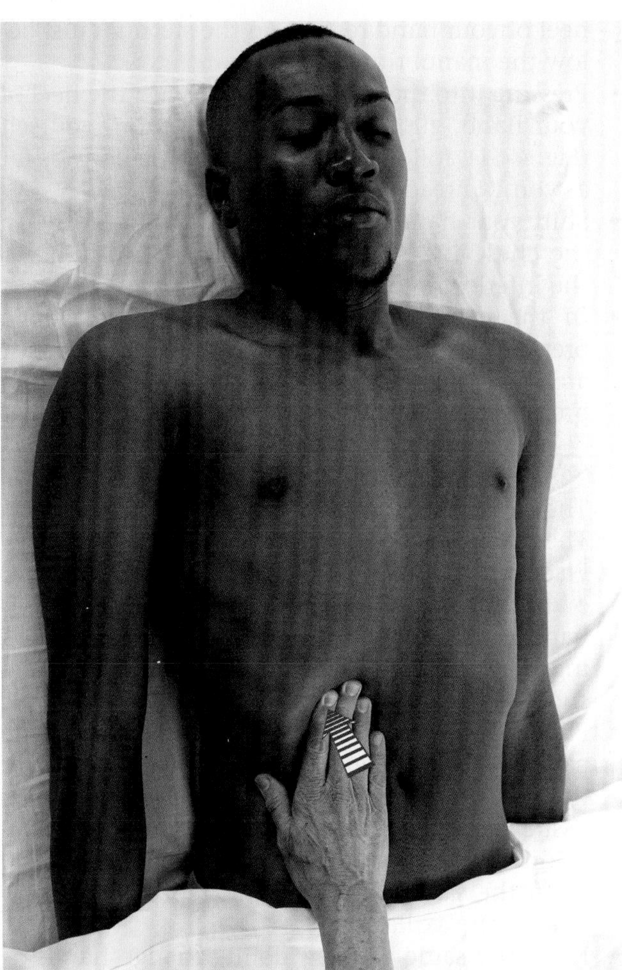

FIGURE 4-56 Examination of the diaphragm

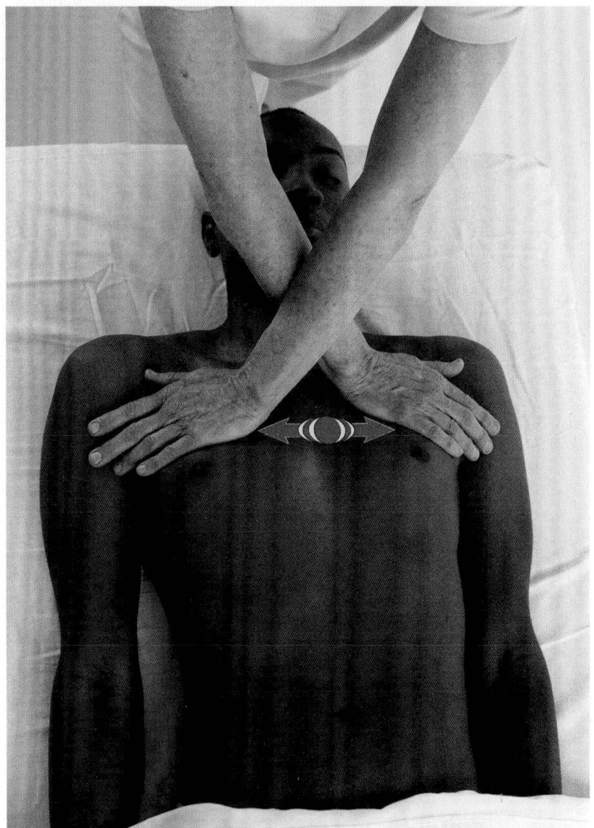

FIGURE 4-58 Myofascial release of the chest (2)

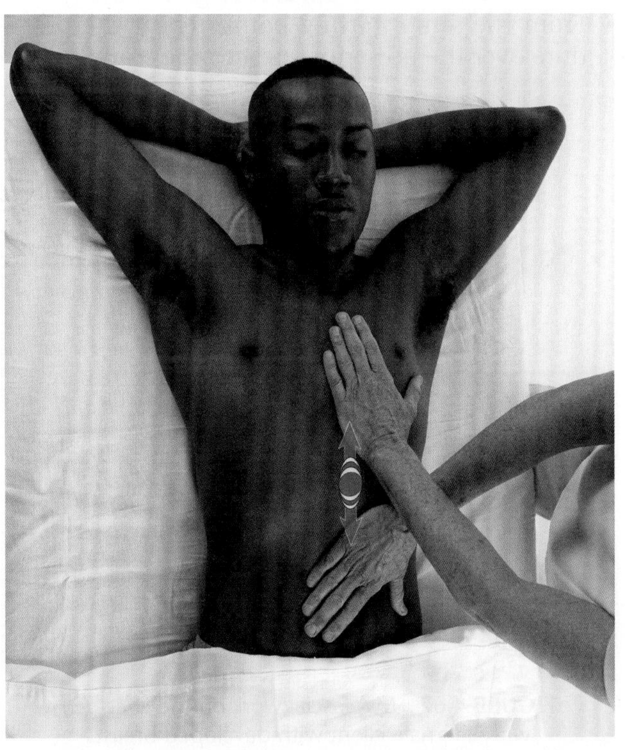

FIGURE 4-57 Myofascial release of the chest (1)

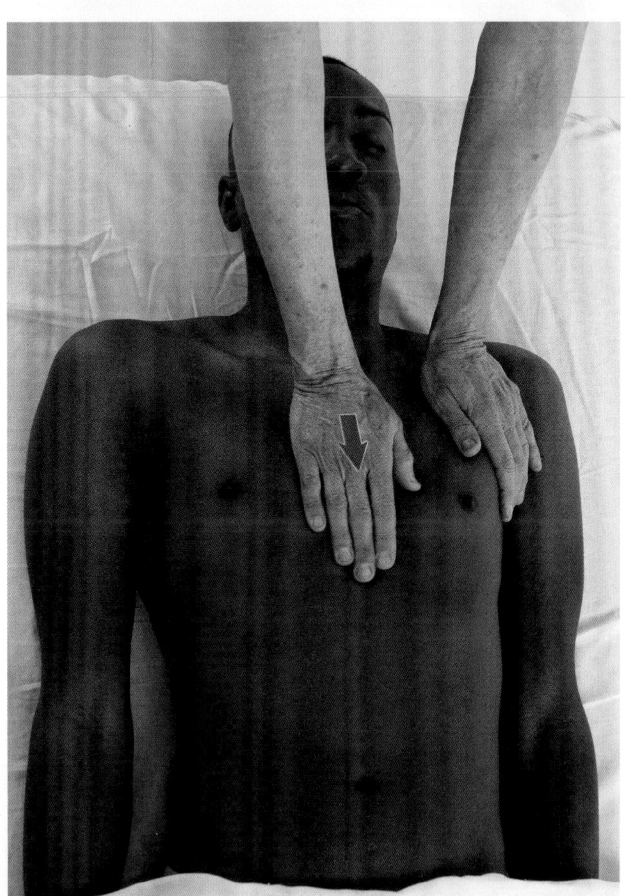

FIGURE 4-59 Myofascial work on the chest (2) with the hand

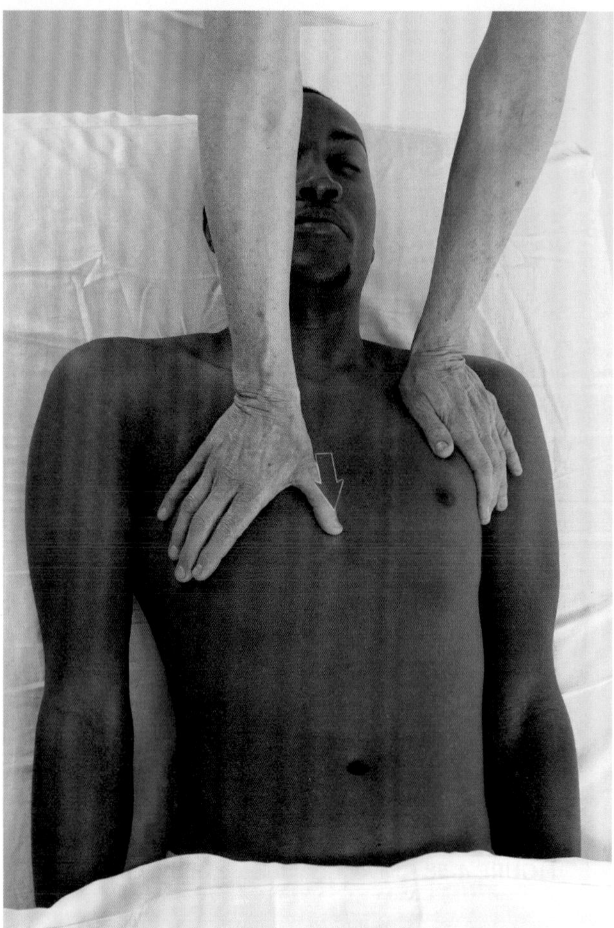

FIGURE 4-60 Myofascial work on the chest (2) with the thumb

heel of your hand resting on the sternum just below the manubrium.

- Pressing into the tissue primarily with the heel of your hand, glide your hand away from yourself (Fig. 4-61), following the curve of the body as far as you can reach comfortably.
- Shift your hand by a hand's width inferiorly on the chest and repeat the process, continuing to the inferior rib cage.
- In the case of female clients with developed breasts, perform this procedure as far as the breast area, and then continue on the chest below the breast (Fig. 4-62).

Myofascial Work on the Chest (4)

- The client is in side-lying position.
- The therapist stands behind the client at waist level.
- Place one hand on the inferior rib cage, iliac crest, or back, to stabilize the client. Place the other hand on the lateral rib cage, the fingers pointing diagonally toward the client's contralateral shoulder (Fig. 4-63A).
- Pressing deeply into the tissue with the whole palm of the hand, glide the hand diagonally over the rib cage as far as the sternum (or until breast tissue is encountered in a female client with developed breasts).
- From the same starting point, repeat the procedure to the axilla.
- From the same starting point, change hands as necessary, and repeat the procedure directly up the client's side and over the posterior border of the axilla to the deltoid area (Fig. 4-63B).
- From the same starting point, repeat the procedure over the posterior chest to the scapula.

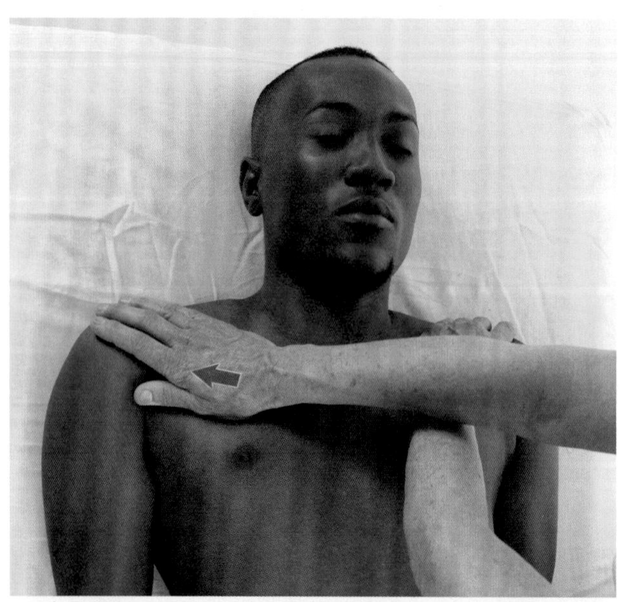

FIGURE 4-61 Myofascial work on the chest (3) with the hand

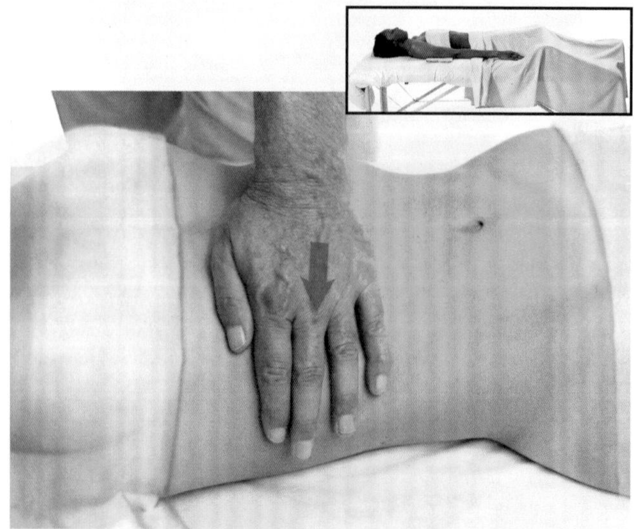

FIGURE 4-62 Myofascial work on the chest (3) with a female client with developed breasts

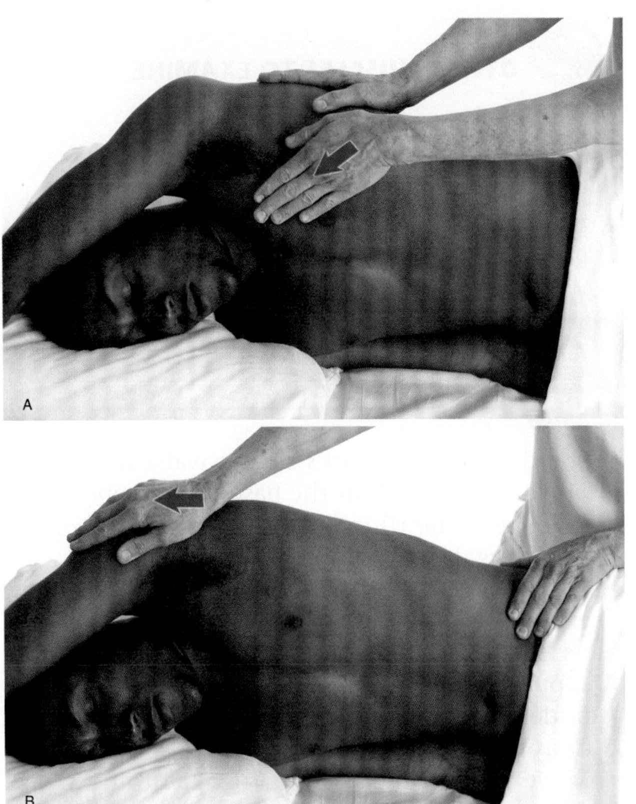

FIGURE 4-63 Myofascial work on the chest (4) with client in side-lying position: **(A)** starting position, **(B)** over shoulder

DIAPHRAGM

DIE-a-fram

ETYMOLOGY Greek ***dia***, through + ***phragma***, enclosure

Overview

The diaphragm (Fig. 4-64) is a dome of muscle and connective tissue separating the thoracic cavity from the abdominal cavity. It is the primary muscle of inspiration and is sometimes referred to as the thoracic diaphragm. The diaphragm has three distinct sections—the sternal, costal, and lumbar—with muscle fibers grouped according to their origin.

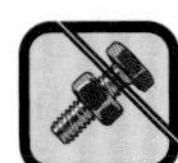

ATTACHMENTS

Origin

- Sternal: two muscular slips from the posterior sternum
- Costal: the inner surface of the cartilage and adjacent portions of the lower six ribs on either side, integrating with transverse abdominus
- Lumbar: lumbocostal arches and lumbar vertebrae

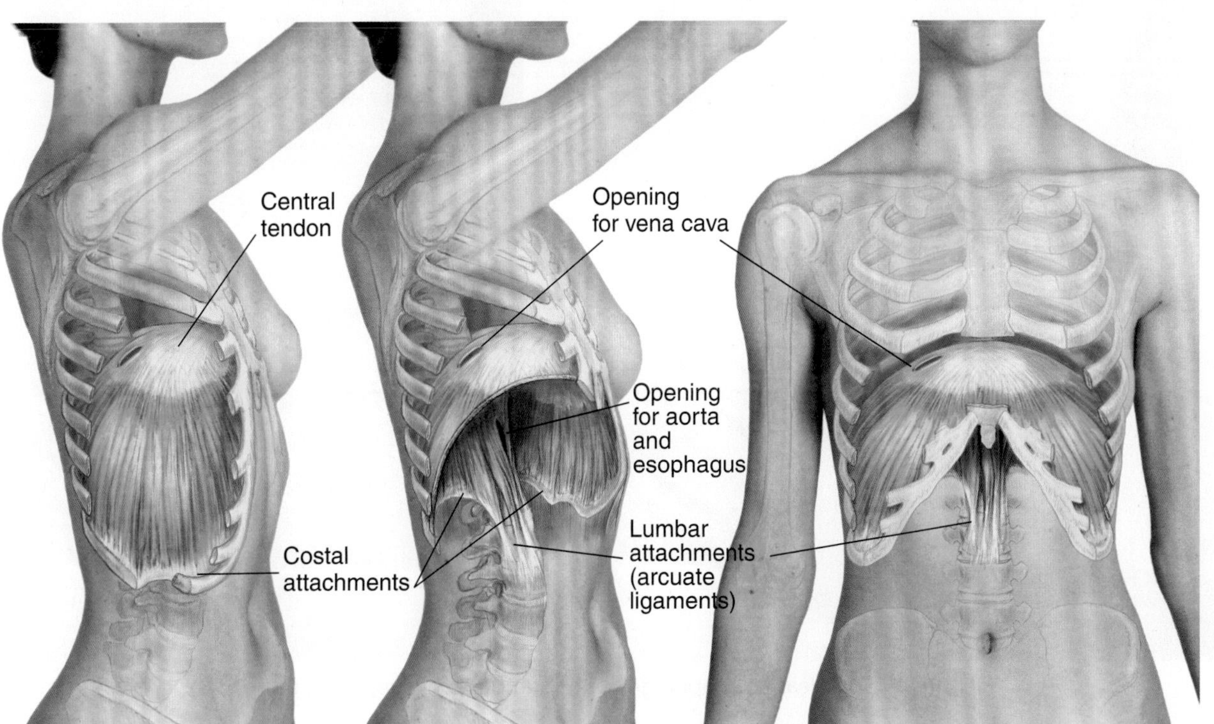

FIGURE 4-64 Anatomy of the diaphragm

- In the center, the central tendon is penetrated by the aorta, vena cava, and esophagus.
- Posteriorly the arcuate ligaments allow passage of psoas major and quadratus lumborum.

Insertion

- Central tendon

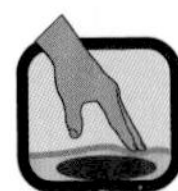

PALPATION

The diaphragm can be palpated by following the instructions for manual therapy described here.

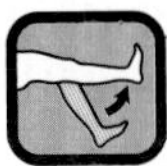

ACTION

Pulls downward, flattening its dome and compressing the abdominal contents, expanding the volume of the thoracic cavity during inhalation (inspiration)

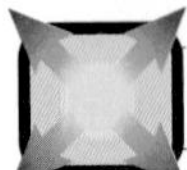

REFERRAL AREA

"Stitch in the side," chest pain, substernal pain, or pain along the lower border of the ribs

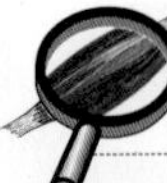

OTHER MUSCLES TO EXAMINE

- Intercostals
- Scalenes
- Pectoralis major
- Pectoralis minor
- Rectus abdominis

MANUAL THERAPY

Release

- Standing at the client's side at waist level, place one or both hands at the base of the opposite rib cage, with the thumb, supported thumb, or fingertips against the lowest rib.
- Ask the client to inhale deeply and then slowly exhale.
- As the client exhales, press the thumb (Fig. 4-65A), supported thumb (Fig. 4-65B), or fingertips deeply under the lower rib cage, lifting it upward and away from yourself.
- Move to the other side of the client and repeat the procedure.

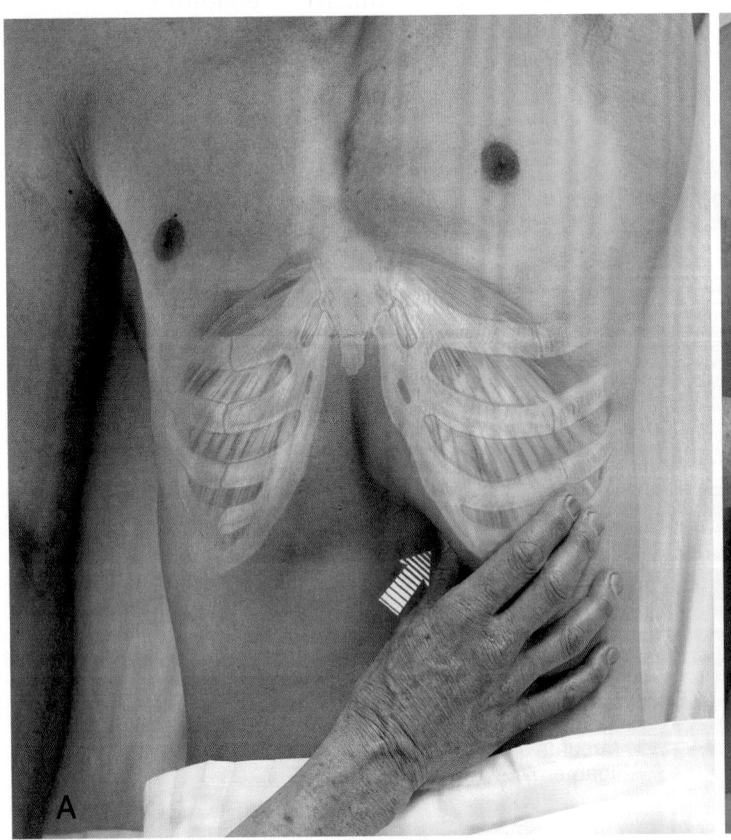

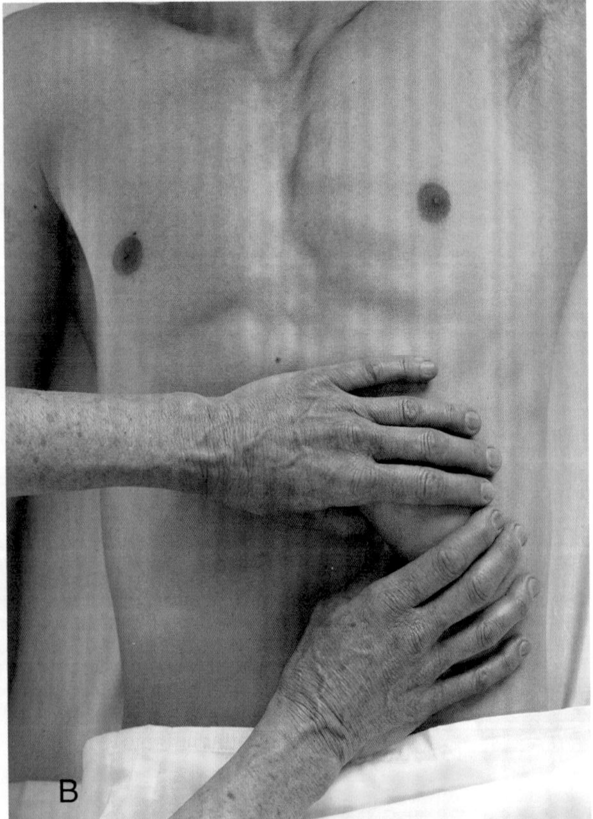

FIGURE 4-65 Release of diaphragm with thumb **(A)** or supported thumb **(B)**

SERRATUS POSTERIOR SUPERIOR

serr-RATE-us poss-TIER-ee-yore sue-PEER-ee-yore

ETYMOLOGY Latin ***serra***, saw + ***posterior***, toward the back + ***superior***, higher

Overview

Serratus posterior superior (Fig. 4-66) assists in breathing by raising the ribs to which it attaches. Note that the client's arm must be raised to access its most common trigger point.

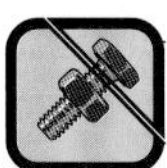

ATTACHMENTS

- Origin: spinous processes of the two lower cervical and two upper thoracic vertebrae
- Insertion: lateral side of angles of second to fifth ribs

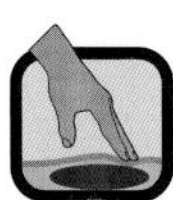

PALPATION

Place hands alongside the spine between the spine and the medial border of the scapula and slide fingers down the serrated edges of the tissue on ribs 2 to 5. Architecture is parallel, and fibers are diagonal.

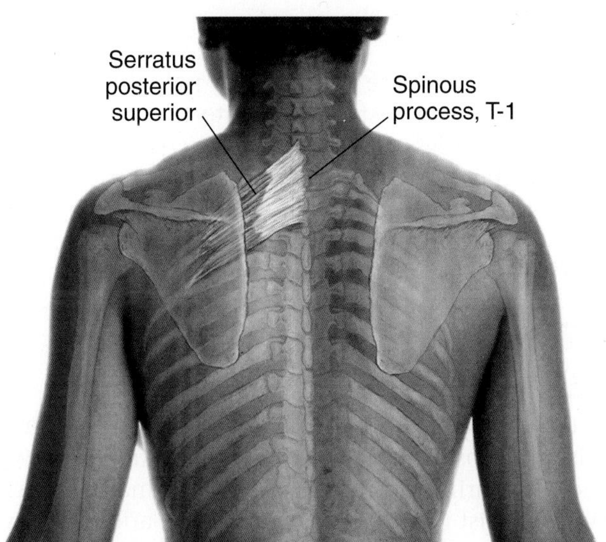

FIGURE 4-66 Anatomy of serratus posterior superior

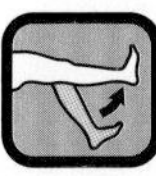

ACTION

Raises the second through fifth ribs to assist inhalation

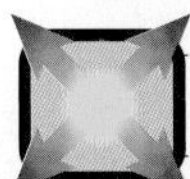

REFERRAL AREA

Over the upper half of the scapula, into the anterior chest, along the dorsal and ulnar aspects of the arm to the little finger

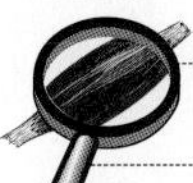

OTHER MUSCLES TO EXAMINE

- Rhomboids
- Rotator cuff muscles
- Teres major
- Pectoralis minor
- Posterior and middle deltoids

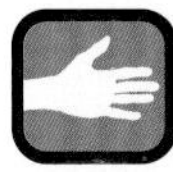

MANUAL THERAPY

Stripping/Compression

- The client lies prone, with the arm on the side to be treated abducted and extended to rotate the superior angle of the scapula downward to expose more of the muscle. The therapist stands beside the client's head contralateral to the side to be treated.
- Place the fingertips or supported thumb just next to the spinous process of the sixth cervical vertebra. Pressing deeply, glide the hand diagonally downward as far as the scapula will permit.
- Repeat the process at the seventh cervical and first two thoracic vertebrae.
- The most common trigger point in this muscle lies in the area nearest the ribs that is uncovered by rotating the scapula. If this trigger point is present, compress and hold until it releases (Fig. 4-67).

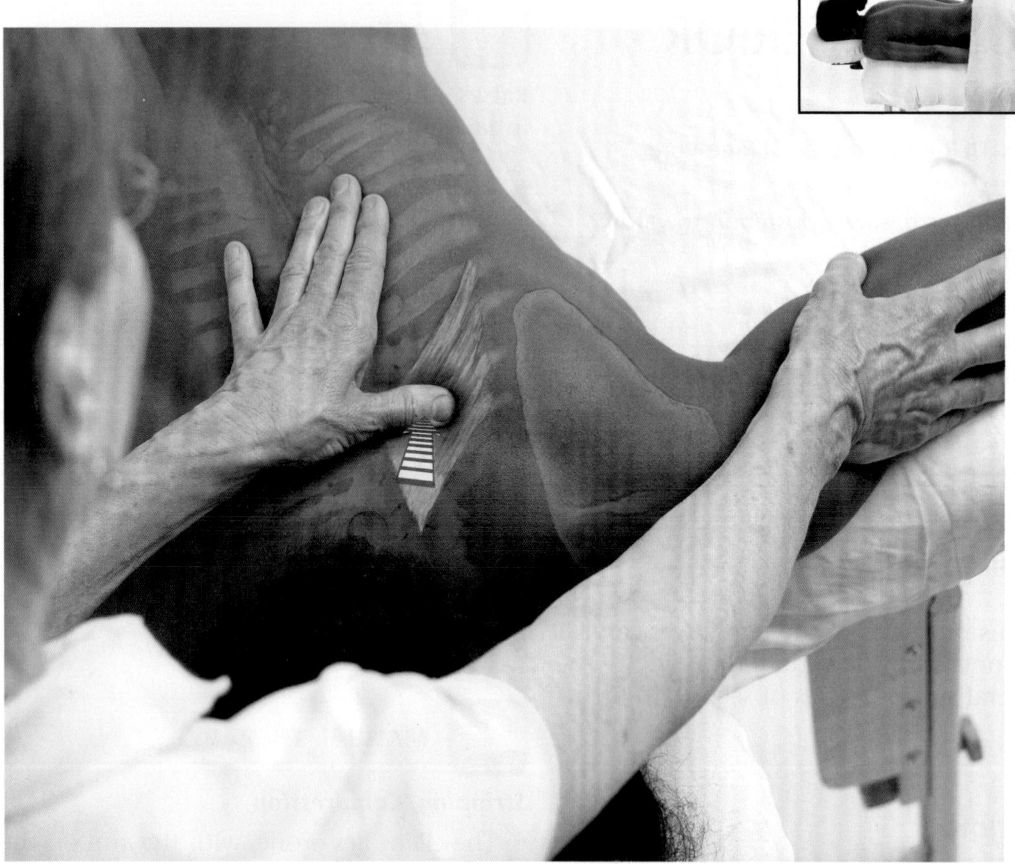

FIGURE 4-67 Compression of trigger point in serratus posterior superior

INTERCOSTALS

In-ter-COST-als

ETYMOLOGY Latin ***inter***, between + ***costa***, rib

Overview

The intercostals (Fig. 4-68) have both respiratory and postural functions, and their precise functions are quite complex. Essentially, they control the activity of the ribs, and thus both inspiration and thoracic rotation. Release of shortened intercostals is therefore an important part of work on the thorax.

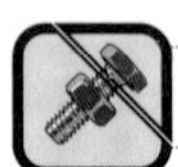

ATTACHMENTS

- Origin: external intercostals: inferior border of ribs 1 to 11 and passes obliquely in an inferior and anterior direction.
- Insertion: superior border of the rib below (ribs 2 to 12).
- Origin: internal intercostals: inferior border of ribs 2 to 12 and passes obliquely in an inferior and posterior direction.
- Insertion: superior border of ribs 1 to 11.
- Note: external intercostals do not extend all the way to the costal cartilages except between the lowest ribs. In their place is fascia.

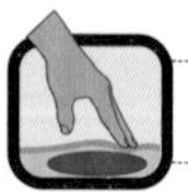

PALPATION

The intercostals are fairly easily palpable between the ribs. It is easiest on the anterior aspect of the chest, where less intervening tissue is present. It is more difficult on the upper anterior chest because of pectoralis major and, in women, because of the breasts. The muscle architecture is parallel and the fibers are diagonal.

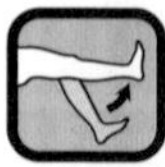

ACTION

External intercostals contract during inspiration to raise the ribs; internal intercostals contract to lower the ribs during expiration. Both also maintain tension to resist mediolateral movement, and are active in rotation of the thoracic spine.

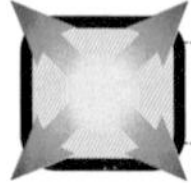

REFERRAL AREA

Locally, tending to extend anteriorly

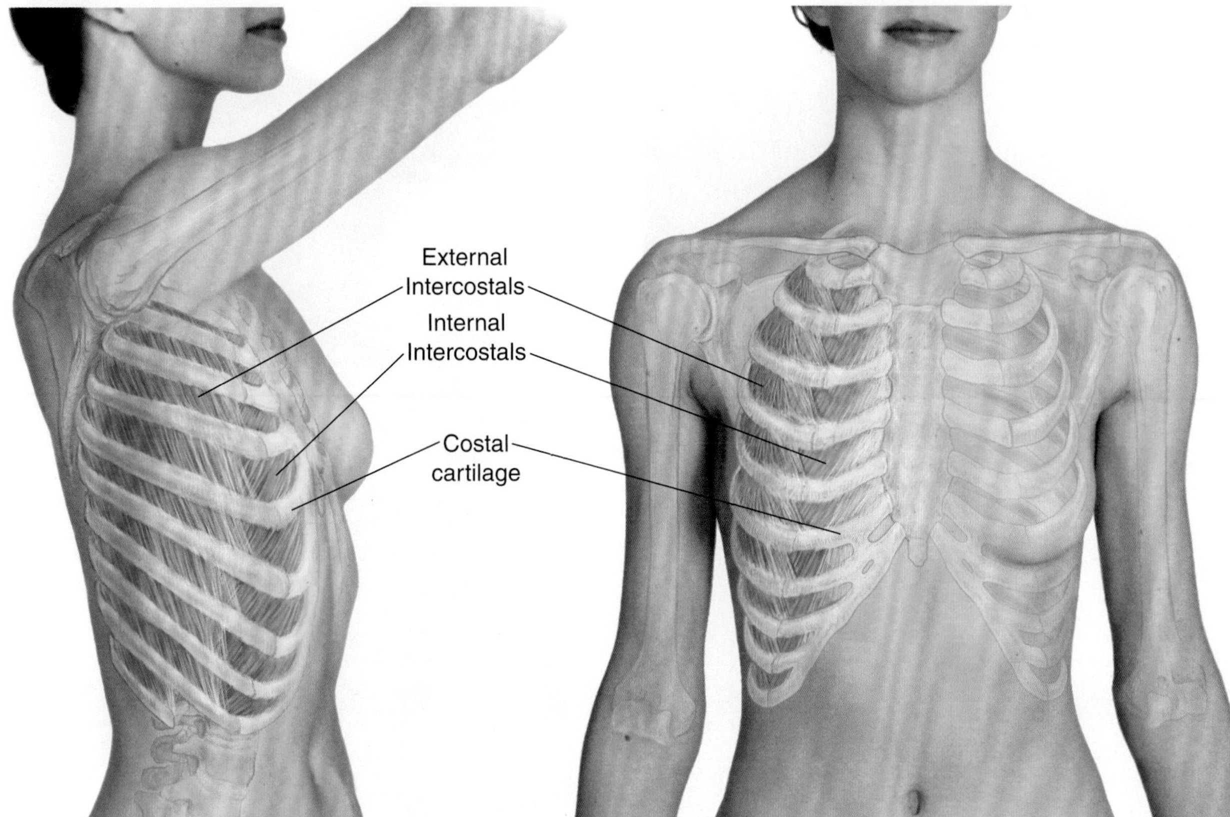

FIGURE 4-68 Anatomy of the intercostals

OTHER MUSCLES TO EXAMINE

- Diaphragm
- Serratus posterior inferior
- Serratus anterior
- Pectoralis major
- Pectoralis minor
- Rectus abdominis
- Transversus abdominis
- External and internal obliques

MANUAL THERAPY

Anterior Treatment

LOWER INTERCOSTALS

Stripping

- The client lies supine.
- Standing beside the client at chest level, place your thumb at the juncture of the eighth and ninth ribs at the costal cartilage on the opposite side of the body.
- Pressing between the ribs and following the curve of the ribs, glide your thumb slowly as far as you can comfortably reach.
- Shift your thumb superiorly to the next intercostal space and repeat the process (Fig. 4-69).
- As you move into the area occupied by the pectoralis major, and the breasts in women, continue your motion only as far as you are able to feel the intercostal space (Fig. 4-70).
- Move to the other side of the client and repeat the process.

Stretch

- The client lies supine.
- Stand next to the client at chest level. Have the client raise the near arm overhead, reaching toward the opposite shoulder.
- Place your hand nearest the client's head on the client's axillary region, maintaining an upward pressure.
- Place your other hand over the client's lower rib cage on the side, maintaining a downward pressure.
- Ask the client to breathe deeply. As the client inhales, use the rib cage hand to resist the elevation of the ribs.
- As the client exhales, press downward on the ribs, and have the client reach toward the opposite shoulder (Fig. 4-71).

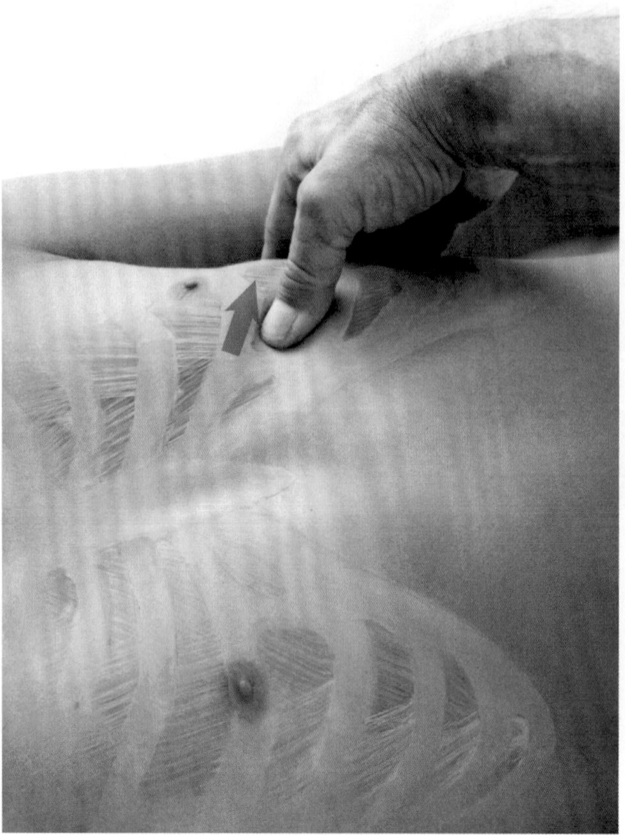

FIGURE 4-69 Stripping massage of intercostals

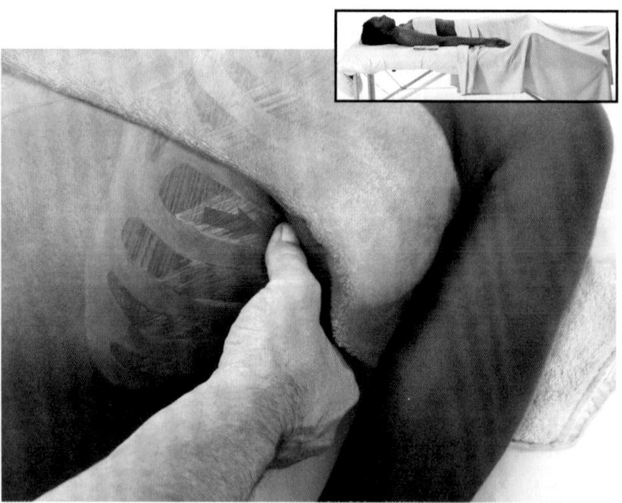

FIGURE 4-70 Stripping massage of intercostals in a female client

- Repeat for two or three cycles, and then move to the other side of the client and repeat the entire process.

UPPER INTERCOSTALS

Stretch

- Stand at the head of the client, who is supine with the hand on the side to be treated raised overhead.

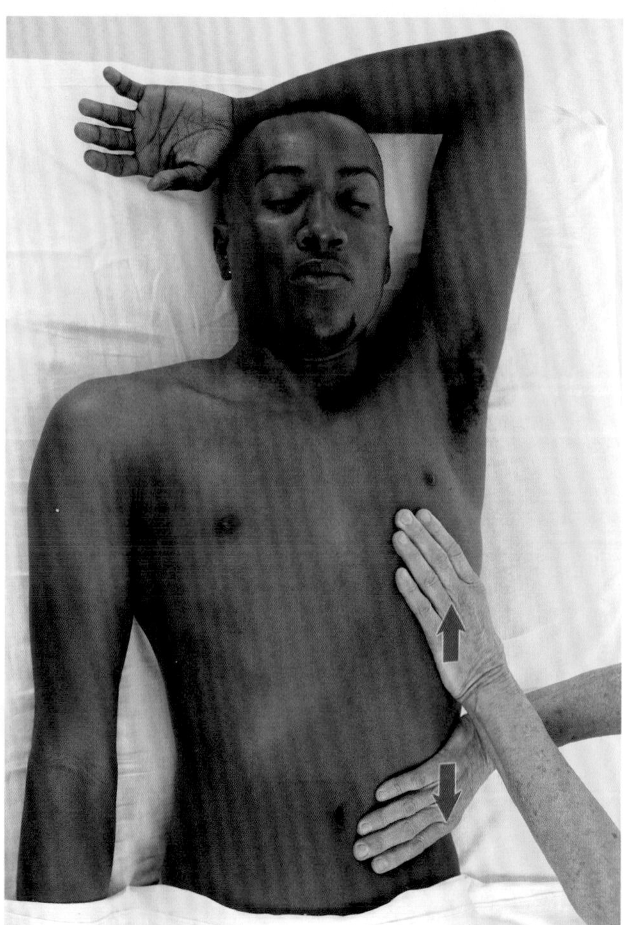

FIGURE 4-71 Lower intercostal stretch

- Place one hand under the client's back on the posterior superior ribs.
- Place the other hand on the client's upper rib cage.
- Ask the client to take slow, deep breaths. Pull the posterior ribs superiorly (toward you) with the hand underneath the client; push the anterior ribs inferiorly (away from you) with the hand on the client's chest (Fig. 4-72).
- Maintain this pressure through five or six breathing cycles, or until you feel release in the rib cage.
- Repeat on the other side.

Posterior Treatment

Posterior trigger points in the intercostals tend to refer anteriorly and should be located and treated individually with compression.

Teaching Diaphragmatic Breathing

Once all the muscles of the breathing apparatus have been released, the client is ready to learn diaphragmatic breathing skills without muscular restrictions. Proceed slowly and patiently; a good rapport with

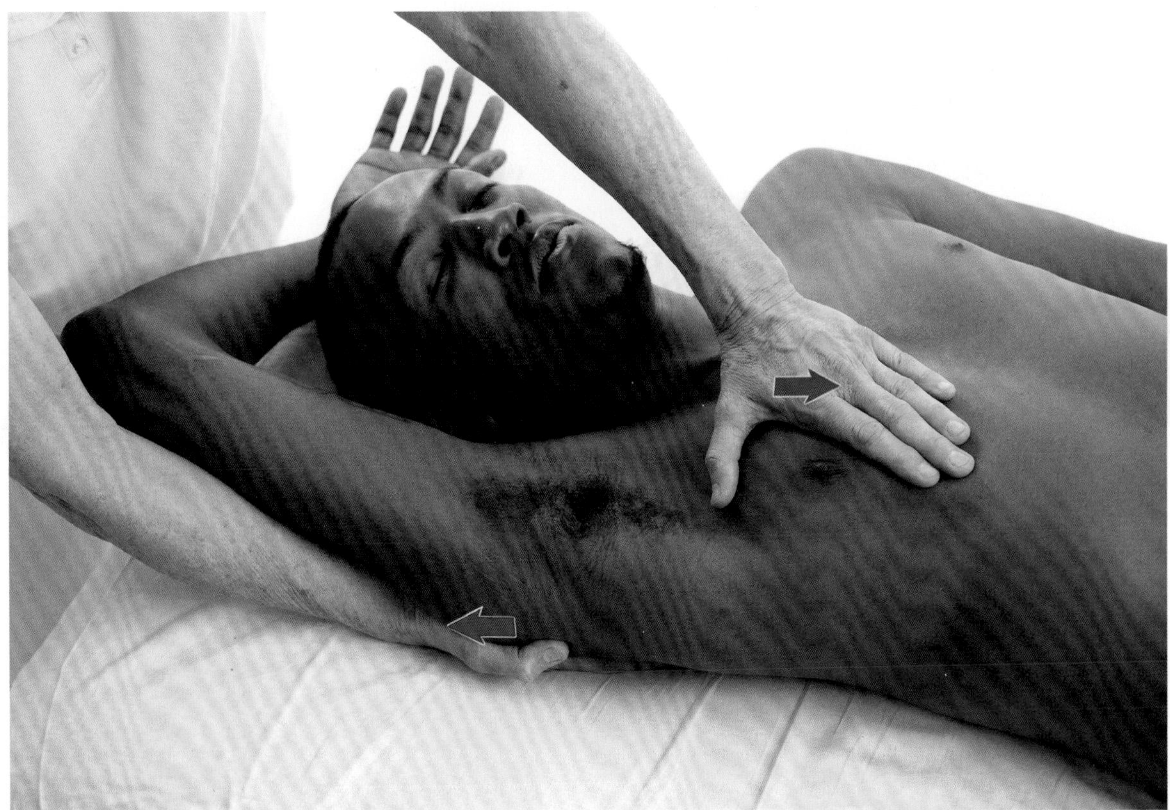

FIGURE 4-72 Upper intercostal stretch

the client is essential. The process will seem awkward and ungainly at first, like any new activity.

The client should experience expansion of the lower rib cage and the abdomen, and then be encouraged to let the expansion move deeply into the pelvic basin. The learning process is kinesthetic, of course, and you can best teach it by placing your hand successively on the lower rib cage, the middle abdomen, and the lower abdomen, and asking the client to direct the breathing expansion into your hand as it lies on each of these areas. Remember that these sensations are new to the client. Be encouraging, patient, and supportive, reinforcing every step in the desired direction.

MANUAL THERAPY

- The client may stand, sit, or lie supine.
- Ask the client to place her or his hands behind the head to neutralize involvement of the shoulders.
- Standing beside the supine client, place one hand (Fig. 4-73A) on the lower anterior rib cage. Alternatively, standing or sitting beside the standing or seated client, place one hand on the lower anterior and the other on the lower posterior rib cage (Fig. 4-74).
- Ask the client to inhale slowly and deeply through the nose, concentrating on breathing into your anterior hand. Continue this until you feel movement in the rib cage (Fig. 4-73B). Verbally reinforce any movement you feel.
- Place one hand on the client's upper abdomen, covering the umbilicus (Fig.4-73C). If the client is standing or seated, place the other hand on the same area of the client's back. Ask the client to inhale slowly and deeply through the nose, concentrating on breathing into your hands. Continue this until you feel the abdomen expand (Fig. 4-73D). Verbally reinforce any movement you feel.
- Place your hand on the lower abdomen just above the pubis (Fig. 4-73E). If the client is standing or seated (Fig. 4-74), place the other hand at the top of the client's sacrum. Ask the client to inhale slowly and deeply through the nose, concentrating on breathing into your hands. Continue this until you feel the abdomen expand (Fig. 4-73F). Verbally reinforce any movement you feel.
- Some people catch on very quickly, whereas others find it more challenging; so work patiently. Urge the client to practice these skills at home. Assure the client that this style of breathing, once mastered, will be far more comfortable and relaxing than his or her previous style.

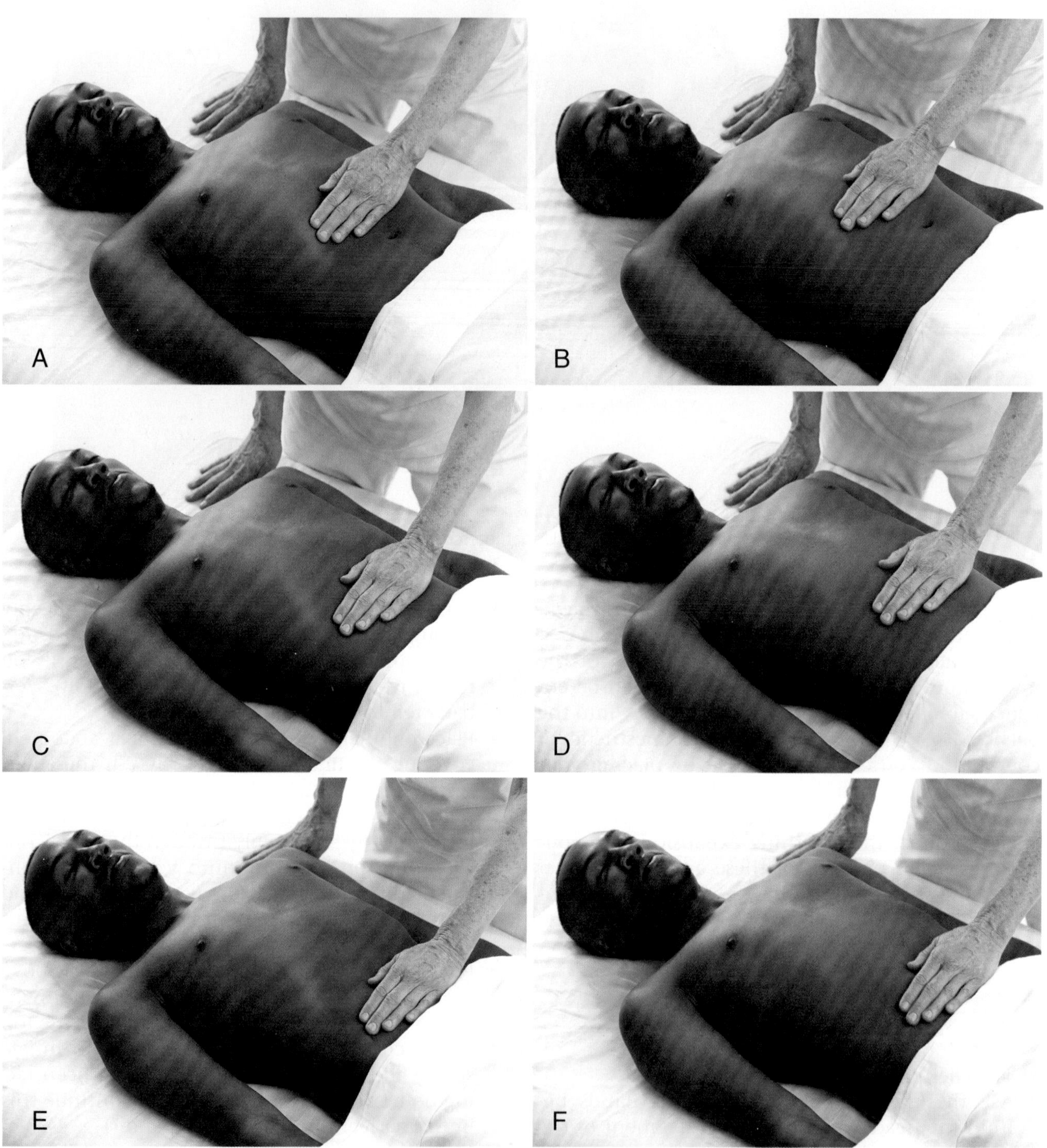

FIGURE 4-73 Teaching diaphragmatic breathing with client supine: **(A)** rib cage neutral, **(B)** rib cage expanded, **(C)** middle abdomen neutral, **(D)** middle abdomen expanded, **(E)** lower abdomen neutral, **(F)** lower abdomen expanded

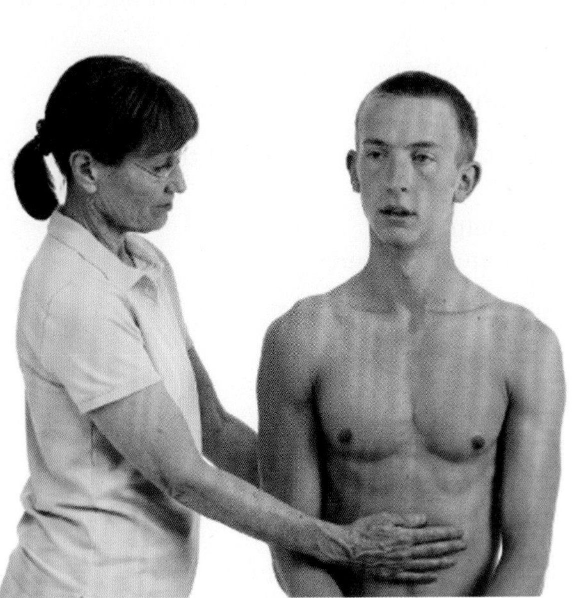
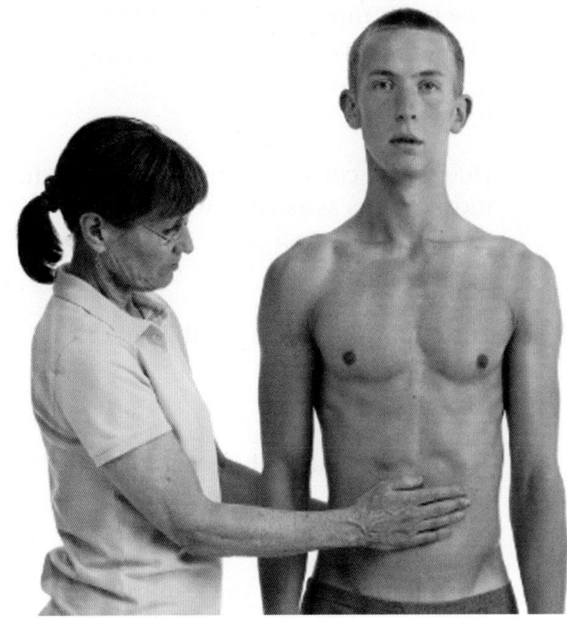

FIGURE 4-74 Teaching diaphragmatic breathing with client standing or seated, with the therapist's hands placed on the anterior and posterior rib cage or abdomen

CHAPTER REVIEW

CASE STUDY

Lou is a 54-year-old professional guitarist and singer; he both performs and gives music lessons. On his first visit, he complained of pain in his right shoulder and upper back. He joked about his "guitaritis" because his guitar strap goes right across the area where he experiences the most pain—the left trapezius muscle, the rhomboids, and all around his right scapula. He has sought massage therapy for relief in the past, but stated that, because of a lot of recent traveling, he has not been on a regular schedule and feels that he has lost some of the progress he had previously made. He stated his pain level was a constant 7 to 8 for the past couple of weeks and that he puts an ice pack on his shoulder after every performance.

The first session began with effleurage to warm the muscles, followed by stripping of the trapezius, the rhomboids, and all the muscles attached around the scapula. The client also received work on the subclavius, pectorals, and axillary muscles, as he tends to "draw in" and rotate the shoulders forward while he is playing. Postsession, he noted his pain level had gone down to 2. He has set up a weekly session for the next 6 weeks, when he has to start traveling again. He is giving me his tour schedule so I can assist him in finding a good therapist when he is on the road. As he is a professional singer, he does breathe correctly and has no issues in that area.

M.H., CMT

REVIEW QUESTIONS

1. The joint that connects the shoulder region and entire upper extremity to the rest of the skeleton is the _______ joint.
   a. Subclavius
   b. Sternoclavicular
   c. Subscapularis
   d. Glenohumeral

2. The shoulder girdle is composed of the manubrium of the sternum, the clavicles, and the _______.
   a. Rotator cuff
   b. Xiphoid process
   c. Two scapulae
   d. Acromion

3. The main muscle that would facilitate pulling yourself up by the arms, such as in doing chin-ups or riding a trapeze, is the _______.
   a. Latissimus dorsi
   b. Pectoralis major
   c. Teres major
   d. Rhomboid

4. Due to the constant tension with the forces of the chest muscles, tautness of the rhomboids is almost always associated with tautness of the _______.
   a. Serratus posterior
   b. Pectorals
   c. Deltoids
   d. Lateral obliques

5. The supraspinatus is a stabilizer of the _______ joint.
   a. Glenohumeral
   b. ASIS
   c. PSIS
   d. Subclavicular

6. The trigger points of teres minor refer to the outer aspect of the _______.
   a. Scapula
   b. Ribs
   c. Chest muscles
   d. Upper arm

7. An inability to raise the arm fully overhead could be a sign of tautness in the _______.
   a. Subscapularis
   b. Erector spinae
   c. Extensor digitorum
   d. Brachioradialis

8. Improper breathing is also referred to as _______ breathing.
   a. Paraclete
   b. Paralyzed
   c. Paradoxical
   d. Paregoric

9. The external intercostals _______ during inspiration.
   a. Prevent rib movement
   b. Relax
   c. Raise the ribs
   d. Lower the ribs

10. Proper breathing is known as _______ breathing.
   a. Thoracic
   b. Diaphragmatic
   c. Harmonic
   d. Paroxysmal

CHAPTER 5

The Arm and Hand

LEARNING OBJECTIVES

At the end of this chapter, the learner will be able to:

- State the correct terminology of the muscles of the arm and hand.
- Palpate the muscles of the arm and hand.
- Identify their attachments at the origins and insertions.
- Explain the actions of the muscles.
- Describe their pain referral areas.
- Recall related muscles.
- Recognize any endangerment sites and ethical cautions for massage therapy.
- Demonstrate proficiency in manual therapy techniques for muscles of the arm and hand.

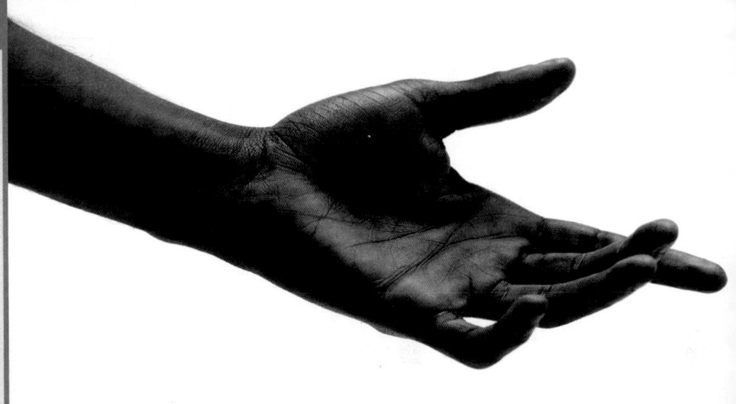

The Overview of the Region begins on page 166, after the anatomy plates.

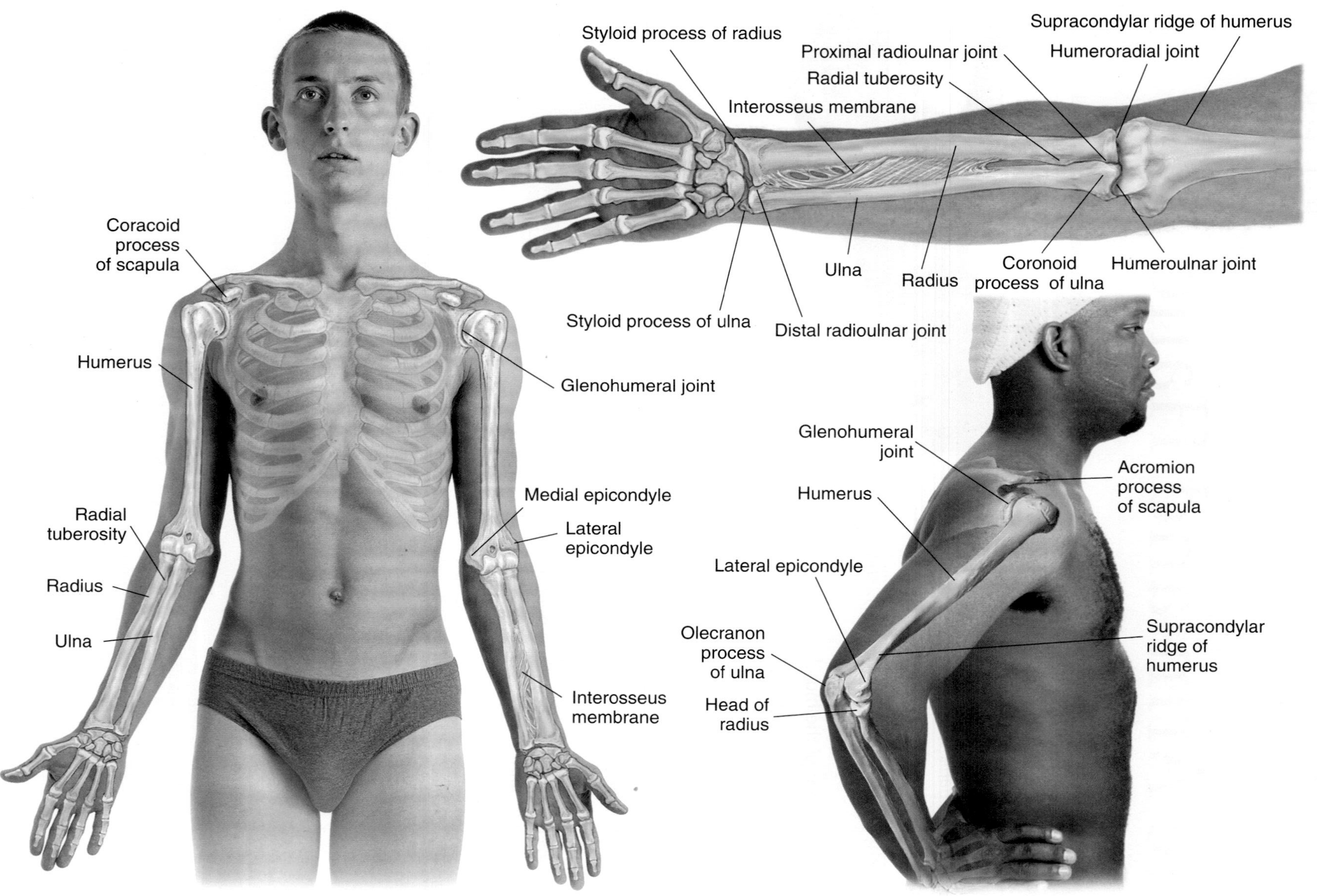

PLATE 5-1 ■ Skeletal features of the arm

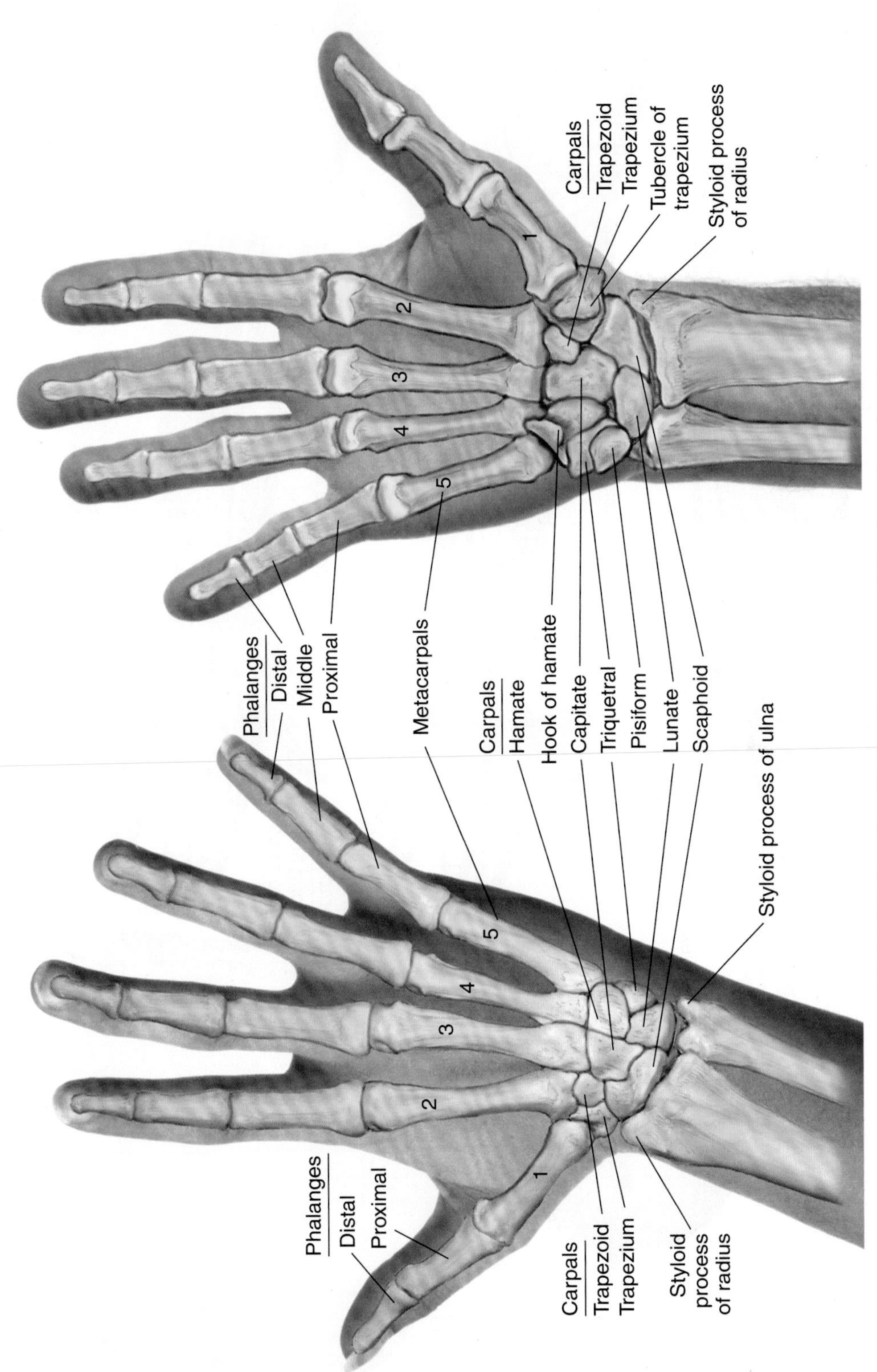

PLATE 5-2 ■ Skeletal features of the hand and wrist

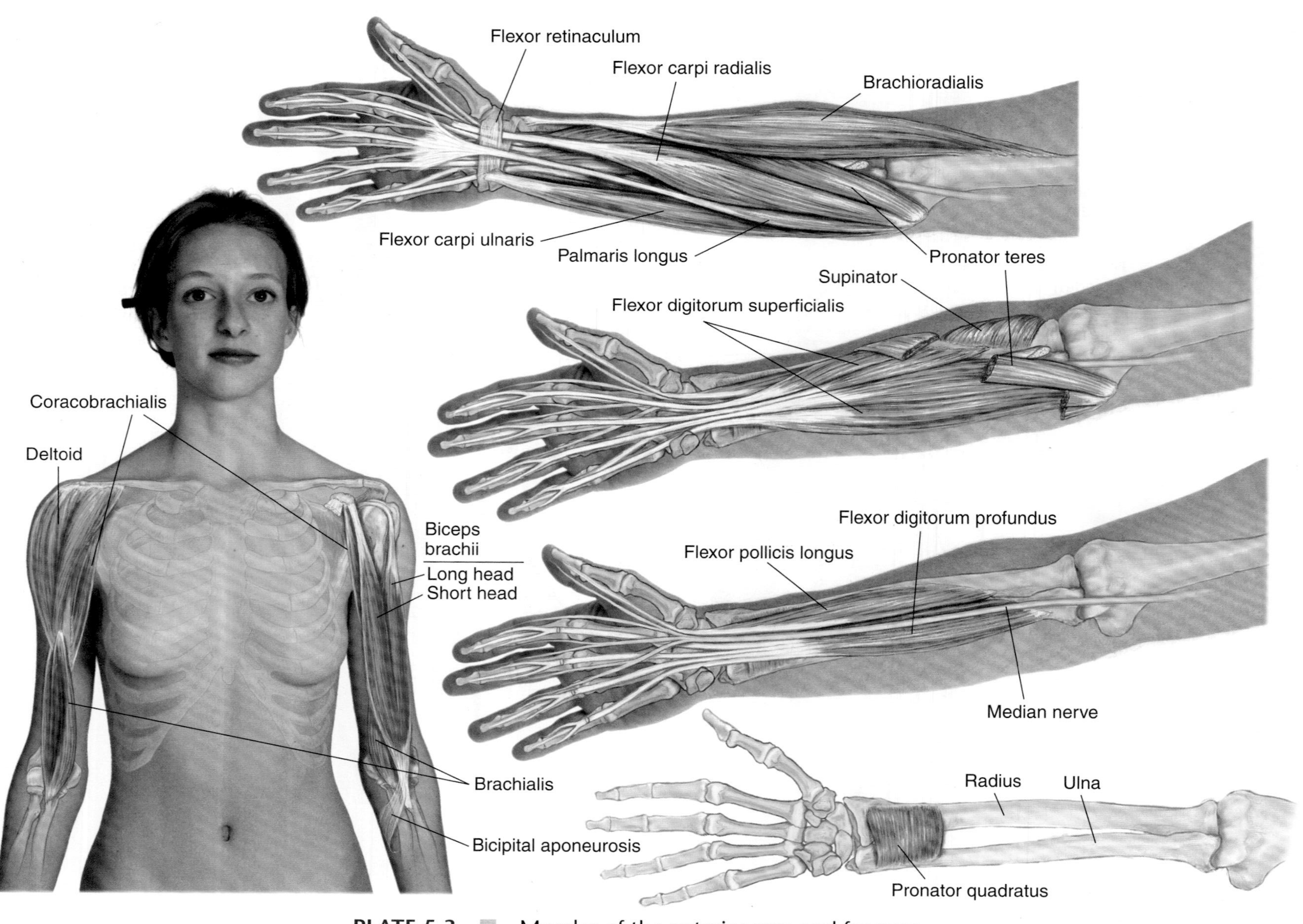

PLATE 5-3 ■ Muscles of the anterior arm and forearm

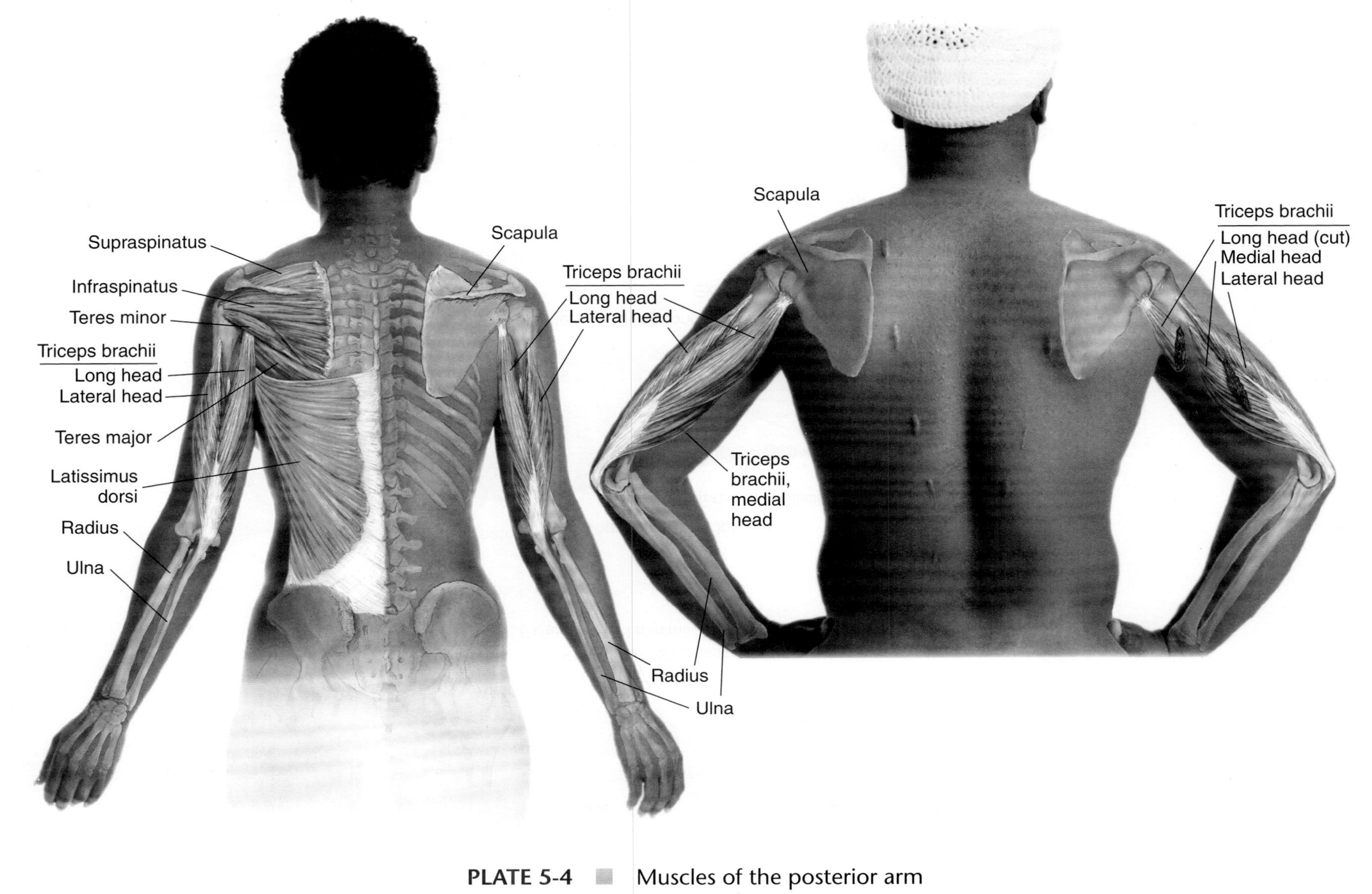

PLATE 5-4 ■ Muscles of the posterior arm

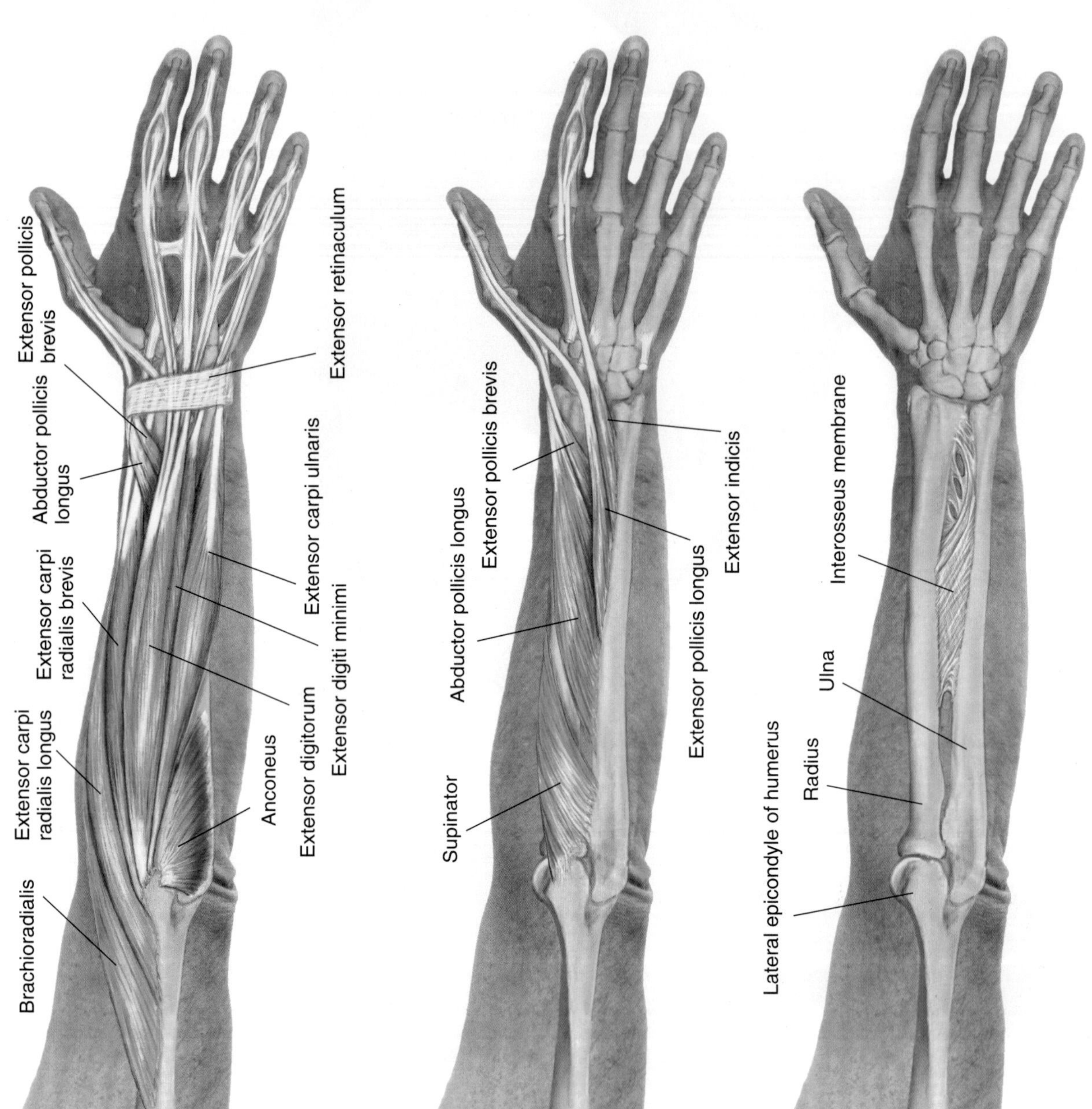

PLATE 5-5 ■ Muscles of the posterior forearm

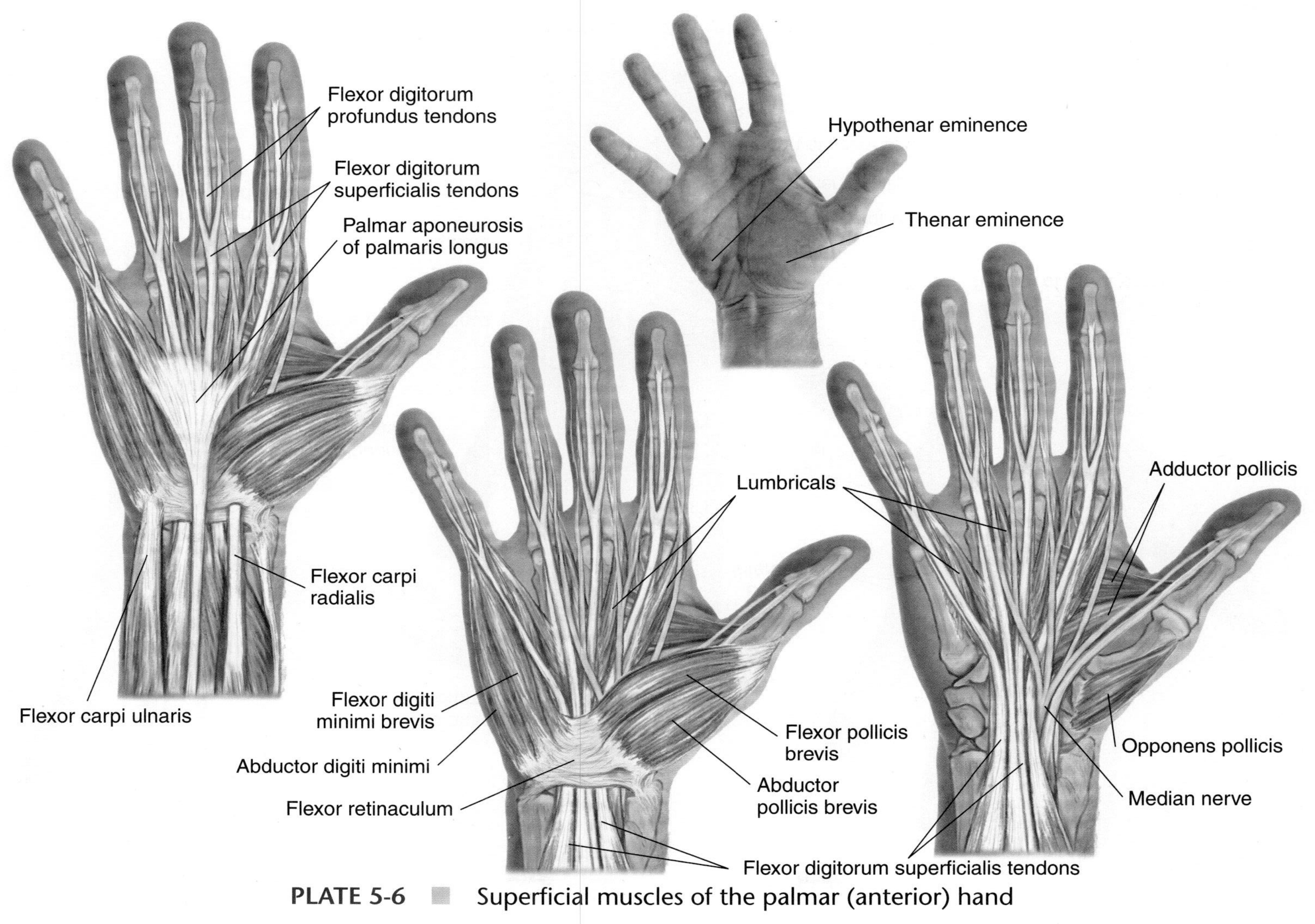

PLATE 5-6 ■ Superficial muscles of the palmar (anterior) hand

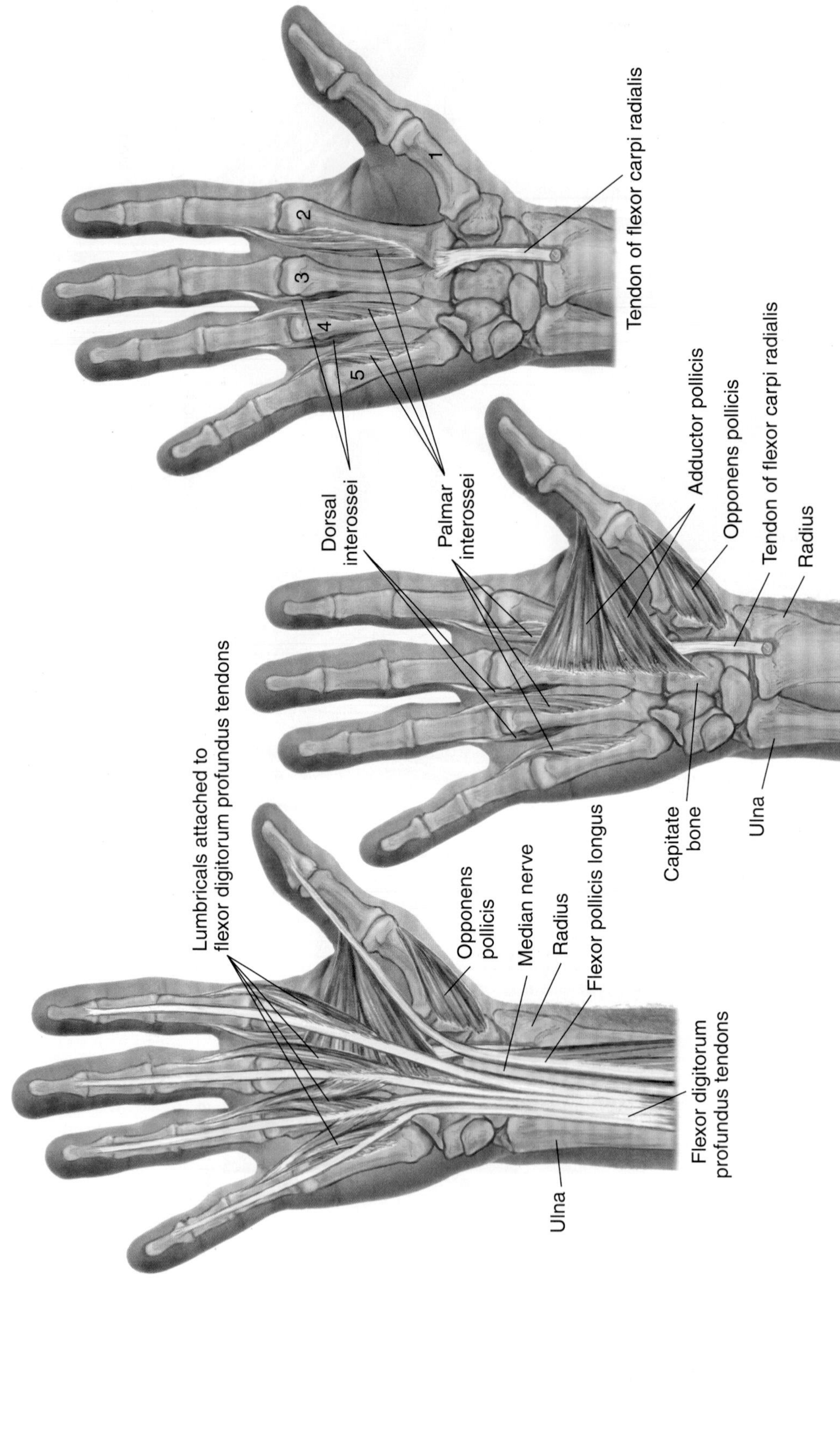

Lumbricals attached to flexor digitorum profundus tendons
Opponens pollicis
Median nerve
Radius
Flexor pollicis longus
Flexor digitorum profundus tendons
Ulna

Dorsal interossei
Palmar interossei
Adductor pollicis
Opponens pollicis
Tendon of flexor carpi radialis
Radius
Capitate bone
Ulna

1
2
3
4
5
Tendon of flexor carpi radialis

PLATE 5-7 ■ Deep muscles of the palmar (anterior) hand

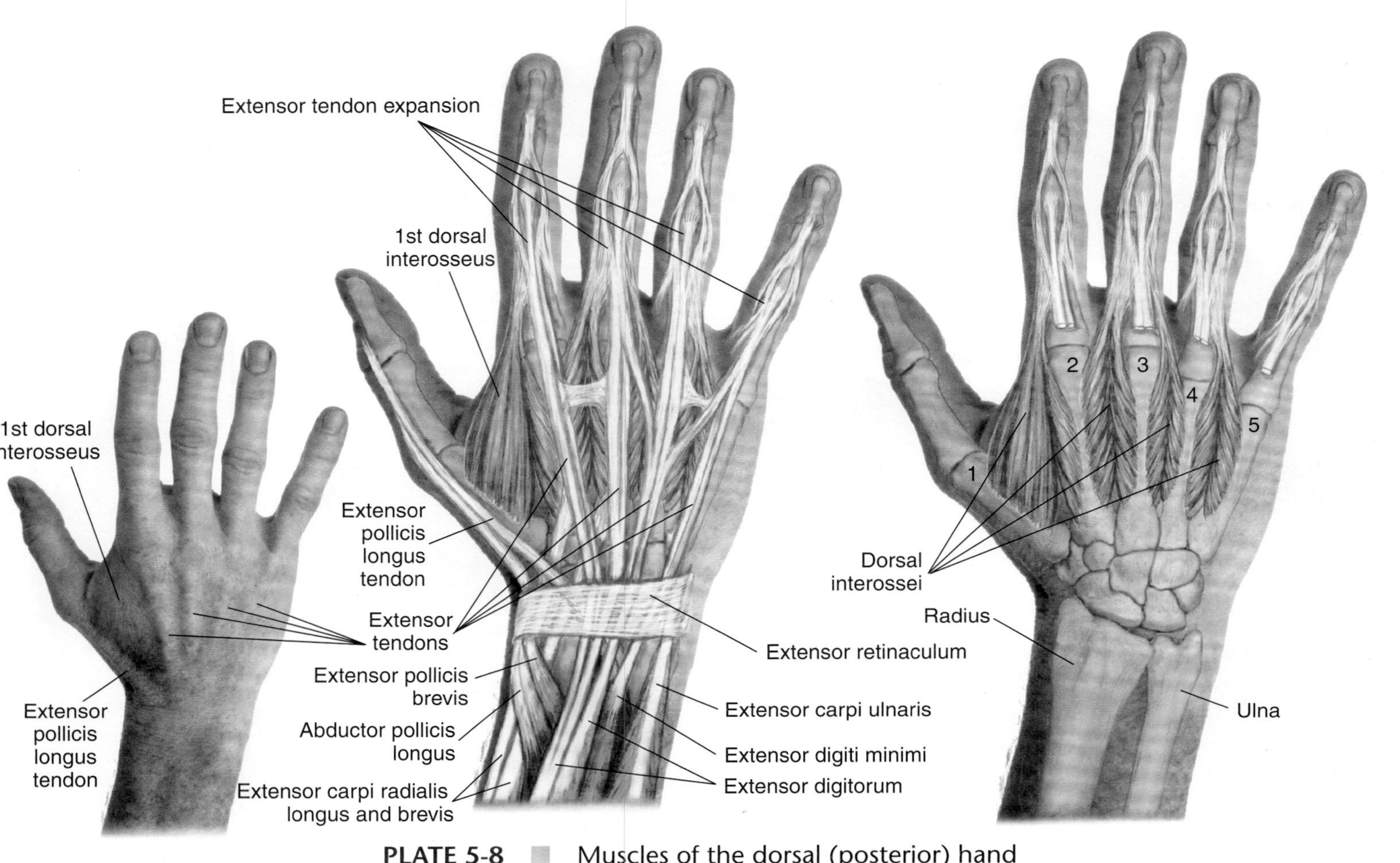

PLATE 5-8 ■ Muscles of the dorsal (posterior) hand

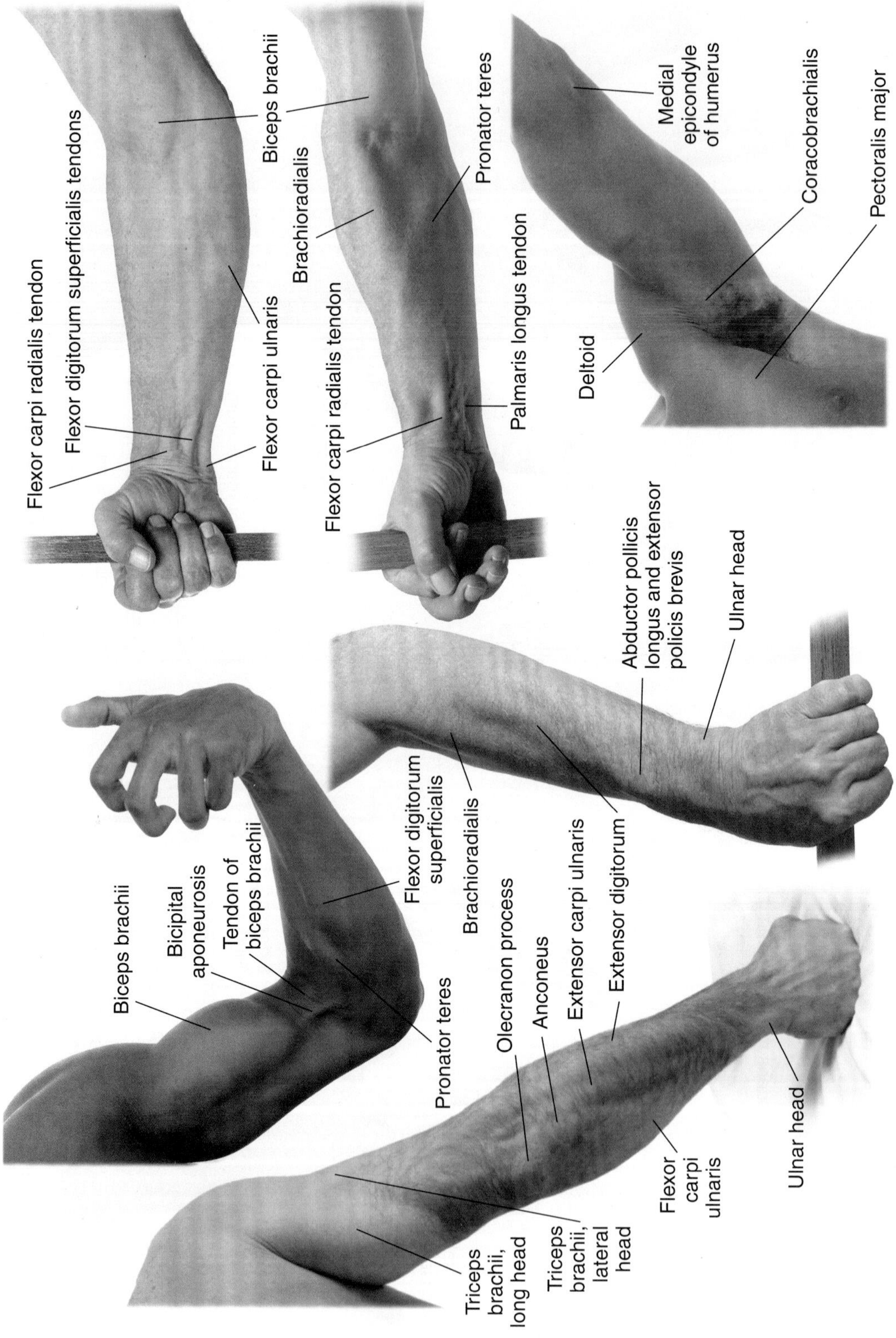

PLATE 5-9 ■ Surface anatomy of the arm and forearm

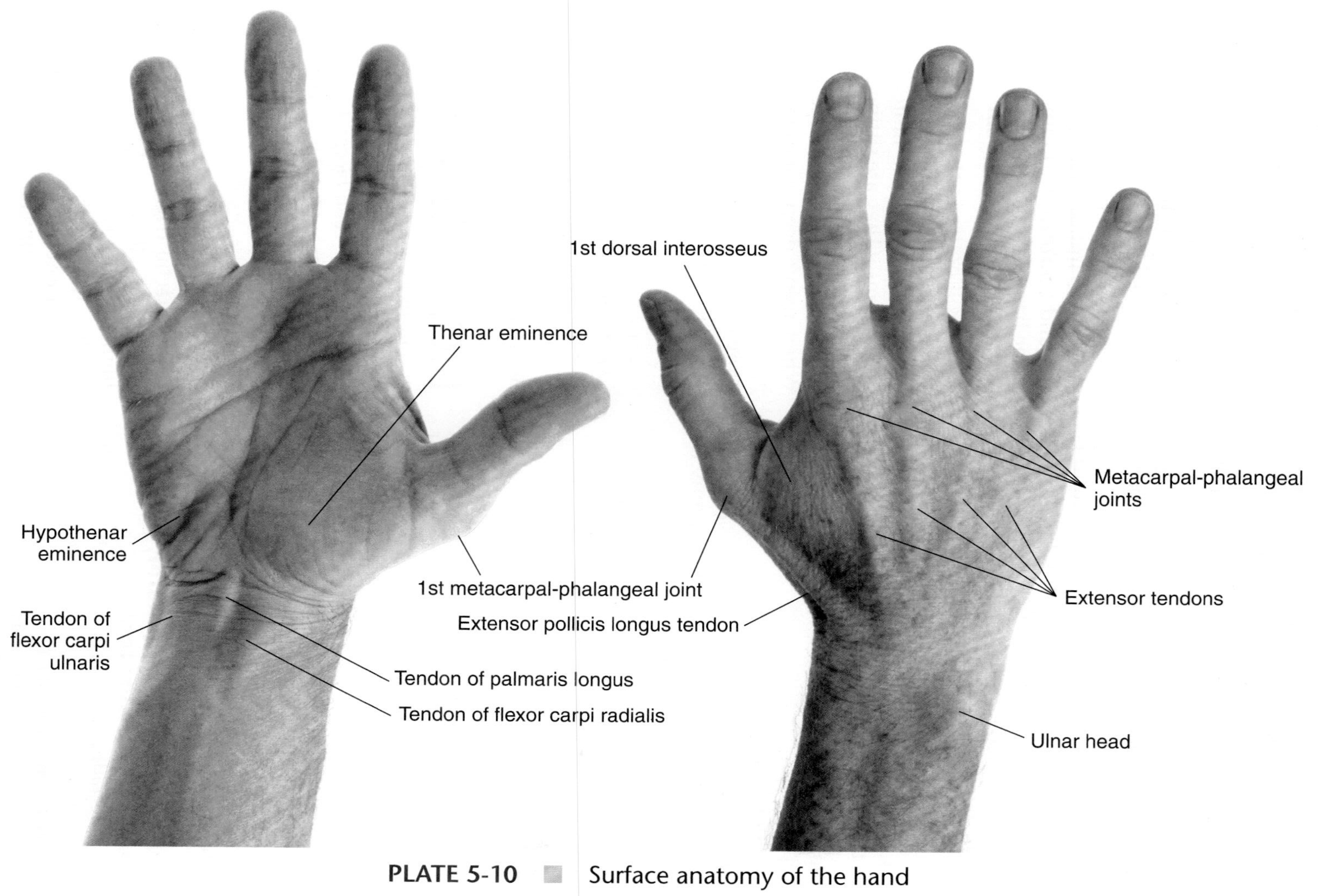

PLATE 5-10 ■ Surface anatomy of the hand

Overview of the Region (Plates 5-1 to 5-10)

Pain in the arm and hand presents a clinical challenge because it can originate in so many different places. Nerve entrapments at the cervical roots, thoracic outlet, pectoralis minor attachment to the coracoid process, or in the arm itself, including the wrist, may be responsible for arm or hand pain. Arm or hand pain may also be referred from trigger points in the muscles of the neck, shoulder, upper arm, or forearm. An assessment of arm or hand pain must include all these possibilities.

In anatomy, the word "arm" (Latin brachium) is reserved for what we normally call the upper arm. The term "forearm" is used to denote the lower arm. The arm consists of a single bone, the *humerus,* which articulates with the scapula via the *glenohumeral joint.* We have already seen the muscles that cross the glenohumeral joint from the scapula in Chapter 4. The muscles that reside on the humerus and cross the glenohumeral joint are:

- biceps brachii
- triceps brachii
- coracobrachialis

The elbow consists of two joints: the *humeroradial* and *humeroulnar* joints. The significant muscles crossing this pair of joints are:

- biceps brachii
- triceps brachii
- brachialis
- anconeus
- brachioradialis

The arm and forearm joints distal to the glenohumeral joint allow several distinct movements, which in combination provide a considerable range of movement. The elbow joint is limited to flexion and extension while the proximal and distal radioulnar joints allow a pivoting rotation of the radius around the ulna, called **supination** ("palm up," lateral or upward rotation) and **pronation** ("palm down," medial or downward rotation). The proximal (or superior) radioulnar joint shares the joint capsule with the elbow joint, but plays no functional role at the elbow. Radioulnar rotation is accomplished primarily by **biceps brachii, supinator, pronator quadratus,** and **pronator teres**.

Distally, the radius and ulna articulate with the carpal bones of the **wrist** and with each other at the **distal radioulnar joint**.

One wrist structure that deserves special clinical attention is the **carpal tunnel**, formed by the carpal bones deep and on either side, and the **flexor retinaculum** superficially. This tunnel permits passage of the flexor tendons and the median nerve to the hand (see Fig. 5-33). When these tendons become inflamed and swollen, they compress the median nerve, producing pain and numbness in its distribution area of the hand, known as **carpal tunnel syndrome**. Numbness and tingling in the extremities can also indicate other conditions, including the peripheral neuropathy that often accompanies diabetes, multiple sclerosis, stroke, transient ischemic attack (TIA, or mini-stroke), an underactive thyroid, or Raynaud's phenomenon.

The muscles that cross the wrist are the flexors and extensors of the hand and fingers, which will be addressed in some detail in this chapter.

Note: Directional terms used in this chapter include **"volar"** to indicate the anterior aspect of the forearm and **"palmar"** to indicate the anterior aspect of the hand in anatomical position. The opposite of both these terms is **"dorsal"** or posterior.

You will notice in the directions for manual therapy, the therapist is always directed to stand. Many massage therapists are more comfortable working on the arms if they are sitting tableside at about hip level to work on the upper arms, and about mid-thigh level to work on the forearms and hands. When using deep compression for myofascial release, standing gives you more leverage. If you are more comfortable sitting for arm work, follow your instincts. Different strokes for different folks!

Etymology

- Latin *vola*, palm of the hand or sole of the foot
- Latin *palma*, palm of the hand
- Latin *dorsum*, back

Muscles of the Upper Arm

BICEPS BRACHII

BI-seps BRAY-kee-eye

ETYMOLOGY Latin ***biceps***, two-headed + ***brachii***, of the arm. Note: in anatomical terminology, the Latin word ***brachium*** and the English word ***arm*** refer technically to the upper arm and do not include the forearm.

Overview

Biceps brachii (Fig. 5-1) crosses three joints: the glenohumeral, elbow, and radioulnar. It resides on the humerus but has no attachments to it. Although we think of it as the flexor of the elbow, biceps brachii is also the most powerful supinator of the forearm and assists glenohumeral movement.

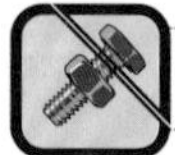

ATTACHMENTS

- Origin: long head from supraglenoid tuberosity of scapula, short head from coracoid process

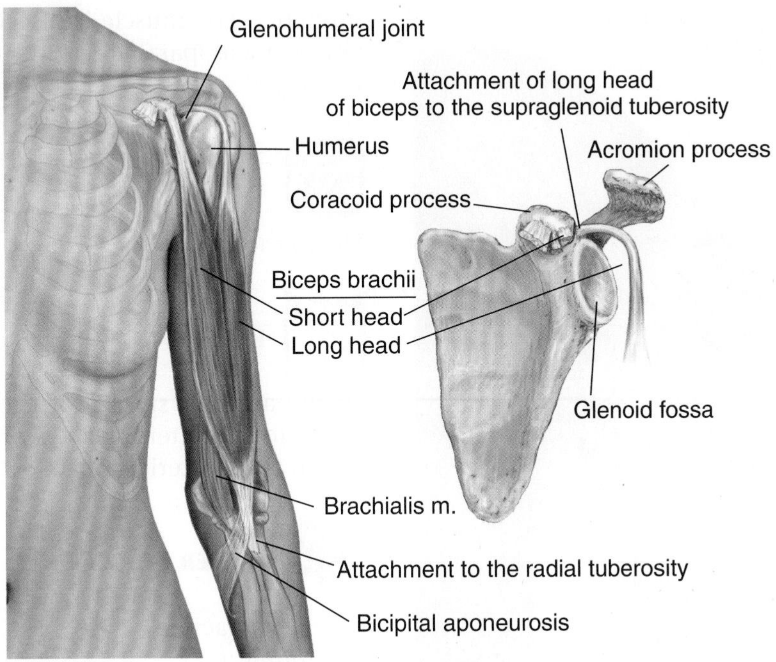

FIGURE 5-1 Anatomy of biceps brachii

- Insertion: tuberosity of radius and antebrachial fascia by the aponeurosis of the biceps brachii

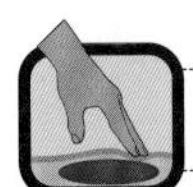

PALPATION

Origin

- Architecture of biceps brachii is parallel, and its fibers are largely parallel to the humerus.
- Long head: follow the muscle up to the intertubercular groove of the humerus, beyond which it passes under the acromion process and is no longer palpable.
- Short head: follow the muscle into the axilla and up to the coracoid process.

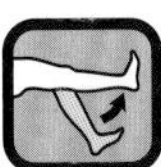

ACTION

Flexes the elbow, supinates the forearm, and assists in glenohumeral flexion, adduction, and abduction

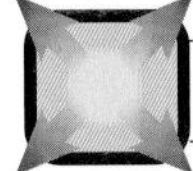

REFERRAL AREA

Over the area of the muscle itself, to the inner aspect of the elbow, to the area of the middle deltoid, and to the area just proximal to supraspinatus

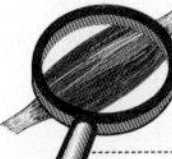

OTHER MUSCLES TO EXAMINE

- Brachialis
- Supinator
- Brachioradialis
- Middle deltoid
- Rotator cuff muscles

MANUAL THERAPY

Stripping

- The client lies supine.
- The therapist stands beside the client at the hip.
- Place the knuckles on the muscle at the elbow.
- Pressing firmly into the tissue, slide the knuckles proximally along the muscle (Fig. 5-2) to the head of the humerus.
- Beginning at the same spot, repeat this procedure, following the short head medially to the axilla.

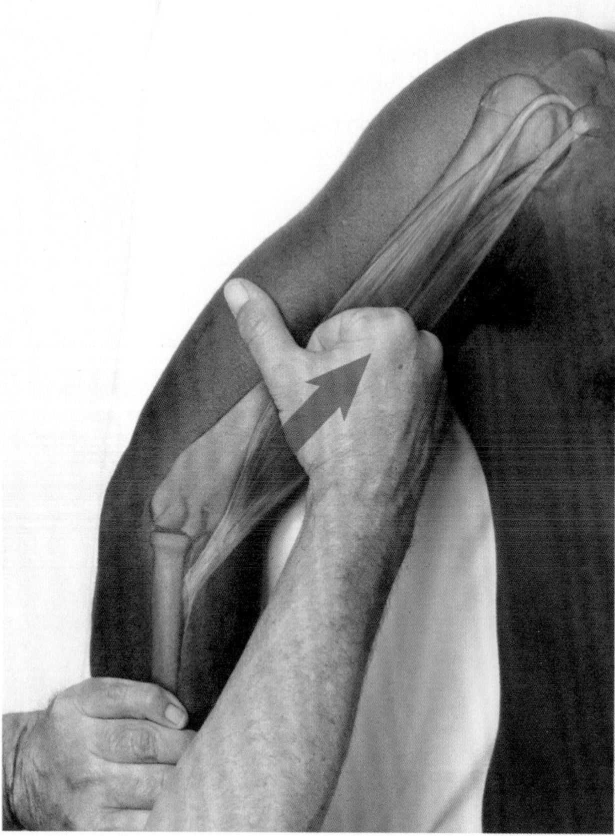

FIGURE 5-2 Stripping massage of biceps using knuckles

BRACHIALIS

BRAY-kee-AL-is

ETYMOLOGY Latin ***brachium***, arm

Overview

Brachialis (Fig. 5-3) is a prime flexor of the elbow. It balances the biceps' pull on the radius with its attachment to the ulna. Biceps brachii must be displaced to work on this muscle.

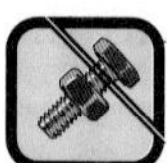

ATTACHMENTS

- Origin: to the lower half of anterior surface of humerus and the associated intermuscular septa
- Insertion: coronoid process of the ulna

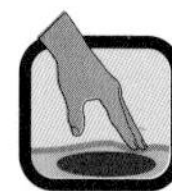

PALPATION

Brachialis can be palpated from the distal half of the medial side of the arm between biceps and the humerus. The muscle is discernible here and its architecture is parallel. Its fibers are parallel to the humerus.

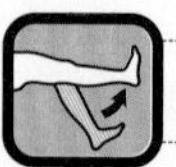

ACTION

Flexes the elbow

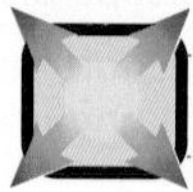

REFERRAL AREA

To the anterior surface of the arm up to the acromion, to the anterior aspect of the elbow, and to the lateral and posterior aspect of the base of the thumb

OTHER MUSCLES TO EXAMINE

- Biceps brachii
- Supinator
- Brachioradialis
- Opponens pollicis
- Adductor pollicis

MANUAL THERAPY

Stripping

- The client lies supine.
- The therapist stands beside the client at the hip.
- Place the thumb on the lateral aspect of the distal extent of brachialis just proximal to the elbow, pushing biceps brachii medially out of the way.

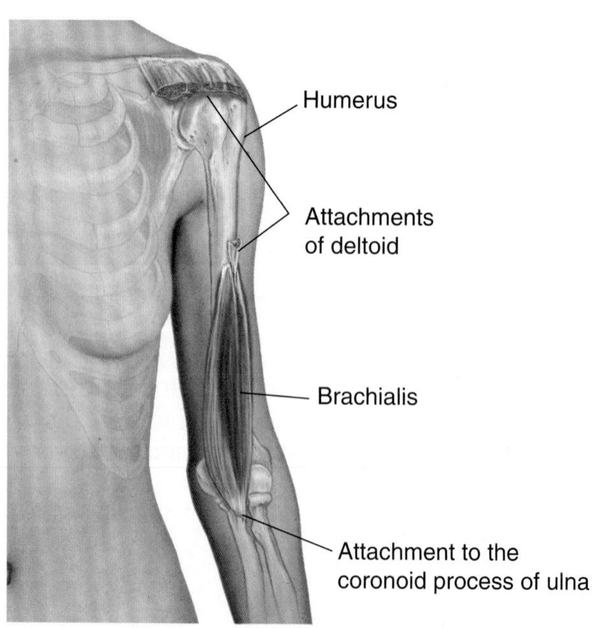

FIGURE 5-3 Anatomy of brachialis

- Pressing firmly into the tissue, slide the thumb along brachialis (Fig. 5-4) to its attachment on the humerus just distal to the attachment of the middle deltoid.
- Repeat the stroke on the medial side of the muscle (Fig. 5-5), continuing about halfway up the humerus.

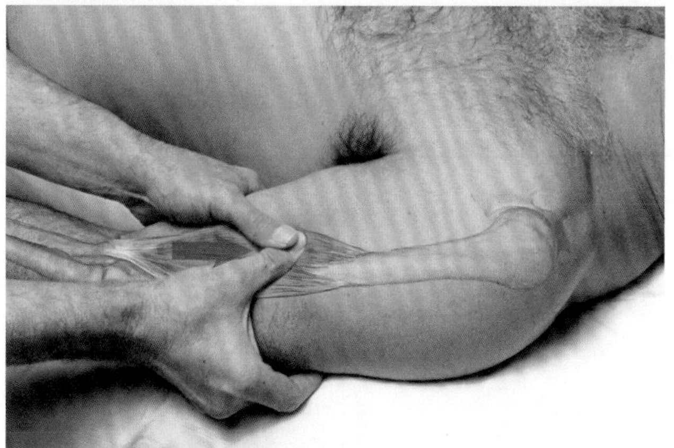

FIGURE 5-4 Stripping massage of brachialis using supported thumb (from lateral side)

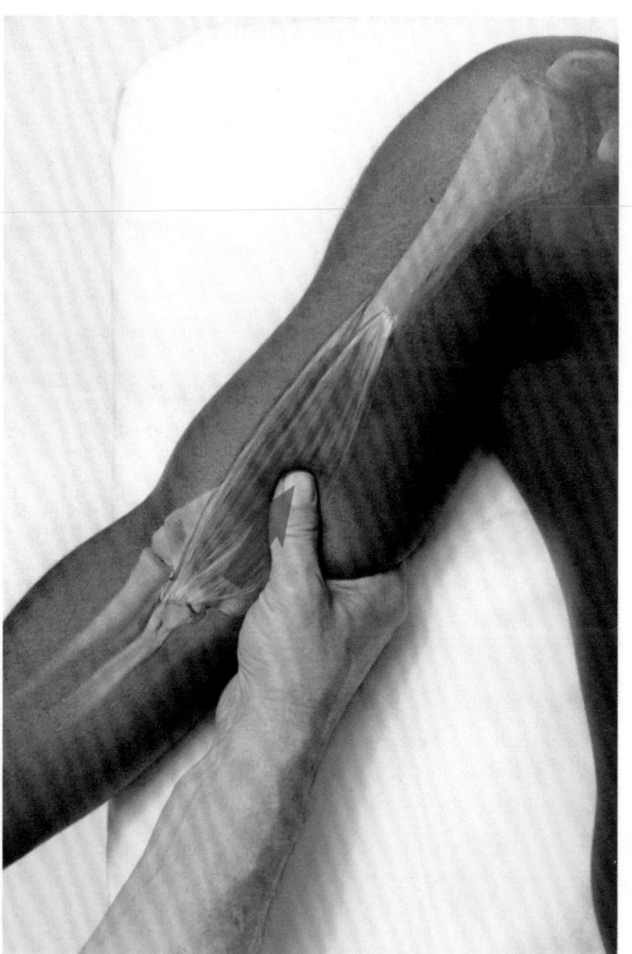

FIGURE 5-5 Stripping massage of brachialis using the thumb (from medial side)

TRICEPS BRACHII

TRY-seps BRAY-kee-eye

ETYMOLOGY Latin ***triceps***, three-headed+ ***brachii***, of the arm

Overview

Two of the three heads of triceps brachii (Fig. 5-6) cross only the elbow joint, while the long head crosses both the elbow and shoulder joints. This muscle opposes biceps brachii and brachialis. Its trigger points can cause pain in an area ranging from the neck to the fingers.

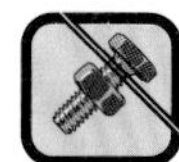

ATTACHMENTS

Origin

- Long or scapular head: infraglenoid tubercle at the lateral border of scapula inferior to the glenoid fossa
- Lateral head: lateral and posterior surface of humerus below greater tubercle
- Medial head: distal posterior surface of humerus

Insertion (all three heads)

- Olecranon of ulna

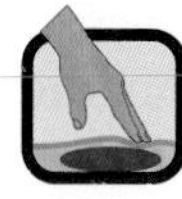

PALPATION

Palpate from the olecranon process to (1) long head: the upper, outer edge of the scapula; (2) medial head: upper posterior surface of humerus; and (3) lateral

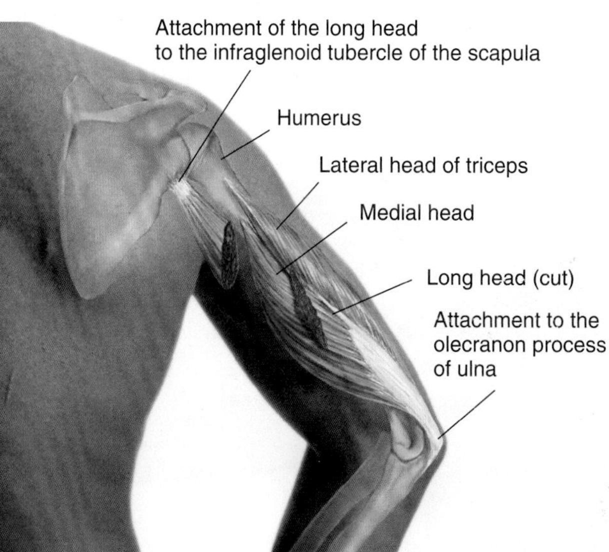

FIGURE 5-6 Anatomy of triceps brachii

head: outer posterior surface of humerus. It is discernible. Its architecture as a whole is bipennate, and fibers of its main body are parallel to the humerus.

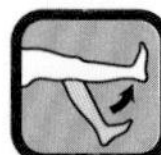

ACTION

Extends elbow; long head assists in glenohumeral extension and adduction

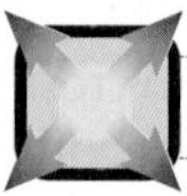

REFERRAL AREA

To the dorsal surface of the arm proximally over the back of the shoulder and distally to the back of the hand into the 4th and 5th fingers; also over the volar surface of the forearm and just proximal to the elbow

OTHER MUSCLES TO EXAMINE

- All the muscles of the arm and forearm
- Rotator cuff muscles
- Pectoralis minor
- Pectoralis major

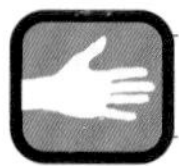

MANUAL THERAPY

Stripping

- The client lies prone.
- The therapist stands beside the client at the waist.
- Place the thumb, knuckles, or fingertips on the muscle just proximal to the olecranon process.
- Pressing firmly into the tissue, slide the thumb, knuckles, or fingertips (Figs. 5-7 and 5-8) along the muscle to the attachment of the posterior deltoid.
- The client lies supine.
- The therapist stands at the client head.
- Position the client's hand under the shoulder (Fig. 5-9A).
- Place the heel of the hand just proximal to the olecranon process.

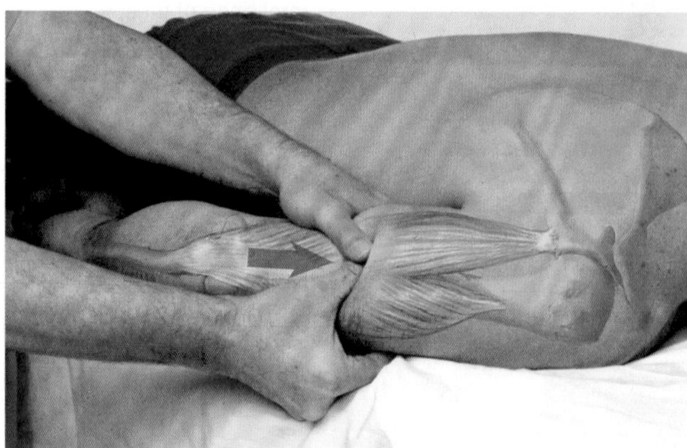

FIGURE 5-7 Stripping massage of triceps using thumbs

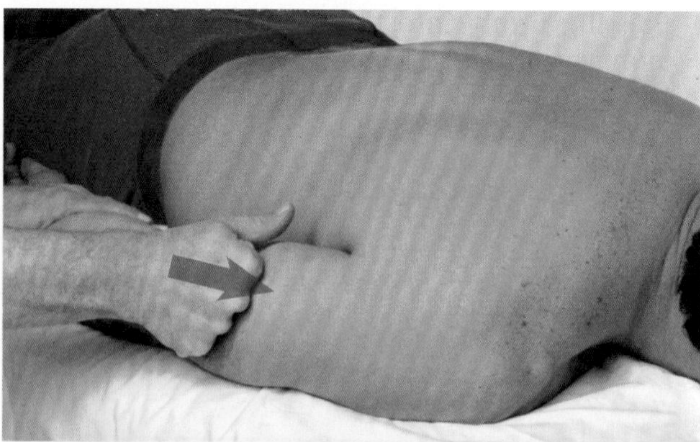

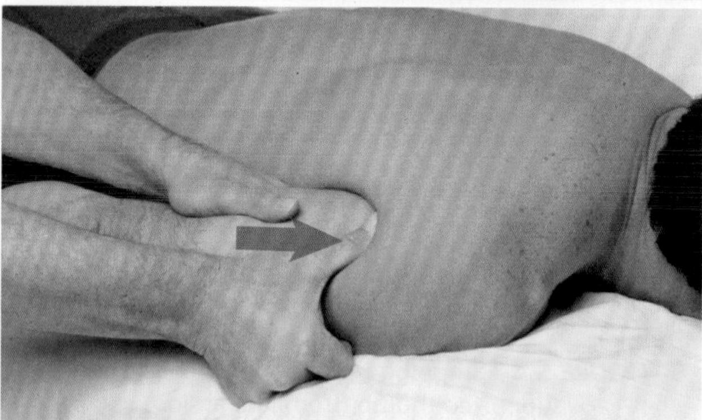

FIGURE 5-8 Stripping massage of triceps using knuckles and the thumb

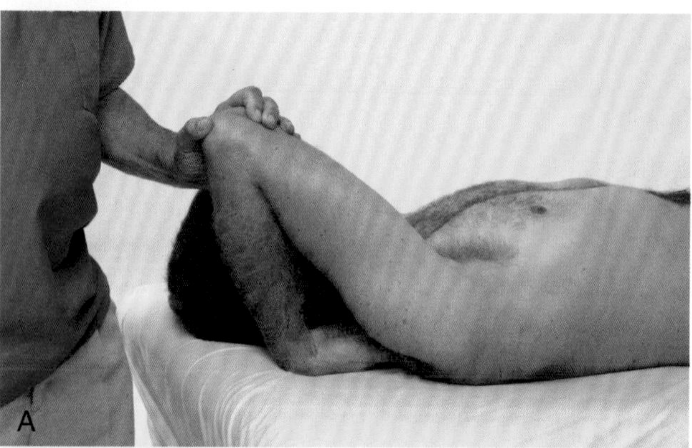

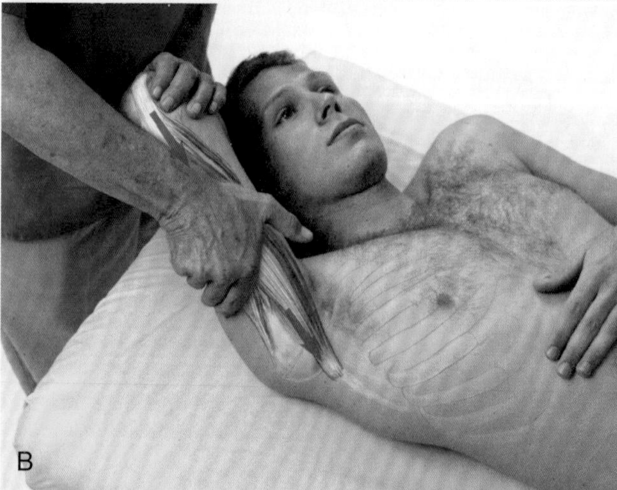

FIGURE 5-9 Stripping massage of triceps in supine position with heel of hand. **(A)** Positioning of client, **(B)** stripping

- Pressing firmly into the tissue, slide the heel of the hand along triceps to the attachment on the scapula (Fig. 5-9B).

ANCONEUS

ang-KO-knee-us, an-KO-knee-us

ETYMOLOGY Latin ***ancon***, from Greek ***ankon***, elbow

Overview

Anconeus (Fig. 5-10) is a small muscle that assists triceps brachii in elbow extension. Its pain referral zone is local.

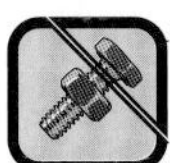

ATTACHMENTS

- Origin: posterior aspect of the lateral epicondyle of the humerus
- Insertion: olecranon process and the posterior surface of the ulna

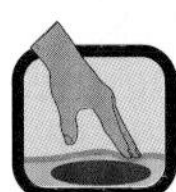

PALPATION

Palpable just distal to the lateral epicondyle of the humerus and the lateral side of the olecranon process of the ulna. Its architecture is convergent, and its fibers are diagonal to the forearm.

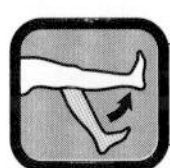

ACTION

Extends elbow

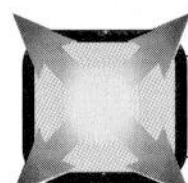

REFERRAL AREA

Area over the lateral epicondyle of humerus

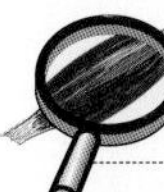

OTHER MUSCLES TO EXAMINE

- Triceps brachii
- Scalenes
- Supraspinatus
- Serratus posterior superior

MANUAL THERAPY

Stripping

- The client may be in any position that makes the dorsal aspect of the elbow easily accessible.
- Place the thumb on the proximal posterior aspect of the ulna just distal to the olecranon.
- Pressing firmly into the tissue, slide the thumb along the muscle (Fig. 5-11) diagonally to its attachment on the lateral epicondyle of the humerus (a very short distance!).

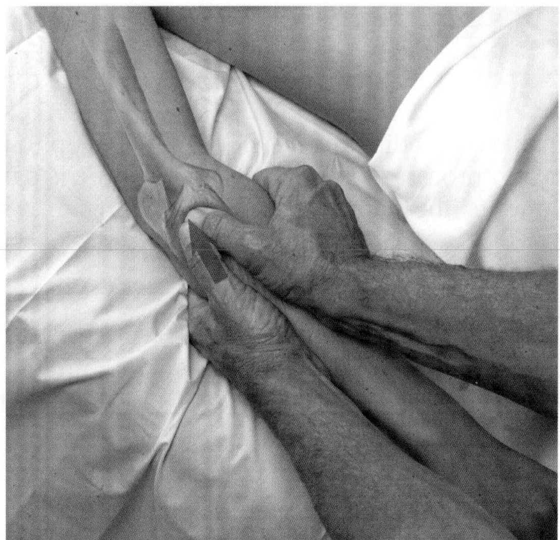

FIGURE 5-11 Stripping massage of anconeus

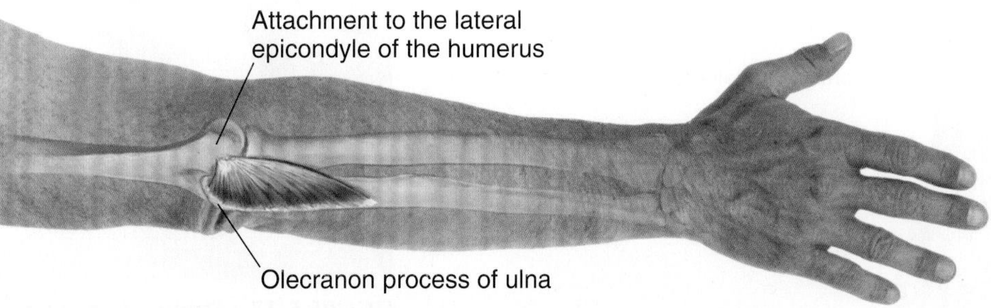

FIGURE 5-10 Anatomy of anconeus, dorsal (posterior) view

CORACOBRACHIALIS

KOR-a-ko-BRAKE-ee-AL-is

ETYMOLOGY From ***coracoid*** (Greek ***korakodes***, like a raven's beak, from ***korax***, raven + ***eidos***, resemblance) + Latin ***brachialis***, relating to the arm ***(brachium)***

Overview

Coracobrachialis (Fig. 5-12) is one of three muscles that attach to the coracoid process of the scapula and that maintain the complex, three-way interaction of the arm, scapula, and chest (rib cage). The other two muscles are biceps brachii and pectoralis minor.

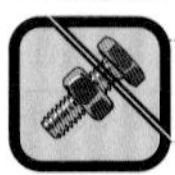

ATTACHMENTS

- Origin: coracoid process of the scapula
- Insertion: middle of the medial border of the humerus

PALPATION

Palpable on medial upper half of humerus up to the coracoid process of scapula. Its architecture is parallel, and its fibers are diagonal.

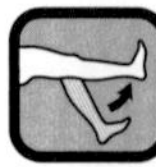

ACTION

- Adducts and flexes the glenohumeral joint
- Resists downward dislocation of shoulder joint

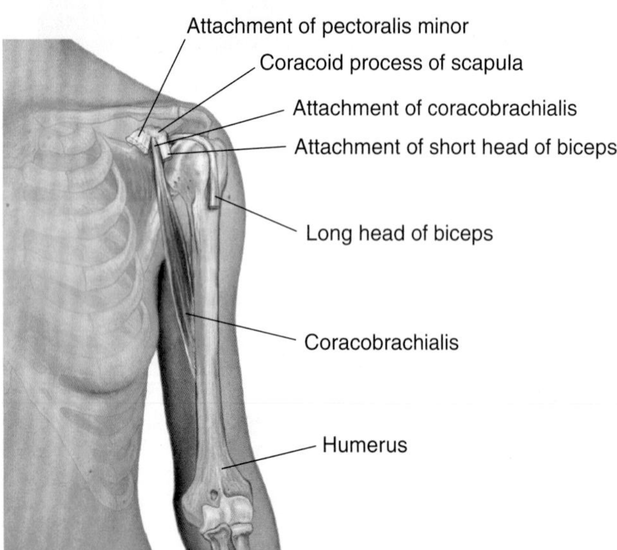

FIGURE 5-12 Anatomy of coracobrachialis

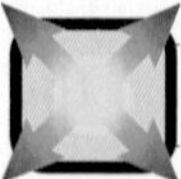

REFERRAL AREA

To the posterior aspect of the upper arm, forearm, and hand and to the area of the middle and anterior deltoid

OTHER MUSCLES TO EXAMINE

- All the muscles of the arm and forearm
- Rotator cuff muscles
- Deltoids

MANUAL THERAPY

Stripping and Compression

- The client lies supine. The therapist stands at the client's side, facing the client's head. The therapist holds the arm to be treated at the elbow with the nontreating hand.
- With the treating hand (i.e., the hand nearest the client), grasp the upper arm from the medial side in such a way that the thumb can comfortably extend along the medial side of the humerus.
- Press the thumb under biceps brachii to the medial side of the humerus about halfway up the humerus, seeking the distal attachment of coracobrachialis. Hold for release.
- Glide the thumb proximally along the muscle, holding for release where tenderness is found (Fig. 5-13).

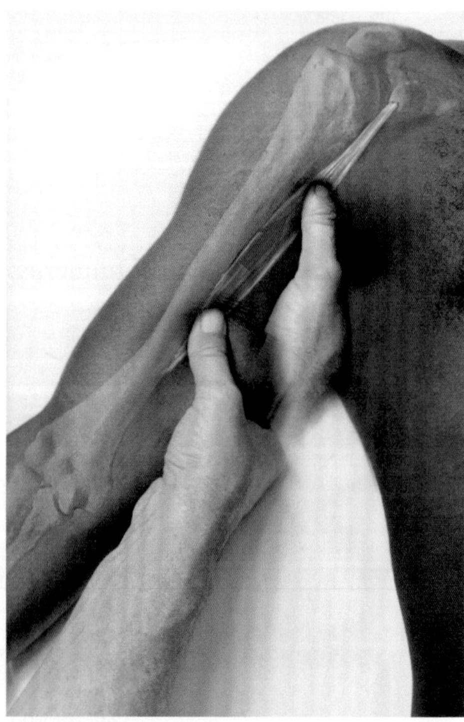

FIGURE 5-13 Stripping and compression of coracobrachialis using the thumb

- The thumb will finally follow the muscle deep into the axilla to the upper attachment to the coracoid process.

CAUTION In working in the axilla, take care to maintain contact with the muscle and avoid the nerves and blood vessels that pass under the coracoid process into the arm.

Muscles of the Forearm and Hand

SUPINATOR

SOUP-in-ay-ter

ETYMOLOGY Latin ***supinare***, to bend backward or place on back (***supinus***, supine)

Overview

Supinator (Fig. 5-14) assists biceps brachii in its supinating function. Supinator is deep, but can be worked by compression through the superficial muscles.

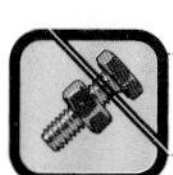

ATTACHMENTS

- Origin: lateral epicondyle of humerus radial collateral and annular ligaments, and to the supinator ridge of ulna
- Insertion: anterior and lateral surface of radius

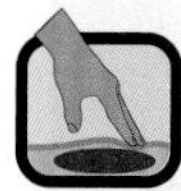

PALPATION

Place the client's elbow in extension and in pronation. Identify the radius from the radial head downward. Identify the ulna from the olecranon downward. The supinator is in the interspace between radius and ulna, between the elbow and mid-forearm. Ask the client to supinate and resist this attempt. Contraction can be felt.

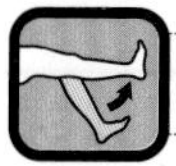

ACTION

Supinates the forearm (radioulnar joints)

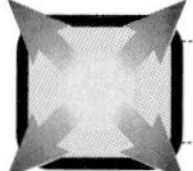

REFERRAL AREA

To the volar elbow and over the lateral epicondyle, and to the dorsal side of the hand at the base of the thumb and index finger

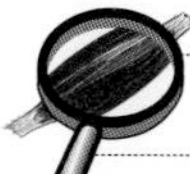

OTHER MUSCLES TO EXAMINE

- Infraspinatus
- Subclavius
- Scalenes
- Brachialis
- Anconeus
- Brachioradialis
- Extensors of the hand

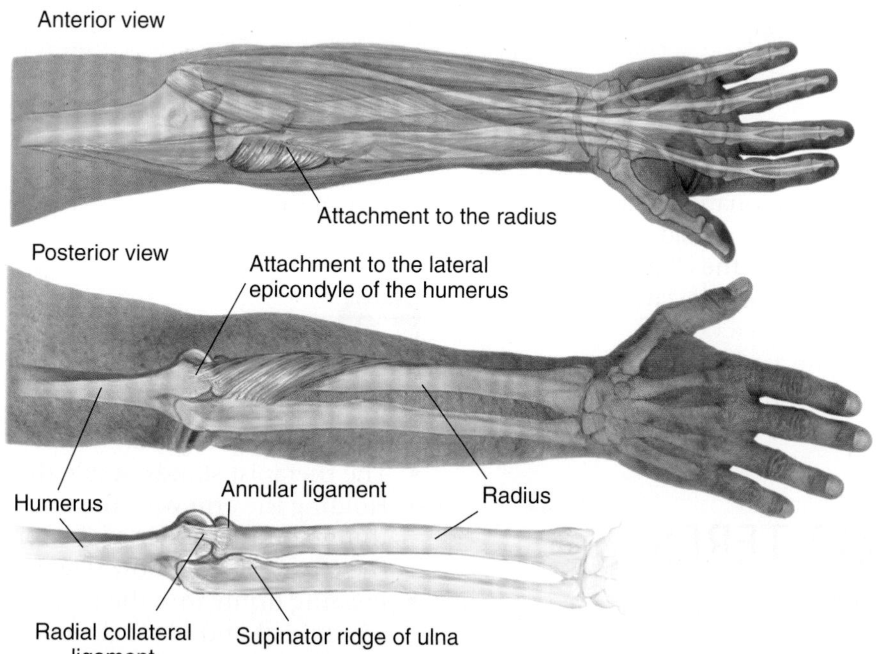

FIGURE 5-14 Anatomy of supinator

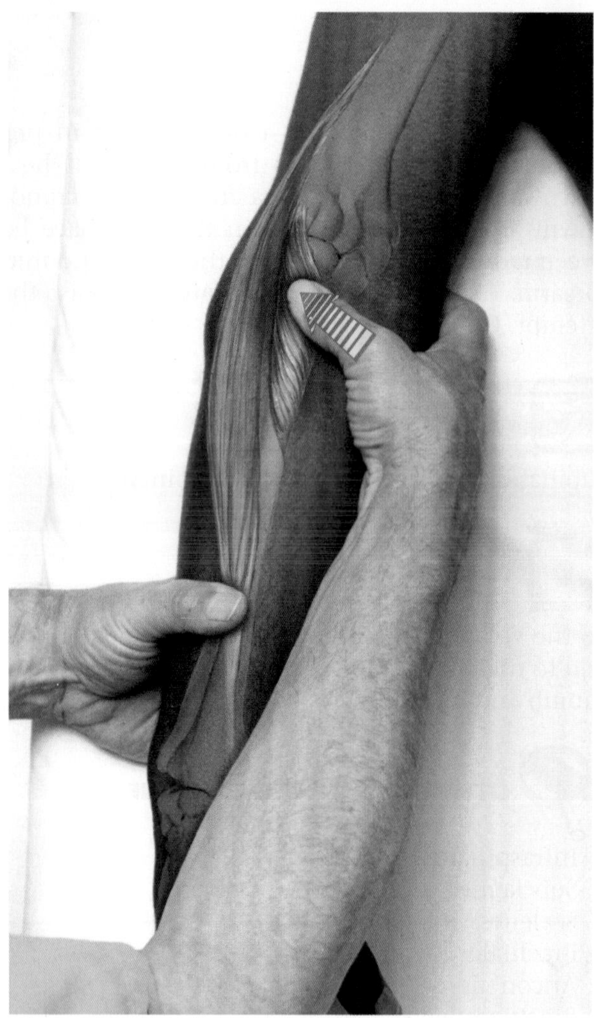

FIGURE 5-15 Compression of trigger point in supinator

MANUAL THERAPY

Compression

- The client lies supine.
- The therapist stands beside the client at the hip.
- Holding the forearm in pronation, place the thumb of the other hand on the ulnar side of the large extensor bundle just distal to the elbow.
- Displace the extensor bundle laterally to press into the interosseous space.
- Press firmly into the tissue, looking for tender spots. Hold for release (Fig. 5-15).

PRONATOR TERES

PRO-nay-ter TERR-ease

ETYMOLOGY Latin, ***pronare***, to bend forward + ***teres***, round, smooth, from ***terere***, to rub

Overview

Pronator teres (Fig. 5-16) is matched to supinator in size and opposing action. Like supinator, it lies deep but can be compressed through the muscles superficial to it.

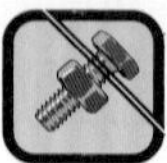

ATTACHMENTS

- Origin: superficial (humeral) head from the common flexor origin on the medial epicondyle of the humerus, deep (ulnar) head from the medial (ulnar) side of the coronoid process of the ulna
- Insertion: middle of the lateral surface of the radius

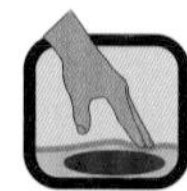

PALPATION

Palpable by pronating the forearm against resistance. Architecture is parallel.

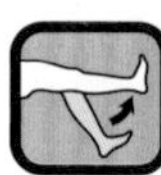

ACTION

- Pronates forearm (radioulnar joints)
- Assists in elbow flexion

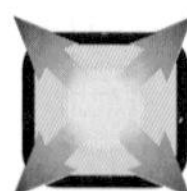

REFERRAL AREA

Over the radial edge of the volar forearm, especially to the wrist, and into the base of the thumb

OTHER MUSCLES TO EXAMINE

- Scalenes
- Infraspinatus
- Subclavius

MANUAL THERAPY

Stripping

- The client lies supine.
- The therapist stands beside the client at the hip.
- Holding the arm with the volar side up, place the thumb on the center of the forearm just distal to the crease of the elbow (Fig. 5-17).
- Pressing firmly into the tissue, glide the thumb in a proximal and ulnar direction across the crease of the elbow to the attachment on the medial epicondyle of the humerus.

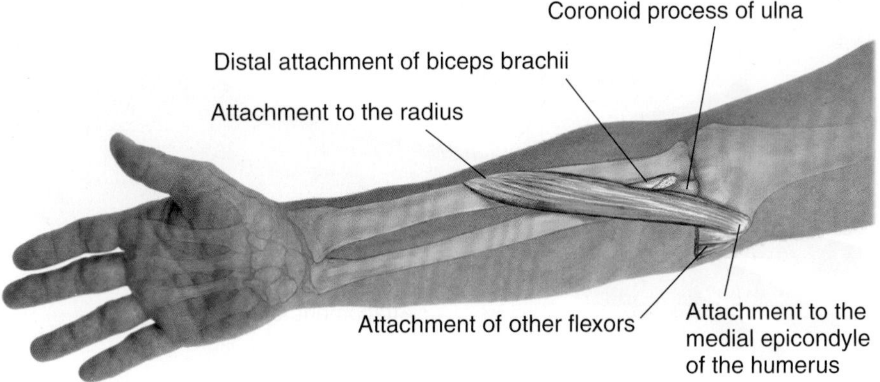

FIGURE 5-16 Anatomy of pronator teres, volar (anterior) view

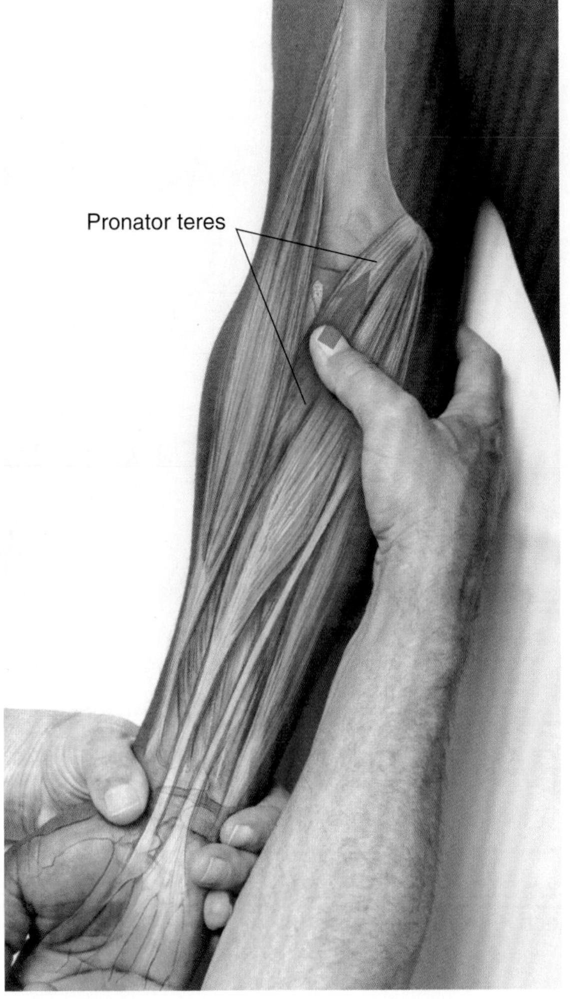

FIGURE 5-17 Stripping of pronator teres

Overview

Any strong repetitive motion of pronation such as might be performed during sports, such as playing tennis, or a factory job could overtire the pronator and set up a trigger point with a referral area between the superior edge of the muscle on the side toward the thumb and the wrist (Fig. 5-18).

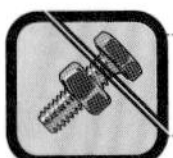

ATTACHMENTS

- Origin: distal fourth of anterior surface of ulna
- Insertion: distal fourth of anterior surface of radius

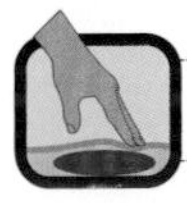

PALPATION

You can test for strength and feel the muscle contraction by having the client completely flex the forearm and then pronate against resistance.

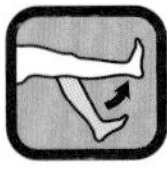

ACTION

Pronates forearm (radioulnar joints)

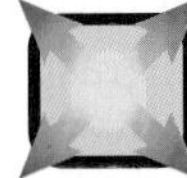

REFERRAL AREA

Between the superior edge of the muscle on the side toward the thumb, and the wrist

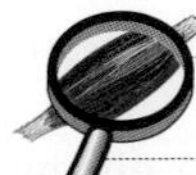

OTHER MUSCLES TO EXAMINE

- Pronator teres

PRONATOR QUADRATUS

PRO-nay-ter qua-DRAY-tus

ETYMOLOGY Latin, ***pronare***, to bend forward + ***quadratus***, four-sided

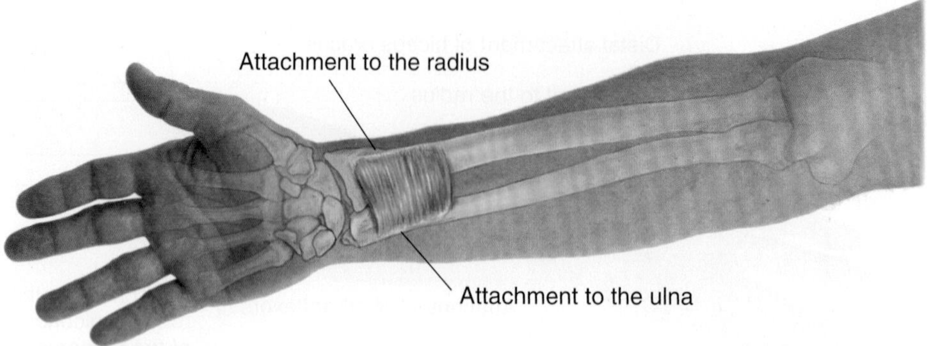

FIGURE 5-18 Anatomy of pronator quadratus, volar (anterior) view

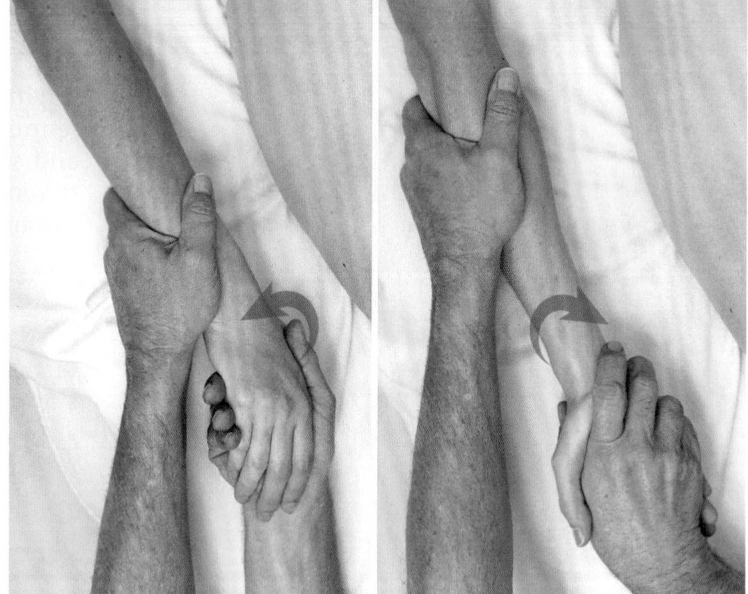

FIGURE 5-19 Stretching the pronator and supinator muscles

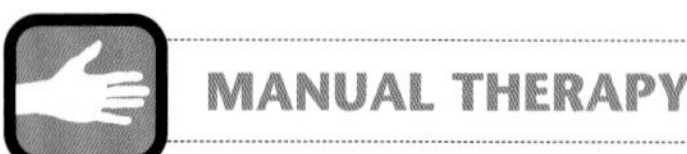

PRONATOR AND SUPINATOR MUSCLES

Stretch and mobilization

- The client lies supine.
- The therapist stands beside the client at the hip.
- With the hand that is further from the client, grasp the client's forearm just proximal to the wrist.
- With the hand that is nearer the client, grasp the client's hand as if shaking hands.
- Turn the hand firmly into supination, then into pronation.
- Shift the other hand to the middle of the forearm and repeat the stretch.
- Shift the other hand to just distal to the elbow and repeat the stretch (Fig. 5-19).

BRACHIORADIALIS

BRAY-key-oh-ray-dee-AL-is

ETYMOLOGY Latin ***brachium***, arm + ***radialis***, adjective from ***radius***, spoke of a wheel

Overview

Brachioradialis (Fig. 5-20) is a flexor of the elbow, effective mainly when the brachialis or biceps have already partially flexed at the elbow or the forearm is in half-pronation. It may assist with both pronation and supination. With the insertion of the muscle so far from the fulcrum of the elbow, the brachioradialis does not generate as much joint torque as the brachialis or the biceps.

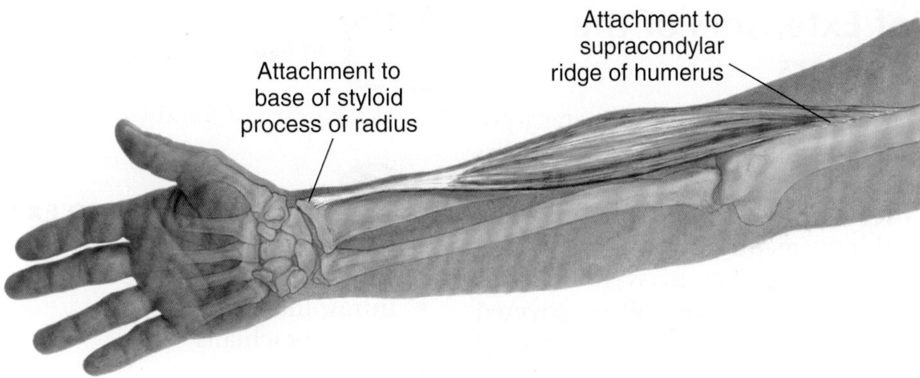

FIGURE 5-20 Anatomy of brachioradialis

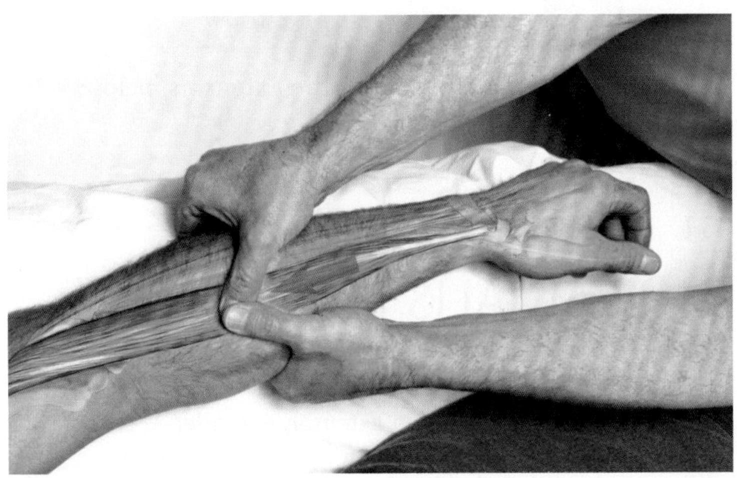

FIGURE 5-21 Stripping of brachioradialis with supported thumb

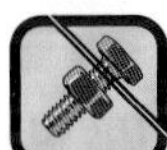

ATTACHMENTS

- Origin: lateral supracondylar ridge of humerus
- Insertion: lateral side of the base of the styloid process of the radius

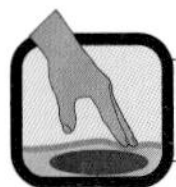

PALPATION

Can be palpated between elbow and radius by flexing the neutral forearm against resistance. Architecture is parallel and fibers are parallel to the muscle.

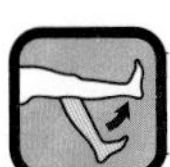

ACTION

Flexes elbow and returns forearm to a neutral position from supination or pronation

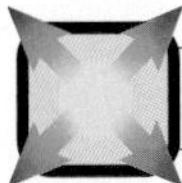

REFERRAL AREA

Radial surface of elbow, dorsal surface of hand between the thumb and the index finger, radial surface of forearm

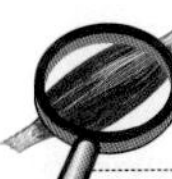

OTHER MUSCLES TO EXAMINE

- Infraspinatus
- Supraspinatus
- Scalenes
- Subclavius

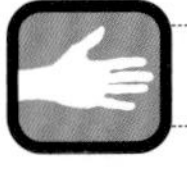

MANUAL THERAPY

Stripping

- The client lies supine.
- The therapist stands beside the client at the hip.
- Using the supported thumb, find the brachioradialis at its attachment near the distal end of the radius.
- Pressing firmly into the tissue, glide the thumb (Fig. 5-21) proximally along the muscle across the elbow to its attachment on the humerus.

Overview of Extensors of the Wrist and Fingers

The muscles that extend the wrist and metacarpophalangeal and interphalangeal joints of the fingers cover the dorsal aspect of the forearm. Along with the flexors on the volar forearm, they stabilize the wrist during hand movements. They can be treated effectively as a group with deep massage. For this reason, manual therapy for them will be covered at the end of the descriptions of all the individual extensors.

EXTENSOR CARPI RADIALIS BREVIS

ex-TEN-ser CAR-pie ray-dee-AL-is BREV-is

ETYMOLOGY Latin ***extensor***, extender + ***carpi***, of the wrist + ***radialis***, adjective from radius, spoke of a wheel + ***brevis***, short

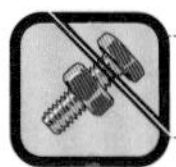

ATTACHMENTS

- Origin: lateral epicondyle of humerus (Fig. 5-22)
- Insertion: base of the 3rd metacarpal bone

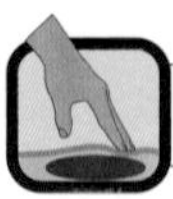

PALPATION

The extensors can be palpated as a group by hyperextending the wrist. Their architecture is unipennate, oriented at one fiber angle to the force-generating axis, and are all on the same side of a tendon.

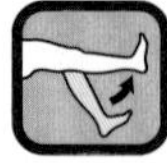

ACTION

Extends and abducts wrist radially

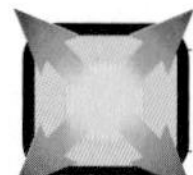

REFERRAL AREA

Dorsal surface of hand

OTHER MUSCLES TO EXAMINE

- Subscapularis
- Infraspinatus
- Coracobrachialis
- Brachialis

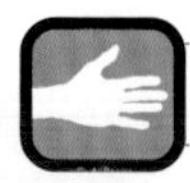

MANUAL THERAPY

See Manual Therapy for the Extensors, below.

EXTENSOR CARPI RADIALIS LONGUS

ex-TEN-ser CAR-pie ray-dee-AL-is LONG-gus

ETYMOLOGY Latin ***extensor***, extender + ***carpi***, of the wrist + ***radialis***, adjective from ***radius***, spoke of a wheel + ***longus***, long

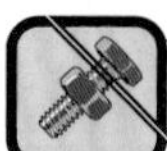

ATTACHMENTS

- Origin: lateral supracondylar ridge of humerus (Fig. 5-23)
- Insertion: dorsal base of 2nd metacarpal bone

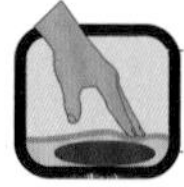

PALPATION

The extensors can be palpated as a group by hyperextending the wrist. Their architecture is unipennate,

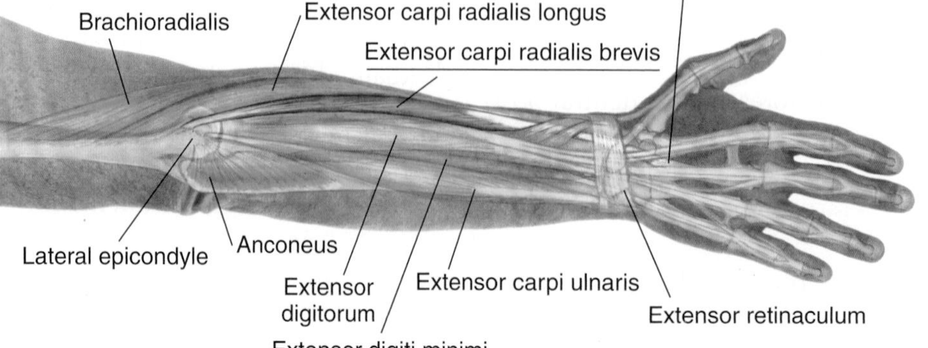

FIGURE 5-22 Anatomy of extensor carpi radialis brevis, dorsal (posterior) view

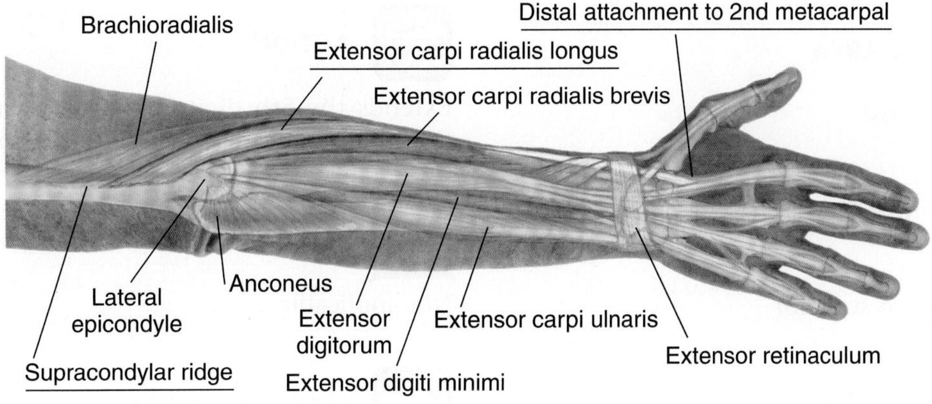

FIGURE 5-23 Anatomy of extensor carpi radialis longus, dorsal (posterior) view

oriented at one fiber angle to the force-generating axis, and are all on the same side of a tendon.

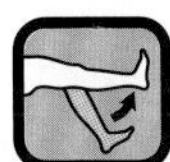

ACTION

Extends and abducts wrist radially

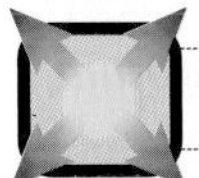

REFERRAL AREA

Surface of elbow, radial aspect of dorsal hand, dorsal forearm

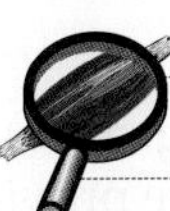

OTHER MUSCLES TO EXAMINE

- Extensor carpi radialis brevis
- Supinator
- Extensor indicis
- Brachialis
- Infraspinatus
- Serratus posterior superior
- Scalenes

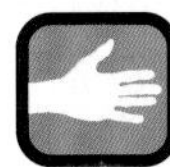

MANUAL THERAPY

See Manual Therapy for the Extensors, below.

EXTENSOR CARPI ULNARIS

ex-TEN-ser CAR-pie ul-NAR-is

ETYMOLOGY Latin ***extensor***, extender + ***carpi***, of the wrist + ***ulnaris***, adjective from ***ulna***, elbow or arm

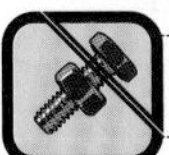

ATTACHMENTS

- Origin: lateral epicondyle of humerus (humeral head) and posterior border of proximal ulna (ulnar head) (Fig. 5-24)
- Insertion: base of the 5th metacarpal bone

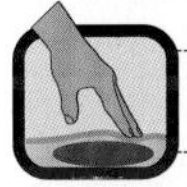

PALPATION

The extensors can be palpated as a group by hyperextending the wrist. Their architecture is bipennate, with fibers at an angle on both sides of the tendon.

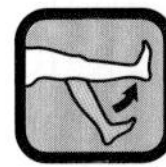

ACTION

Extends and adducts wrist ulnarly

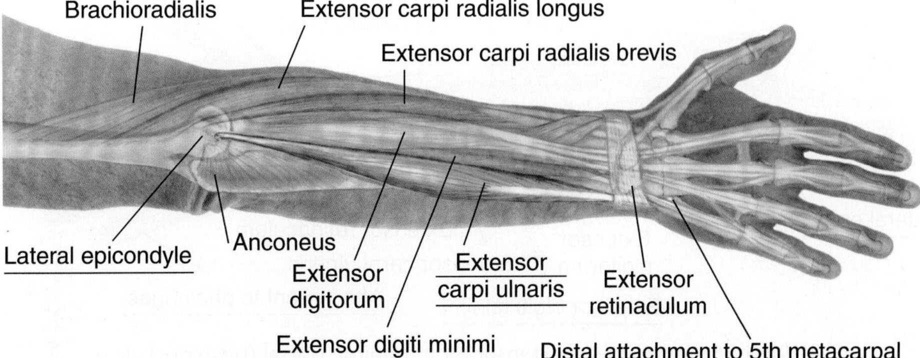

FIGURE 5-24 Anatomy of extensor carpi ulnaris, dorsal (posterior) view

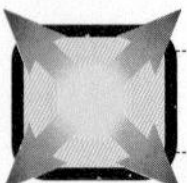

REFERRAL AREA

Ulnar surface of wrist

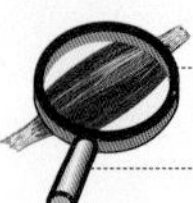

OTHER MUSCLES TO EXAMINE

- Subscapularis
- Serratus posterior superior

MANUAL THERAPY

See Manual Therapy for the Extensors, below.

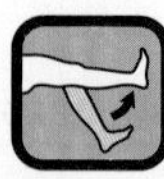

ACTION

Extends the 5th digit at the metacarpophalangeal (MP) joint and interphalangeal (IP) joints

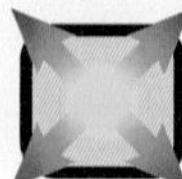

REFERRAL AREA

Not applicable

MANUAL THERAPY

See Manual Therapy for the Extensors, below.

EXTENSOR DIGITI MINIMI

ex-TEN-ser DIH-jih-tea MIH-nih-mee

ETYMOLOGY Latin ***extensor,*** extender + ***digiti,*** of the finger + ***minimi,*** smallest

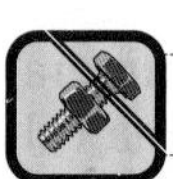

ATTACHMENTS

- Origin: lateral epicondyle of the humerus (Fig. 5-25)
- Insertion: dorsum of the proximal, middle, and distal phalanges of little finger

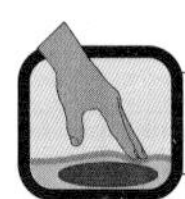

PALPATION

The extensors can be palpated as a group by extending the flexed fingers against resistance. Their architecture is unipennate, oriented at one fiber angle to the force-generating axis, and are all on the same side of a tendon.

EXTENSOR DIGITORUM

ex-TEN-ser dih-jih-TOR-um

ETYMOLOGY Latin ***extensor,*** extender + ***digitorum,*** of the fingers

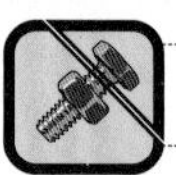

ATTACHMENTS

- Origin: lateral epicondyle of humerus (Fig. 5-26)
- Insertion: four tendons into the base of the proximal and middle and base of the distal phalanges of digits 2 through 5 (not the thumb)

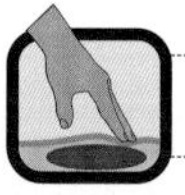

PALPATION

The extensors can be palpated as a group by extending the flexed fingers against resistance. Their architecture is unipennate, oriented at one fiber angle to the force-generating axis, and are all on the same side of a tendon.

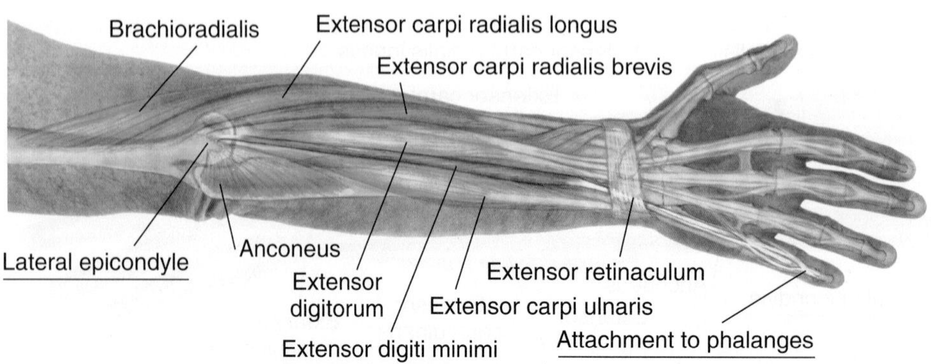

FIGURE 5-25 Anatomy of extensor digiti minimi, dorsal (posterior) view

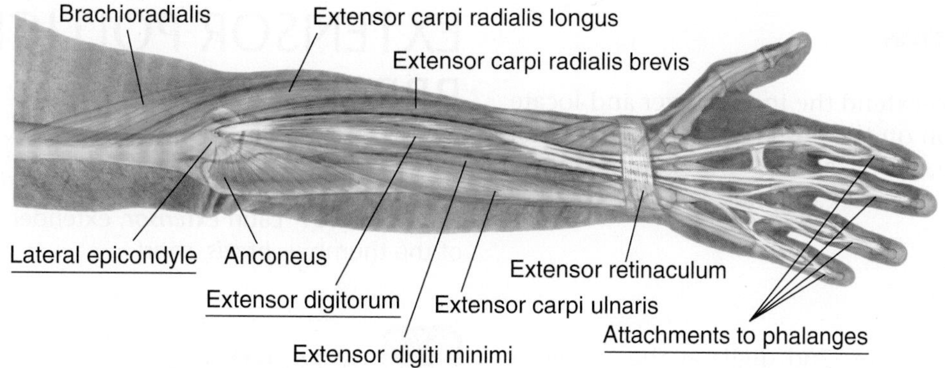

FIGURE 5-26 Anatomy of extensor digitorum, dorsal (posterior) view

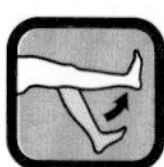

ACTION

Extends digits 2 through 5 (not the thumb) at the MP joints and IP joints

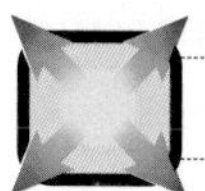

REFERRAL AREA

Not applicable

MANUAL THERAPY

See Manual Therapy for the Extensors, below.

EXTENSOR INDICIS

ex-TEN-ser IN-dis-sis

ETYMOLOGY Latin ***extensor***, extender + ***indicis***, of the forefinger

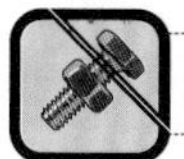

ATTACHMENTS

- Origin: posterior surface of the ulna and interosseous membrane (Fig. 5-27)
- Insertion: dorsal extensor aponeurosis of index finger

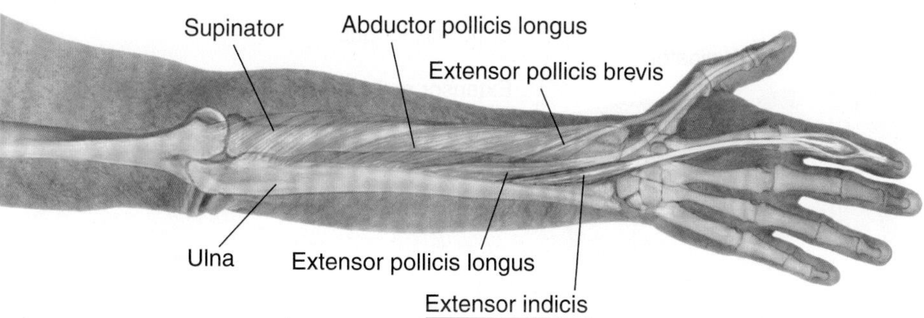

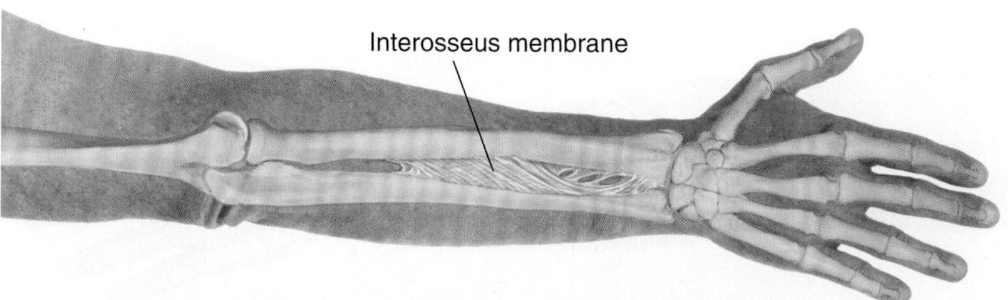

FIGURE 5-27 Anatomy of extensor indicis, dorsal (posterior) view

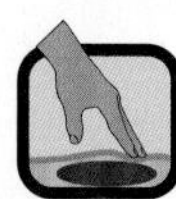

PALPATION

Ask the client to extend the index finger and locate the distal tendon on the posterior side of the hand; palpate proximally by asking the client to alternately contract and relax the muscle.

ACTION

Extends the forefinger (2nd digit) at the MP joint and IP joints

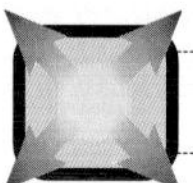

REFERRAL AREA

Dorsal surface of the hand to the dorsal forefinger

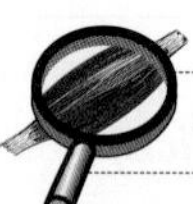

OTHER MUSCLES TO EXAMINE

- Coracobrachialis
- Subclavius

MANUAL THERAPY

See Manual Therapy for the Extensors, below.

EXTENSOR POLLICIS BREVIS

ex-TEN-ser PAHL-iss-iss BREV-iss

ETYMOLOGY Latin ***extensor***, extender + ***pollicis***, of the thumb + ***brevis***, short

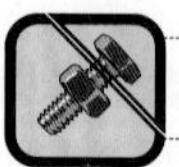

ATTACHMENTS

- Origin: posterior surface of radius and interosseous membrane (Fig. 5-28)
- Insertion: base of proximal phalanx of the thumb

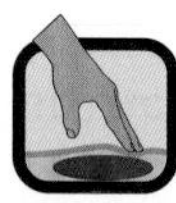

PALPATION

Tendon can be palpated at the dorsal base of the extended thumb. Architecture is convergent, and fibers are parallel to the muscle.

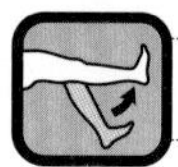

ACTION

Extends and abducts the thumb

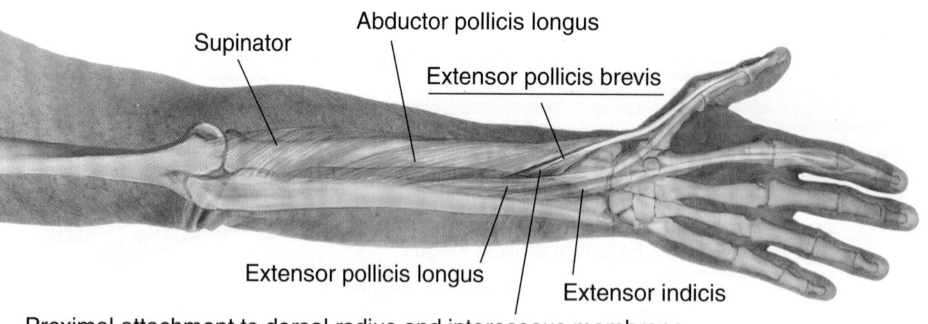

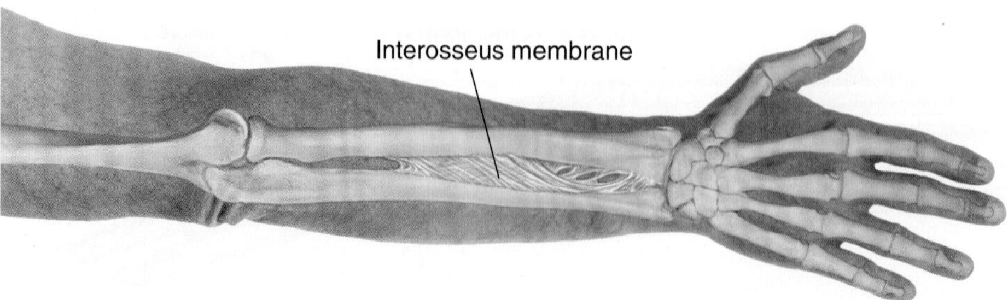

FIGURE 5-28 Anatomy of extensor pollicis brevis, dorsal (posterior) view

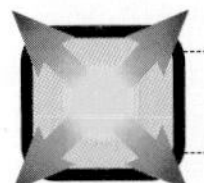

REFERRAL AREA

Not applicable

OTHER MUSCLES TO EXAMINE

Not applicable

MANUAL THERAPY

See Manual Therapy for the Extensors, below.

EXTENSOR POLLICIS LONGUS

Ex-TEN-ser PAHL-iss-iss LONG-gus

ETYMOLOGY Latin ***extensor***, extender + ***pollicis***, of the thumb + ***longus***, long

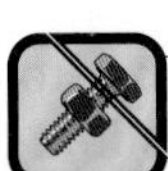

ATTACHMENTS

- Origin: posterior surface of the ulna and middle third of the interosseous membrane (Fig. 5-29)
- Insertion: base of distal phalanx of the thumb at the IP joint

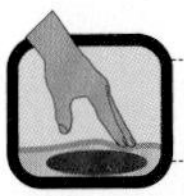

PALPATION

Tendon can be palpated on the back of the hand about an inch from extensor pollicis brevis with the thumb extended. Architecture is convergent, and fibers are parallel to the muscle.

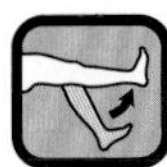

ACTION

Extends MP and IP joint of the thumb

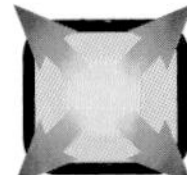

REFERRAL AREA

Not applicable

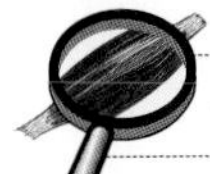

OTHER MUSCLES TO EXAMINE

Not applicable

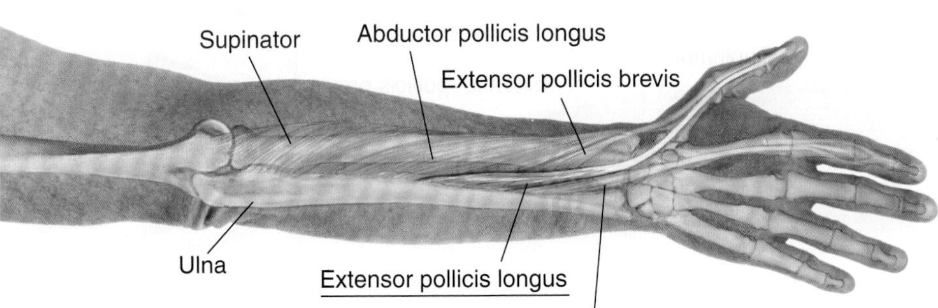

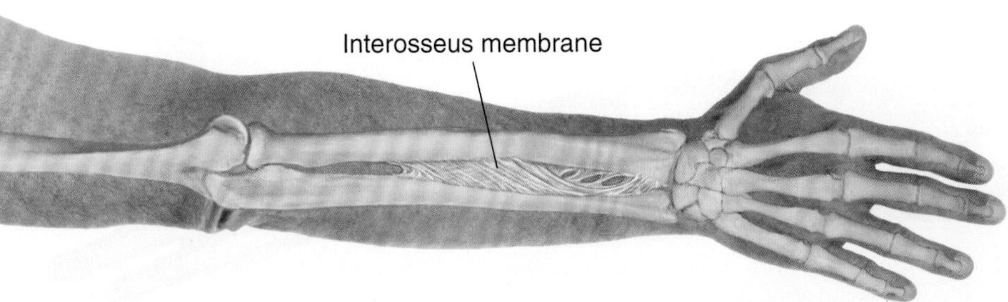

FIGURE 5-29 Anatomy of extensor pollicis longus, dorsal (posterior) view

ABDUCTOR POLLICIS LONGUS

ab-DUCK-ter PAHL-iss-iss LONG-gus

ETYMOLOGY Latin ***abductor***, that which draws away from + ***pollicis***, of the thumb + ***longus***, long

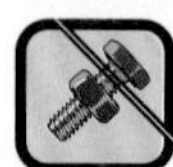

ATTACHMENTS

- Origin: posterior surfaces of radius and ulna and the interosseous membrane (Fig. 5-30)
- Insertion: lateral side of the base of the 1st metacarpal bone

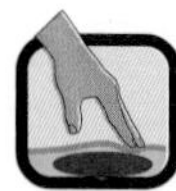

PALPATION

Tendon is palpable on 1st metacarpal. Architecture is convergent, and fibers are parallel to the muscle.

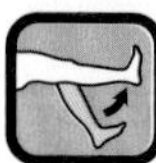

ACTION

Abducts and assists in extending the thumb

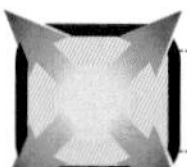

REFERRAL AREA

Not applicable

OTHER MUSCLES TO EXAMINE

Not applicable

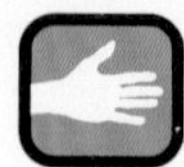

MANUAL THERAPY

See Manual Therapy for the Extensors, below.

Manual Therapy for the Extensors of the Wrist and Fingers

Stripping Massage of Individual Extensor Muscles

- The client lies supine with the forearm and hand pronated and slightly flexed at the elbow.
- The therapist stands beside the client at the hip.
- With the nontreating hand, hold the client's hand to steady the arm and wrist.
- Place the thumb on the wrist next to the head of the ulna.
- Pressing firmly into the tissue, glide the thumb proximally (Fig. 5-31) to the lateral epicondyle of the humerus.
- Shifting the thumb to a point slightly farther toward the radius, repeat this movement, sliding along a line parallel to the last motion to the distal humerus.
- Repeat the same procedure, following parallel lines, until the whole extensor (dorsal) aspect of the forearm has been covered.

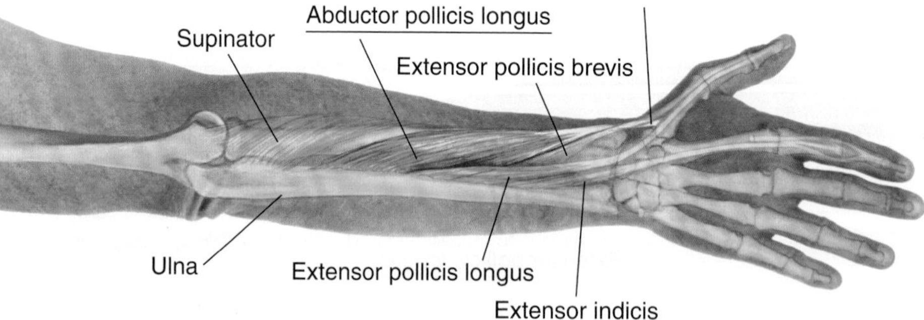

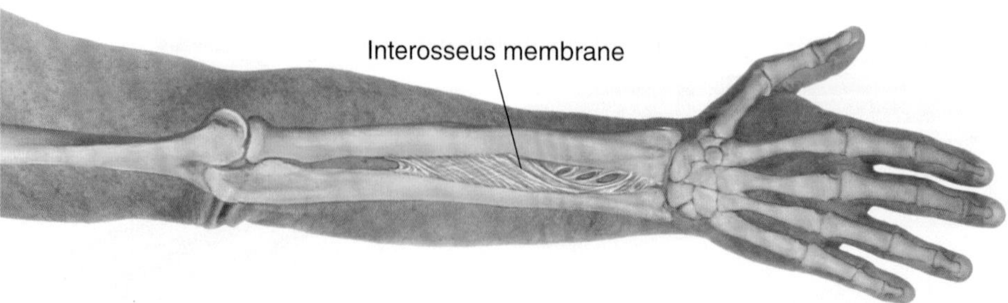

FIGURE 5-30 Anatomy of abductor pollicis longus, dorsal (posterior) view

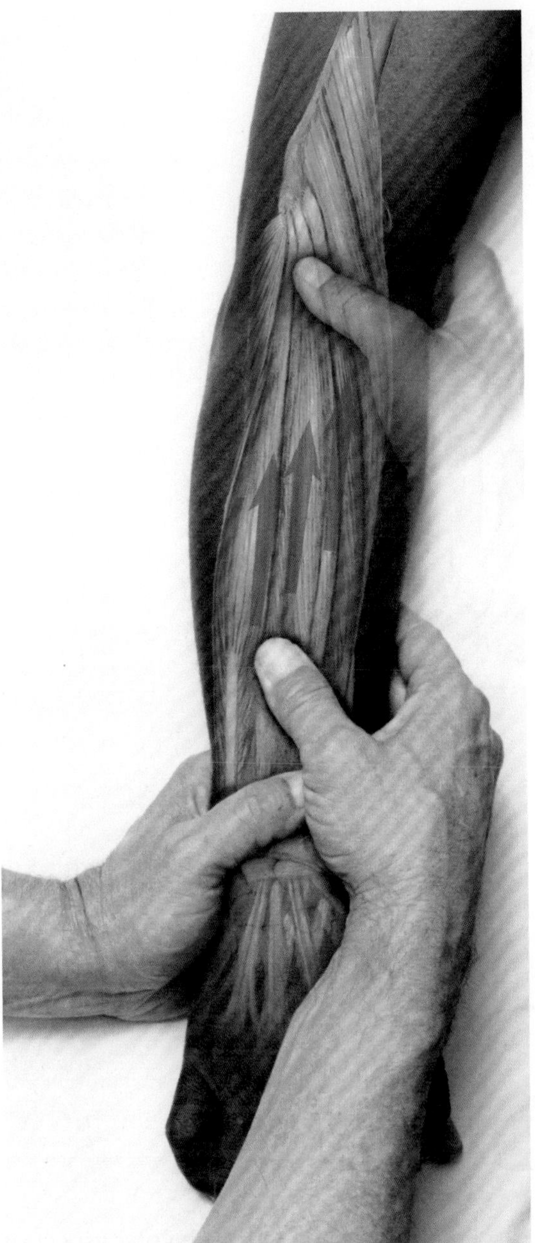

FIGURE 5-31 Stripping massage of the extensors using the thumb

Stripping Massage of the Extensor Group

- The client lies supine.
- The therapist stands beside the client at the hip.
- Place the knuckles or the heel of the hand on the dorsal wrist.
- Pressing firmly into the tissue, glide the knuckles (Fig. 5-32) or heel of the hand slowly along the muscle group across the elbow to the distal humerus.

Overview of Flexors of the Wrist and Fingers

Most of the tendons of the flexors of the wrist and fingers pass through the carpal tunnel, a passage formed by the carpal bones and the flexor retinaculum (Fig. 5-33). When these tendons are swollen, they can entrap and irritate the median nerve, causing carpal tunnel syndrome. Keeping the flexor muscles in the forearm relaxed can help prevent this condition. Like the extensors, the flexors can be massaged deeply as a group. Manual therapy will follow individual descriptions of all the muscles.

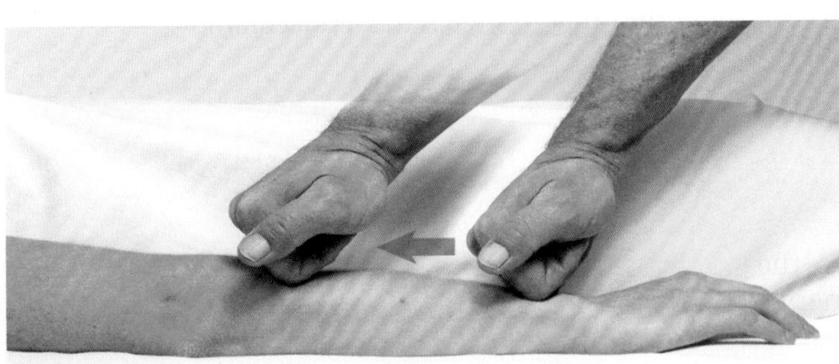

FIGURE 5-32 Stripping massage of the extensor muscles using the knuckles

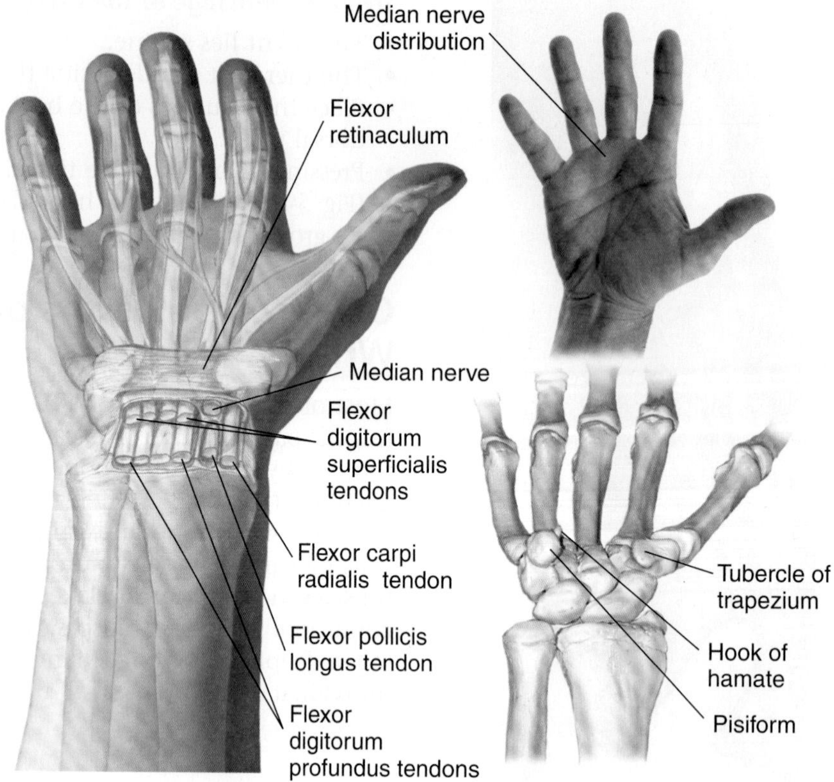

FIGURE 5-33 Carpal tunnel and flexor retinaculum, volar (anterior) view

FLEXOR RETINACULUM (TRANSVERSE CARPAL LIGAMENT)

FLEX-er ret-in-ACK-yu-lum

ETYMOLOGY Latin ***flexor***, bender + ***retinaculum***, band or halter (from retinere, to hold back)

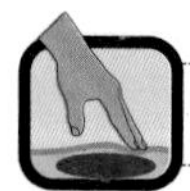

PALPATION

Palpable between the hook of the hamate and pisiform on the ulnar side and the tubercle of the trapezium on the radial side.

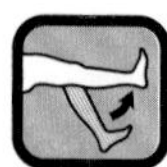

ACTION

Binds down the flexor tendons of the digits, the flexor carpi radialis tendon, and the median nerve, creating the carpal tunnel

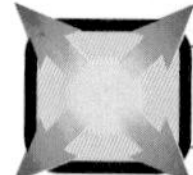

REFERRAL AREA

Not applicable

MANUAL THERAPY

Deep Cross-fiber Stroking

- The client lies supine with the volar aspect of the forearm facing up.
- Place the thumbs on the palmar surface of the hand about an inch distal to the wrist.
- Slide proximally in a series of parallel lines (Fig. 5-34) shifting gradually from one side of the volar wrist to the other to stretch the retinaculum.

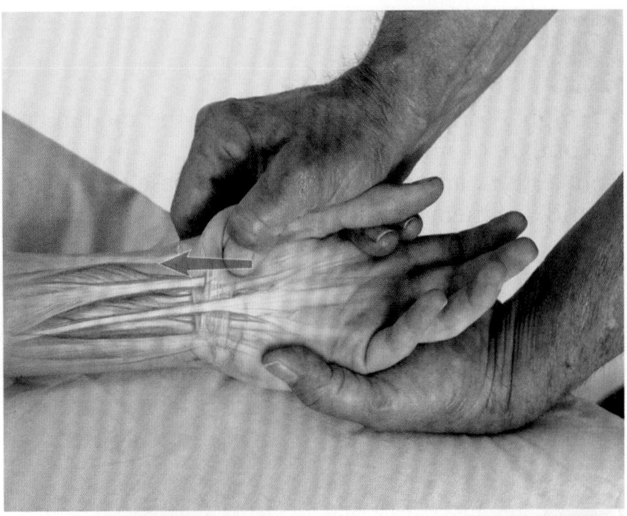

FIGURE 5-34 Stretching the flexor retinaculum using the thumb and elbow

PALMARIS LONGUS

pal-MAR-is LONG-gus

ETYMOLOGY Latin ***palmaris,*** relating to the palm + ***longus,*** long

Overview

Palmaris longus (Fig. 5-35) is the only hand flexor whose tendon lies superficial to the flexor retinaculum. It stands out prominently when the hand is cupped and flexed at the wrist. The palmaris longus is variably absent on one or both sides in some people. Since flexion is handled by other muscles, it is not a "necessary" muscle, and surgeons sometimes harvest the tendon to use for tendon repairs in other areas of the body.

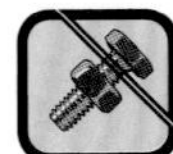

ATTACHMENTS

- Origin: medial epicondyle of the humerus
- Insertion: flexor retinaculum of the wrist and palmar fascia

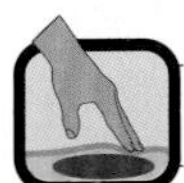

PALPATION

Tendon can be palpated by cupping the hand and flexing the wrist. Architecture is parallel, and fibers are parallel to the muscle.

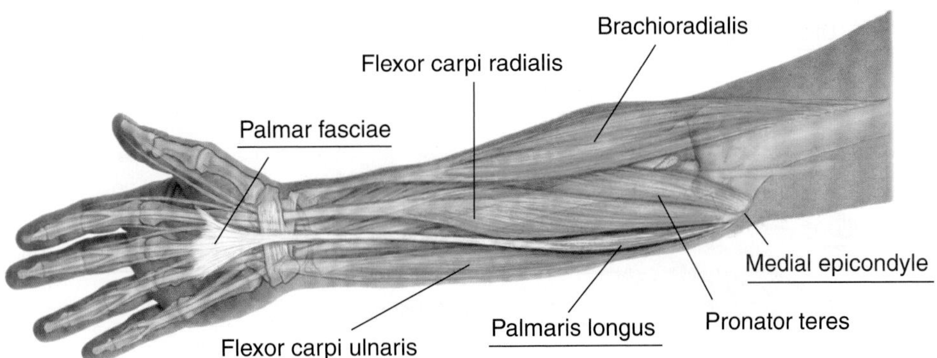

FIGURE 5-35 Anatomy of palmaris longus, volar (anterior) view

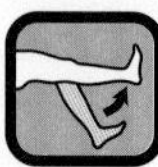

ACTION

- Tenses palmar fascia
- Flexes the hand at the wrist

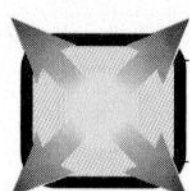

REFERRAL AREA

Prickling pain along the volar surface of the forearm and concentrated in the palm

OTHER MUSCLES TO EXAMINE

- All other flexors in the forearm
- Pronator teres
- Serratus anterior
- Pectoralis major and minor

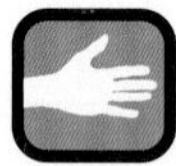

MANUAL THERAPY

See Manual Therapy for the Flexors, below.

FLEXOR CARPI RADIALIS

FLEX-er CAR-pie ray-dee-AL-iss

ETYMOLOGY Latin flexor, ***bender*** + ***carpi***, of the wrist + ***radialis***, adjective from ***radius***, spoke of a wheel

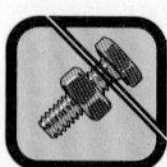

ATTACHMENTS

- Origin: common flexor origin of the medial epicondyle of humerus (Fig. 5-36)
- Insertion: anterior surface of the base of the 2nd and 3rd metacarpal bones

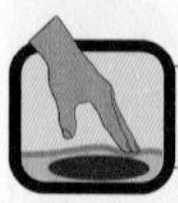

PALPATION

The flexors can be palpated as a group by flexing the wrist and fingers against resistance. Architecture is bipennate, and fibers are angled out from a central tendon.

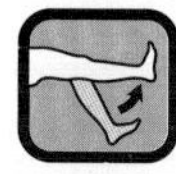

ACTION

Flexes wrist and abducts wrist radially

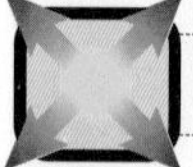

REFERRAL AREA

Middle of the volar wrist toward the radial side

OTHER MUSCLES TO EXAMINE

Pronator teres

MANUAL THERAPY

See Manual Therapy for the Flexors, below.

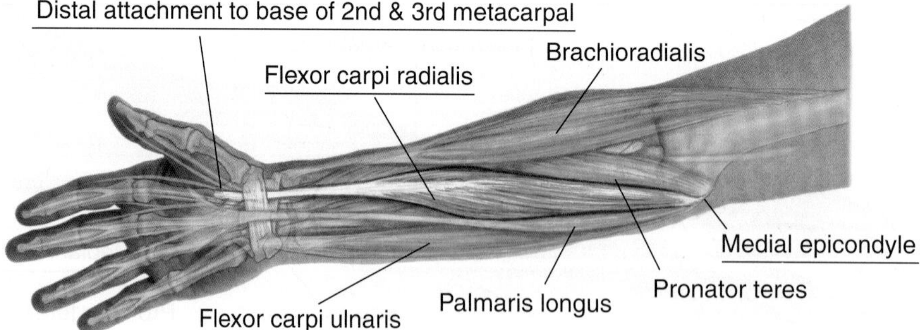

FIGURE 5-36 Anatomy of flexor carpi radialis, volar (anterior) view

FLEXOR CARPI ULNARIS

FLEX-er CAR-pie ul-NAR-iss

ETYMOLOGY Latin ***flexor***, bender + ***carpi***, of the wrist + ***ulnaris***, adjective from ***ulna***, elbow or arm

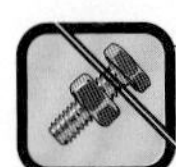

ATTACHMENTS

- Origin: humeral head of the muscle to the medial epicondyle of humerus; ulnar head of the muscle to the olecranon process, and upper three-fifths of posterior border of ulna (Fig. 5-37)
- Insertion: pisiform bone, the pisometacarpal ligament, and base of the 5th metacarpal

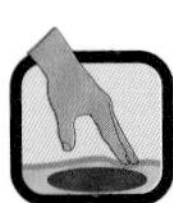

PALPATION

The flexors can be palpated as a group by flexing the wrist and fingers against resistance. Architecture is parallel, and fibers are unipennate to the muscle.

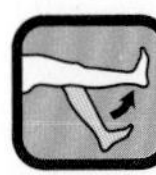

ACTION

Flexes wrist and adducts wrist ulnarly

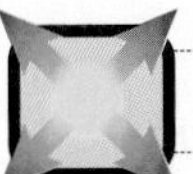

REFERRAL AREA

Ulnar and volar wrist

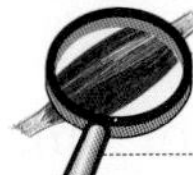

OTHER MUSCLES TO EXAMINE

- Pectoralis minor
- Serratus posterior superior

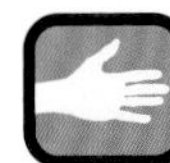

MANUAL THERAPY

See Manual Therapy for the Flexors, below.

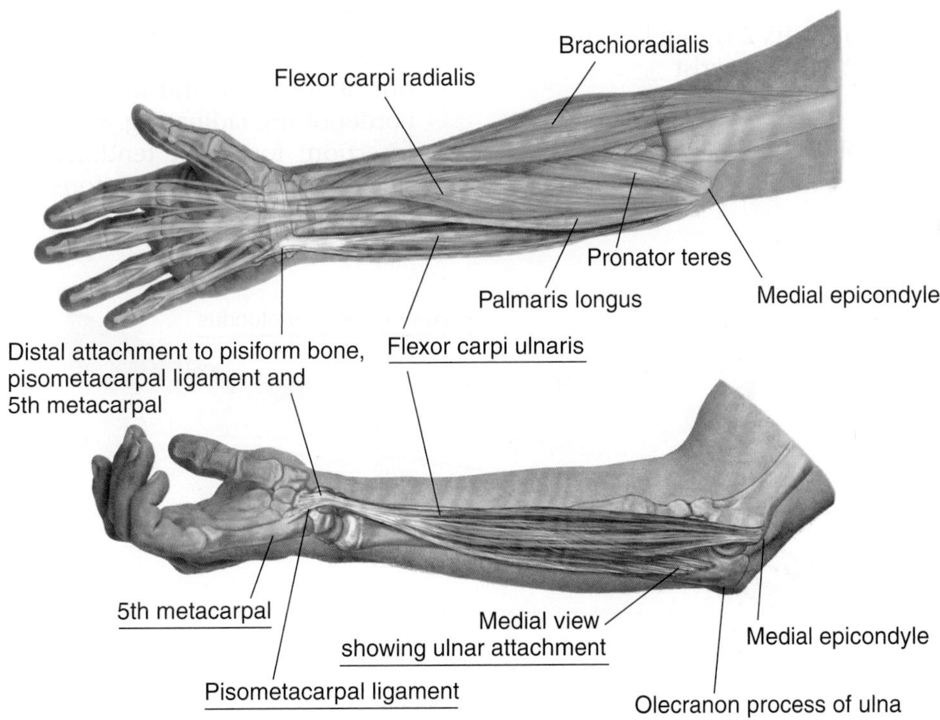

FIGURE 5-37 Anatomy of flexor carpi ulnaris, volar (anterior) and ulnar (medial) view

FLEXOR DIGITORUM PROFUNDUS

FLEX-er dih-jih-TOR-um pro-FUN-dus

ETYMOLOGY Latin ***flexor***, bender + ***digitorum***, of the fingers + ***profundus***, deep

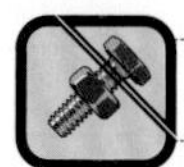

ATTACHMENTS

- Origin: anterior surface of upper third of ulna and interosseous membrane (Fig. 5-38)
- Insertion: four tendons into the base of distal phalanx of each finger except the thumb

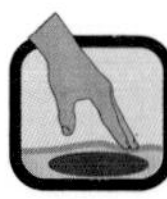

PALPATION

The flexors can be palpated as a group by flexing the wrist and fingers against resistance. Architecture is parallel, and fibers are bipennate to the muscle.

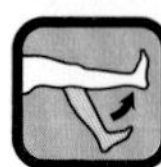

ACTION

Flexes distal IP joint of digits 2 through 5; assists in flexion of proximal IP, MP, and wrist

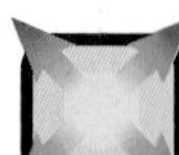

REFERRAL AREA

Not applicable

OTHER MUSCLES TO EXAMINE

Not applicable

MANUAL THERAPY

See Manual Therapy for the Flexors, below.

FLEXOR DIGITORUM SUPERFICIALIS

FLEX-er dih-jih-TOR-um SOUP-or-fishy-Alice

ETYMOLOGY Latin ***flexor***, bender + ***digitorum***, of the fingers + ***superficialis***, superficial

ATTACHMENTS

- Origin: humeroulnar head to the medial epicondyle of the humerus, the medial border of the coronoid process, and a tendinous arch between these points; the radial head to the anterior oblique line and middle third of the lateral border of the radius (Fig. 5-39)
- Insertion: four split tendons, passing to either side of the profundus tendons, into sides of middle phalanx of digits 2 through 5

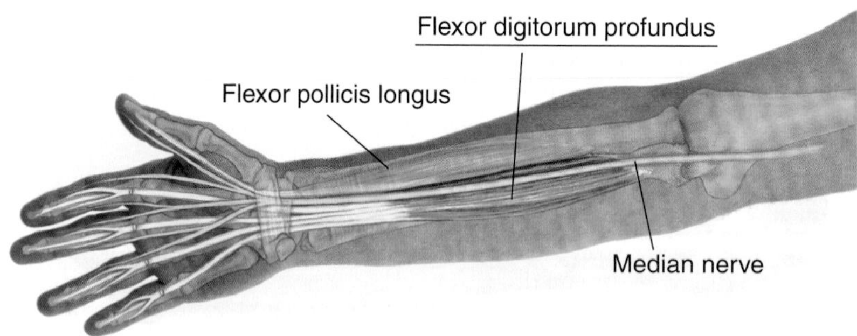

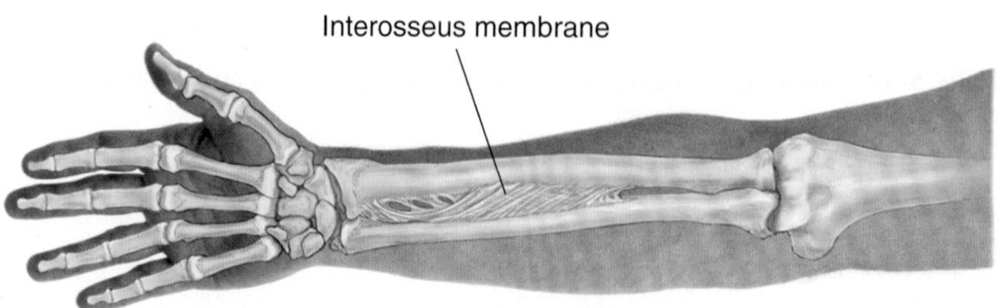

FIGURE 5-38 Anatomy of flexor digitorum profundus, volar (anterior) view

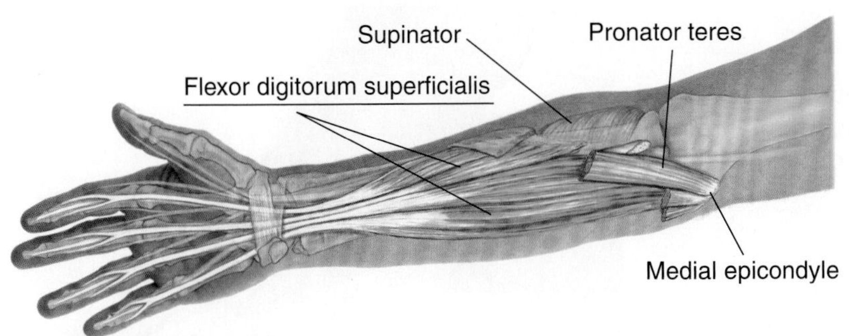

FIGURE 5-39 Anatomy of flexor digitorum superficialis, volar (anterior) view

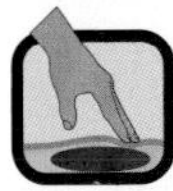

PALPATION

The flexors can be palpated as a group by flexing the wrist and fingers against resistance. Architecture is parallel, and fibers are unipennate to the muscle.

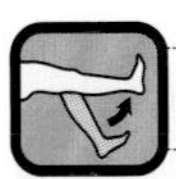

ACTION

Flexes proximal IP joint of digits 2 through 5; assists in flexion of MP and wrist

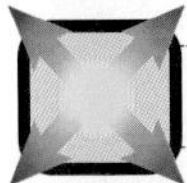

REFERRAL AREA

Not applicable

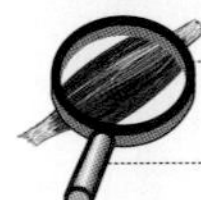

OTHER MUSCLES TO EXAMINE

Not applicable

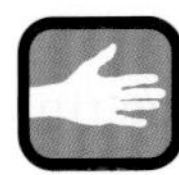

MANUAL THERAPY

See Manual Therapy for the Flexors, below.

FLEXOR POLLICIS LONGUS

FLEX-er PAHL-iss-iss LONG-gus

ETYMOLOGY Latin ***flexor***, bender + ***pollicis***, of the thumb + ***longus***, long

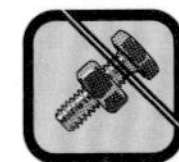

ATTACHMENTS

- Origin: anterior surface of the middle third of the radius and interosseous membrane (Fig. 5-40)
- Insertion: distal phalanx of the thumb

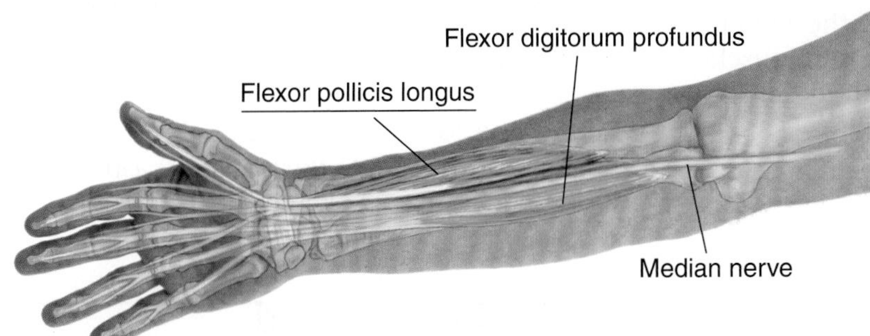

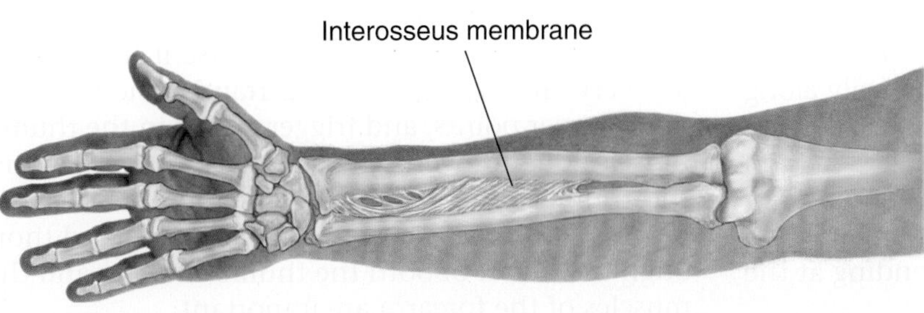

FIGURE 5-40 Anatomy of flexor pollicis longus, volar (anterior) view

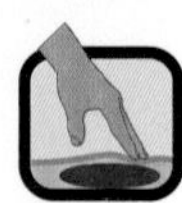

PALPATION

The flexors can be palpated as a group by flexing the wrist and fingers against resistance. Architecture is unipennate, and fibers are parallel to the muscle.

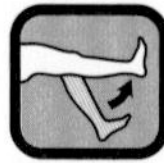

ACTION

Flexes distal phalanx of the thumb at IP joint

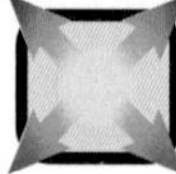

REFERRAL AREA

Through the palmar aspect of the thumb to the tip

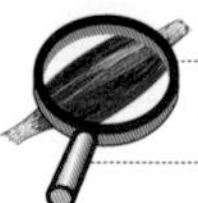

OTHER MUSCLES TO EXAMINE

- Scalenes
- Subclavius

MANUAL THERAPY

See Manual Therapy for the Flexors, below.

Manual Therapy for the Flexor Muscles of the Hand, Wrist, and Fingers

Stripping Massage of the Flexor Group

- The client lies supine.
- The therapist stands beside the client at the hip.
- With the nontreating hand, hold the client's hand to stabilize the arm.
- Place the knuckles or the heel of the hand on the volar wrist.
- Pressing firmly into the tissue, slide the knuckles or heel of the hand slowly along the muscle group (Fig. 5-41) across the elbow onto the distal end of biceps brachii.

Stripping Massage of Individual Extensor Muscles

- The client lies supine.
- The therapist stands beside the client at the hip.
- With the nontreating hand, hold the client's hand to stabilize the arm.
- Place the thumb, knuckles, or fingertips on the wrist just to the ulnar side of and proximal to the distal end of the radius.
- Pressing firmly into the tissue, slide the thumb, knuckles, or fingertips (Fig. 5-42) proximally along the radius to the volar aspect of the lateral epicondyle of the humerus.
- Beginning at a point slightly nearer the center of the wrist, repeat this movement, sliding along a line parallel to the last motion and ending at the base of biceps brachii.

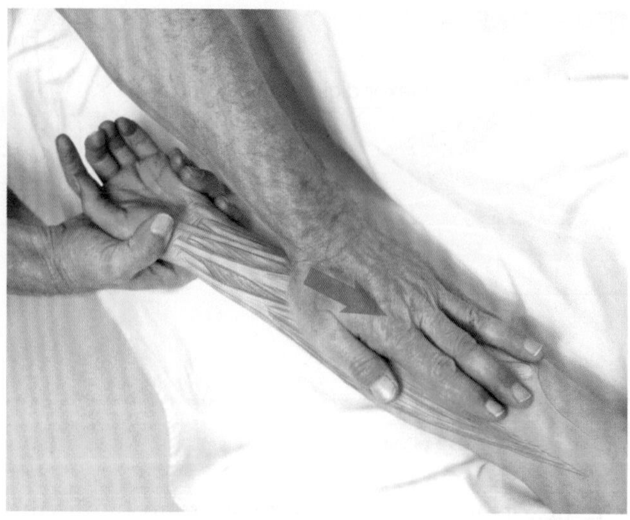

FIGURE 5-41 Moving compression of the flexors

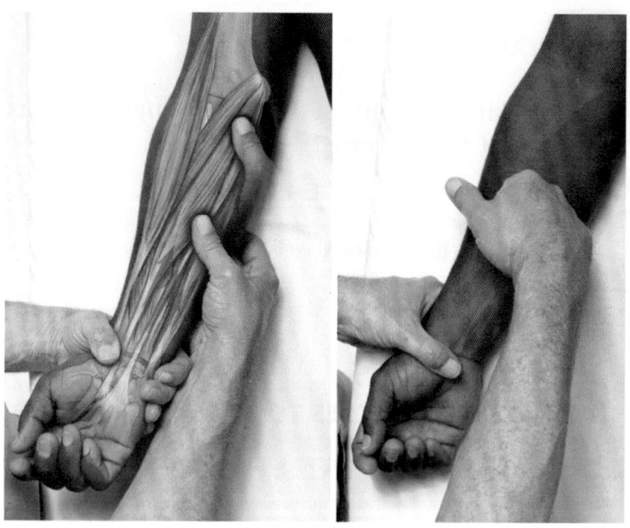

FIGURE 5-42 Stripping massage of the flexors using the thumb and the knuckles

- Repeat the same movement, following parallel lines, until the whole flexor (volar) aspect of the forearm has been covered (the last movement should be along the ulna).

Muscles in the Hand

Muscles of the Thumb

One of the distinguishing characteristics of humans is the opposable thumb, and we use it intensively, as every massage therapist certainly knows. Soreness, tender points, and trigger points in the thumb muscles due to overuse are quite common. Pain in the thumb area can also be a symptom of carpal tunnel syndrome, so careful examination and thorough treatment of both the thumb muscles and the muscles of the forearm are important.

The principal muscles of the thumb (abductor pollicis and opponens pollicis) form a thick, muscular bundle at the base of the thumb just distal to the wrist. These muscles comprise the *thenar eminence* (see plates 5-6 and 5-10), commonly called the ball of the thumb.

ADDUCTOR POLLICIS

ad-DUCK-ter POL-ly-sis

ETYMOLOGY Latin ***adductor*** (***ad***, to or toward + ***ducere***, to lead), that which draws toward + ***pollex***, thumb

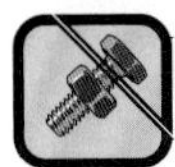

ATTACHMENTS

BY TWO HEADS

Origin

- The transverse head from the shaft of the 3rd metacarpal (Fig. 5-43)
- The oblique head from the front of the base of the 1st, 2nd, and 3rd metacarpals

Insertion

- Both heads to the medial side of base of proximal phalanx of the thumb and medial sesamoid at the MP joint

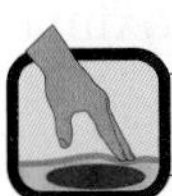

PALPATION

Palpable distal to the thenar eminence; architecture is slightly convergent, and fibers are parallel to the muscle.

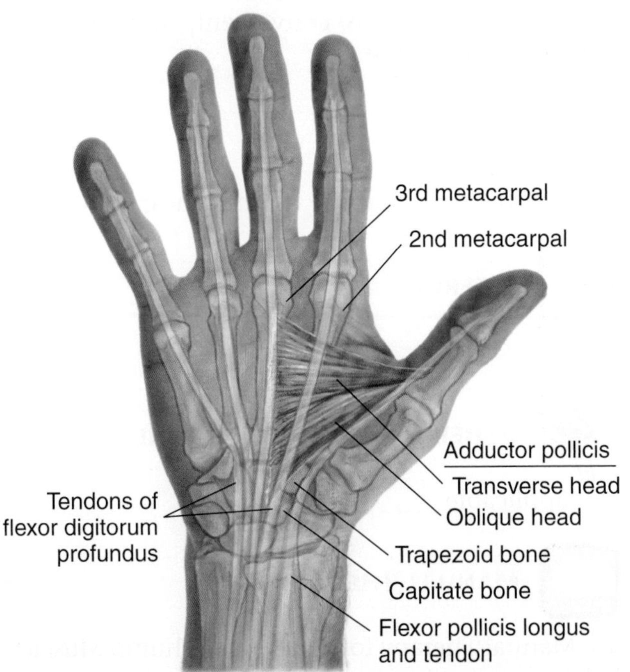

FIGURE 5-43 Anatomy of adductor pollicis

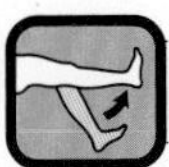

ACTION

Adducts the thumb at carpometacarpal joint and assists in flexion at the MP joint

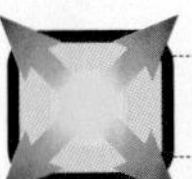

REFERRAL AREA

The base of the thumb on both the palmar and dorsal sides

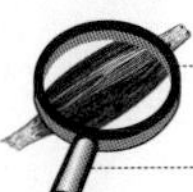

OTHER MUSCLES TO EXAMINE

- Opponens pollicis
- Supinator
- Brachioradialis
- Brachialis
- Infraspinatus
- Subclavius
- Scalenes

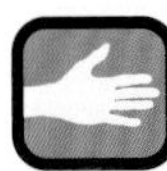

MANUAL THERAPY

See Manual Therapy for the Palmar Thumb Muscles, below

FLEXOR POLLICIS BREVIS

FLEX-er PAHL-iss-iss BREV-iss

ETYMOLOGY Latin ***flexor***, bender + ***pollicis***, of the thumb + ***brevis***, short

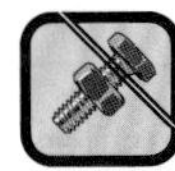

ATTACHMENTS

- Origin: superficial portion to the trapezium and the flexor retinaculum of the wrist, deep portion from trapezoid and capitate bones (Fig. 5-44)
- Insertion: base of the proximal phalanx of the thumb

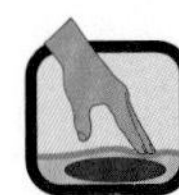

PALPATION

Palpable as the most distal muscle in the thenar eminence. Architecture is parallel, and fibers are parallel to the muscle.

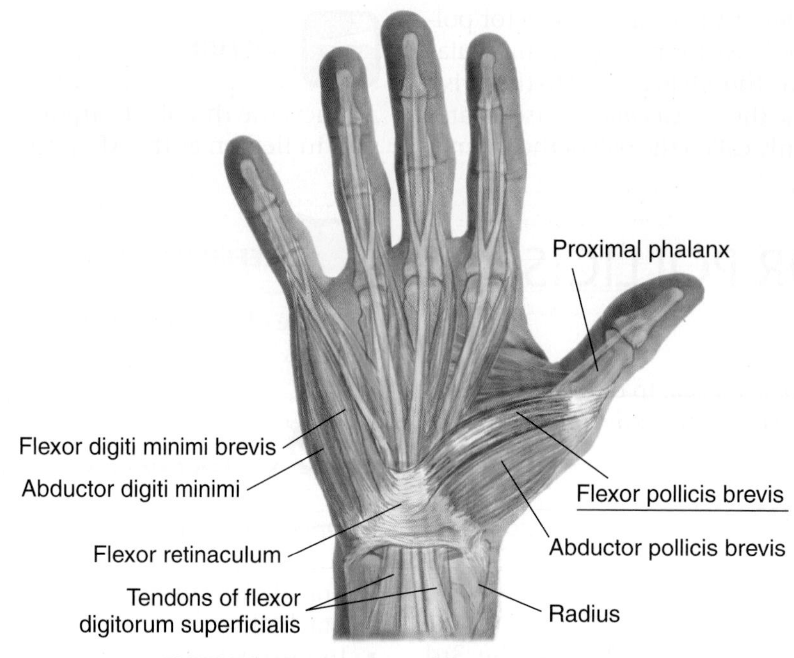

FIGURE 5-44 Anatomy of flexor pollicis brevis

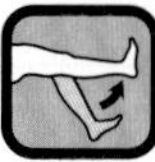

ACTION

Flexes MP joint of the thumb

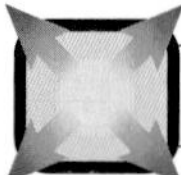

REFERRAL AREA

Not applicable

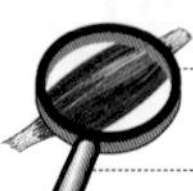

OTHER MUSCLES TO EXAMINE

Not applicable

MANUAL THERAPY

See Manual Therapy for the Palmar Thumb Muscles, below.

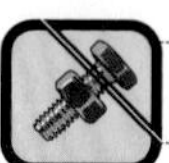

ATTACHMENTS

- Origin: tubercle of the trapezium and flexor retinaculum (Fig. 5-45)
- Insertion: base of the lateral side of the proximal phalanx of the thumb

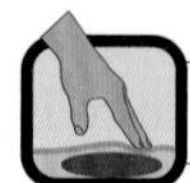

PALPATION

Palpable as the central muscle in the thenar eminence. Architecture is convergent, and fibers are parallel to the muscle.

ABDUCTOR POLLICIS BREVIS

ab-DUCK-ter POL-ly-sis BREV-iss

ETYMOLOGY Latin ***abductor*** (***ab***, from + ***ducere***, to lead), that which draws away from + ***pollex***, thumb

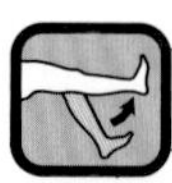

ACTION

Abducts the thumb at the carpometacarpal joint

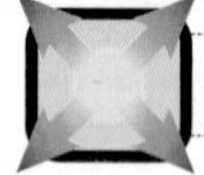

REFERRAL AREA

None

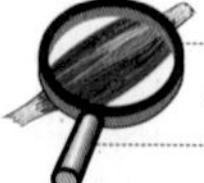

OTHER MUSCLES TO EXAMINE

Not applicable

MANUAL THERAPY

See Manual Therapy for the Palmar Thumb Muscles, below.

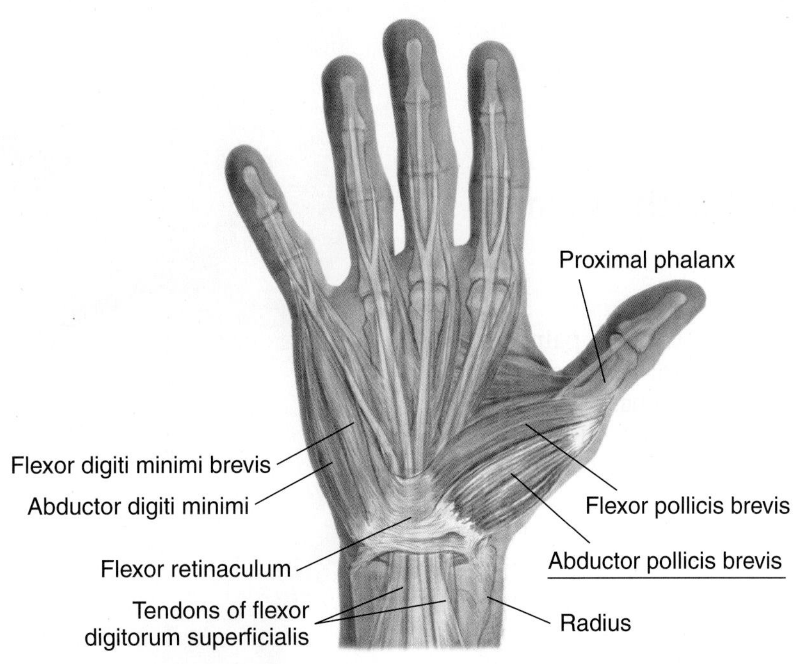

FIGURE 5-45 Anatomy of abductor pollicis brevis

OPPONENS POLLICIS

op-POE-nens POL-ly-sis

ETYMOLOGY Latin ***opponere***, to place against, oppose

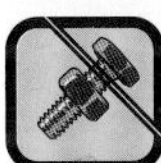

ATTACHMENTS

- Origin: ridge of the trapezium and flexor retinaculum (Fig. 5-46)
- Insertion: lateral side of the full length of the shaft of the 1st metacarpal bone

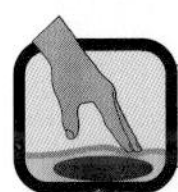

PALPATION

Palpable as the most proximal muscle in the thenar eminence. Architecture is convergent, and fibers are parallel to the muscle.

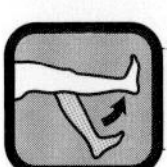

ACTION

Puts the thumb in opposition to the other fingers by drawing the base of the thumb toward the palm at the carpometacarpal joint

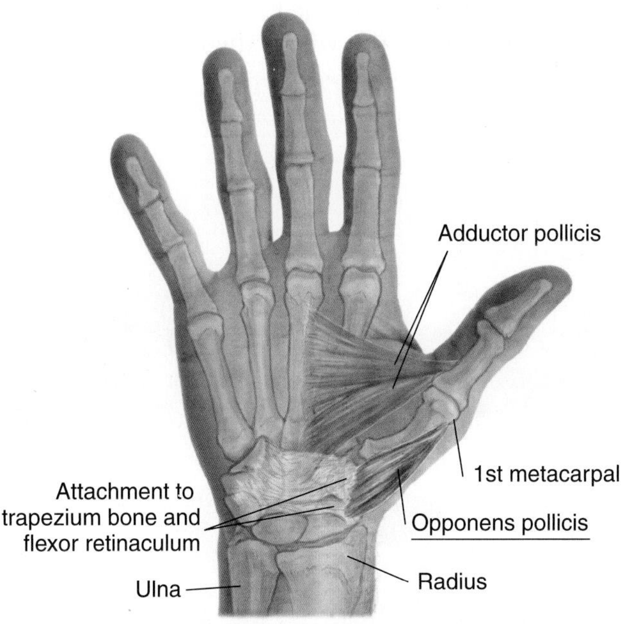

FIGURE 5-46 Anatomy of opponens pollicis

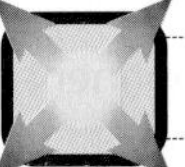

REFERRAL AREA

Lateral surface of thumb, wrist at the head of the radius

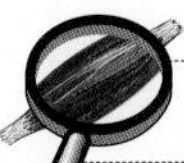

OTHER MUSCLES TO EXAMINE

- Adductor pollicis
- Infraspinatus

- Brachialis
- Subscapularis
- Subclavius
- Scalenes
- Serratus posterior superior

Manual Therapy for the Palmar Thumb Muscles

Trigger Point Compression

- Holding the client's hand with the palm up, use the other thumb to search for a trigger point on the thenar eminence near the base (Fig. 5-47).
- Compress with the thumb and hold for release.

Stripping

- The client may be in any position that gives easy access to the palm of the hand.
- Holding the hand firmly with the palm facing you, place your supported or unsupported thumb at the base of the thenar eminence (Fig. 5-48).
- Pressing firmly, slide your thumb radially to the 1st MP joint.
- Repeat this procedure (Fig. 5-49) on a line just distal and parallel to the first.
- Continue until the whole thenar eminence has been treated.

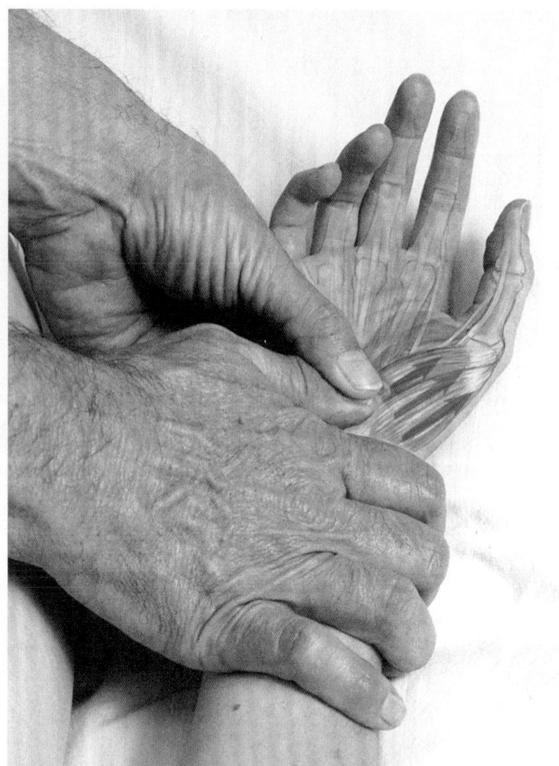

FIGURE 5-48 Stripping massage of the thenar eminence beginning at opponens pollicis (with supported thumb)

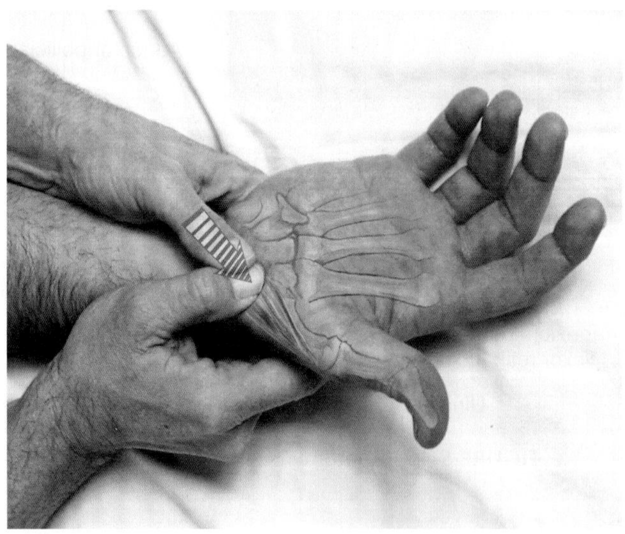

FIGURE 5-47 Compression of trigger point in opponens pollicis

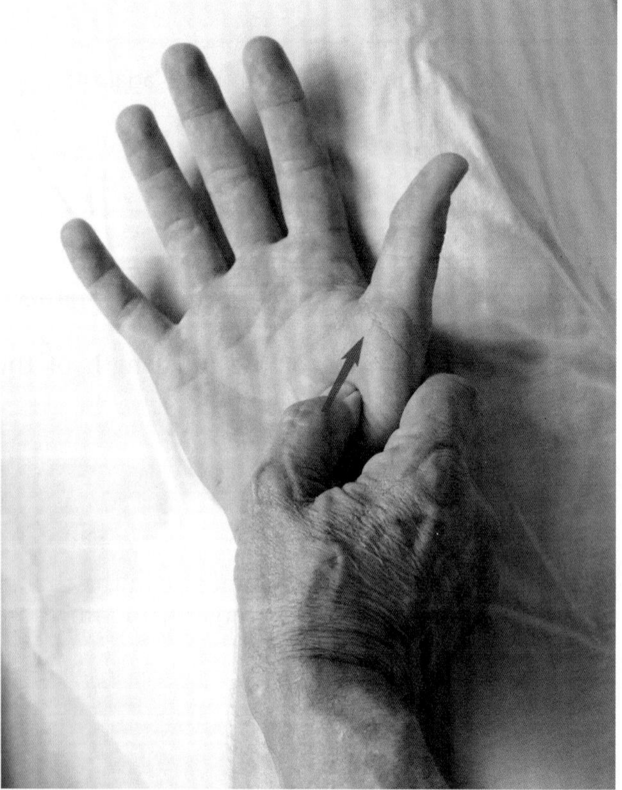

FIGURE 5-49 Stripping massage of the muscles of the thenar eminence (with unsupported thumb)

INTEROSSEUS MUSCLES OF THE HAND

IN-ter-OSS-see-us

ETYMOLOGY Latin ***inter***, between + ***os***, bone

Overview

The palmar interosseous muscles adduct the fingers toward the midline of the hand, and the dorsal interosseous muscles abduct the fingers from the midline.

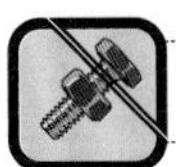

ATTACHMENTS

Dorsal interosseous muscles (four) (Fig. 5-50):

- Origin: sides of adjacent metacarpal bones
- Insertion: base of the proximal phalanges and extensor expansion, first on radial side of 2nd digit, second on radial side of 3rd digit, third on ulnar side of 3rd digit, and fourth on ulnar side of 4th digit

Palmar interosseous muscles (three) (Fig. 5-51):

- Origin: palmar surface of the 2nd, 4th, and 5th metacarpal bones
- Insertion: 1st palmar interosseous muscle into the base of the ulnar side of the 2nd digit, the 2nd and 3rd palmar interosseous muscles into radial sides of 4th and 5th digits.

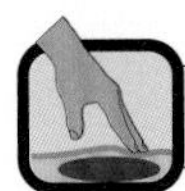

PALPATION

Palpable between the metacarpals on the front and back of the hand. Architecture varies from unipennate (all on the same side of the tendon) to bipennate (fibers are at an angle to the force-generating axis [pennation angle] and insert into a central tendon).

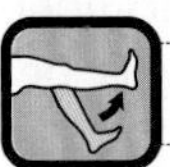

ACTION

Dorsal: abduct 2nd through 4th digits from the midline of the hand (axis of the 3rd digit and adduct third and fourth digits); note that the 2nd and 3rd interosseous muscles can abduct the 3rd digit in two directions from the midline but only when acting alone

Palmar: adduct 2nd, 4th, and 5th digits toward the midline of the hand (axis of the 3rd digit)

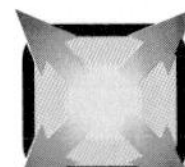

REFERRAL AREA

Edges of corresponding fingers

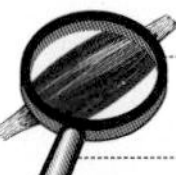

OTHER MUSCLES TO EXAMINE

- Infraspinatus
- Scalenes
- Subclavius
- Pectoralis major
- Pectoralis minor
- Coracobrachialis
- Serratus anterior

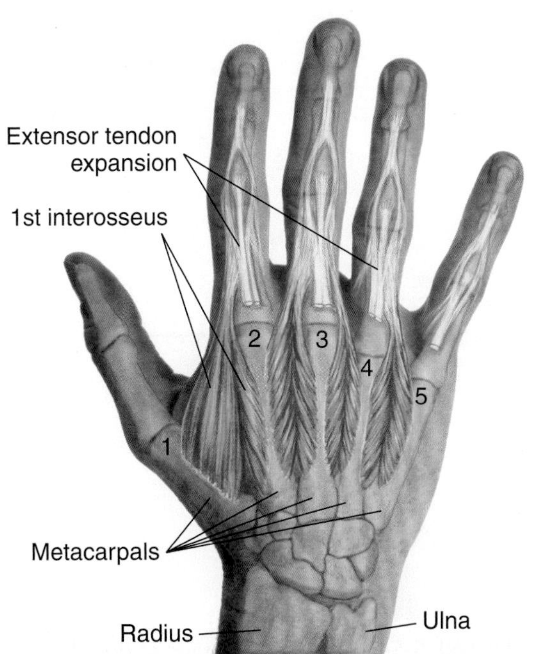

FIGURE 5-50 Anatomy of the dorsal interosseous muscles

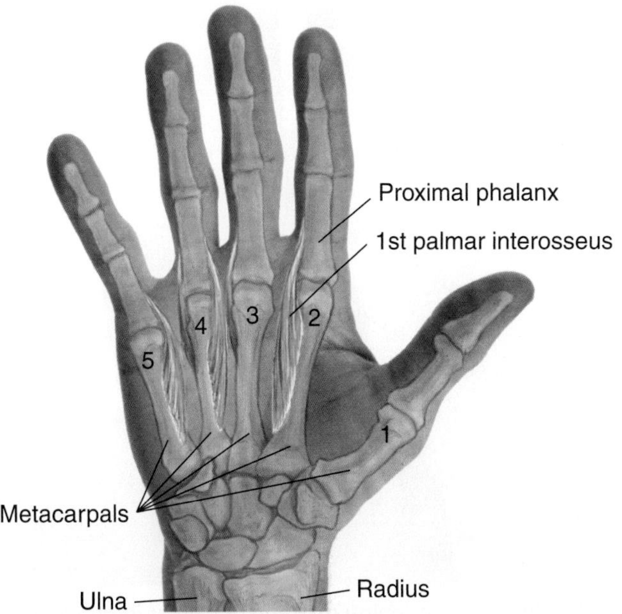

FIGURE 5-51 Anatomy of the palmar interosseous muscles

MANUAL THERAPY

PALMAR INTEROSSEOUS MUSCLES OF THE HAND

Stripping

- The client lies supine. (The client may also be seated, or in any position that makes the palmar aspect of the hand accessible.)
- The therapist stands beside the client at the shoulder.
- Place the thumb on the palm of the hand between the 1st and 2nd MP joints.
- Pressing firmly into the tissue, slide the thumb proximally between the 1st and 2nd fingers to the thenar eminence.
- Repeat this procedure between each pair of metacarpals (Fig. 5-52), shifting the thumb ulnarly, until the entire hand has been treated.

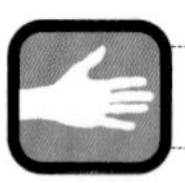

MANUAL THERAPY

DORSAL INTEROSSEOUS MUSCLES OF THE HAND

Stripping

- The client lies supine. (The client may also be seated, or in any position that allows access to the dorsal aspect of the hand.)
- The therapist stands beside the client at the hips.
- Hold and stabilize the client's hand with your nontreating hand.
- Place the thumb on the dorsal aspect of the hand between the 1st and 2nd metacarpals (i.e., between the thumb and forefinger) just next to the MP joint.
- Pressing firmly into the tissue, slide the thumb proximally between the thumb and forefinger (Fig. 5-53) to the end of the tissue.
- Repeat this procedure between each pair of metacarpals until the entire hand has been treated (Fig. 5-54).

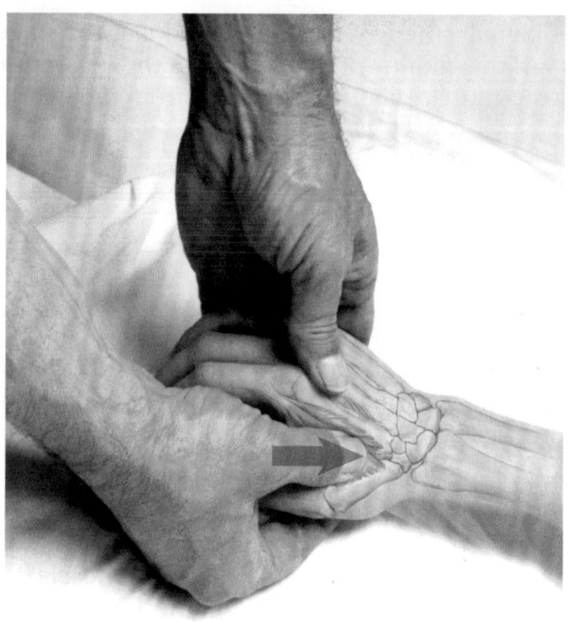

FIGURE 5-53 Stripping massage of first dorsal interosseous muscle

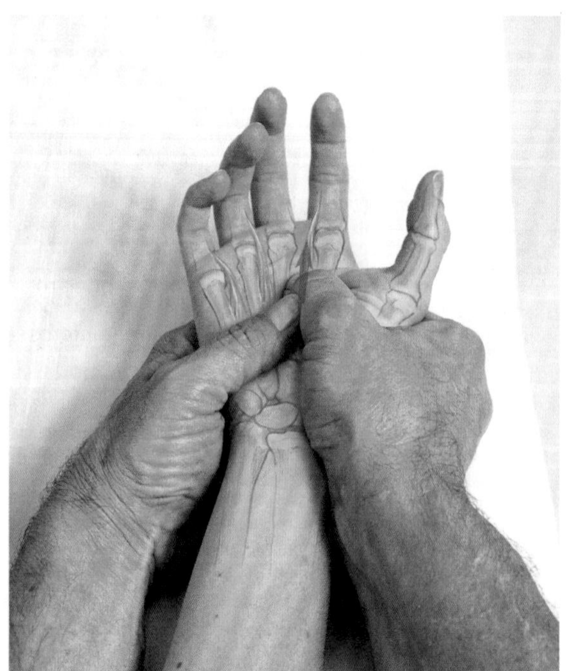

FIGURE 5-52 Stripping massage of palmar interosseous muscles between 2nd and 3rd metacarpals

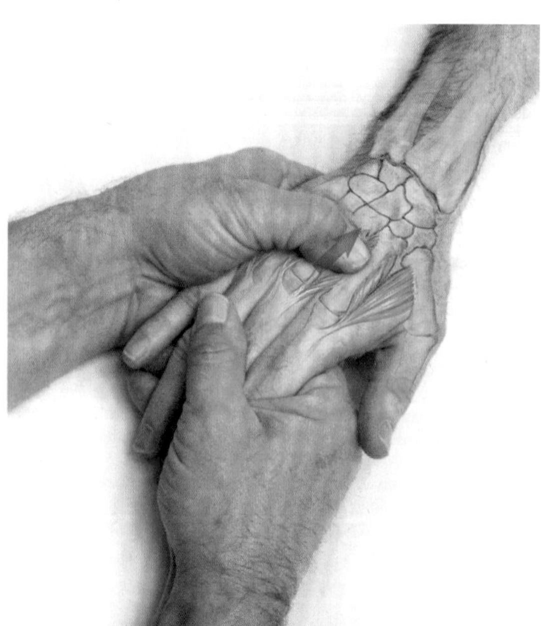

FIGURE 5-54 Stripping massage of dorsal interosseous muscles

LUMBRICAL MUSCLES OF THE HAND

LUM-bri-cal

ETYMOLOGY Latin ***lumbricus***, earthworm

The lumbricals (Fig. 5-55) work with the interossei in refining actions of the fingers, particularly in strong grasping. They are unusual in that they attach only to tendons, rather than bones.

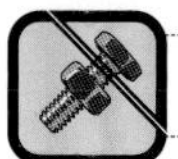

ATTACHMENTS

Origin

- The two lateral (radial): from the radial side of the tendons of the flexor digitorum profundus going to the 2nd and 3rd digits
- The two medial (ulnar): from the adjacent sides of the 2nd and 3rd, and 3rd and 4th tendons

Insertion

- Radial side of extensor tendon on dorsum of each of the four fingers (not including the thumb) at the proximal phalanges

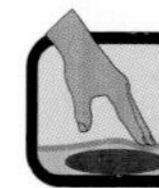

PALPATION

Neither palpable nor discernible.

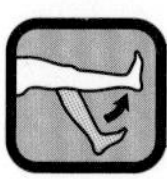

ACTION

Flex MP joint and extend the proximal and distal IP joint of digits 2 through 5.

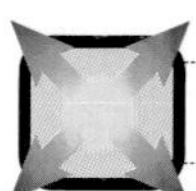

REFERRAL AREA

No specific trigger points have been documented in the lumbrical muscles. They are included here for completeness.

OTHER MUSCLES TO EXAMINE

None

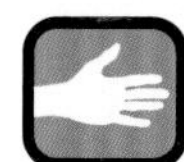

MANUAL THERAPY

These muscles are treated with the interossei, above.

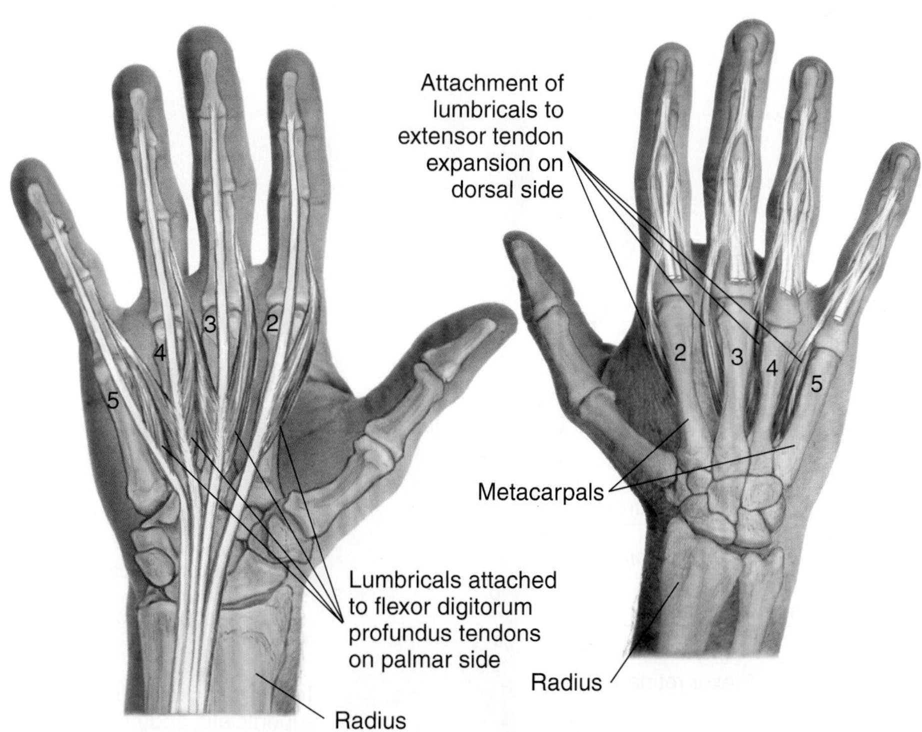

FIGURE 5-55 Anatomy of lumbricals

FLEXOR DIGITI MINIMI BREVIS

FLEX-er DIJ-it-tea MIN-im-me BREV-is

ETYMOLOGY Latin ***flexor***, flexor + ***digiti***, of the finger + ***minimi***, smallest + ***brevis***, short

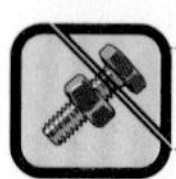

ATTACHMENTS

- Origin: hamulus of the hamate bone (Fig. 5-56)
- Insertion: lateral side of the proximal 5th phalanx

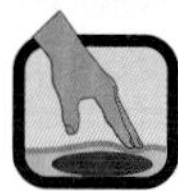

PALPATION

Palpable on the palm between the hamate and the base of the 5th digit. Architecture is parallel, and fibers are parallel to the muscle.

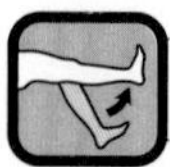

ACTION

Flexes the MP joint of the 5th digit

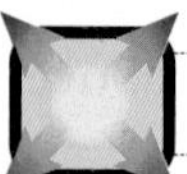

REFERRAL AREA

No trigger points have been documented for this muscle.

OTHER MUSCLES TO EXAMINE

None

MANUAL THERAPY

Not applicable

ABDUCTOR DIGITI MINIMI

ab-DUCK-ter DIJ-it-tea MIN-im-me

ETYMOLOGY Latin ***abductor*** (***ab***, away from + ***ducere***, to lead), that which draws away + ***digiti***, of the finger + ***minimi***, smallest

Overview

If there were a 6th digit, abductor digiti minimi (Fig. 5-57) would be half of its dorsal interosseous muscle. It typically develops a trigger point at the center of the belly, palpable on the dorsal side.

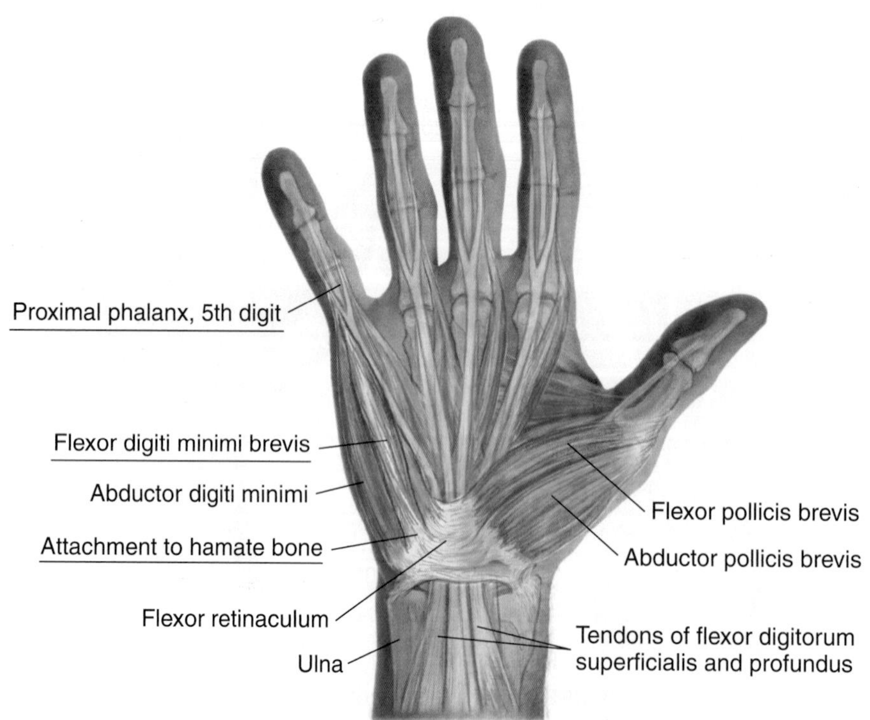

FIGURE 5-56 Anatomy of flexor digiti minimi brevis

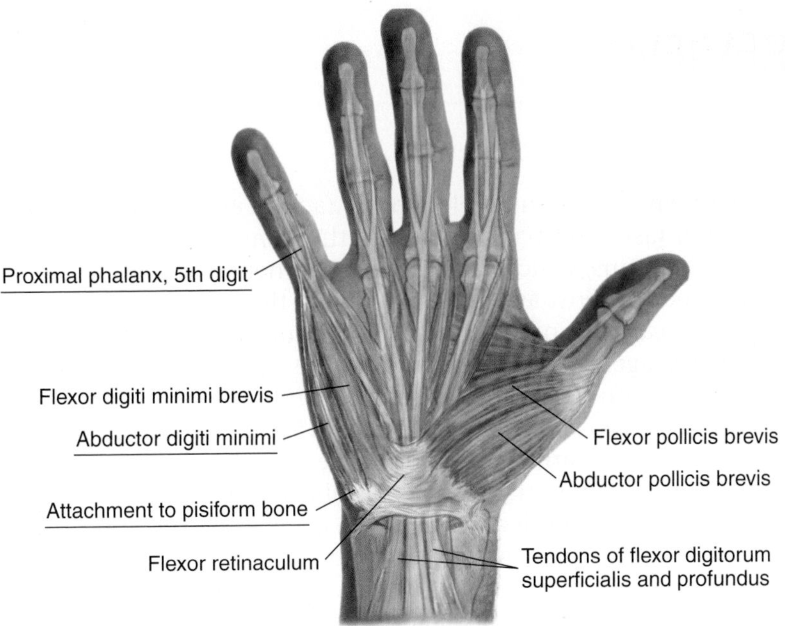

FIGURE 5-57 Anatomy of abductor digiti minimi

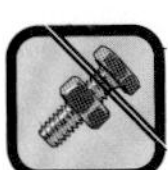

ATTACHMENTS

- Origin: pisiform bone and pisohamate ligament
- Insertion: lateral side of the base of the proximal 5th phalanx

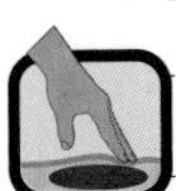

PALPATION

Palpable on the ulnar edge of the hand. Architecture is parallel, and fibers are parallel to the muscle.

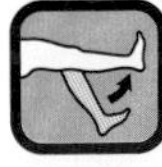

ACTION

Abducts and flexes the MP joint of the 5th digit

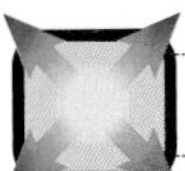

REFERRAL AREA

Lateral and dorsal aspects of the little finger

OTHER MUSCLES TO EXAMINE

- Pectoralis minor
- Serratus posterior superior
- Latissimus dorsi
- Triceps brachii
- Flexor digitorum

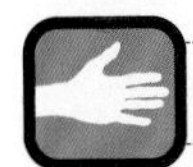

MANUAL THERAPY

Pincer Compression

- The client is in any position that allows access to the ulnar edge of the hand.
- With the nontreating hand, hold and stabilize the client's hand.
- Using the thumb and index finger, explore the dorsal aspect of abductor digiti minimi looking for tender spots (Fig. 5-58).
- Hold for release.

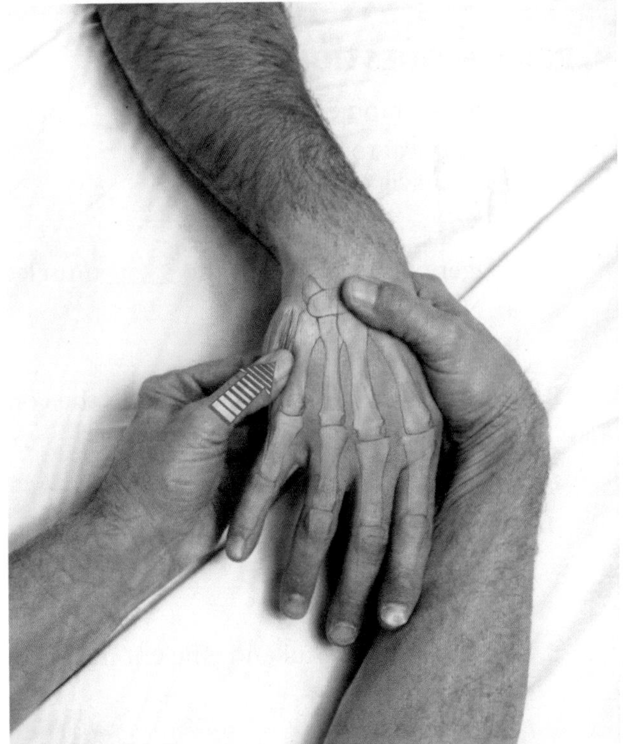

FIGURE 5-58 Pincer compression of trigger point in abductor digiti minimi

CHAPTER REVIEW

CASE STUDY

S.H. is a 30-year old woman who works in an electronics factory as a packer; she spends 8 hours a day performing repetitive motion tasks and has been doing the same job for the past 6 years. She is seeking massage for the pain in her arms, which radiates down to her hands. She is also experiencing some tingling and numbness around the wrist area and says that at times she has difficulty making a fist; she states that she thinks she has carpal tunnel syndrome, although she has not seen a doctor for a diagnosis. She was referred for massage by a coworker and has never experienced massage. Her first session began with basic Swedish strokes on the head, neck, shoulders, and upper extremities to help the client relax and acclimate to massage. Deep tissue was applied for 15 minutes on upper back/shoulder muscles prior to beginning stripping work on arms and hands. The right brachialis was very tender just below the origin of brachioradialis and had referred pain at the elbow and radiating down the arm. Deep compression and stripping within her pain tolerance resulted in relief by the end of the session. The need for her to see her doctor was discussed, as she intends to continue with the job she is on; she agreed to see him before the next visit, scheduled 2 weeks from today. She was suggested that in the meantime she may want to use ice for pain. Based on the relief she felt at the end of the session, she has agreed to twice-monthly appointments for the foreseeable future.

M.O., LMBT

REVIEW QUESTIONS

1. Nerve entrapments at the __________ may be responsible for arm and hand pain.
   a. Cervical roots
   b. Thoracic outlet
   c. Pectoralis minor attachment at the coracoid process
   d. All of the above

2. Trigger points located in the ______muscles may refer pain to the arm and/or hand.
   a. Neck
   b. Lumbar
   c. Quadricep
   d. PSIS

3. Which of the following attaches to the coracoid process of the scapula?
   a. Subclavius
   b. Pectoralis major
   c. Pectoralis minor
   d. Serratus anterior

4. *Volar* refers to the _______ aspect of the forearm.
   a. Posterior
   b. Anterior
   c. Superior
   d. Inferior

5. One of the powerful and efficient flexors of the elbow is the _______.
   a. Subclavius
   b. Teres major
   c. Biceps femoris
   d. Brachialis

6. The condition of tendons becoming inflamed and swollen, thereby compressing the median nerve, is referred to as _________.
   a. Media otitis
   b. Thoracic outlet syndrome
   c. Carpal tunnel syndrome
   d. Phlebitis

7. One of the distinguishing characteristics of humans that sets them apart from other species is the ________.
   a. Opposable thumb
   b. Mammary glands
   c. Pennate muscle fibers
   d. Fascia

8. The thenar eminence is located ________.
   a. At the base of the thumb
   b. On the fingertips
   c. At the first joint of the little finger
   d. On the medial side of the palm

9. The lumbrical muscles of the hand are attached to the ________.
   a. Metacarpophalangeal joint
   b. Tendons only
   c. Coracoid process
   d. First two phalanges

10. Extensors can be palpated as a group by __________.
   a. Cracking the knuckles
   b. Flexing the triceps
   c. Hyperextending the wrist
   d. Hyperflexing the wrist

thePoint Additional helpful resources are available at http://thePoint.lww.com.

CHAPTER 6

The Vertebral Column

LEARNING OBJECTIVES

At the end of this chapter, the learner will be able to:

- State the anatomical names of the muscles of the vertebral column.
- Palpate the muscles of the vertebral column.
- Identify the origins and insertions of the spinal muscles.
- Explain the actions of the muscles.
- Describe their pain referral areas.
- Recall related muscles that are synergists and antagonists of spinal muscles.
- Recognize any endangerment sites of the vertebral column, contraindications, and ethical cautions for massage therapy.
- Demonstrate proficiency in manual therapy techniques on muscles of the vertebral column.

The Overview of the Region begins on page 209, after the anatomy plates.

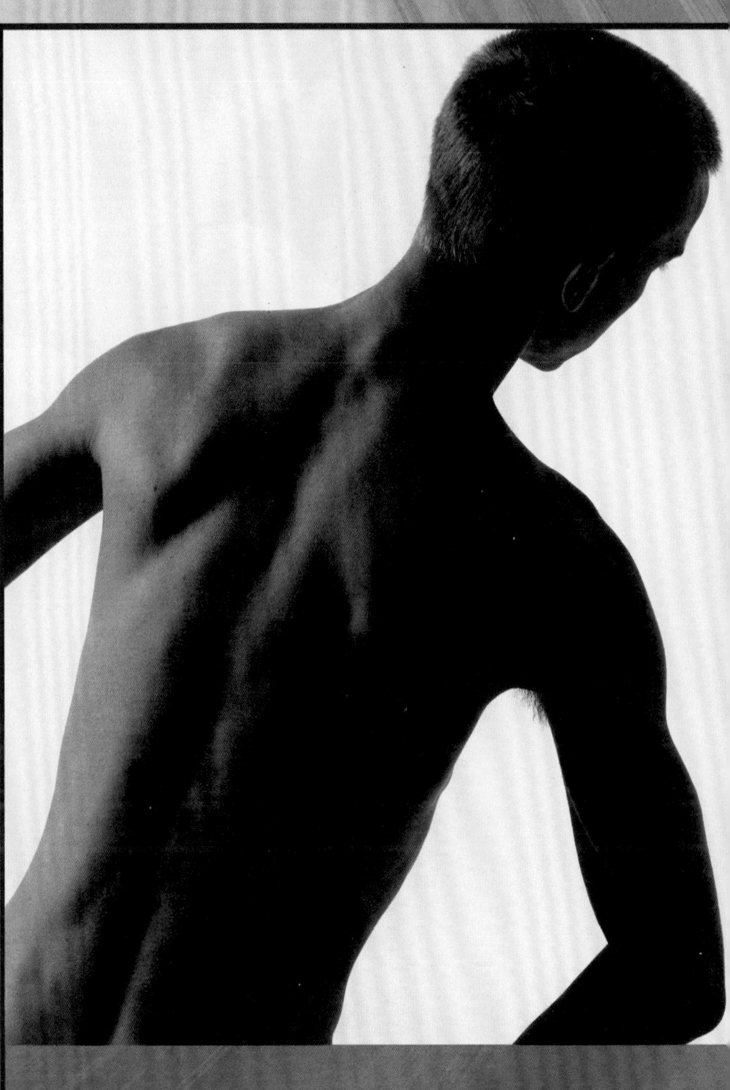

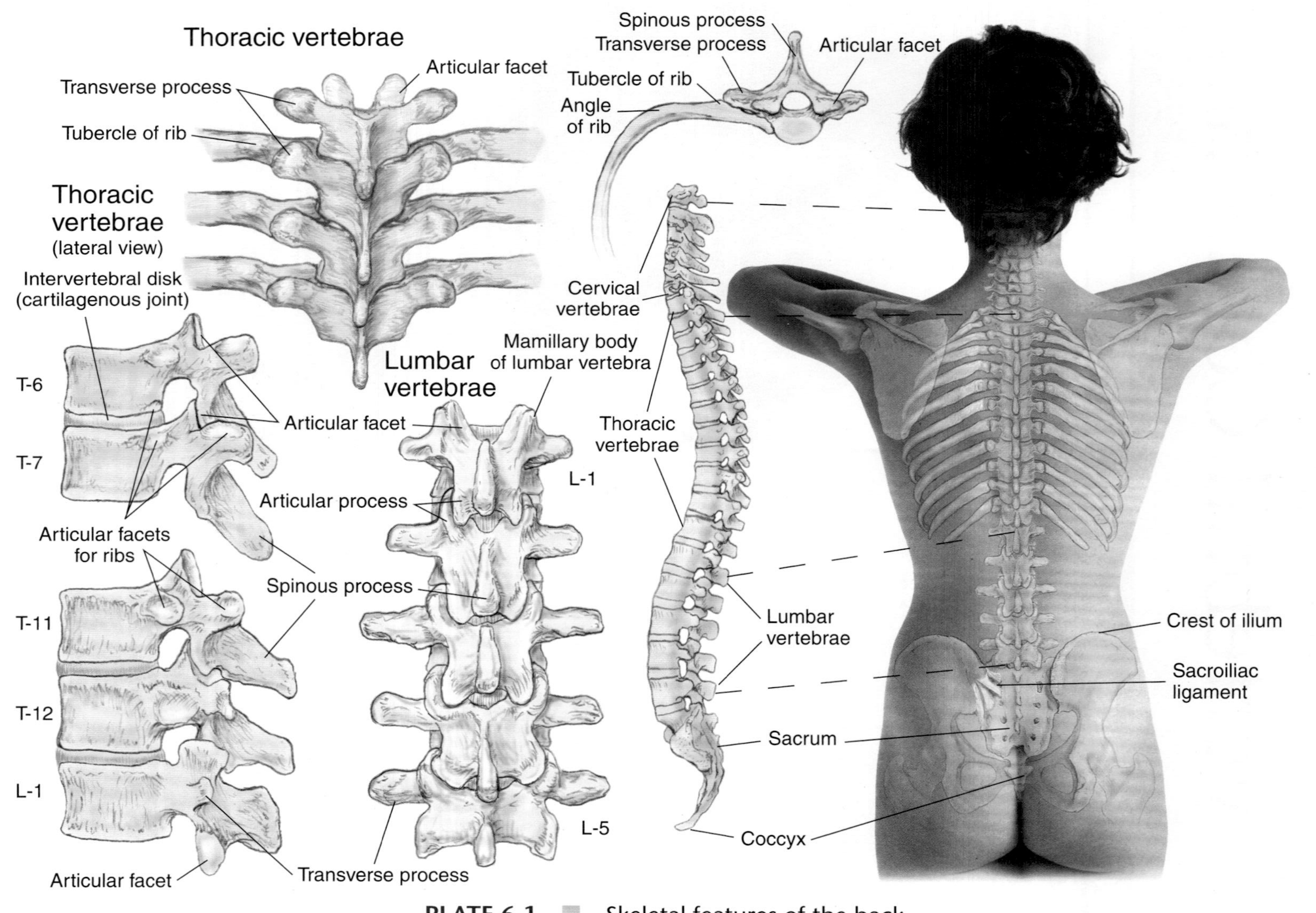

PLATE 6-1 ■ Skeletal features of the back

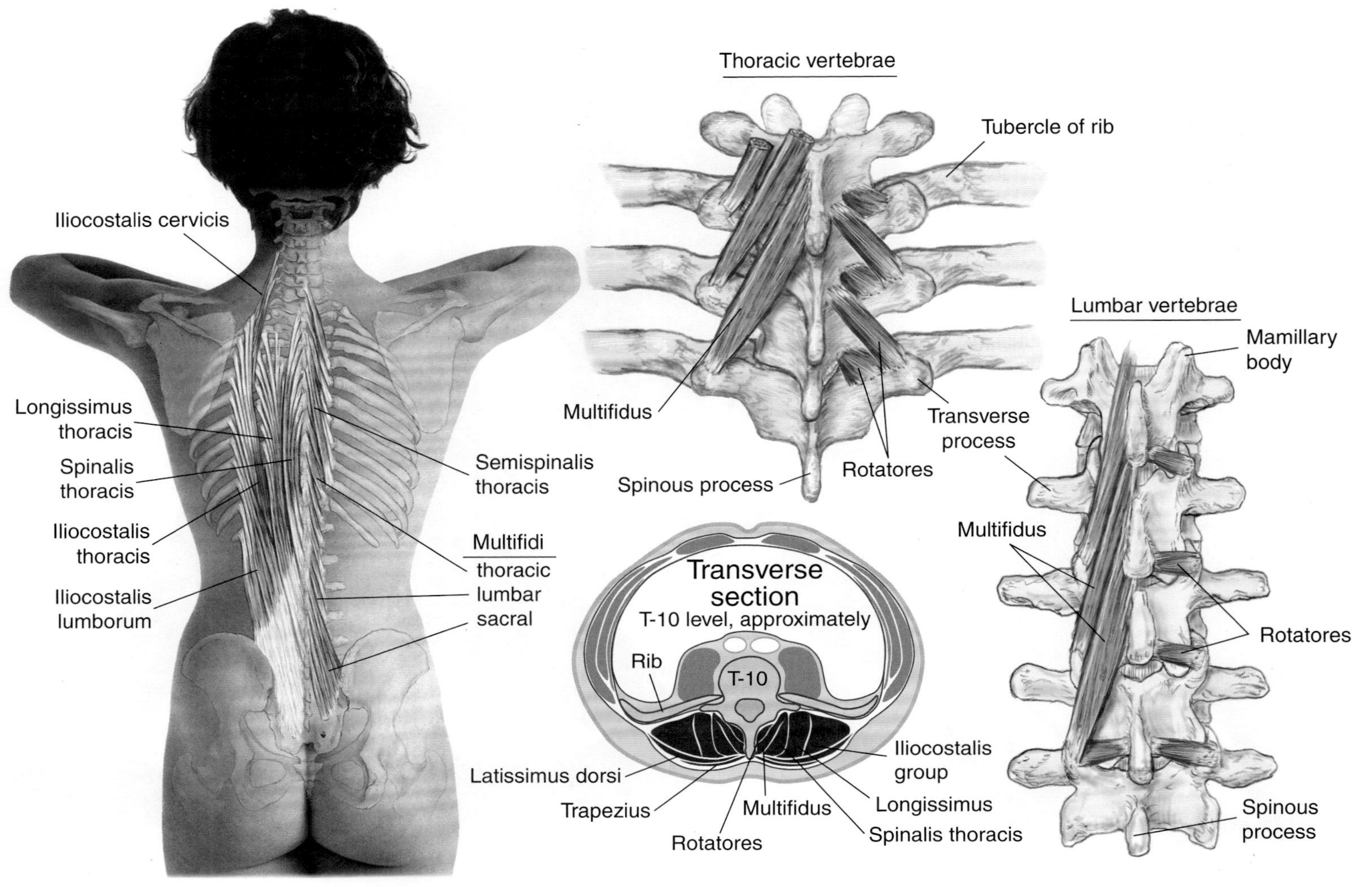

PLATE 6-2 ■ Muscles of the back

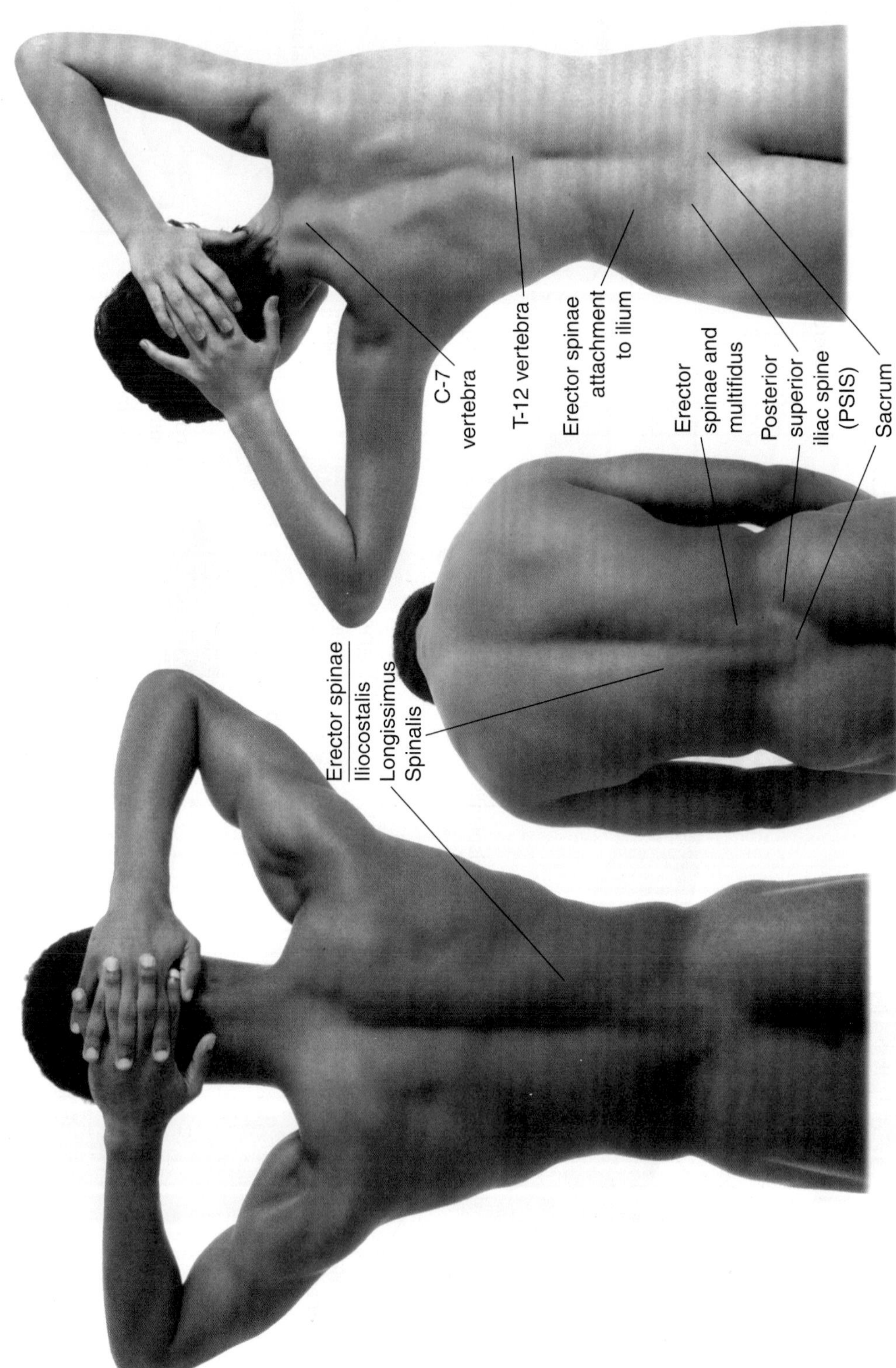

PLATE 6-3 ■ Surface anatomy of the back

Overview of the Region (Plates 6-1 to 6-3)

The vertebral column, or spine, is divided into five regions:

- The cervical spine, with seven vertebrae (C1 through C7)
- The thoracic spine, with twelve vertebrae and attached ribs (T1 through T12)
- The lumbar spine, with five vertebrae (L1 through L5)
- The sacrum, with five fused vertebrae
- The coccyx, usually consisting of four fused vertebrae

Though similar in basic structure and function, the vertebrae vary considerably in size and shape in the different regions, the cervical vertebrae being the smallest and the lumbar vertebrae being the largest.

At birth the spine has a single posterior curvature forming the typical "C" shape of the newborn infant. As the child begins to hold the head erect, sit up, and learn to stand, additional spinal curvatures develop. The five regions of the adult spine include four normal curvatures. The cervical and lumbar regions have an anterior curvature while the thoracic, sacral, and coccygeal regions retain their original posterior curvature. Excessive increases or decreases in these curves (**kyphosis, lordosis**) or abnormalities such as scoliosis, threaten postural integrity, and the restoration of good posture and maintenance is one of the aims of posturally oriented bodywork. However, we must remember that we are just massage therapists, not miracle workers. We cannot "fix" every problem resulting from postural deviations; furthermore, not everyone who has a deviation has pain related to it—and plenty of people who *are* in pain may not have any postural deviations. It is much easier to achieve postural corrections on a child who is still growing—in some cases. It is beyond our ability to correct structural issues that have to do with actual bone deformities, although massage can certainly help with decreasing resulting muscular pain and increasing mobility. Once adulthood has been achieved and growth has stopped, we may not have the success we hope for in treating postural problems. We may be able to relieve pain where it exists, but it is less than realistic to think we can correct every posture-impaired person who comes in the door.

There are two types of joints between most of the vertebrae of the spine:

- Cartilaginous joints between the broad vertebral bodies of adjoining vertebrae are known as intervertebral disks. They are composed of fibrocartilage surrounding a gel-filled disk and support most of the weight
- Synovial facet joints between the articular processes of adjacent vertebrae guide most of the movement

There are two facet joints on each superior and inferior side, articulating with the facets of the two adjoining vertebrae. In addition, the thoracic vertebrae also articulate with the ribs and accordingly have synovial facet joints for them on the right and left sides.

The variations in shape and orientation between the facet joints of the vertebrae in different spinal regions determine the type and range of movement of the spine.

These movements are:

- Flexion
- Extension (and hyperextension)
- Lateral flexion (to the left and right; sometimes called lateral bending)
- Rotation (to the left and right)

The cervical region is the only one capable of the full range of spinal movement. All other regions are limited in one or more movements. The spinous processes of the thoracic vertebrae are angled sharply in an inferior direction and prevent hyperextension of this region in most individuals. The articular facets of the lumbar region are nearly vertical in the sagittal plane, "locked" to the sacrum and thus limit rotation. Since the vertebrae are usually fused in the sacrum and coccyx by 18 to 30 years of age (and for all practical purposes much earlier), there is no movement possible within those regions, although they do move relative to adjoining regions. For example, the coccyx is joined to the sacrum by ligaments and can move in relation to it in response to pressure.

The lumbar region of the back is the most frequently injured; it bears more weight than the rest of the spine. However, the cervical vertebrae are the most delicate, the most mobile, and surrounded by complex anatomy (see chapter 3). They are also quite vulnerable to injury.

Contraindications for massage around the vertebral column are the same as general contraindications elsewhere in the body (no massage in areas of broken bones, no massage when communicable sickness and/or fever is present, no massage if bleeding is present, and so forth). Avoid performing deep massage when working with anyone who has osteoporosis or other conditions that may contribute to brittleness of bones. It's always better to err on the side of caution.

Note: The directional terms **"cephalad"** (toward the head) and **"caudad"** (toward the tail, i.e., coccyx) are used in this chapter.

Etymology Greek ***kephal***, head, Latin ***cauda***, tail

It is helpful to do some general work on the back before treating specific areas in order to stimulate local blood flow and relax the superficial musculature. This may include effleurage, petrissage, kneading, and percussion, but be careful not to use excessive lubrication, as it will hinder work in specific areas afterward. One helpful technique for preparatory treatment of the back is myofascial stretching.

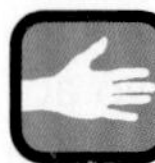

MANUAL THERAPY

Myofascial Stretching for the Back

- The client lies prone.
- The therapist stands beside the client at the torso.
- Place the hand nearest the client's head flat on the lumbar area lateral to the vertebrae with the fingers over the iliac crest just lateral to the sacrum.
- Crossing the other hand over or under the first, place it flat on the thoracic area over the lowest three or four ribs.
- Let your hands sink into the tissue until you feel contact with the superficial myofascial tissue.
- Press the hands in opposite directions, with enough downward pressure to engage and stretch the superficial myofascial tissue (Fig. 6-1).
- Hold until you feel significant release in the tissue.
- Shift both hands laterally (toward yourself) by one hand's width and repeat the technique.
- Shift the hands cephalad, so that the caudad hand rests on the lower three or four ribs and the cephalad hand rests on the 3rd through the 6th ribs, both hands just lateral to the vertebrae.
- Repeat the technique.
- Repeat the technique at this level, shifting the hands laterally.
- Repeat the entire procedure on the opposite side.

The Superficial Paraspinal Muscles

We need to keep two facts in mind when viewing the vertebral column in the context of the whole body:

- The center of gravity of the body is in the pelvic region, well forward of the spine.
- As we noted in Chapter 4 (page 127), the entire arm and shoulder structure is attached to the skeleton by only one joint, the sternoclavicular joint, also well forward of the spine.
- Most of the weight of the skull, ribs, and thoracic contents are also well forward of the spine.

The implication is that the spine and the muscles that attach to it must maintain the integrity of the posture

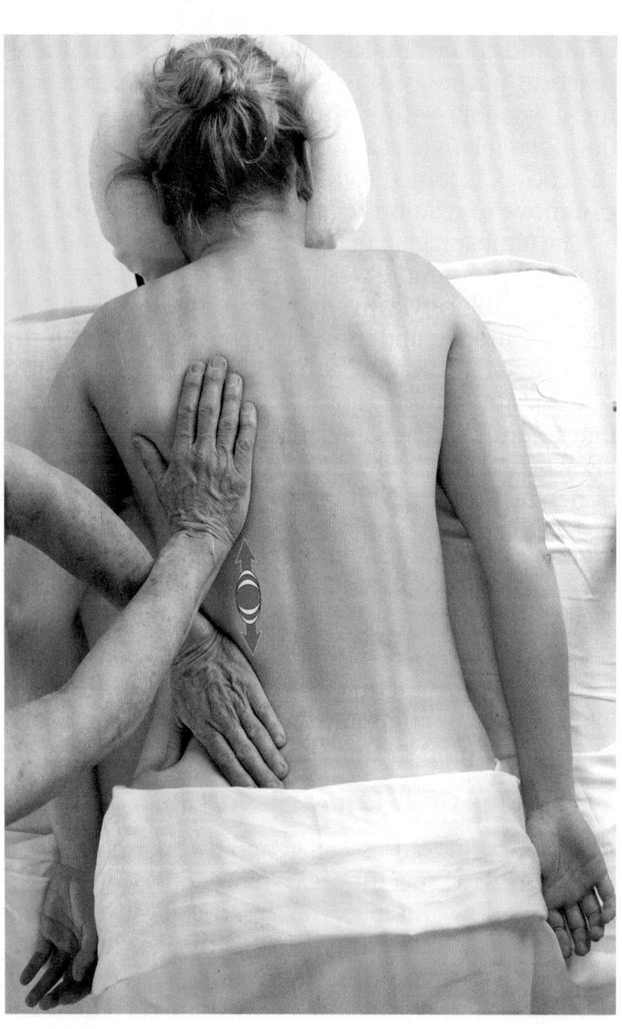

FIGURE 6-1 Myofascial stretch for the back

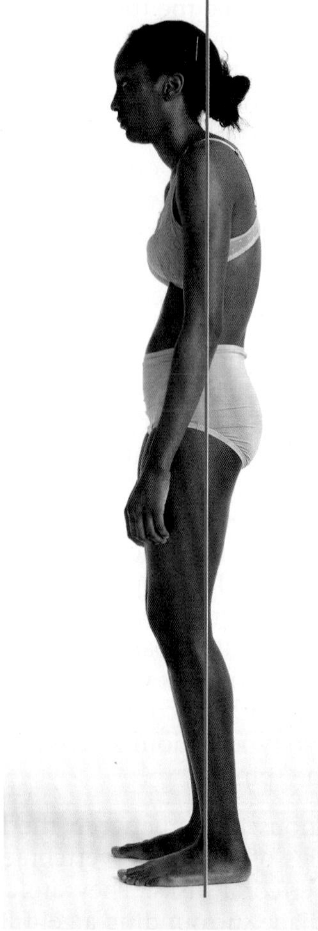

FIGURE 6-2 Posture with head forward and shoulders medially rotated

against a strong anterior pull. Because of the location of our eyes and the construction of our shoulders and arms, virtually everything that we do requires us to move our heads, arms, and torsos forward, down, and inward. It is the task of the superficial muscles of the vertebral column (along with the muscles of the low back) to stabilize us in such activities. Poor posture—that is, posture in which the head is carried forward of the sagittal midline, and/or the shoulders are medially rotated, and/or the anterior intercostal and abdominal muscles are habitually shortened (Fig. 6-2)—places a severe strain on the superficial muscles of the spine and posterior neck, resulting in the development of active trigger points and pain. Although, according to David G. Simons, MD (private communication, September 25, 2001), "there are no hard scientific data as to when and how latent MTrPs [myofascial trigger points] start,"[1] we do know that "by correcting the postural problem the MTrP either clears up or is much more treatable."

ERECTOR SPINAE

e-REK-tor SPEE-nuh

ETYMOLOGY Latin ***erector,*** straightener + ***spinae,*** of the spine

Overview

Erector spinae (Fig. 6-3) is a collective term for the group of muscles that extend and maintain the balance of the vertebral column and the rib cage. They also contract strongly in coughing and in straining during bowel movements.

These muscles originate from the sacrum, ilium, and the processes of the lumbar and the lower thoracic vertebrae. They are divided into three groups: iliocostalis, longissimus, and spinalis. Their branches attach to the vertebrae and ribs at ascending levels.

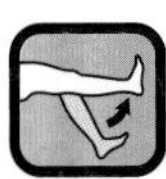

ACTION

The action is the same for all erector spinae, in their respective regions:

- Bilateral
  - Extension and hyperextension (in regions where possible) of vertebral column
  - Isometrically oppose gravity to maintain erect posture (mnemonic = *I* Like Standing)
  - Contract eccentrically to stabilize the vertebral column during flexion, acting in opposition to abdominal muscles and the action of gravity
- Unilateral
  - Lateral bending to the same side
  - Assist rotation in complex ways; often to the same side
  - Opposite muscles contract eccentrically for stabilization during lateral bending

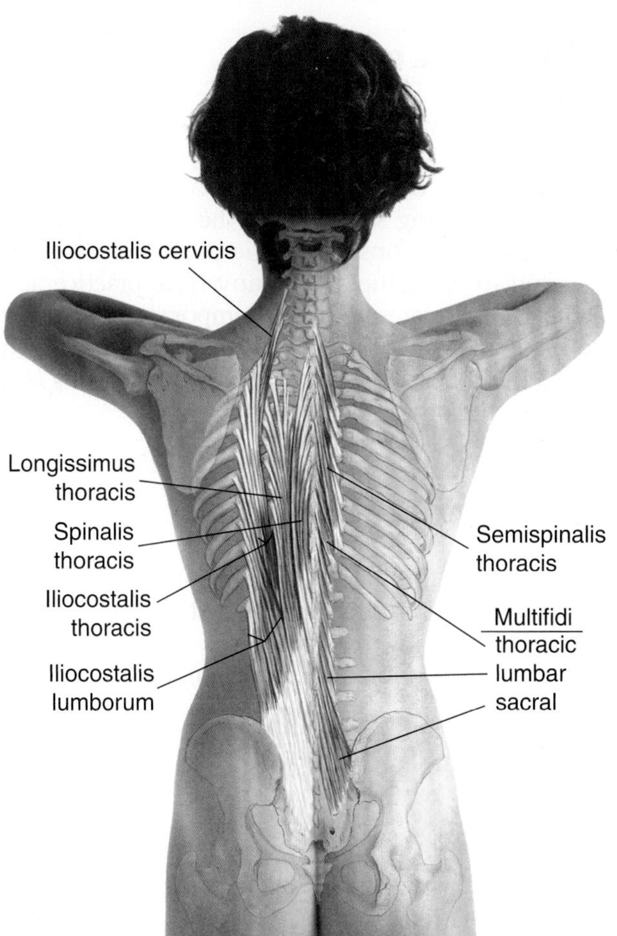

FIGURE 6-3 Anatomy of the erector spinae muscles

Overview of the Iliocostalis Group

The iliocostalis group represents the most lateral column of the erector spinae. It comprises three divisions: iliocostalis lumborum, iliocostalis thoracis, and iliocostalis cervicis.

ILIOCOSTALIS LUMBORUM

ILL-ee-oh-kos-TAL-is lum-BOR-um

ETYMOLOGY Latin ***ilio-***, relating to the ilium + ***costalis,*** relating to the ribs (costa, rib) + ***lumborum,*** of the loins

ETHICAL CAUTION

Working the lower back usually requires working the gluteal muscles. Always properly drape the client, and always educate the client about what you're doing. Abruptly touching someone in the sacral or gluteal area could be misconstrued if the client is unaware of the need to work the area. Many state practice acts in the United States allow for temporary removal of the drape in order to apply treatment, but the client should never be fully exposed; if you are working one side, keep the other side covered.

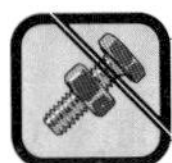

ATTACHMENTS

- Origin: sacrum, iliac crest, and spinous processes of the lower thoracic and most of the lumbar vertebrae
- Insertion: inferior borders of angles of ribs 6 to 12 (Fig. 6-4)

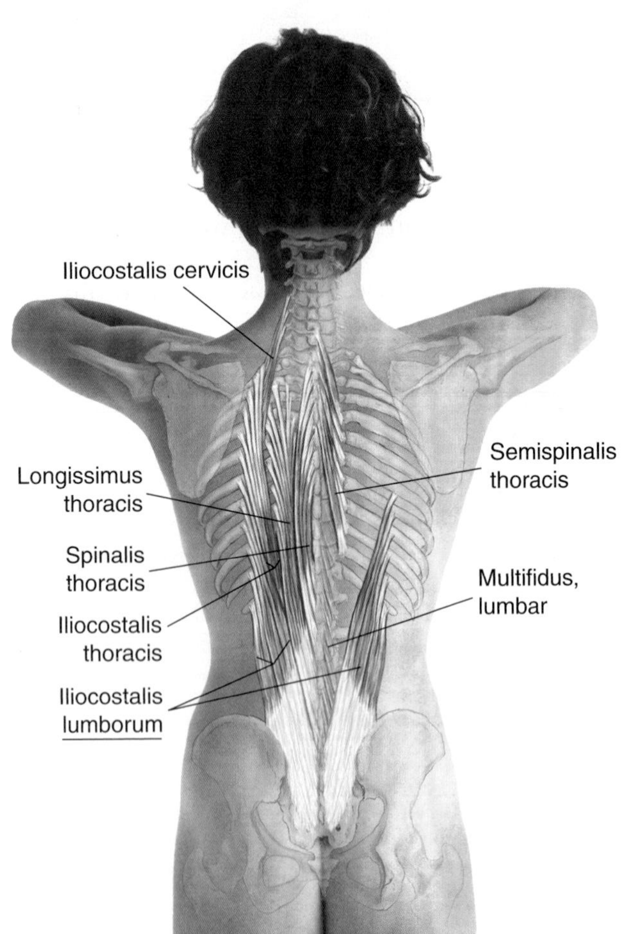

FIGURE 6-4 Anatomy of iliocostalis lumborum

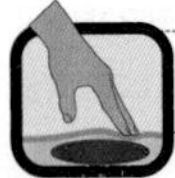

PALPATION

Discernible by cross-fiber stroking if pathologically hypercontracted. Architecture is parallel, and fibers are parallel to the muscle.

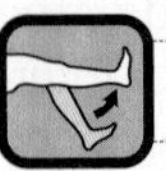

ACTION

Extends and laterally flexes thoracic and lumbar vertebrae; rotates thoracic vertebrae

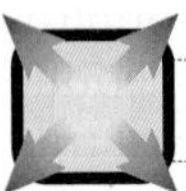

REFERRAL AREA

Over the lumbar region into the center of the buttock

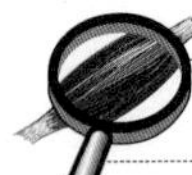

OTHER MUSCLES TO EXAMINE

- Iliocostalis thoracis
- Longissimus
- Quadratus lumborum
- Gluteals
- Piriformis and other lateral hip rotators

MANUAL THERAPY

Stripping

- The client lies prone.
- The therapist stands beside the client at the torso.
- Place the heel of the hand on the muscles at the waist of the client just lateral to the lumbar vertebrae.
- Pressing firmly into the tissue, slide the heel of the hand inferiorly over the sacrum to its base (Fig. 6-5).
- Repeat the procedure on the opposite side.

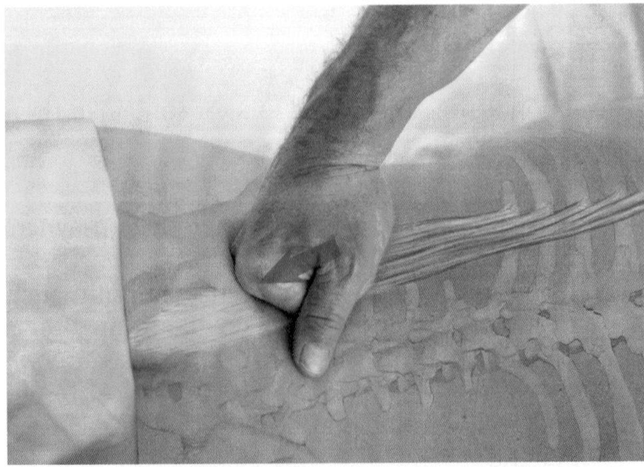

FIGURE 6-5 Stripping of origins of iliocostalis lumborum

ILIOCOSTALIS THORACIS

ILL-ee-oh-kos-TAL-is THOR-as-iss

ETYMOLOGY Latin *ilio-*, relating to the ilium + ***costalis***, relating to the ribs (costa, rib) + ***thoracis***, of the chest

Overview

Because of our extensive use of our arms and hands, our need to look down at what our hands are doing, and the prevalence of poor posture, iliocostalis thoracis (Fig. 6-6) frequently develops painful trigger point activity in branches of the muscle that extend under the scapulae. This area just inferior and medial to the scapula is one of the most common areas in need of trigger point release. Pain here often accompanies pain in the muscles of the shoulders.

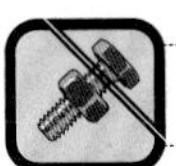

ATTACHMENTS

- Origin: superior borders ribs 6 to 12
- Insertion: inferior borders of the upper six ribs and sometimes transverse process of C-7

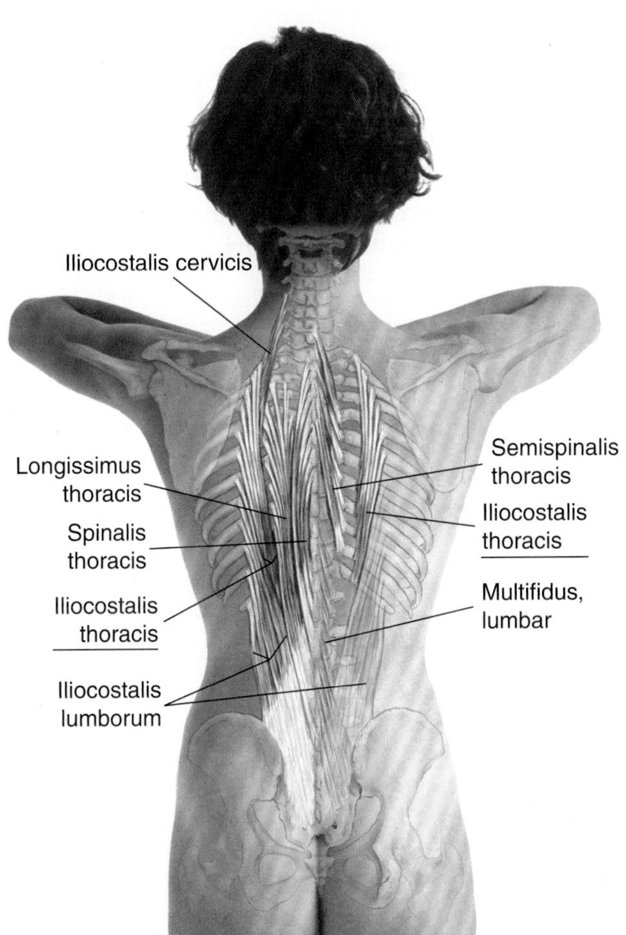

FIGURE 6-6 Anatomy of iliocostalis thoracis

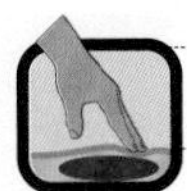

PALPATION

Discernible if pathologically hypercontracted, by cross-fiber stroking, particularly in the area of the inferior angle of the scapula. Architecture is parallel, and fibers are parallel to the muscle.

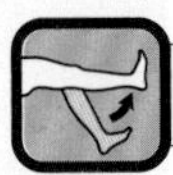

ACTION

Extends, laterally flexes, and rotates thoracic vertebrae

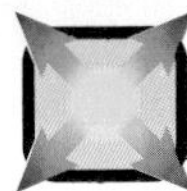

REFERRAL AREAS

- Inferior angle of the scapula, inside the medial border of the scapula to the superior angle; anterior chest over the angle of the sternum and the costal arch
- Over the lumbar region, into the lateral inferior thoracic region, up across the scapula; lower ipsilateral quadrant of the abdomen

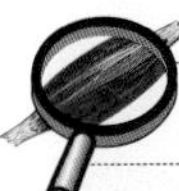

OTHER MUSCLES TO EXAMINE

- Trapezius, rotator cuff muscles, teres major, rhomboids
- Pectoralis major, intercostals
- Serratus posterior inferior, quadratus lumborum, iliocostalis lumborum
- Abdominal obliques, iliopsoas

MANUAL THERAPY

Stripping

- The client lies prone.
- The therapist stands beside the client at the head.
- Palpate for a distinct muscular band running diagonally in a superolateral direction under the inferomedial border of the scapula. Explore this band just inferior to the scapula for tenderness.
- Place the supported thumb on the tender spot and press firmly into the tissue.
- Glide the thumb diagonally along the muscle to the erector bundle (Fig. 6-7).
- Beginning at the same spot, repeat this procedure 2 or 3 times.

Cross-fiber Stroking

- The client lies prone.
- The therapist stands beside the client at the head.

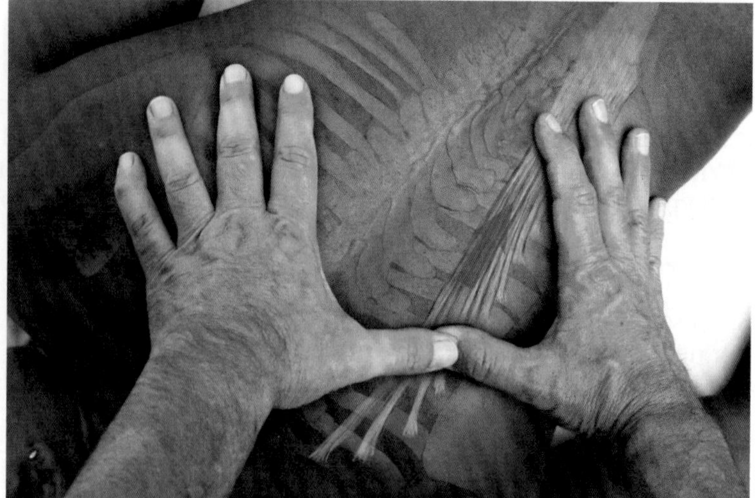

FIGURE 6-7 Stripping of iliocostalis thoracis with supported thumb

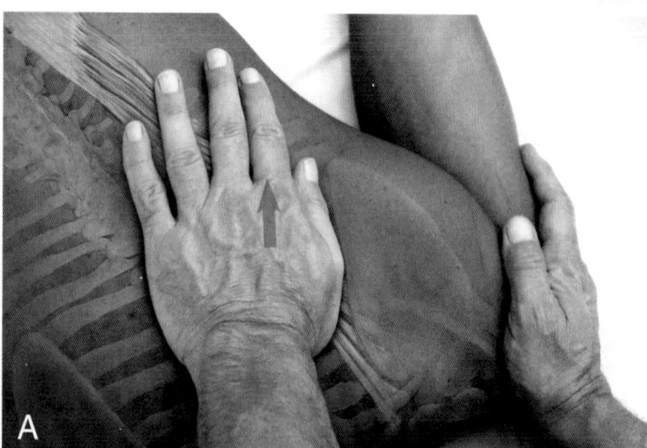

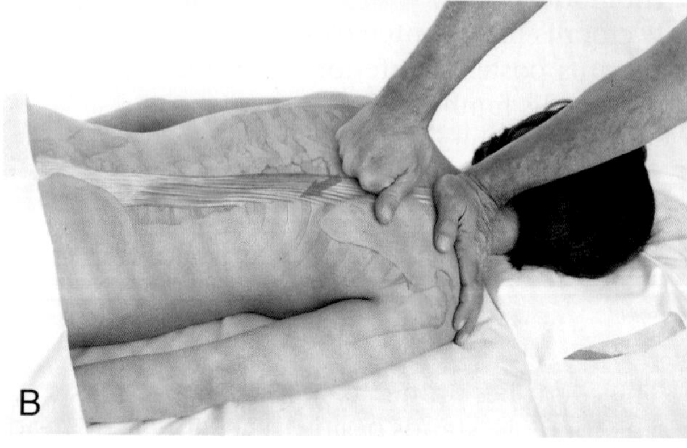

FIGURE 6-8 Cross-fiber stroking of iliocostalis thoracis with heel of hand **(A)** or knuckles **(B)**

- Place the hand (Fig. 6-8A) or the knuckles (Fig. 6-8B) on the upper back medial to the superior angle of the scapula.
- Pressing firmly into the tissue with the heel of your hand or your knuckles, slide your hand diagonally along the medial border of the scapula past the inferior angle.
- Beginning at the same spot, repeat this procedure 2 or 3 times.

Cross-fiber Friction

- The client lies prone.
- The therapist stands beside the client at the head.
- Place the fingertips or the knuckles next to the muscular band at the inferomedial border of the scapula.
- Move the fingertips or knuckles back and forth across the band at a rate of about twice per second.
- Continue until you feel release in the tissue.

ILIOCOSTALIS CERVICIS

ILL-ee-oh-kos-TAL-is SERV-iss-iss

ETYMOLOGY Latin *ilio-*, relating to the ***ilium*** + ***costalis,*** relating to the ribs (costa, rib) + *cervicis*, of the neck

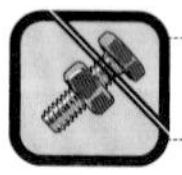

ATTACHMENTS

- Origin: angles of the upper six ribs (Fig. 6-9)
- Insertion: transverse processes of C4-C6

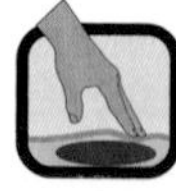

PALPATION

Discernable by cross-fiber stroking if pathologically hypercontracted. Architecture is parallel, and fibers are parallel to the muscle.

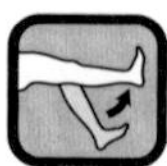

ACTION

Extends, laterally flexes, and rotates cervical vertebrae

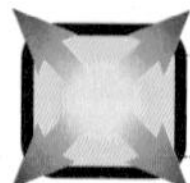

REFERRAL AREAS

No trigger points have been recorded for this muscle; it is included here for completeness.

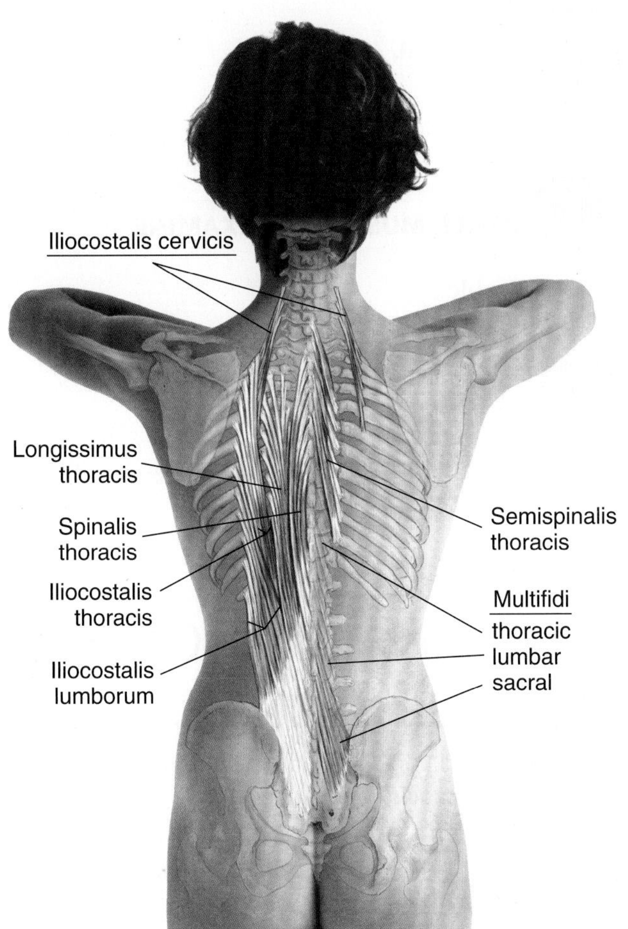

FIGURE 6-9 Anatomy of iliocostalis cervicis

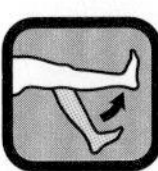

ACTION

Extends vertebral column

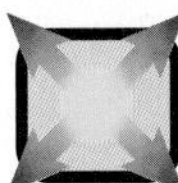

REFERRAL AREA

Over the lumbar region into the superior aspect of the buttock; over the buttock to the inferior aspect

OTHER MUSCLES TO EXAMINE

- Serratus posterior inferior
- Quadratus lumborum
- Iliocostalis lumborum and thoracis
- Gluteal muscles
- Piriformis and other lateral hip rotators
- Hamstrings

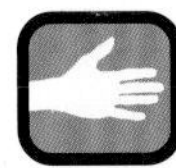

MANUAL THERAPY

See Manual Therapy for the Erector Spinae, below.

LONGISSIMUS THORACIS

long-GISS-i-mus THOR-as-iss

ETYMOLOGY Latin, ***longissimus***, longest + ***thoracis***, of the chest

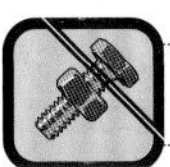

ATTACHMENTS

- Origin: sacrum and spinous processes of lower thoracic and most lumbar vertebrae (Fig. 6-10)
- Insertion: tips of the transverse processes of all thoracic vertebrae and the last 9 or 10 ribs between their tubercles and angles

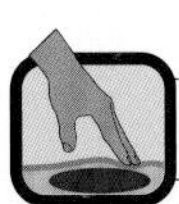

PALPATION

Discernible by cross-fiber stroking if pathologically hypercontracted. Architecture is parallel, and fibers are parallel to the muscle.

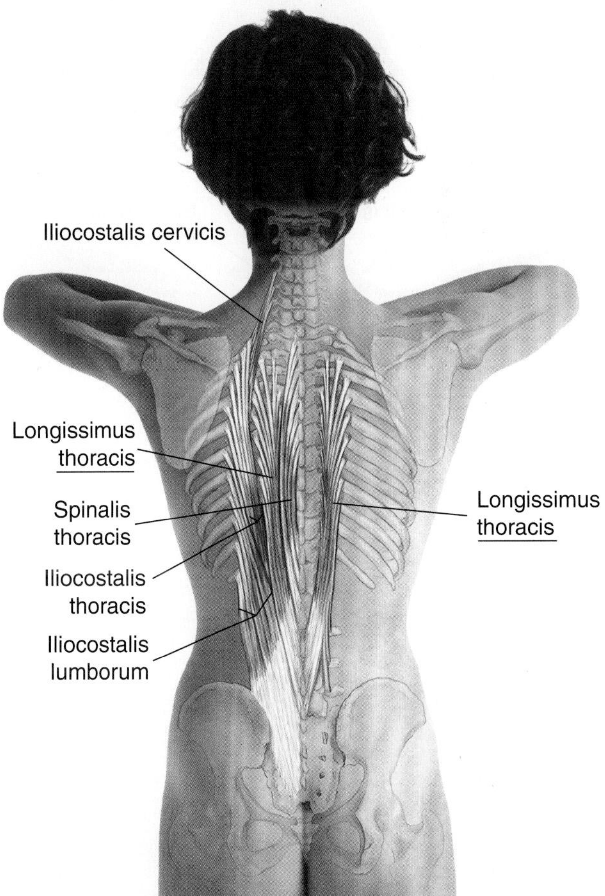

FIGURE 6-10 Anatomy of longissimus thoracis

SPINALIS THORACIS

spin-AL-iss THOR-as-iss

ETYMOLOGY Latin ***spinalis***, relating to the spine

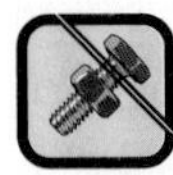

ATTACHMENTS

- Origin: spinous processes of T11, T12, L1, and L2 vertebrae (Fig. 6-11)
- Insertion: spinous processes of upper 4 to 8 thoracic vertebrae

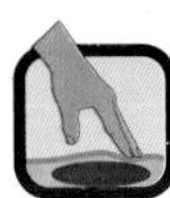

PALPATION

Discernible by cross-fiber stroking, if pathologically hypercontracted. Architecture is parallel, and fibers are parallel to the muscle.

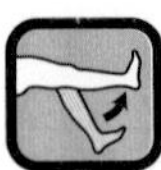

ACTION

Extends the vertebral column

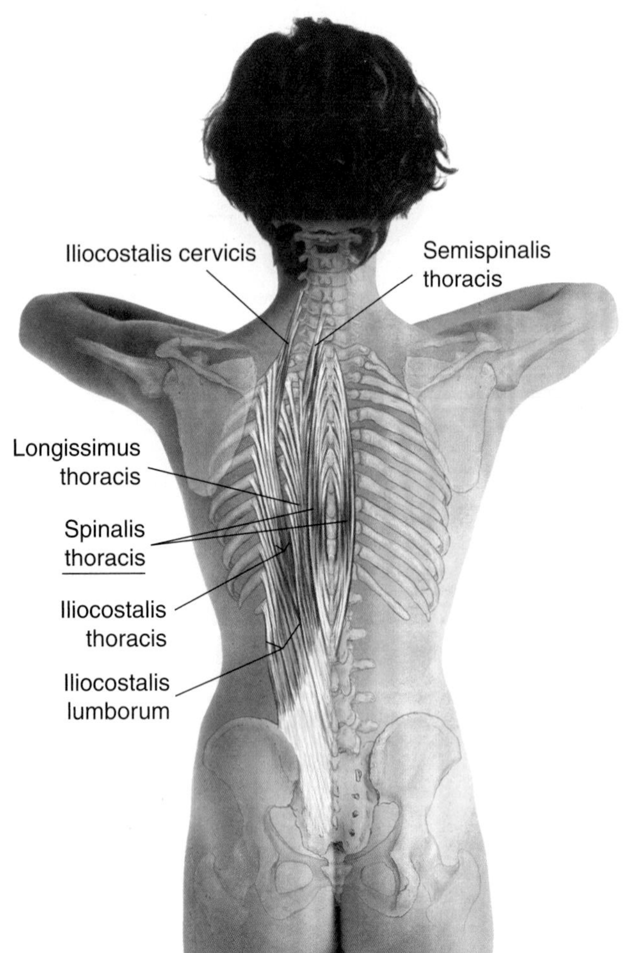

FIGURE 6-11 Anatomy of spinalis thoracis

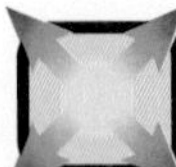

REFERRAL AREA

Not applicable

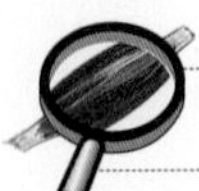

OTHER MUSCLES TO EXAMINE

Not applicable

MANUAL THERAPY

See Manual Therapy for the Erector Spinae, below.

SEMISPINALIS THORACIS

SEM-i-spin-AL-iss THOR-as-iss

ETYMOLOGY Latin ***semi***, half + ***spinalis***, relating to the spine + ***thoracis***, of the chest

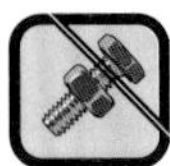

ATTACHMENTS

- Origin: transverse processes of T5 through T10 vertebrae (Fig. 6-12)
- Insertion: spinous processes of C7 through T4

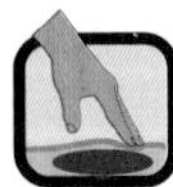

PALPATION

Architecture is parallel, and fibers are parallel to the muscle. Discernible if pathologically hypercontracted, by cross-fiber stroking.

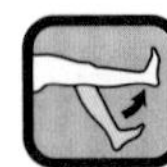

ACTION

Extends vertebral column.

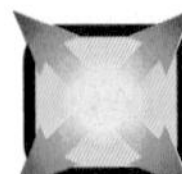

REFERRAL AREA

Not applicable

OTHER MUSCLES TO EXAMINE

Not applicable

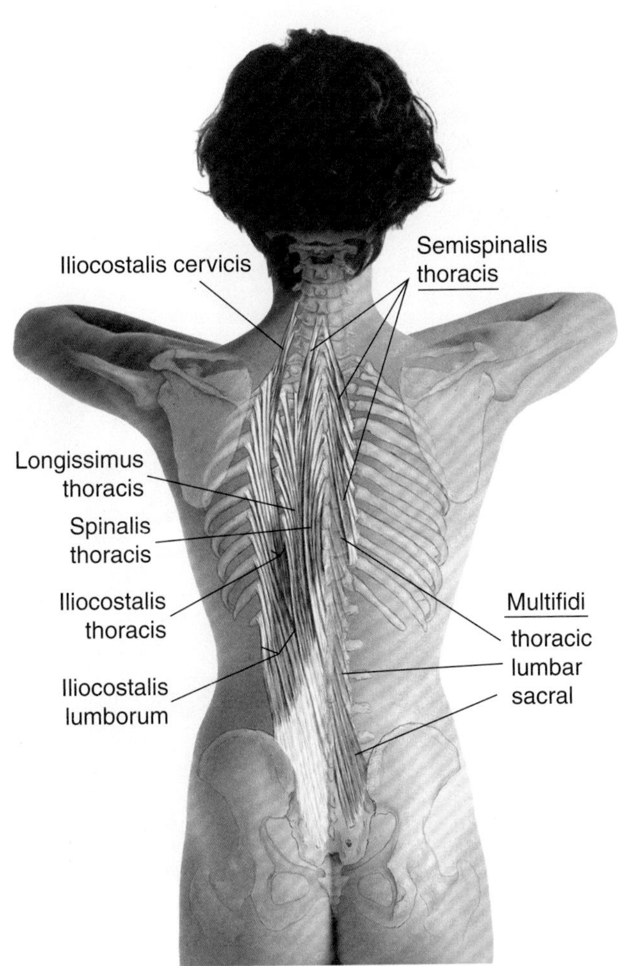

FIGURE 6-12 Anatomy of semispinalis thoracis

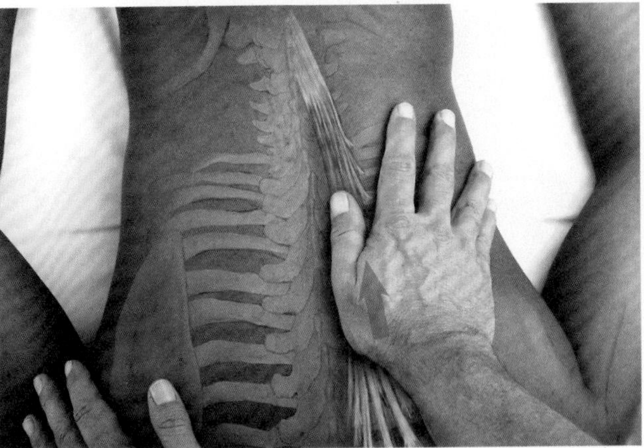

FIGURE 6-13 Stripping of erector spinae bundle with heel of hand (longissimus is shown)

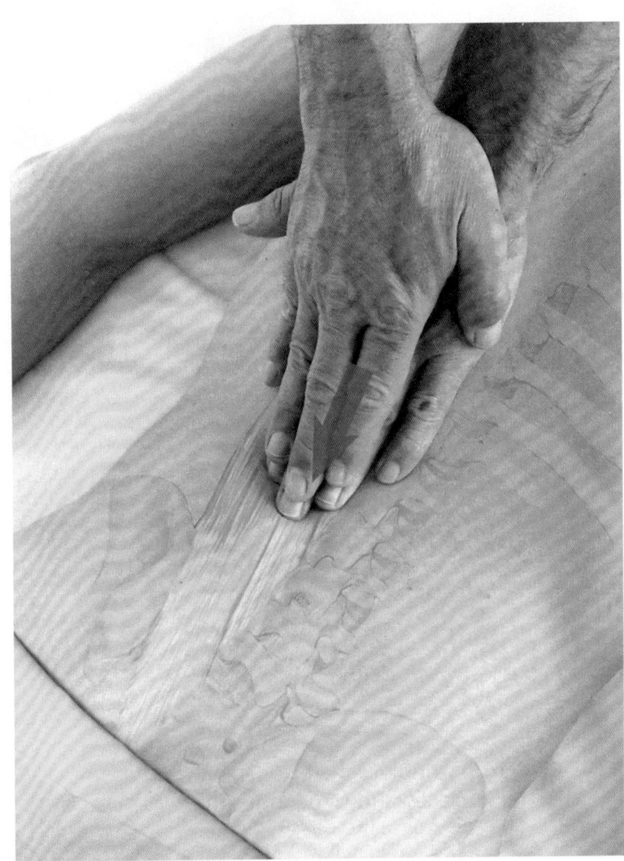

FIGURE 6-14 Stripping of erector spinae bundle with supported fingertips (longissimus is shown)

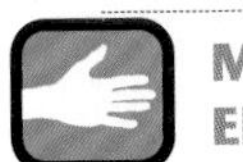

MANUAL THERAPY FOR THE ERECTOR SPINAE

Because the erector spinae muscles are gathered together in a paraspinal bundle, they can most easily be treated as a group. Stripping massage may be applied in either a caudad or cephalad direction. It is helpful to do both, as different trigger points may be accessed in each direction. You may use the hand, thumb, knuckles, fingertips, or elbow.

Stripping

- The client lies prone.
- The therapist stands beside the client at either the head or shoulder (to work in a caudad direction) or at the hips (to work in a cephalad direction).
- Place the heel of the hand (Fig. 6-13), the supported fingertips (Fig. 6-14), the supported thumbs (Fig. 6-15), the knuckles (Fig. 6-16), or the elbow (Fig. 6-17) on the muscle bundle near C7 (to work caudad) or at the sacrum (to work cephalad).
- Pressing firmly into the tissue, slide the body part you are using along the entire length of the muscle bundle.

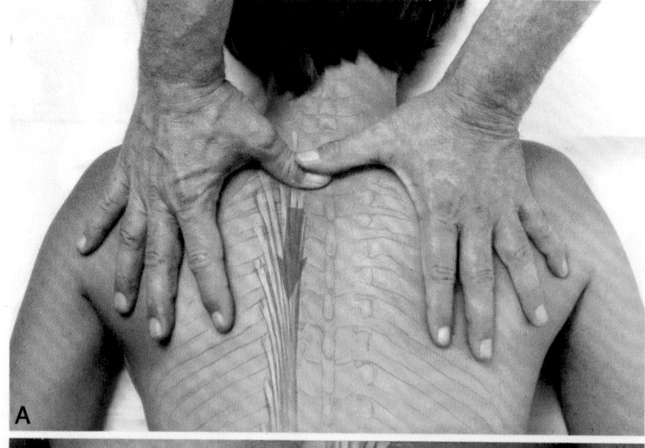

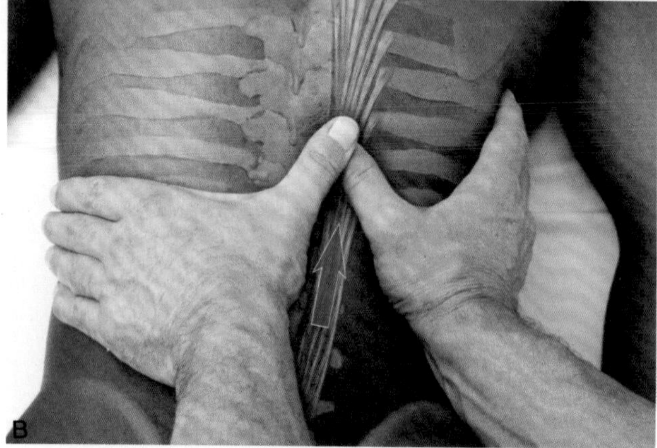

FIGURE 6-15 Stripping of erector spinae bundle with supported thumb both caudad and cephalad, showing longissimus. Starting position stripping caudad **(A)** and midway position stripping cephalad **(B)**

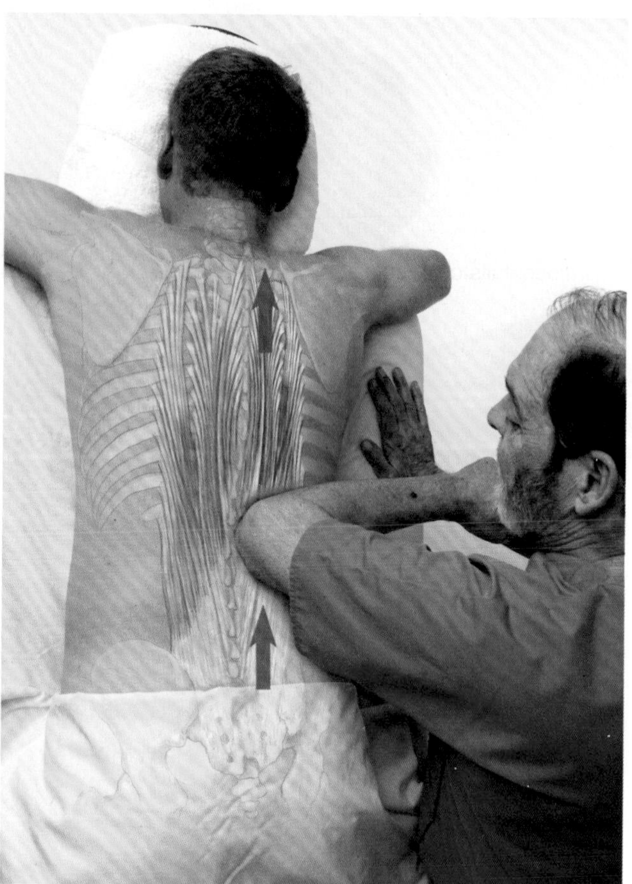

FIGURE 6-17 Stripping of erector spinae bundle with elbow, showing longissimus.

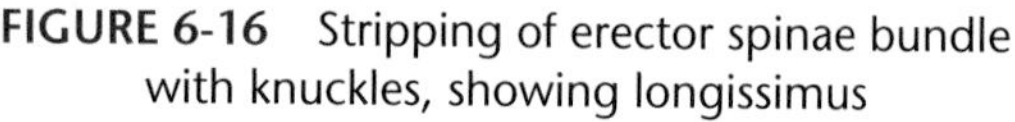

FIGURE 6-16 Stripping of erector spinae bundle with knuckles, showing longissimus

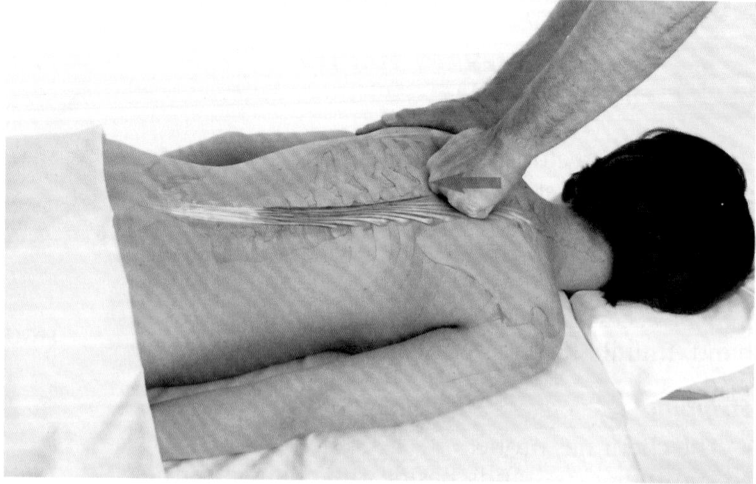

The Deep Muscles of the Vertebral Column

MULTIFIDUS (PLURAL MULTIFIDI)

mul-TIFF-I-duss

ETYMOLOGY Latin ***multi***, many + ***fidus***, divided, thus "divided into many segments"

Overview

This group of muscles (Fig. 6-18) is located all along the vertebral column, from the cervical region to the base of the spine. The lower segments of multifidus that reach from the sacrum to the lumbar vertebrae are very strong and prominent, resembling the stays on the mast of a sailboat. In fact multifidus is one of the strongest muscles in the body. You will frequently find tenderness over the sacrum in clients with low back pain.

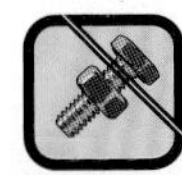

ATTACHMENTS

Origin

- Cervical region: from articular processes of lower cervical vertebrae
- Thoracic region: from transverse processes of all thoracic vertebrae
- Lumbar region: lower portion of dorsal sacrum, PSIS, deep surface of tendinous origin of erector spinae, and mammillary processes of all lumbar vertebrae

Insertion

- Spinous process of all vertebrae extending from L5 through C2 (spanning 2 to 4 vertebrae)

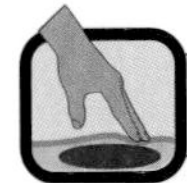

PALPATION

Discernible between the transverse processes of the vertebrae, but most easily on the sacrum. Architecture is parallel, and fibers are parallel to the muscle.

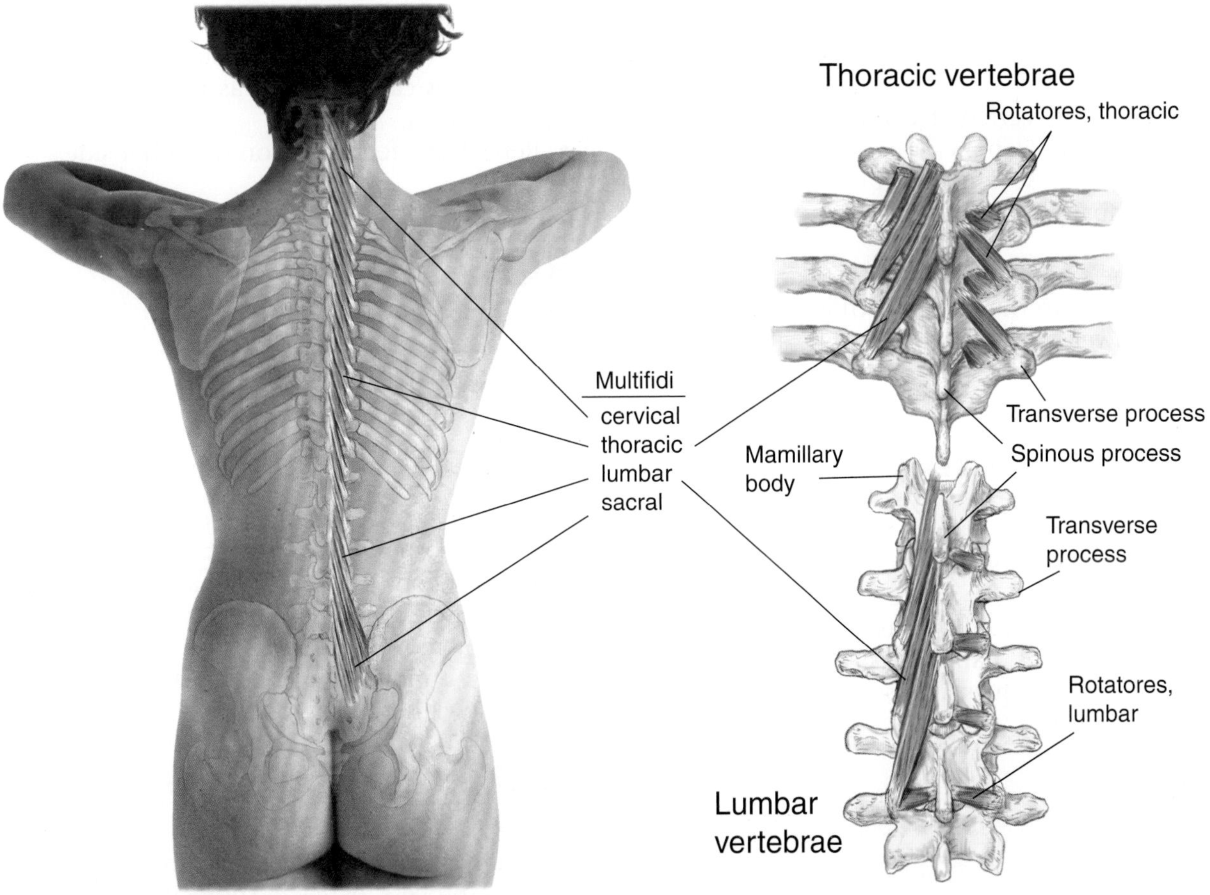

FIGURE 6-18 Anatomy of multifidi

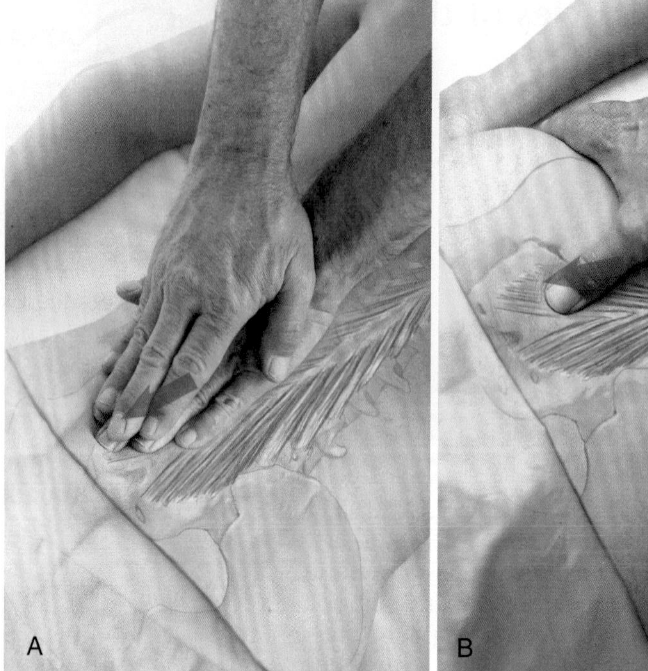

FIGURE 6-19 Stripping of multifidus at inferior attachments with fingertips **(A)** and thumb **(B)**

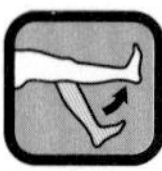

ACTION

Extends, rotates, and stabilizes the vertebral column

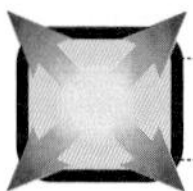

REFERRAL AREA

- Between the vertebral column and the medial border of the scapula
- The region just lateral to T12 and L1, and over the lumbar region; upper lateral quadrant of the abdomen
- Over the sacrum, into the buttock along the gluteal cleft, into the posterior thigh below the buttock; lower lateral quadrant of the abdomen
- Around the coccyx

OTHER MUSCLES TO EXAMINE

- Iliocostalis thoracis, rhomboids
- Quadratus lumborum, serratus posterior inferior, iliocostalis thoracis, and lumborum
- Rectus abdominis, iliopsoas
- Gluteal muscles, hamstrings
- Abdominal obliques, iliopsoas
- Levator ani

MANUAL THERAPY

Stripping

- The client lies prone.
- The therapist stands at the client's side at the chest, facing caudad.
- Place the fingertips (Fig. 6-19A) or thumb (Fig. 6-19B), supported or unsupported, at the superior aspect of the sacrum just lateral to the spinal column, pointing caudad (inferiorly).
- Pressing firmly into the tissue, glide the thumbor fingertips caudad as far as the inferior aspect of the sacrum.
- Repeat this technique on the other side.

ROTATORES

RO-ta-TOR-ace

ETYMOLOGY Latin ***rotatores***, rotators

Overview

Rotatores (Fig. 6-20) are the deepest of the three layers of transversospinalis muscles, chiefly developed in the thoracic region. Because they have a very high density of muscle spindles, they may function to provide important movement sensory feedback (proprioception). Their motor function appears to be in fine adjustments rather than gross movements of the spine.

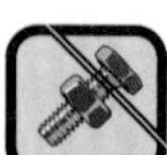

ATTACHMENTS

- Origin: articular process of most cervical, transverse process of each thoracic, and mamillary process of each lumbar vertebra

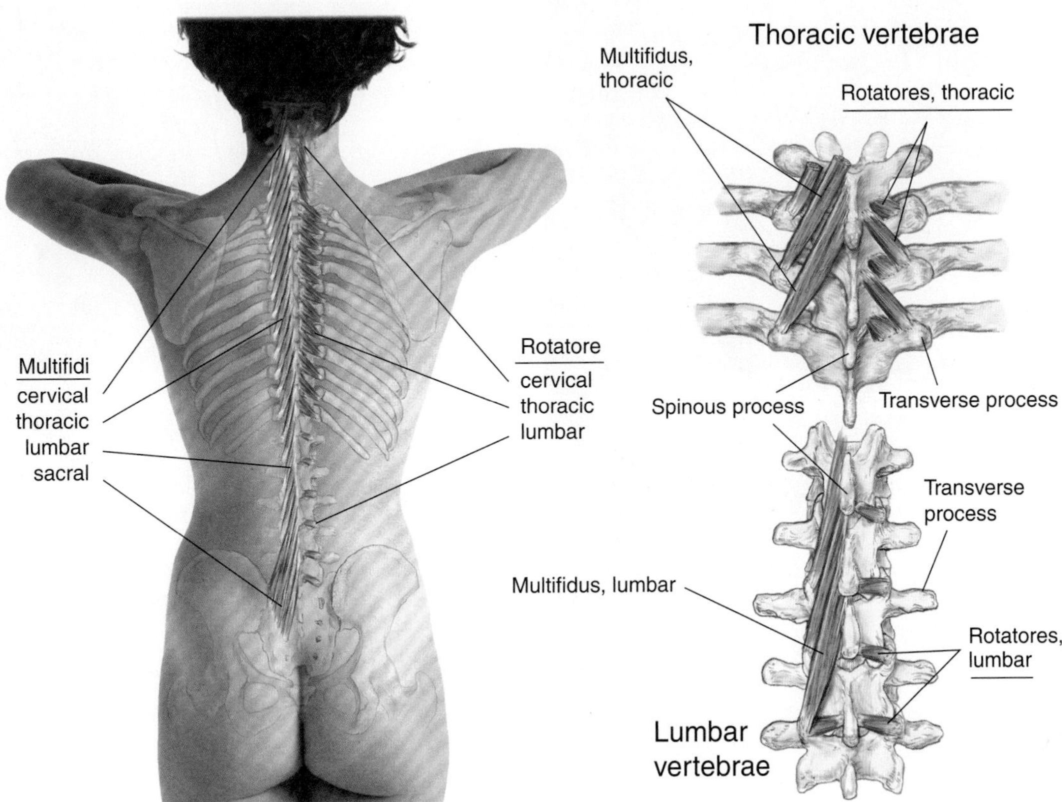

FIGURE 6-20 Anatomy of rotatores

- Insertion: root of the spinous process of the vertebrae above

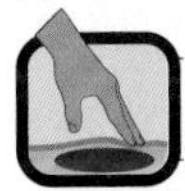

PALPATION

Discernible between the transverse processes of the vertebrae. Architecture is parallel, and fibers are parallel to the muscle.

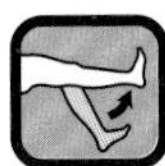

ACTION

- Bilaterally, extension of the spine
- Unilaterally, rotation in the thoracic region
- Proprioception (see overview)

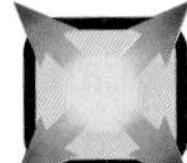

REFERRAL AREA

Along the midline of the spine

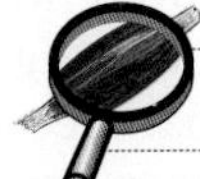

OTHER MUSCLES TO EXAMINE

Other superficial and deep paraspinal muscles

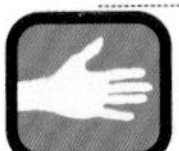

MANUAL THERAPY FOR MULTIFIDI AND ROTATORES

Cross-fiber Stroking

- The client lies prone.
- The therapist stands at the client's side, beginning at the waist.
- Place the thumb or fingertip (supported or unsupported) on the space between the spinous process of L5 and the sacrum (Fig. 6-21).
- Press laterally (away from yourself) and diagonally caudad, pushing the superficial muscles out of the way to reach the intrinsic muscles.
- If the client reports tenderness, hold for release.
- Shifting cephalad, repeat this technique between each two spinous processes as far as the space between T12 and L1.
- Beginning with the space between T11 and T12, perform the same technique gliding the thumb into the space between the ribs.
- Repeat this technique (Fig. 6-22) as far as C7.
- From C7 to the cranial base, use your unsupported thumb.
- This technique is contraindicated in any area of the spine where there is diagnosed or suspected spinal pathology.

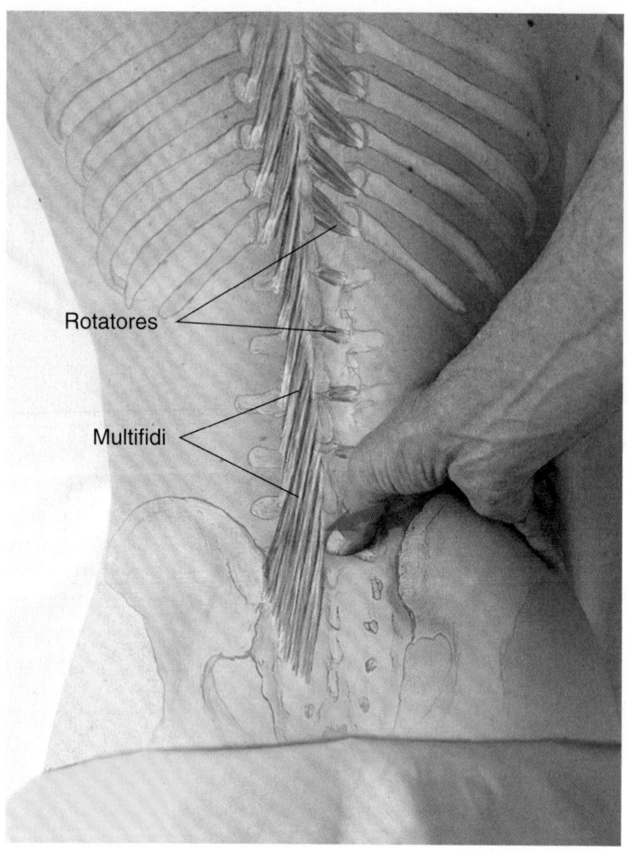

FIGURE 6-21 Cross-fiber stroking of rotatores in lumbar region using thumb.

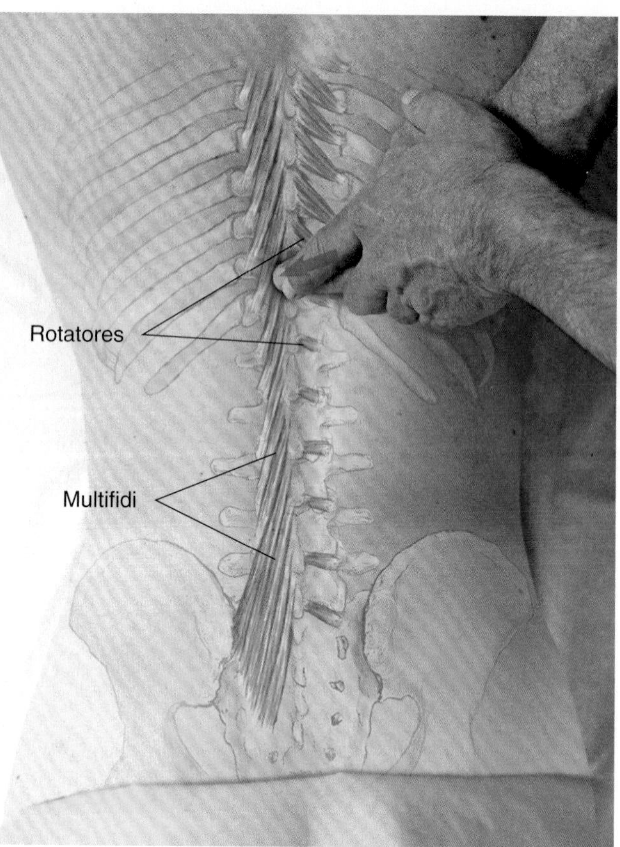

FIGURE 6-22 Cross-fiber stroking of rotatores in thoracic region using support fingertips

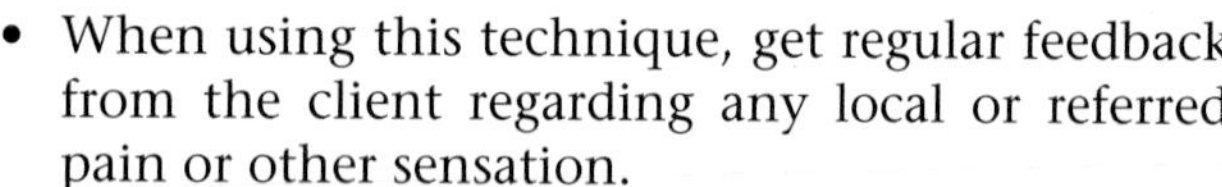

- When using this technique, get regular feedback from the client regarding any local or referred pain or other sensation.

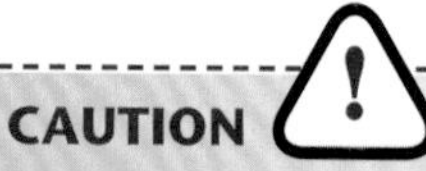

CAUTION

- Use this technique with great care in the cervical region and only after other work has been performed in that area as described in Chapter 3 to release the more superficial posterior neck muscles.

CHAPTER REVIEW

CASE STUDY

G.Q. is a 63-year-old male, retired from the military. He is otherwise in good health and very physically active, plays golf several days a week, and works out daily in a gym. He states he has rarely had any back pain, but that he feels he strained his back a couple of days ago while picking up his grandchild. He said he of course knew to bend at the knee, but that the child unexpectedly jumped up on him and when he bent over to lift him, he felt a strain in his low back. A postural and gait assessment showed no deviations; palpation revealed that he had trigger points active in the iliocostalis lumborum, radiating down to the glutes. Deep Swedish strokes to warm the muscle, followed by stripping of the lumbar erectors, myofascial release in the iliocostalis and quadratus lumborum areas, and deep compression in the gluteals brought total relief by the end of the session.

G.Q. stated that he had never had massage and that it was recommended to him by his neighbor, who is a client. He felt so good after the session he decided to purchase a package and come every other week. He was reminded that he may feel some soreness for a day or two due to the deep tissue work and that, if he noticed any residual pain in his back, to call and get worked in instead of waiting 2 weeks for his next appointment. Two weeks later, at his next appointment, he stated that he had been a little sore but that it had dissipated within a day and that he had felt well in the interim. He stated that he felt so good that he had recommended massage to all his golf and gym buddies and asked for a stack of business cards to share.

K.M., LMT

REVIEW QUESTIONS

1. The ______ region is the only one capable of the full range of possible spinal movements, including anterior and lateral flexion, extension, and rotation.
   a. Lumbar
   b. Sacral
   c. Cervical
   d. Thoracic
2. There are ________curvatures in the normal adult spine.
   a. 5
   b. 4
   c. 3
   d. 2
3. The three groups of erector spinae are ________.
   a. Coracobrachialis, latissimus, and spinalis
   b. Iliocostalis, quadratus, and lumbar
   c. Multifidus, longissimus, and thoracic
   d. Iliocostalis, longissimus, and spinalis
4. The deepest of the three layers of transversospinalis muscles are the ________.
   a. Rotatores
   b. Rhomboids
   c. Multifidi
   d. Intercostals
5. The muscle that originates on the transverse process of a vertebra and inserts on the spinous process of the vertebrae above it is the ________.
   a. Coronoid process
   b. Subscapularis
   c. Rotatores
   d. Serratus
6. The muscles named ________ means "divided into many segments."
   a. Teres minor and major
   b. Infraspinatus
   c. Piriformis
   d. Multifidus
7. A muscle with trigger points that frequently refer pain to the buttocks are the ________.
   a. Iliocostalis cervicis
   b. Iliocostalis thoracis
   c. Spinalis thoracis
   d. Iliocostalis lumborum
8. The center of gravity of the body is in the _______ region.
   a. Thoracic
   b. Cervical
   c. Pelvic
   d. Lumbar
9. The muscles that collectively extend and maintain the balance of the vertebral column and the rib cage are the _________.
   a. Rotatores
   b. Erector spinae
   c. Quadratus
   d. Multifidus
10. The two types of joints between moveable vertebrae in the spine are _____ and ______.
    a. Cartilaginous and synovial
    b. Cartilaginous and diarthrotic
    c. Diarthrotic and synarthrotic
    d. Synovial and fibrous

thePoint Additional helpful resources are available at http://thePoint.lww.com.

CHAPTER 7

The Low Back and Abdomen

LEARNING OBJECTIVES

At the end of this chapter, the learner will be able to:

- State the correct terminology of the muscles of the low back and abdomen.
- Palpate the muscles of the low back and abdomen.
- Identify their attachments at the origins and insertions.
- Explain the actions of the muscles.
- Describe their pain referral areas.
- Recall related muscles.
- Recognize any endangerment sites and ethical cautions for massage therapy.
- Demonstrate proficiency in manual therapy techniques for muscles of the low back and abdomen.

The Overview of the Region begins on page 231, after the anatomy plates.

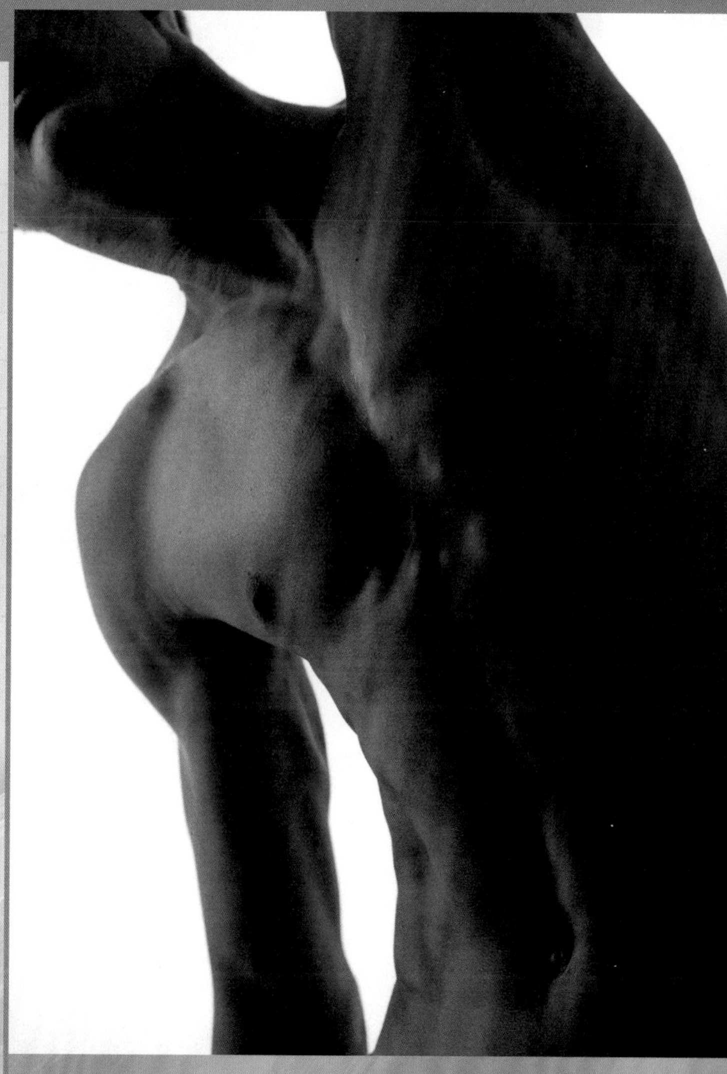

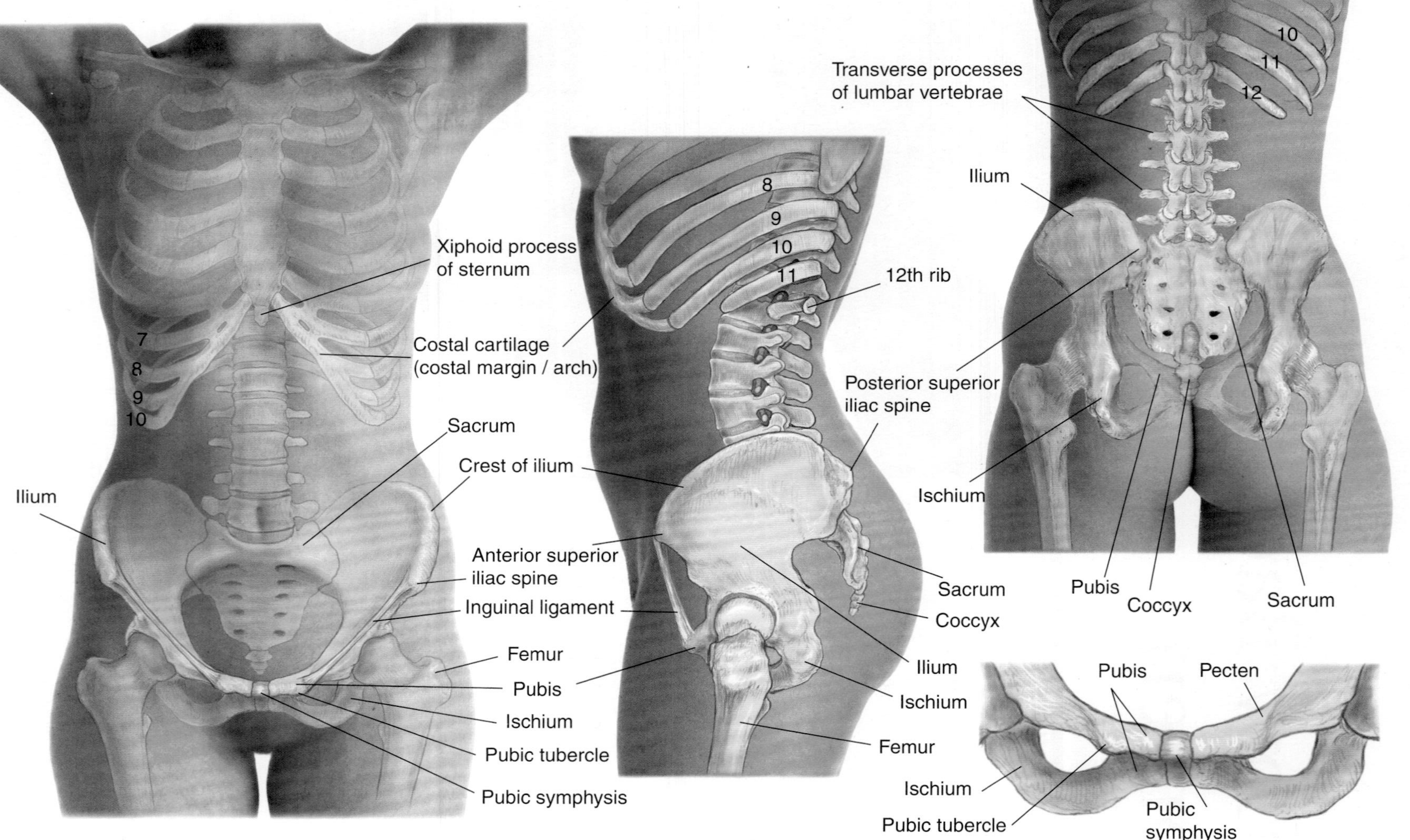

PLATE 7-1 ■ Skeletal features of the abdominal region and lower back

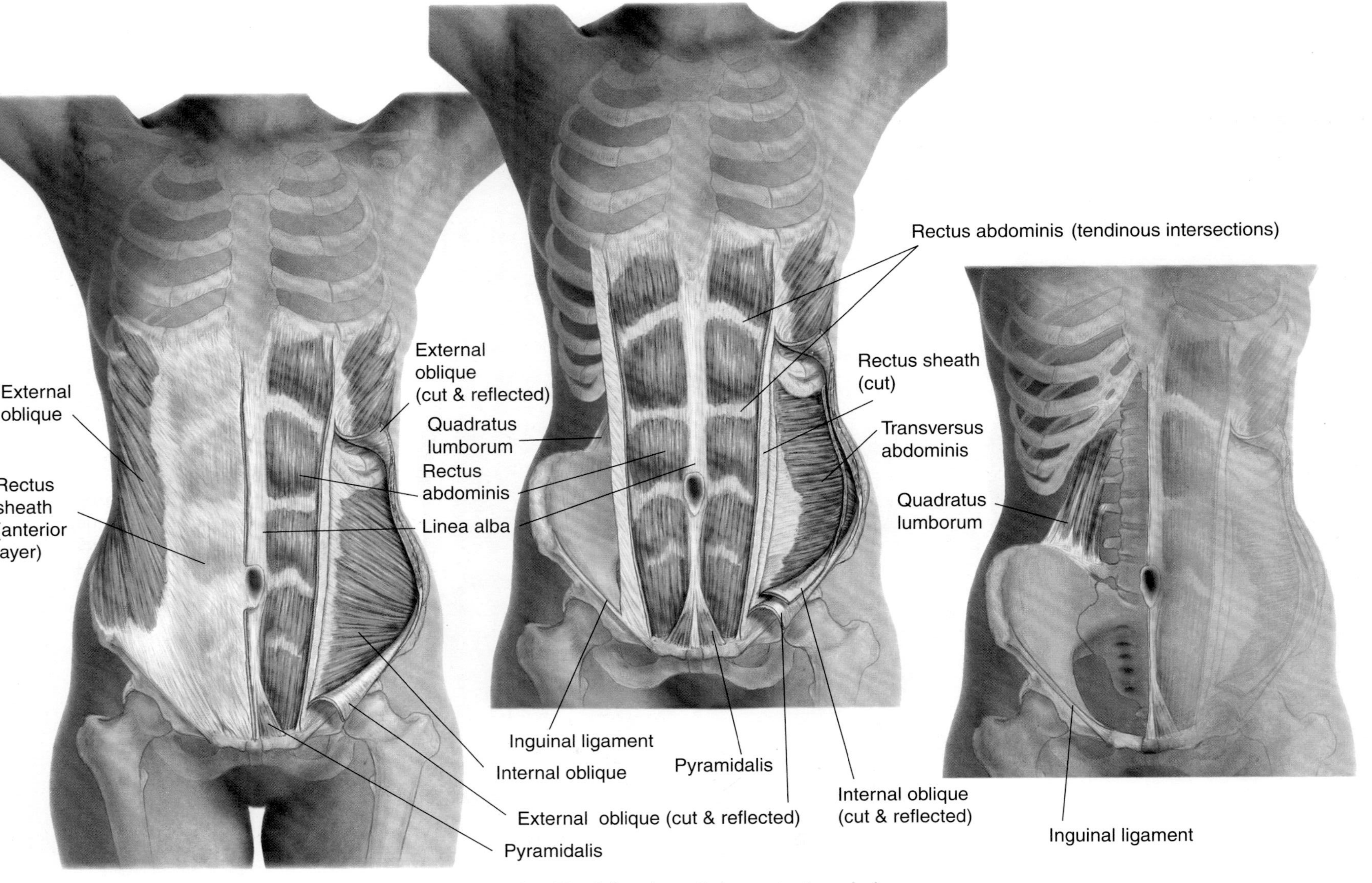

PLATE 7-2 ■ Muscles of the anterior abdomen

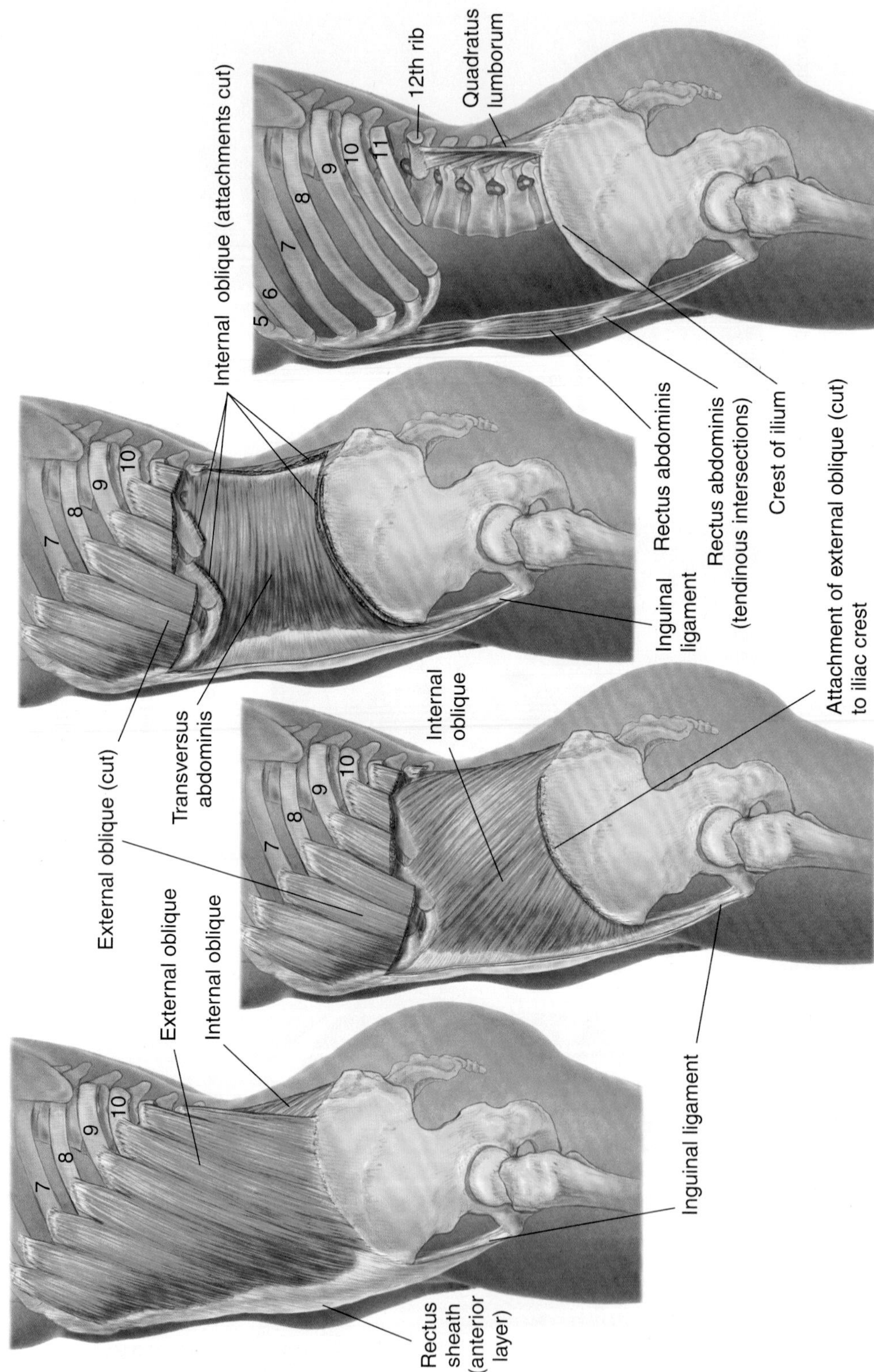

PLATE 7-3 ■ Abdominal and lower back muscles, lateral view

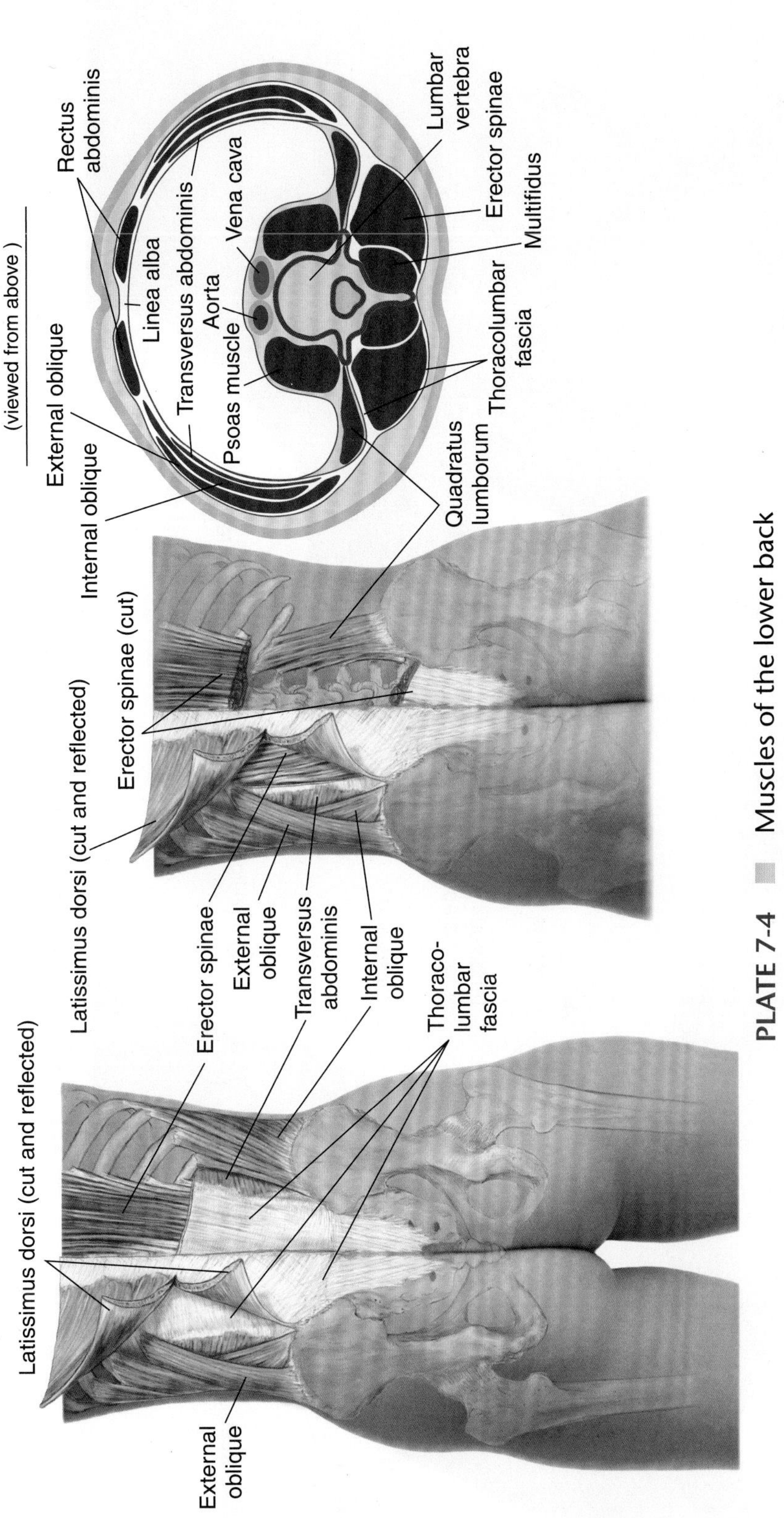

PLATE 7-4 ■ Muscles of the lower back

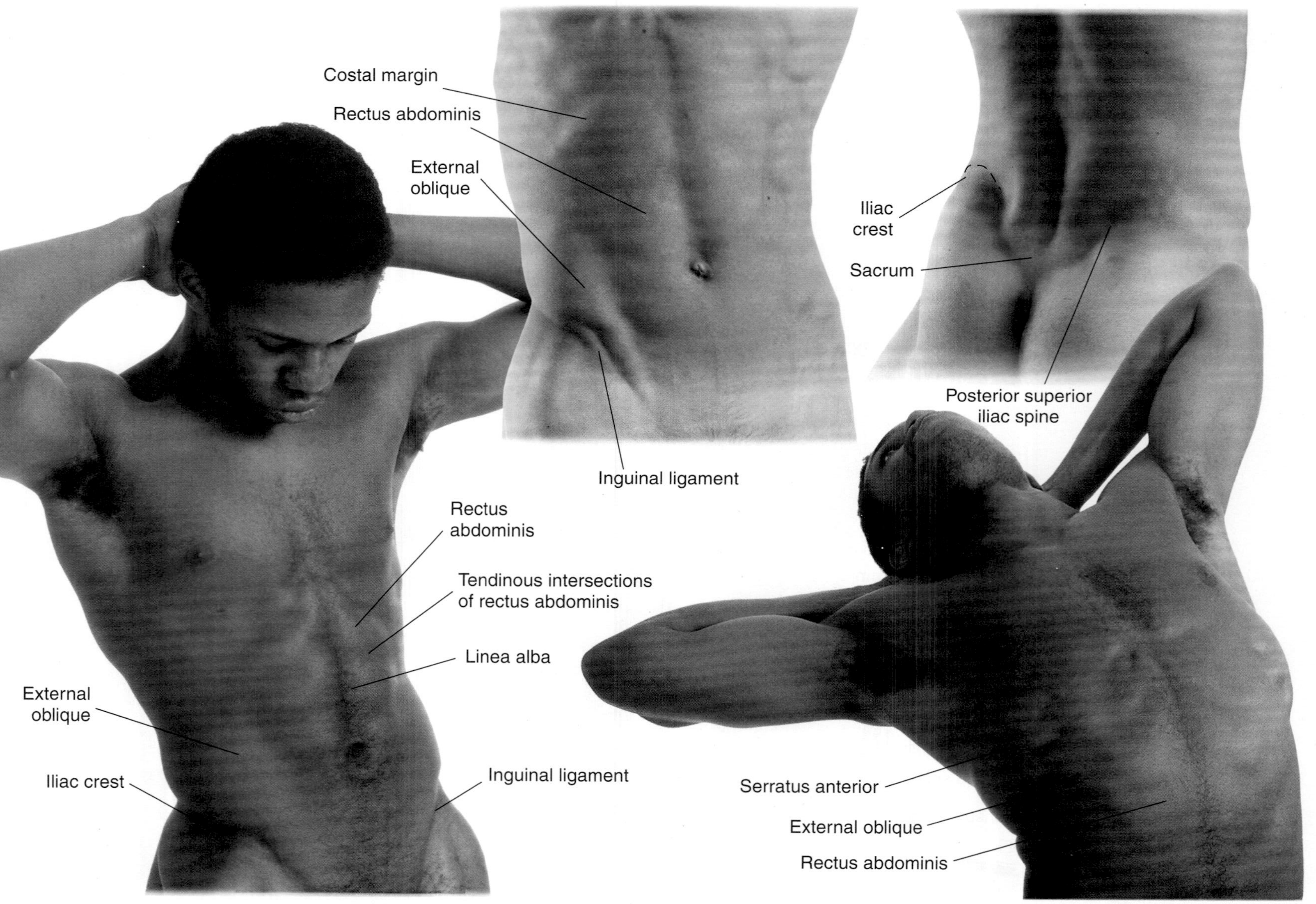

PLATE 7-5 ■ Surface anatomy of the abdomen and lower back

Overview of the Region (Plates 7-1 to 7-5)

The waist, which includes the low back (lumbar region) and middle abdomen, is a very vulnerable area because of its lack of bony armor and support. Above, the torso and spine are stabilized and the internal organs protected by the rib cage. Below, the pelvis—the body's center of gravity—provides stability and protection. In between, however, our need for flexibility and mobility require a space with very little support or protection. The muscles of this region, therefore, have a lot of work to do and are easily stressed or injured. Their primary actions are movement of the upper body in relation to the lower and vice versa: anterior flexion, lateral flexion, and rotation of the torso. Trigger points in these muscles refer to an extensive territory: upward into the back and chest; inward into the viscera; and downward into the buttocks, lower abdomen, groin, genitals, and legs.

The lower back region is characterized by several layers of thick, strong tendinous and fascial tissue, including the thoracolumbar fascia and tendinous portions of the erector spinae and latissimus dorsi. These connective tissues may themselves become tight, congested, and tender, and they should be treated along with the muscles. The lumbar/abdominal muscles constitute one of the muscle groups chiefly implicated in complaints of low back pain—the most common back pain—because of the workload they carry. The others are the buttock muscles, pelvic floor muscles, and iliopsoas, all of which are addressed in the next chapter.

Overview of the Muscles of the Abdomen

These muscles form the wall of the abdomen and include **rectus abdominis, transversus abdominis,** and the **external** and **internal oblique muscles**. Aside from their various primary functions, all of these muscles assist in forced exhalation through compression of the abdominal cavity. They are extremely important clinically, as trigger points in these muscles can refer pain into the viscera and even cause visceral problems, such as somatovisceral disease, which can occur when a pinched nerve travels to and from internal organs, causing pain and/or dysfunction. Likewise, visceral disorders can cause pain in the abdominal musculature that can persist even after the disorder is resolved. They can also refer pain into the low back.

It is helpful to do some preparatory work on the abdomen prior to deeper manual therapy on specific muscles in order to stimulate local blood flow and relax the superficial musculature. This work may include general massage techniques such as effleurage as well as deeper myofascial work. Remember not to work counterclockwise on the abdomen. Clients who may suffer from constipation can be helped by applying abdominal massage in a clockwise direction. Be sure that any pressure applied in the abdominal area is slow and gradual, and be aware that people who are suffering visceral pain may have an undiagnosed pathology present. Anyone who has visceral pain should be referred to a physician for proper diagnosis.

ETHICAL CAUTION

Some people are sensitive to having their abdomen worked on. Always ask the client's permission before touching the abdomen and use proper draping techniques. Of course, be careful to avoid exposing or touching the breasts, pubic hair, and genitals.

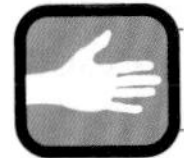

MANUAL THERAPY

ABDOMEN MYOFASCIAL STRETCHING

- The client lies supine.
- The therapist stands beside the client at the hips.
- Place one hand flat on the upper abdomen on the near side of the client, the fingers resting just inferior to the rib cage.
- Cross the other hand over the first and place it on the lower abdomen on the far side of the client, the fingers over the anterior superior iliac spine (ASIS) (Fig. 7-1).

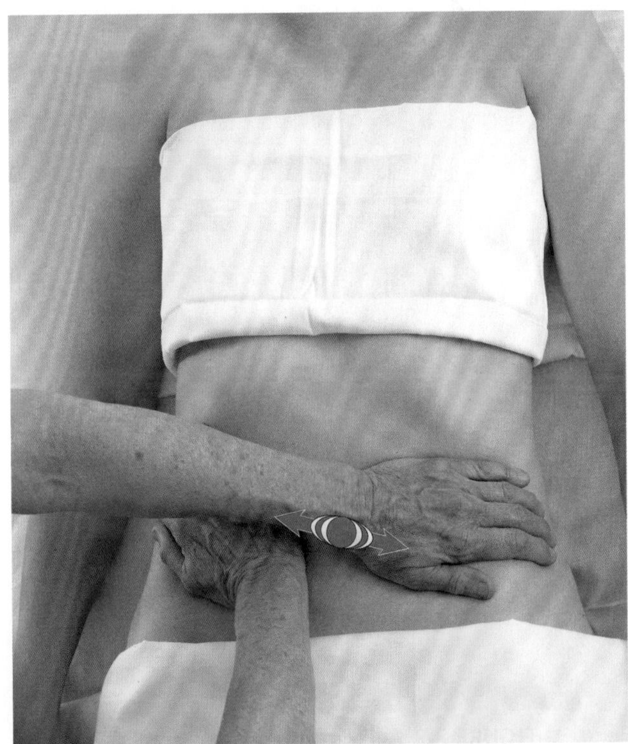

FIGURE 7-1 Myofascial stretch of abdomen

- Let the hands sink into the tissue until they engage the superficial myofascial tissue of the abdomen.
- Press the hands apart without allowing them to glide on the skin. Hold for release.
- Repeat on the opposite side.

RECTUS ABDOMINIS

REK-tus ab-DAHM-in-iss

ETYMOLOGY Latin ***rectus***, straight, upright + ***abdominis***, of the abdomen

Overview

Rectus abdominis (Fig. 7-2) is composed of a series of muscle bodies separated by tendinous intersections, covered by a fascial sheath (rectus sheath) and divided in the center by the **linea alba** (Latin *linea,* line + *alba,* white). This muscle connects the anterior thorax (rib cage) to the anterior pelvis (pubis). It flexes the spine and resists extension of the spine. It is the only muscle in most of the anterior abdomen. Lateral to it, the abdominal muscles are arranged in layers.

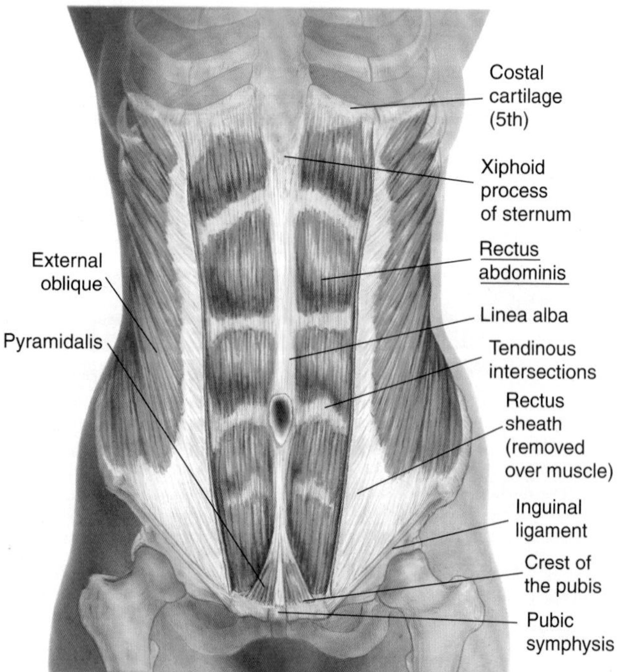

FIGURE 7-2 Anatomy of rectus abdominis

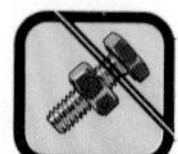

ATTACHMENTS

- Origin: crest and symphysis of the pubis
- Insertion: xiphoid process and 5th to 7th costal cartilages

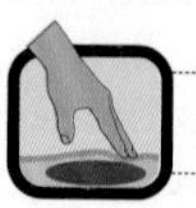

PALPATION

Discernible at the pubis; discernible at the edges with the fingertips from the pubis to the rib cage, although difficult to distinguish in obese clients. Its architecture is parallel, and the fibers are superior-inferior.

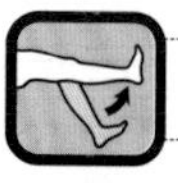

ACTION

- Flexes the thoracic and lumbar vertebral regions
- Draws the thorax inferiorly toward the pubis or the pubis toward the thorax

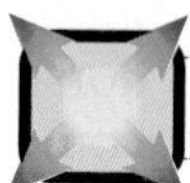

REFERRAL AREAS

- Over the abdomen from the xiphoid process to the pubis
- Across the back just below the scapulae; the region around the xiphoid process (epigastrium, precordium)
- Across the top of the buttocks (iliac crest) and sacrum
- Into the lower lateral quadrant of the abdomen
- Mid-abdomen just inferior to umbilicus
- Also abdominal fullness, dysmenorrhea

OTHER MUSCLES TO EXAMINE

- Pyramidalis
- Serratus posterior inferior
- Iliopsoas
- Abdominal obliques
- Transversus abdominis
- Gluteal muscles
- Quadratus lumborum

MANUAL THERAPY

Stripping (1)

- The client lies supine.
- The therapist stands beside the client at the hip.
- Place the fingertips on one side of the rectus just superior to the pubis.

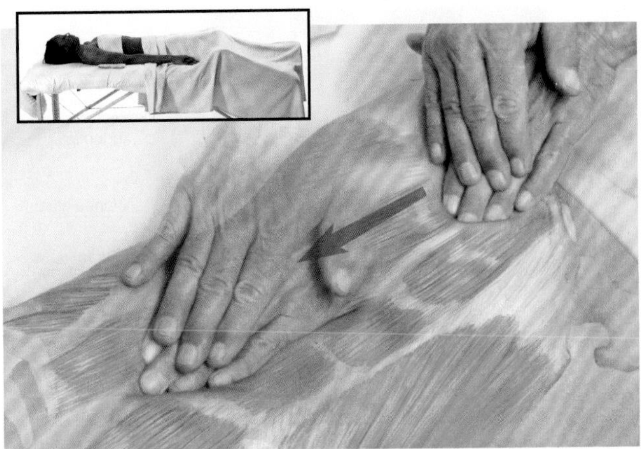

FIGURE 7-3 Stripping of rectus abdominis

- Pressing firmly into the tissue, slide the fingertips superiorly along the muscle to its attachments on the ribs (Fig. 7-3).
- Repeat the same procedure on the other side.

Stripping (2)

- The client lies supine.
- The therapist stands beside the client at the waist.
- Place the fingertips on the lateral border of the rectus just above the pubis. Pressing firmly into the tissue, rotate the hand so that the fingertips move superiorly along the edge of the muscle (Fig. 7-4).
- Beginning just superior to the previous spot, repeat this procedure all the way along the muscle to the rib cage.
- Repeat the same procedure on the other side.

Stripping (3)

- The client lies supine.
- The therapist stands beside the client at the hip.
  - Place the fingertips (Fig. 7-5A) or supported thumb (Fig. 7-5B) on the lateral border of the rectus just above the pubis.

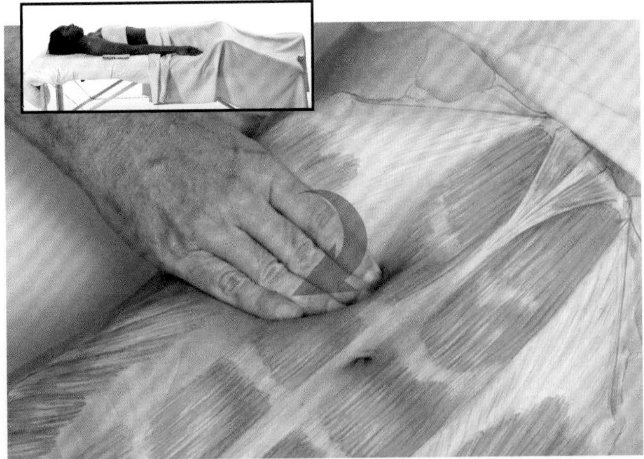

FIGURE 7-4 Stripping of lateral border of rectus abdominis

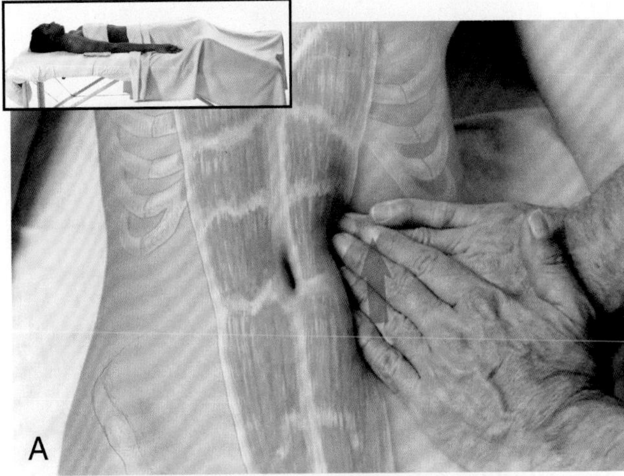

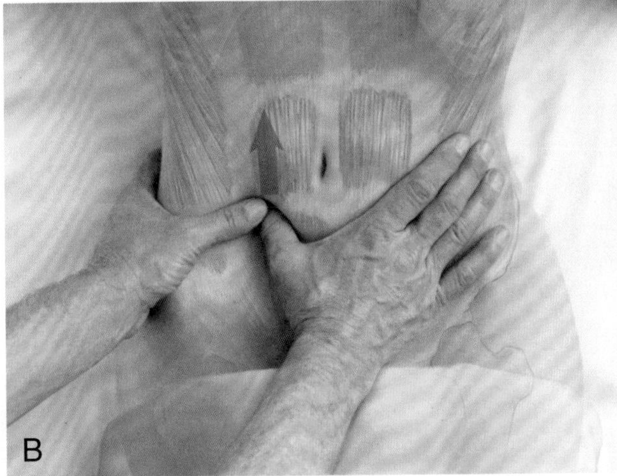

FIGURE 7-5 Stripping of lateral border of rectus abdominis with fingertips **(A)** or supported thumb **(B)**

  - Pressing firmly into the tissue, slide the fingertips or thumb along the muscle to its attachments on the rib cage.
- Repeat the same procedure on the other side.

Compression

- The client lies supine.
- The therapist stands beside the client at the chest.
- Place the supported thumb at the attachment of the rectus to the pubis at the side nearest you.
- Press the muscle firmly against the bone, looking for tender spots. Hold for release.
  - Move the hand medially to the next spot and repeat until you reach the linea alba at the center (Fig. 7-6).
- Repeat this procedure on the other side.

Cross-fiber Stroking

- The client lies supine.
- The therapist stands beside the client at the waist.
- Place the tip of the thumb on rectus abdominis at the linea alba (center line) just superior to the pubic symphysis, with the fingertips resting on the abdomen laterally.

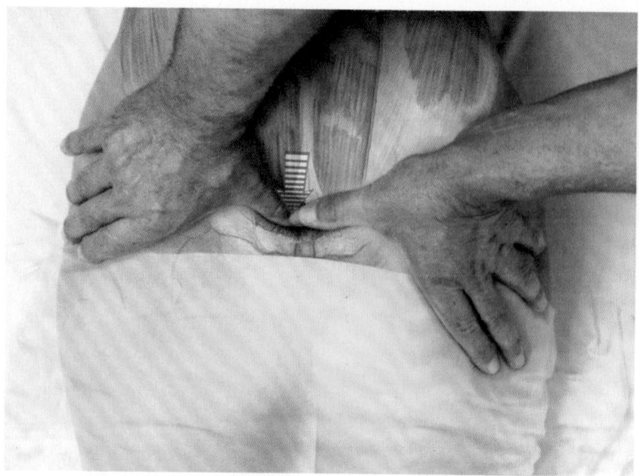

FIGURE 7-6 Compression of rectus abdominis attachments at the pubis

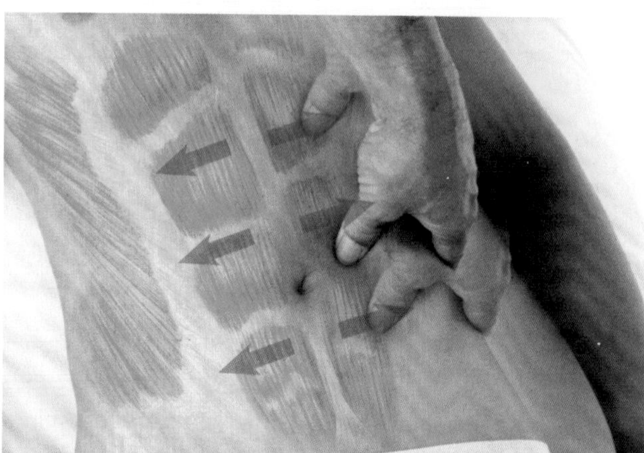

FIGURE 7-7 Cross-fiber stroking of rectus abdominis

- Pressing firmly into the tissue, slide the tip of the thumb laterally toward the fingertips.
- Beginning just superior to the previous point, repeat this procedure.
- Repeat the same procedure (Fig. 7-7), continuing along the rectus until you reach the rib cage.
- Repeat this procedure on the other side.

PYRAMIDALIS

pi-RAM-I-DAL-iss

ETYMOLOGY Latin ***pyramidalis***, shaped like a pyramid

Overview

Pyramidalis (Fig. 7-8) very commonly occurs on one side only and may be absent in many people. It is the only other anterior abdominal muscle (after rectus abdominis) and may harbor a trigger point at its attachment to the pubis.

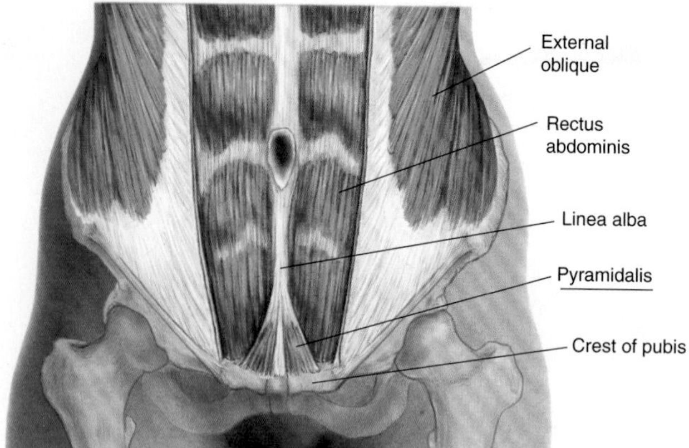

FIGURE 7-8 Anatomy of pyramidalis

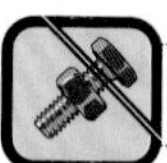

ATTACHMENTS

- Origin: crest of the pubis anterior to origin of rectus abdominis
- Insertion: lower portion of the linea alba

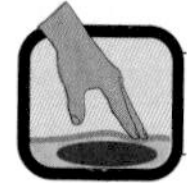

PALPATION

Not normally distinguishable from rectus abdominis

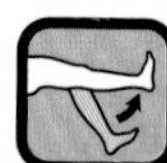

ACTION

Tenses the linea alba

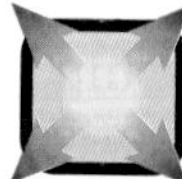

REFERRAL AREAS

- To its attachment to the pubis
- Along the midline to the umbilicus

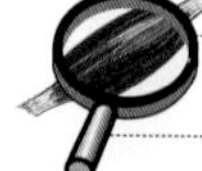

OTHER MUSCLES TO EXAMINE

- Rectus abdominis
- Iliopsoas
- Abdominal obliques

MANUAL THERAPY

Compression

- The client lies supine.
- The therapist stands beside the client at the hip.
- Place the thumb on pyramidalis, just superior and lateral to the symphysis pubis (Fig. 7-9).

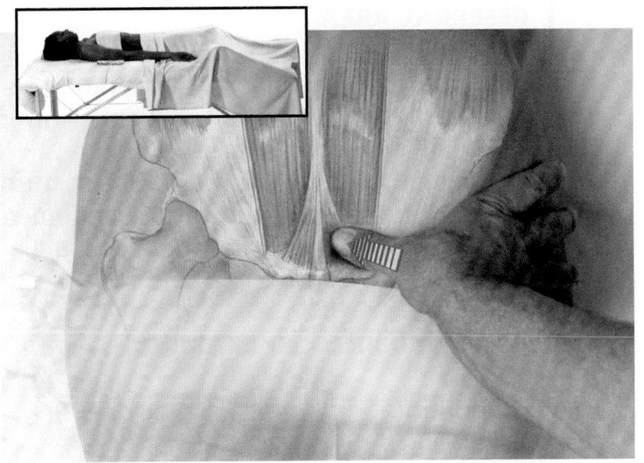

FIGURE 7-9 Compression of pyramidalis

- Press firmly into the tissue, examining for tenderness. Hold for release.
- Repeat this procedure on the other side.

ABDOMINAL OBLIQUES

ab-DAHM-in-al oh-BLEEKS

ETYMOLOGY Latin ***obliquus***, slanting, diagonal

Overview

The external and internal abdominal obliques (Figs. 7-10 and 7-11) are paired on each side of the abdominal wall, and form the first two of three muscle layers lateral to the rectus abdominis. Their fibers run in the same respective directions as the external and internal intercostals. A good way to remember their directions is to place one hand on the opposite side of the abdomen with your fingers pointing diagonally downward, then place the other hand on top of it pointing perpendicularly. The top hand represents the externals, and the bottom hand the internals (Fig. 7-12).

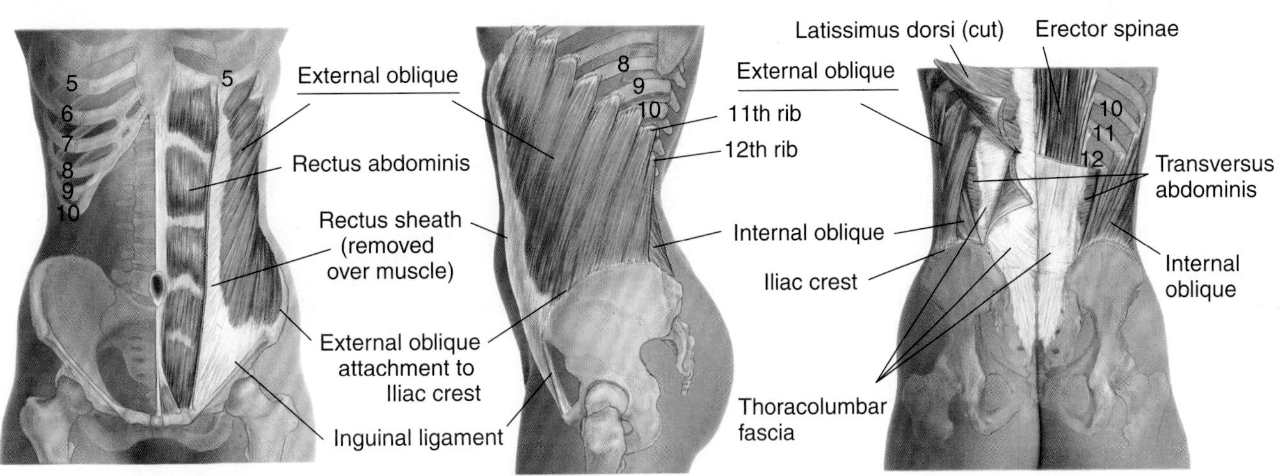

FIGURE 7-10 Anatomy of external oblique

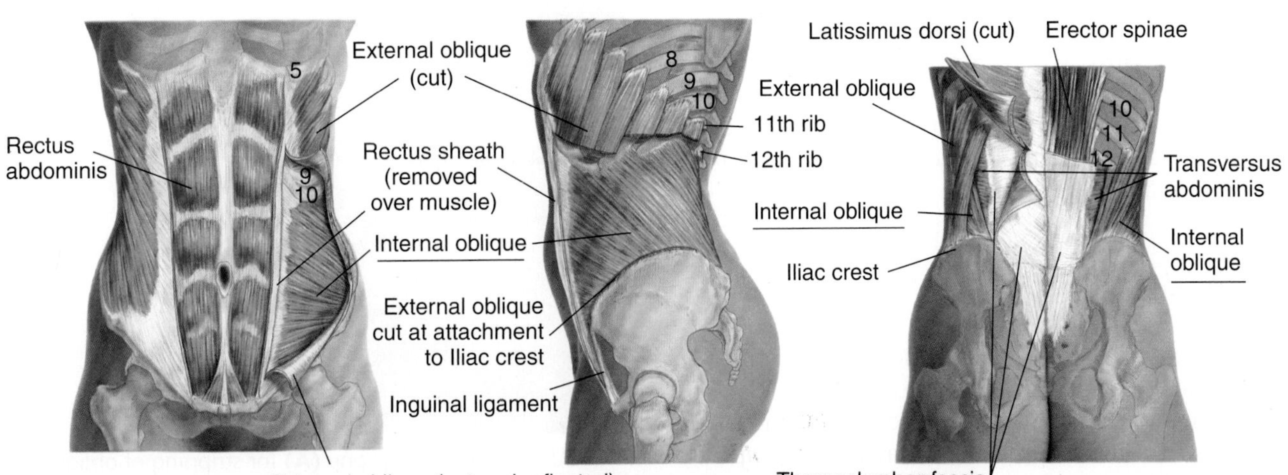

FIGURE 7-11 Anatomy of internal oblique

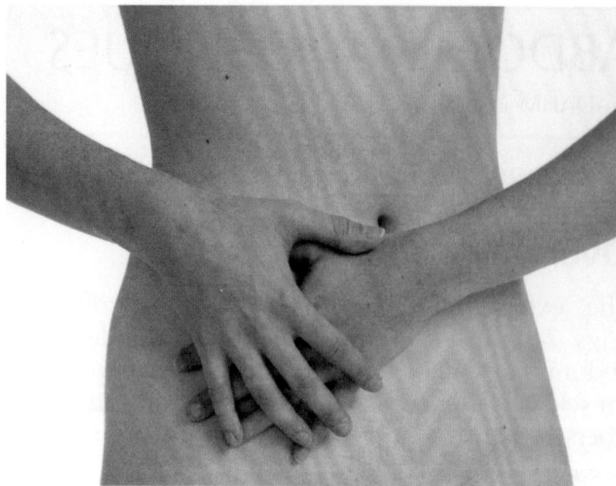

FIGURE 7-12 Mnemonic hand position for direction of external and internal obliques (top hand, external; bottom hand, internal)

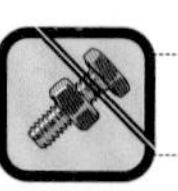

ATTACHMENTS

External:

- Origin: external surfaces and inferior borders of the 5th to 12th ribs
- Insertion: anterior half of the lateral lip of the iliac crest, the inguinal ligament, and the anterior layer of the rectus sheath (lateral edge of the rectus abdominis)

Internal:

- Origin: iliac fascia deep to the lateral part of inguinal ligament, to the anterior half of the crest of the ilium, and to the lumbar fascia
- Insertion: along the bottom of the rib cage (10th to 12th ribs) and the sheath of the rectus abdominis deep to the external oblique

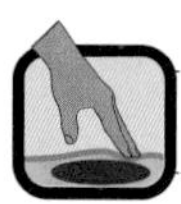

PALPATION

Discernible only when contracted by having the supine client raise one shoulder toward the opposite side of the body. Architecture is parallel and the fibers are, as the name implies, oblique in two opposed directions (Fig. 7-12).

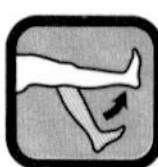

ACTION

- Bilaterally, increase intra-abdominal pressure to assist exhalation, and flex the spine.
- Unilaterally, assist in lateral flexion and rotation of the thoracic spine; external to the opposite side, internal to the same side.

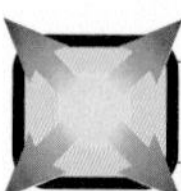

REFERRAL AREA

- To the epigastric region (below the xiphoid process between the costal arches), over the lower chest, and diagonally below the costal arch
- The lower lateral quadrant of the abdomen, into the groin and the testicle, up over the abdomen to the pubis, the umbilicus, and the costal arch

OTHER MUSCLES TO EXAMINE

- Rectus abdominis
- Iliopsoas
- Quadratus lumborum

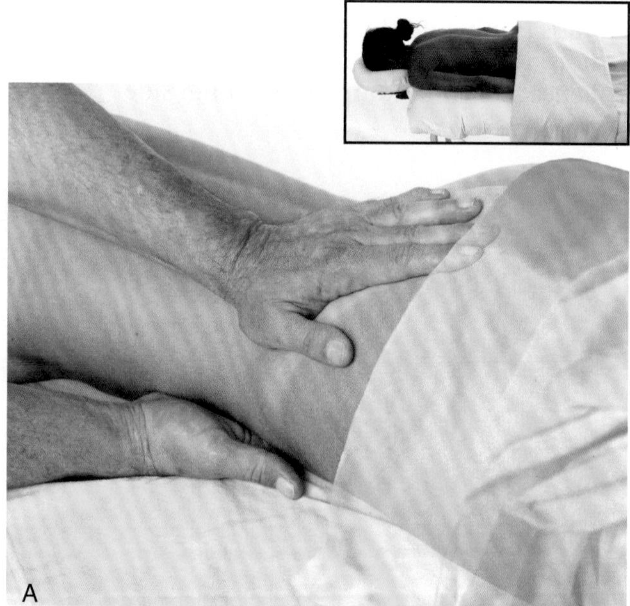

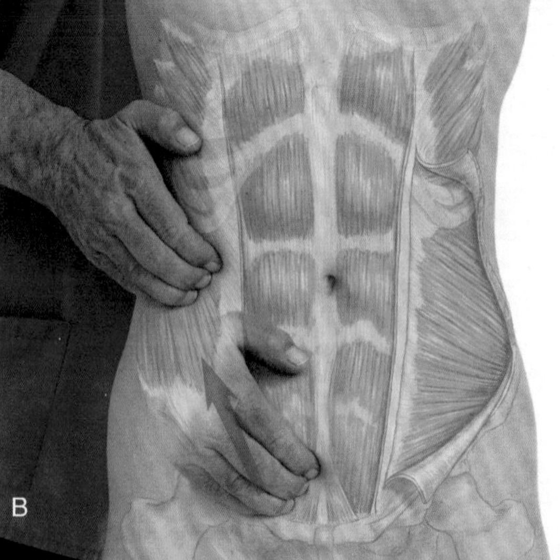

FIGURE 7-13 Client prone **(A)** for stripping of obliques with fingertips **(B)** position for demonstration as if prone

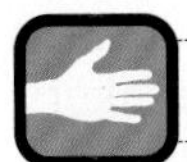

MANUAL THERAPY

Stripping

- The client lies prone.
- The therapist stands beside the client at the chest.
  - Place the hand between the client's abdomen and the table (Fig. 7-13A) with the palm on the abdomen and the fingertips just superior to the pubis at the attachment of the inguinal ligament.
  - Pressing firmly upward into the tissue, slide the fingertips superolaterally along the muscle to the rib cage (Fig. 7-13B). (Note: the client is shown standing in the photograph for illustration of the procedure.)
  - Beginning at the same spot, repeat this procedure at a more oblique angle until the whole surface of the abdomen has been treated.
- Repeat the same procedure on the other side.

TRANSVERSUS ABDOMINIS

trans-VERS-us ab-DOM-in-iss

ETYMOLOGY Latin ***trans***, across + ***versus***, turned

Overview

Transversus abdominis (Fig. 7-14) lies deep to the other abdominal muscles lateral to the rectus abdominis. It is an important muscle of breathing as it compresses the abdomen in forced exhalation.

There is no separate manual treatment for it that is appropriate to this book.

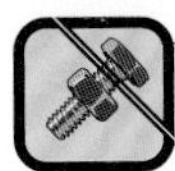

ATTACHMENTS

- Origin: along the inner bottom of the ribcage (7th to 12th ribs and costal cartilages, interdigitating with fibers of the diaphragm), lumbar fascia, iliac crest, and inguinal ligament
- Insertion: aponeurosis of posterior and anterior rectus sheath and conjoint tendon to pubic crest and pectineal line

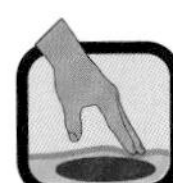

PALPATION

Not palpable

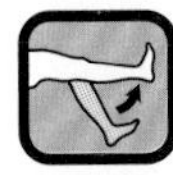

ACTION

Compresses the abdomen, important in forced exhalation

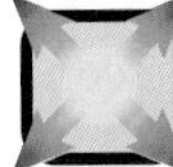

REFERRAL AREA

Along and between the anterior costal margins

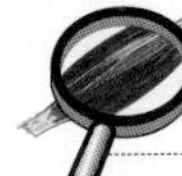

OTHER MUSCLES TO EXAMINE

- Rectus abdominis
- Abdominal obliques

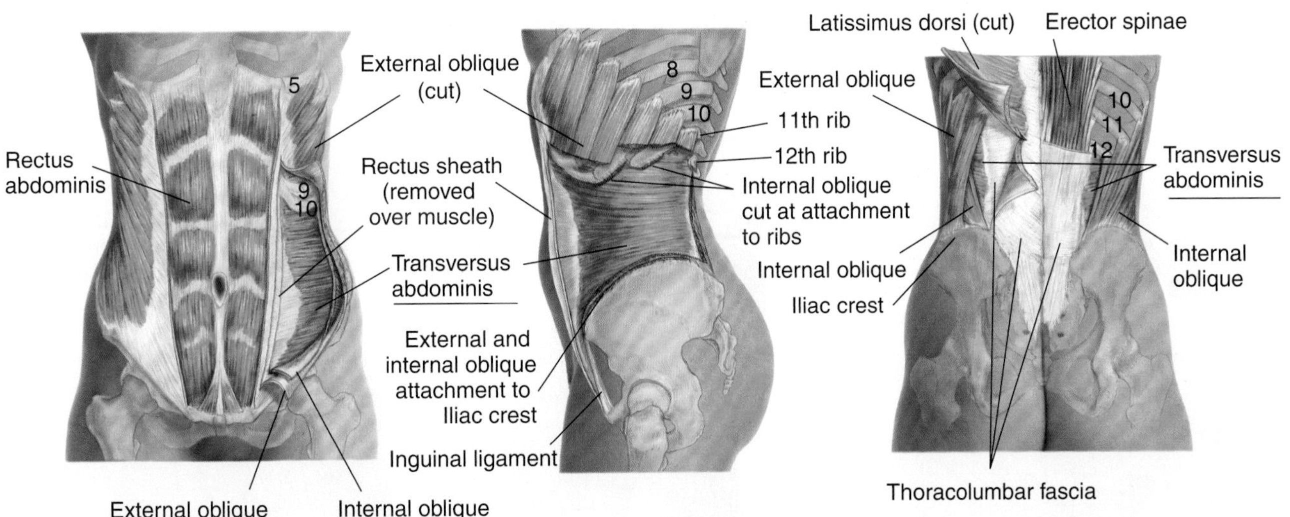

FIGURE 7-14 Anatomy of transversus abdominis

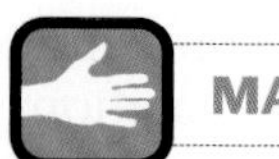

MANUAL THERAPY

Not applicable

Overview of the Muscles of the Lower Back

Shoulder muscles in the lower back, such as the latissimus dorsi, are covered in Chapter 4. Vertebral muscles in the lower back are covered in Chapter 6.

QUADRATUS LUMBORUM

kwa-DRAY-tus lum-BOR-um

ETYMOLOGY Latin *quadratus*, four-sided + *lumborum*, of the loins

Overview

When cinematographers have to shoot a scene in which the camera is moving around, either on someone's back or on a truck, they use a device called Steadicam™—to prevent the movement of the carrier being transferred to the camera. The same coordination between our upper and lower bodies is needed when we perform complex actions with our eyes and hands while running or riding on horseback, or keep our feet and legs steady while performing actions with our arms. In addition to its responsibility for lateral bending, **quadratus lumborum** performs this stabilizing service.

For this reason, you will often find quadratus lumborum problems in horseback riders, kayakers, golfers, and anyone whose activities involve separation of movement between the upper and lower body.

Quadratus lumborum (Fig. 7-15, see also plate 7-4) is not an easy muscle to access manually, as it lies deep to the lumbar paraspinal muscles (erector spinae) and the thick layers of fascia and aponeurotic tissue of the lumbar region. It can be approached obliquely with the elbow just adjacent to the lumbar paraspinal muscles or laterally with the fingers or thumbs.

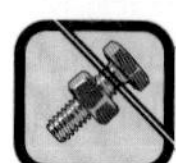

ATTACHMENTS

- Origin: posterior third of iliac crest and iliolumbar ligament
- Inferior: transverse processes of L1-L4 vertebrae and inferior border of the 12th rib

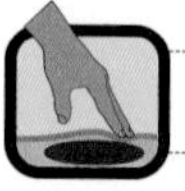

PALPATION

Can be palpated with thumb or fingertips from the side underneath the paraspinal muscles and lumbar aponeurosis between the last rib and the iliac crest. The fibers are oblique, the upper fibers from lateral to medial, lower fibers medial to lateral, and the architecture is parallel.

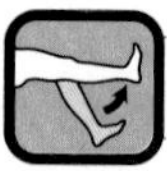

ACTION

- Lateral flexion of the spine (unilaterally)
- Assists extension of the spine (bilaterally)
- Stabilization of the lumbar spine during other movements
- Fixes the 12th rib during respiration

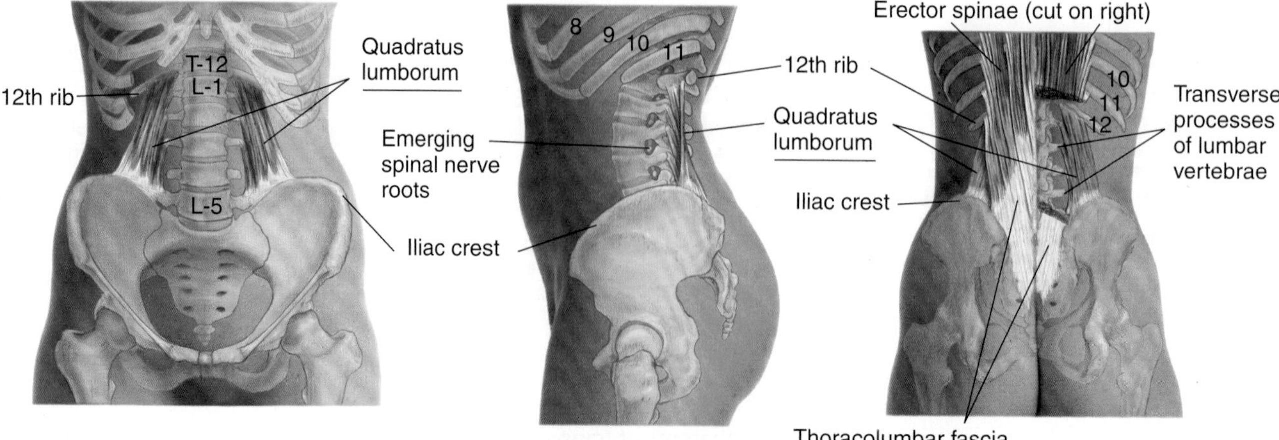

FIGURE 7-15 Anatomy of quadratus lumborum

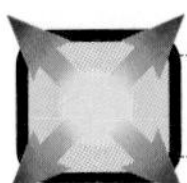

REFERRAL AREAS

- Into the buttock
- Over the hip
- Down the back of the leg
- Over the iliac crest
- Into the groin and sometimes the testicle
- Into the lower lateral quadrant of the abdomen

OTHER MUSCLES TO EXAMINE

- Iliopsoas
- Lumbar paraspinal muscles
- Gluteal muscles
- Piriformis and other deep lateral rotators
- Rectus abdominis and pyramidalis

CAUTION In working in a superior direction on quadratus lumborum, do not place excessive pressure on the last rib. It is joined only to T12, overlies the kidney and can be broken with pressure.

MANUAL THERAPY

MYOFASCIAL STRETCH

- The client lies prone.
- The therapist stands beside the client at the waist.
  - Place the hand near the client's head flat on the lumbar area lateral to the vertebrae with the fingers over the iliac crest just lateral to the sacrum.
- Crossing the other hand over or under the first, place it flat on the thoracic area over the lowest three or four ribs.
- Let your hands sink into the tissue until you feel contact with the superficial myofascial tissue.
  - Press the hands in opposite directions, with enough downward pressure to engage and stretch the superficial tissue (Fig. 7-16).
- Hold until you feel significant release in the myofascial tissue.
- Shift both hands laterally (toward yourself) by one hand's width and repeat the technique.

Compression (1)

- The client lies prone or on one side.
- The therapist stands beside the client at the waist.
  - Grasp the client's waist laterally, with either the thumb (Figs. 7-17, 7-18A) or the fingertips (Fig. 7-18B) pressing under the erector spinae bundle into quadratus lumborum.

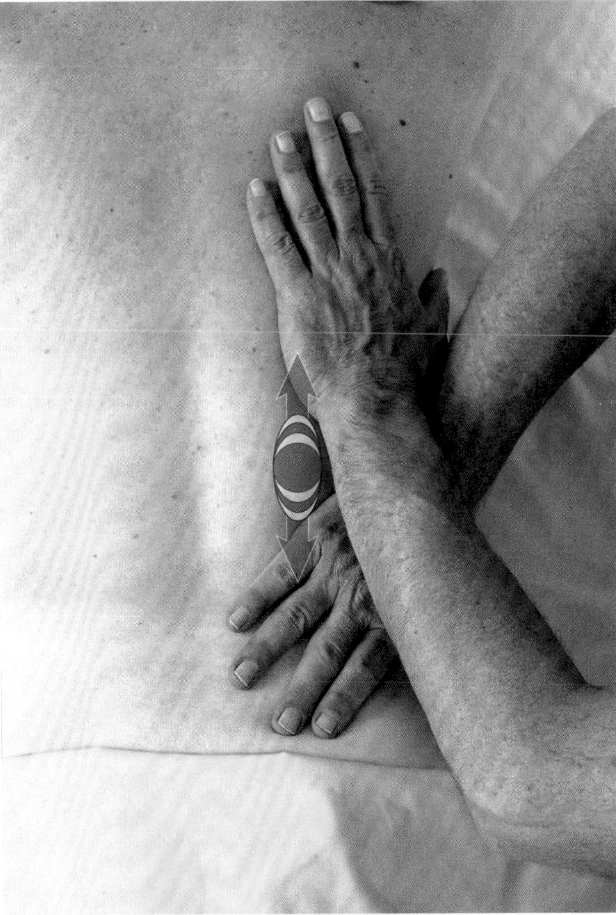

FIGURE 7-16 Myofascial stretch of low back

  - Press firmly into the muscle, looking for tender spots, which may range from the attachments to the ilium to the attachments to the last rib. Hold for release.

Compression (2)

- The client lies prone.
- The therapist stands beside the client at the waist.
- Place the elbow just lateral to the erector spinae bundle.
- Press firmly into the tissue, obliquely in a deep and medial direction. Hold for release.
  - Repeat this procedure, first pressing superiorly toward the muscle's attachment to the last rib (Fig. 7-19A), then inferiorly toward the muscle's attachment to the ilium (Fig. 7-19B).

Stretch

- The client lies prone.
- The therapist stands beside the client at the waist.
  - Place the heel of the hand just lateral to the erector spinae bundle on the opposite side of the client's body, between the ilium and the last rib.

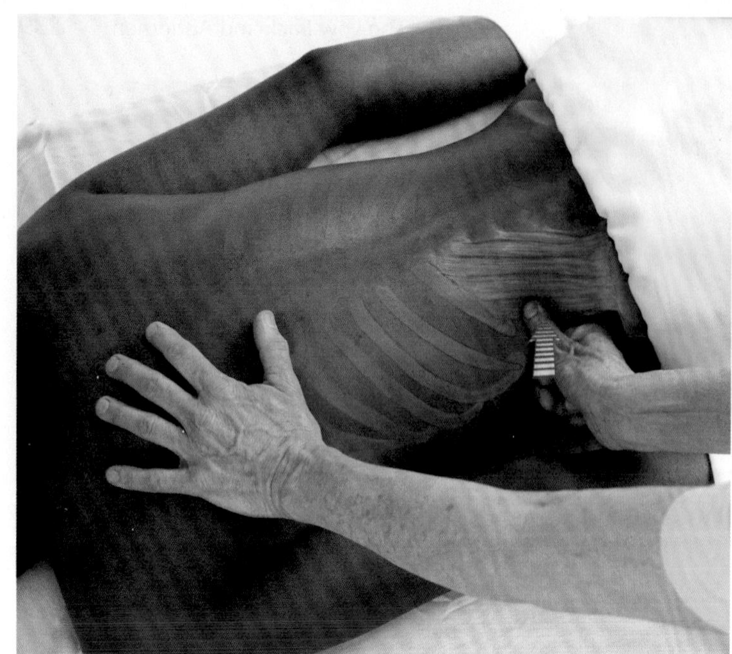

FIGURE 7-17 Compression of quadratus lumborum with the thumb, client prone

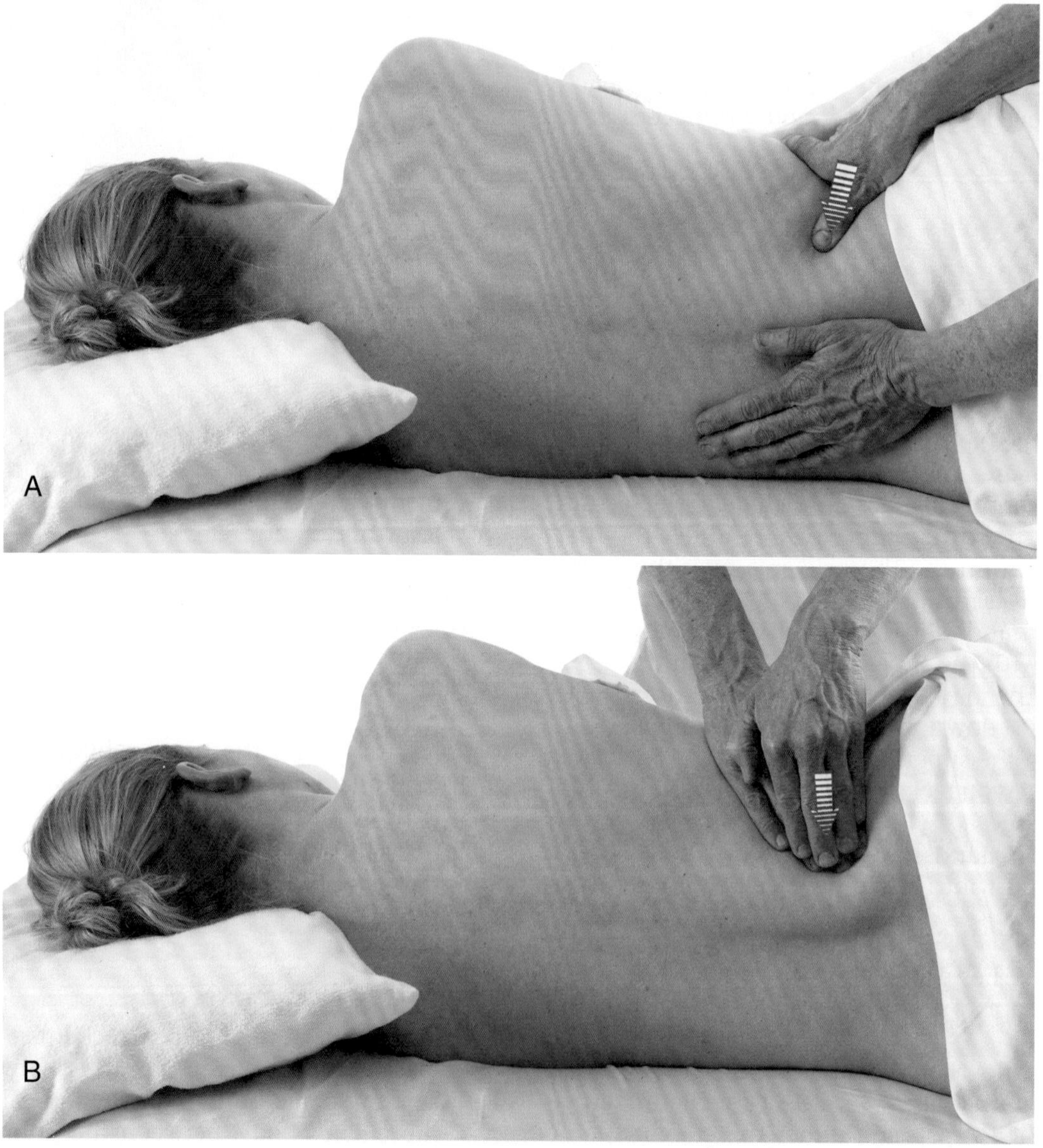

A

B

FIGURE 7-18 Compression of quadratus lumborum with the client sidelying, using the thumb **(A)** or fingertips **(B)**

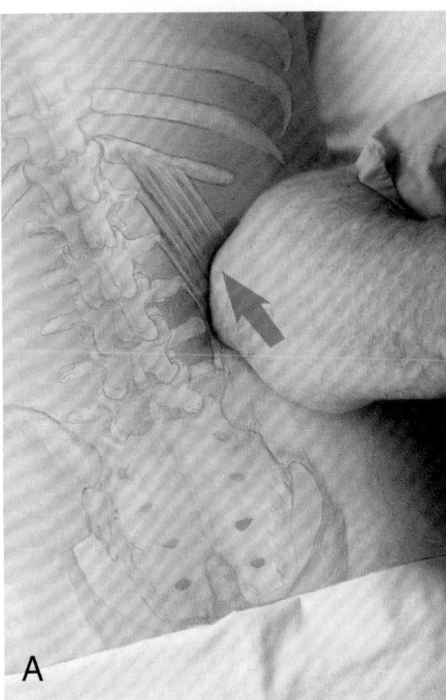

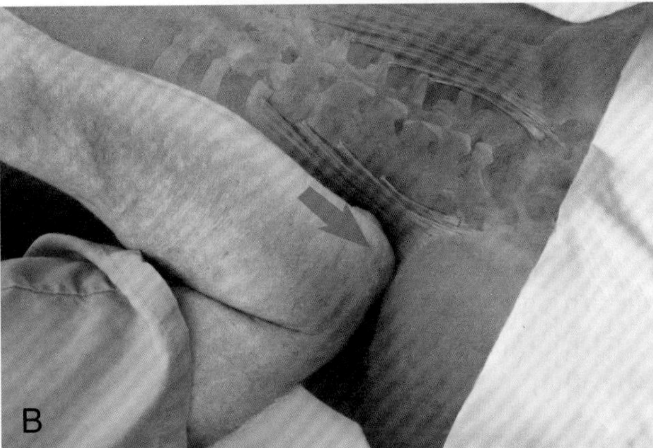

FIGURE 7-19 Compression of quadratus lumborum with the elbow superiorly **(A)** and inferiorly **(B)**

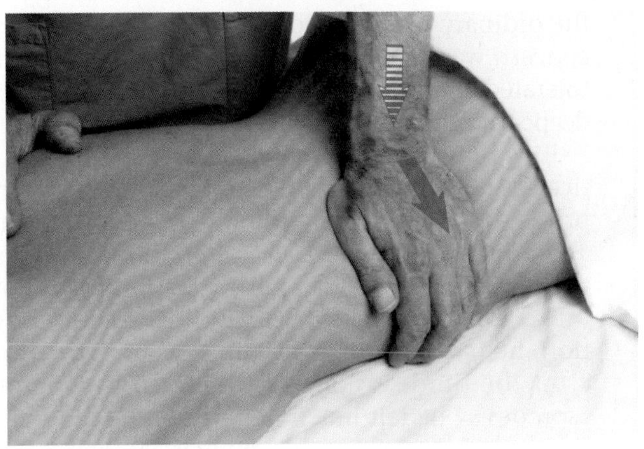

FIGURE 7-20 Stretch of quadratus lumborum with the hand

- Pressing deeply toward the table, let the heel of your hand slide slowly away from you (Fig. 7-20), compressing all the muscles between the pelvis and the last rib, dragging your hand off the client's side.

CHAPTER REVIEW

CASE STUDY

R.G. is a 50-year-old golf pro who owns a local driving range. He stated that he is seeking massage therapy because he has tried everything else, and a cousin of his who is an MT in another state recommended that he get massage. R.G. stated that he has had pain in his lower abdomen for about a year. He is in top physical condition and appears much younger than his age. His recall of the beginning of his pain is that he was doing kettlebell exercise when he felt a big pain in his abdomen. Assuming that he had just strained a muscle, he left off exercising for a few days, and when the pain persisted, went to the doctor. Palpation and an MRI revealed no abnormalities. After several months had passed and he was still experiencing the same level of pain, he sought a second opinion. The doctor said "strained muscle" and advised him to take it easy for a few weeks, although he had already been doing so since the injury. R.G. took it on himself to obtain an elasticized back brace, not for his back but to support his abdominal muscles, and a year later, is still wearing it every day. He no longer does the kettlebell training and states that he has always done stomach crunches as part of his exercise routine, but he is no longer doing those, either. He is still lean and muscular from playing golf and walking the course daily. He states that he feels like he has a "horizontal line" of pain in his abdomen. Posture and gait appear normal. Palpation did not reveal any "knots" or anything out of the ordinary. I proceeded very slowly and cautiously with effleurage, starting with very light pressure. My concern was not to cause him further pain. I performed compression on the rectus abdominis, which he tolerated, and muscle stripping on lateral muscles. My instinct was to wait until the second session to do deep stripping on the actual rectus abdominis—the area of the actual pain.

R.G. returned one week later and stated that he felt a little "looser" in the area and that he had noticed a moderate difference in the pain, although he is continuing to wear the brace. The second session proceeded like the first, but at the end I had him lie supine while I did deep muscle stripping on rectus abdominis, resulting in several profound releases. He stated feeling a significant difference at the end of the session. I suggested another session the following week that would incorporate the abdominal work into a full-body massage, reasoning that although his posture did not appear to suffer from his condition, he had been in a "holding pattern" for a year, and he agreed.

At the third session, R.G. reported leaving off the brace. He stated that although he still felt some "soreness," he felt much better than he did before the first session. He received a 90-minute session of deep Swedish massage and myofascial release, including another stripping session on rectus abdominis. As he has taken good care of himself, he actually appeared to have no other significant body issues or pain elsewhere . . . no active trigger points, taut bands or sore spots, other than the residual abdominal pain, which he says is about 75% better. We will continue with another session in 1 week.

At the end of the fourth session, R.G. stated that if he had known how much relief he would get, he would have sought the massage long ago. As he is in otherwise great physical condition, he stated that he had decided not to return to his kettlebell workout, as he feels that was the cause to start with and that he still didn't feel as if he wanted to do any crunches, and he really has no reason to. He stated that he is now a firm believer in massage and made an appointment 1 month out. He intends to make regular massage a part of his wellness plan.

L.E.A., LMT

REVIEW QUESTIONS

1. The abdominal muscles assist in forced exhalation through _______ of the abdominal cavity.
   a. Inspiration
   b. Stretching
   c. Decompression
   d. Compression
2. Chronic constipation could be an example of a symptom of _______ disease.
   a. Asperger's syndrome
   b. Somatovisceral disease
   c. Diptheria
   d. Poliomyelitis
3. Linea alba divides the _________.
   a. Quadratus lumborum
   b. External obliques from the internal obliques
   c. Rectus abdominis
   d. Diaphragm from the other organs
4. The last rib is joined only to ______.
   a. T-1
   b. T-6
   c. T-12
   d. L-1
5. A muscle that is absent in many people is the ______.
   a. Pyramidalis
   b. Internal oblique
   c. Intercostal
   d. Linea alba
6. When working on muscles that attach to the pubis, it is important to ______.
   a. Be sure the client is undraped
   b. Only use compression
   c. Stay away from the ASIS
   d. Avoid touching pubic hair
7. The _____ may be palpated by having the client raise one shoulder toward the opposite side of the body.
   a. Serratus
   b. Iliopsoas
   c. Diaphragm
   d. Obliques

8. A significant action muscle for lateral bending and lumbar stabilization is the _______.

   a. Quadratus lumborum
   b. Rectus abdominis
   c. Pyramidalis
   d. Serratus anterior

9. Problems in the _______ are common in horseback riders, kayakers, and anyone whose activities involved separation between the upper and lower bodies.

   a. Quadratus lumborum
   b. Diaphragm
   c. Xiphoid process
   d. Rectus abdominis

10. You should avoid applying deep pressure to the _______.

   a. Paraspinal muscles
   b. Last rib
   c. Sacrum
   d. Iliacus

thePoint Additional helpful resources are available at http://thePoint.lww.com.

CHAPTER 8

The Pelvis

LEARNING OBJECTIVES

At the end of this chapter, the learner will be able to:

- State the correct anatomical names of the muscles of the pelvis.
- Palpate the muscles of the pelvis.
- Identify their attachments at the origins and insertions.
- Explain the actions of the muscles.
- Describe their pain referral areas.
- Recall related muscles.
- Recognize any endangerment sites and ethical cautions for massage therapy.
- Demonstrate proficiency in manual therapy techniques for muscles of the pelvis.

The Overview of the Region begins on page 253, after the anatomy plates.

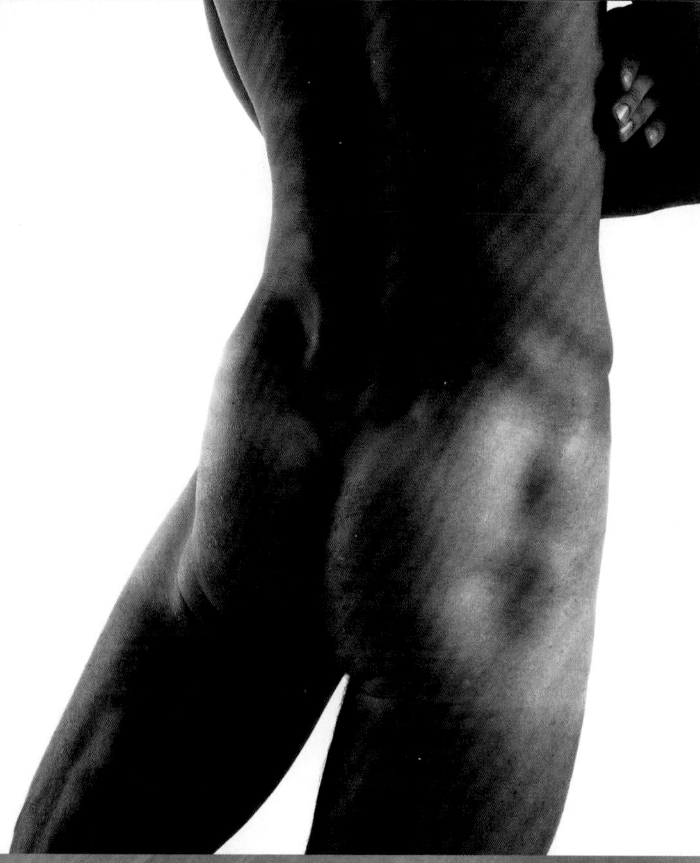

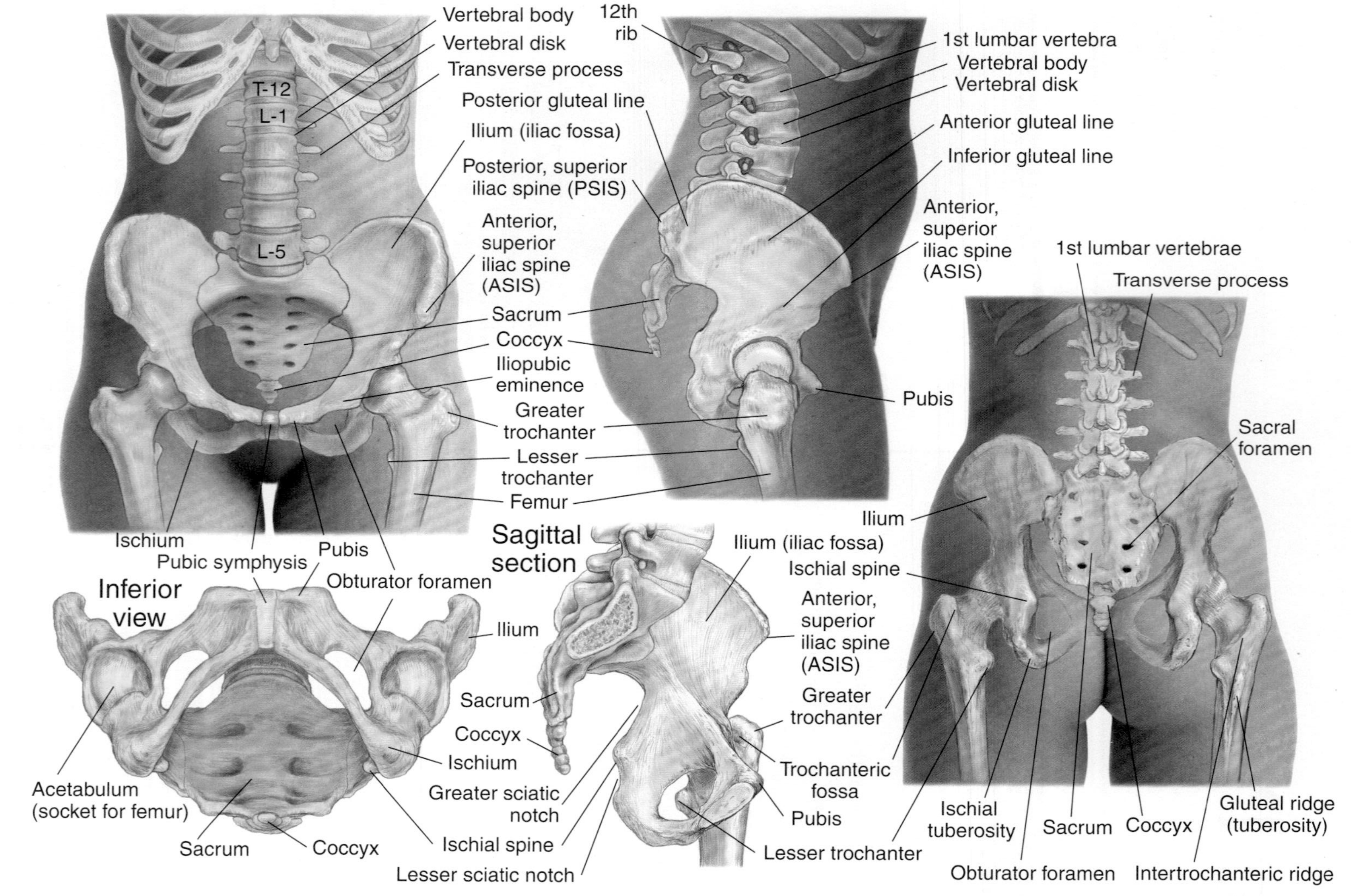

PLATE 8-1 ■ Skeletal features of the pelvic region

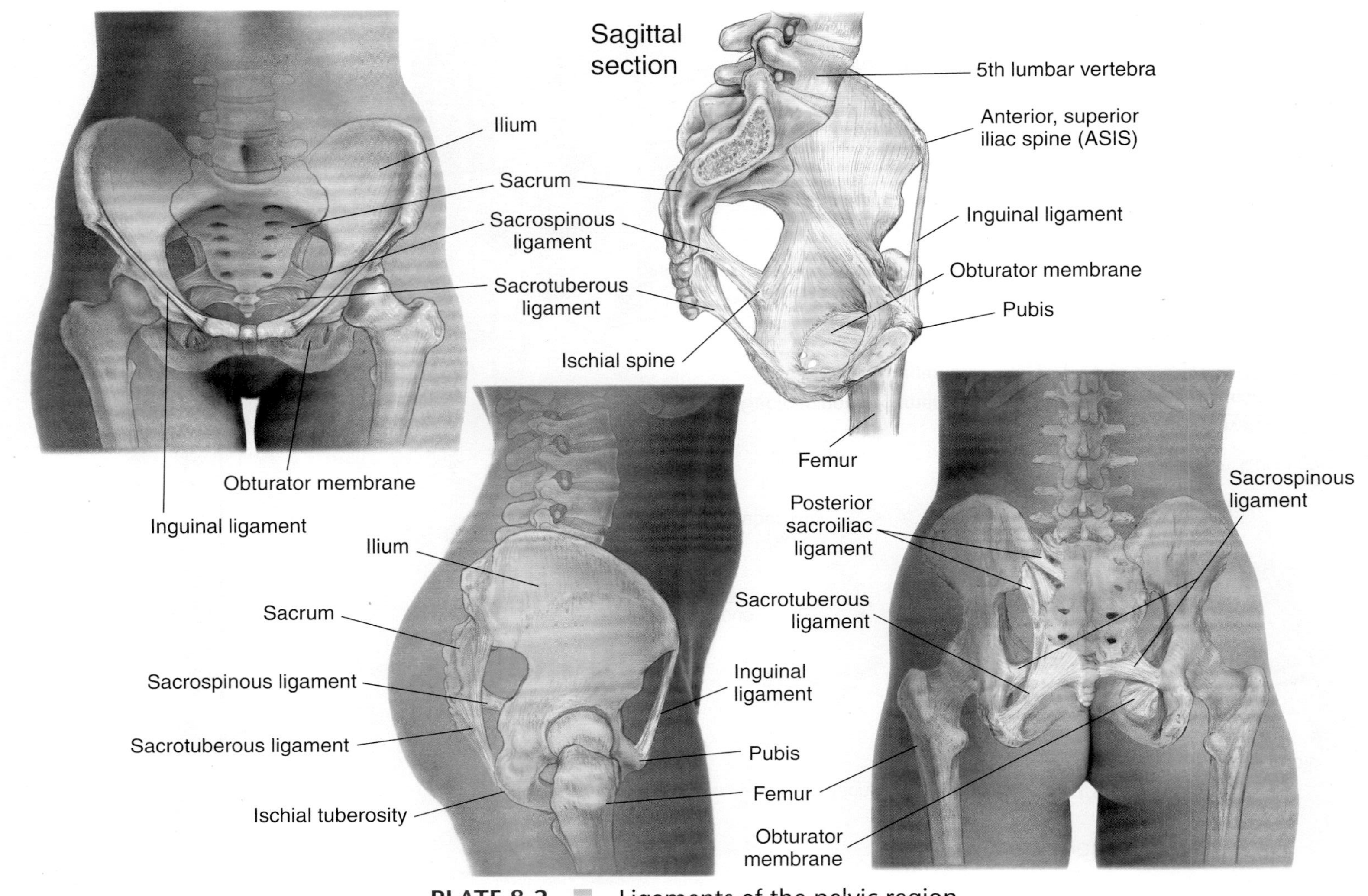

PLATE 8-2 ■ Ligaments of the pelvic region

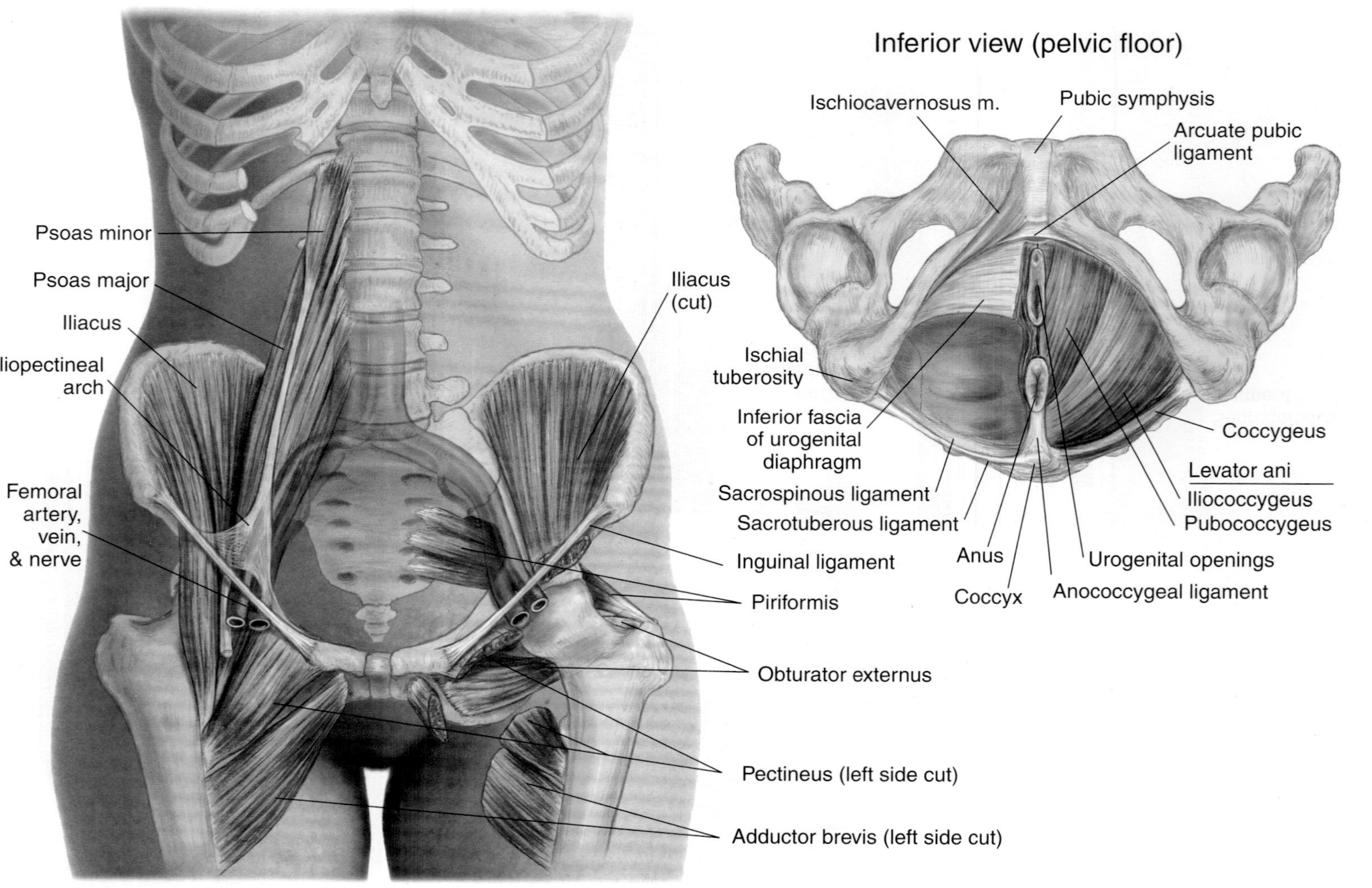

PLATE 8-3 ■ Muscles of the anterior pelvis and pelvic floor

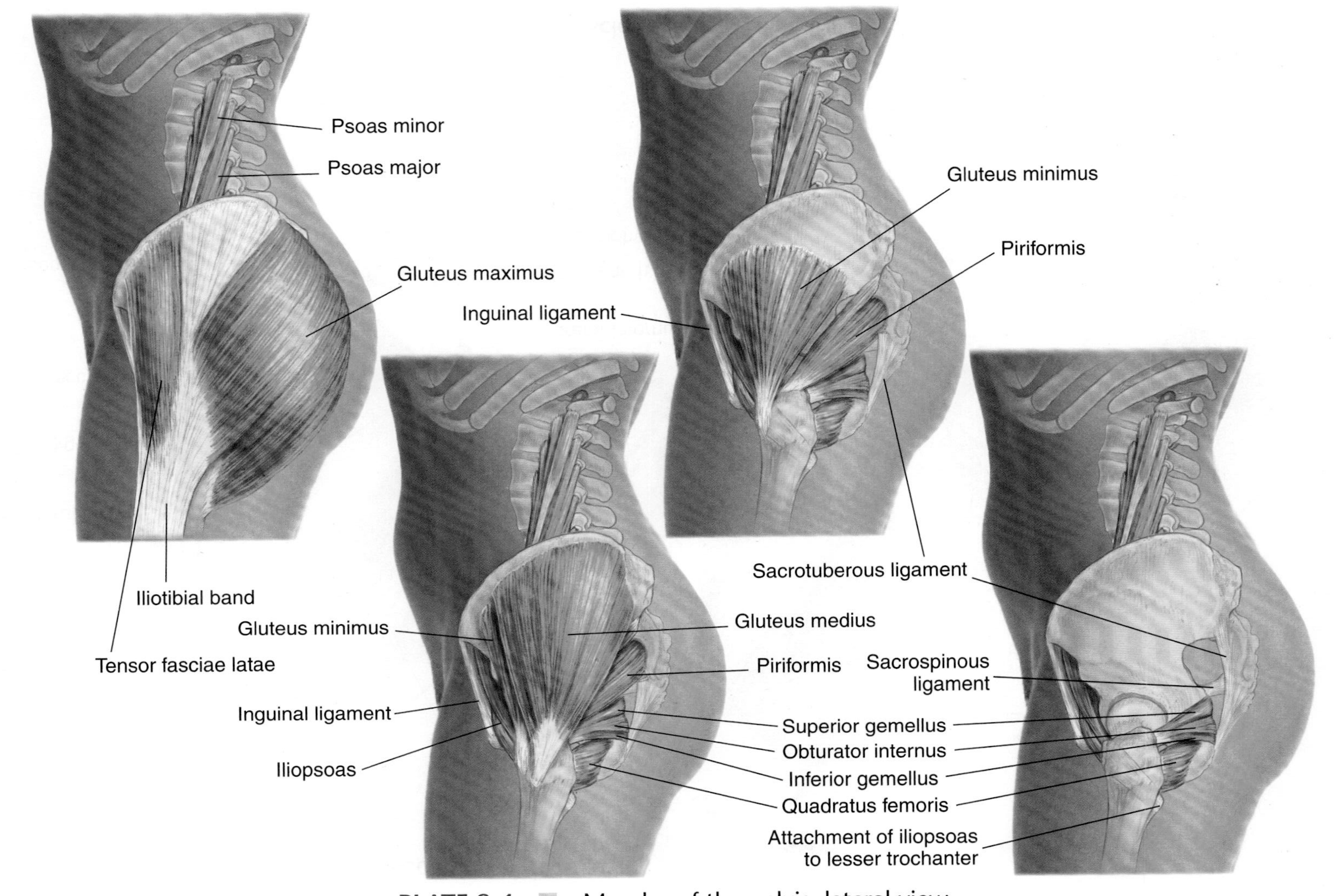

PLATE 8-4 ■ Muscles of the pelvis, lateral view

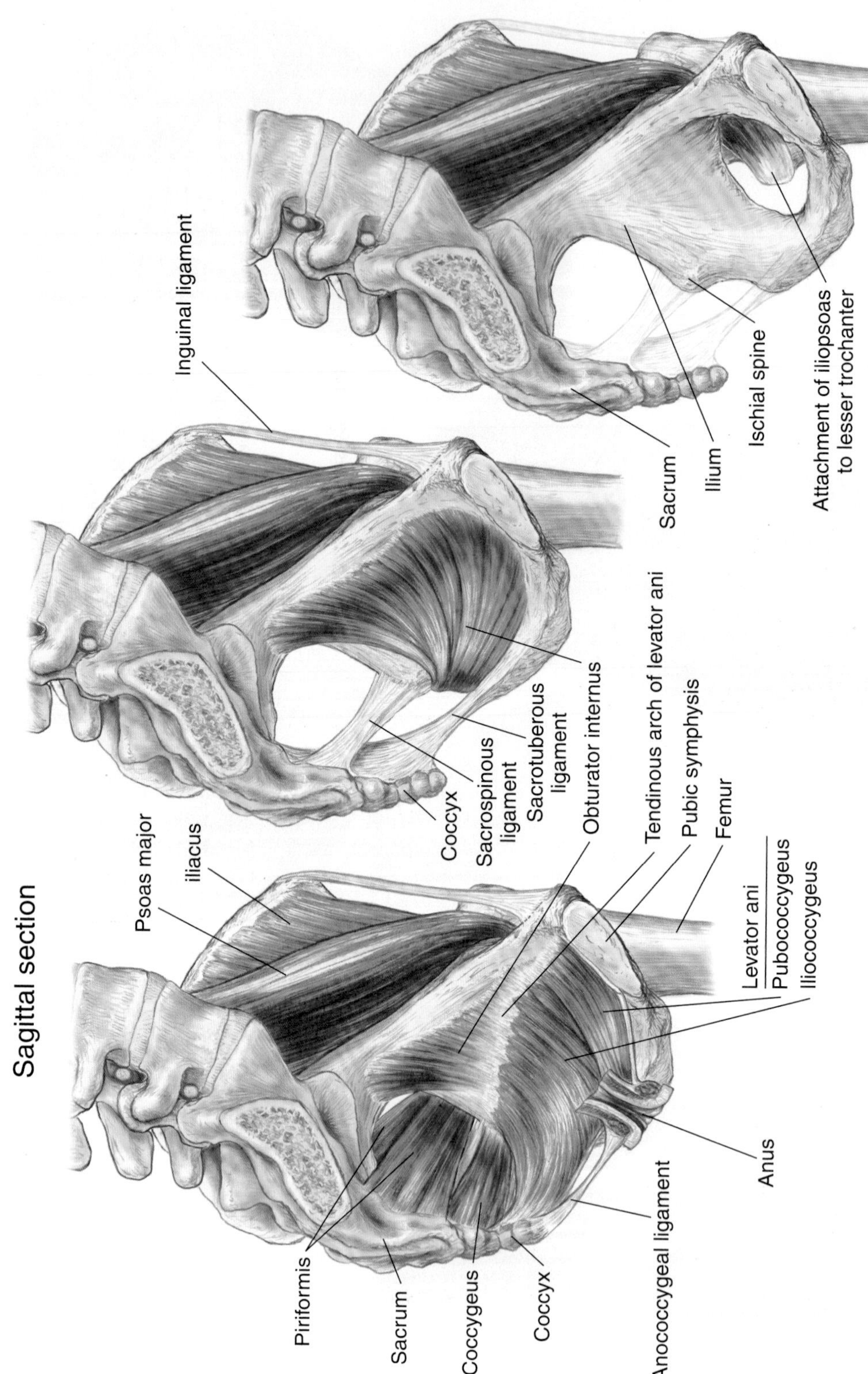

PLATE 8-5 ■ Muscles of the pelvis, sagittal section

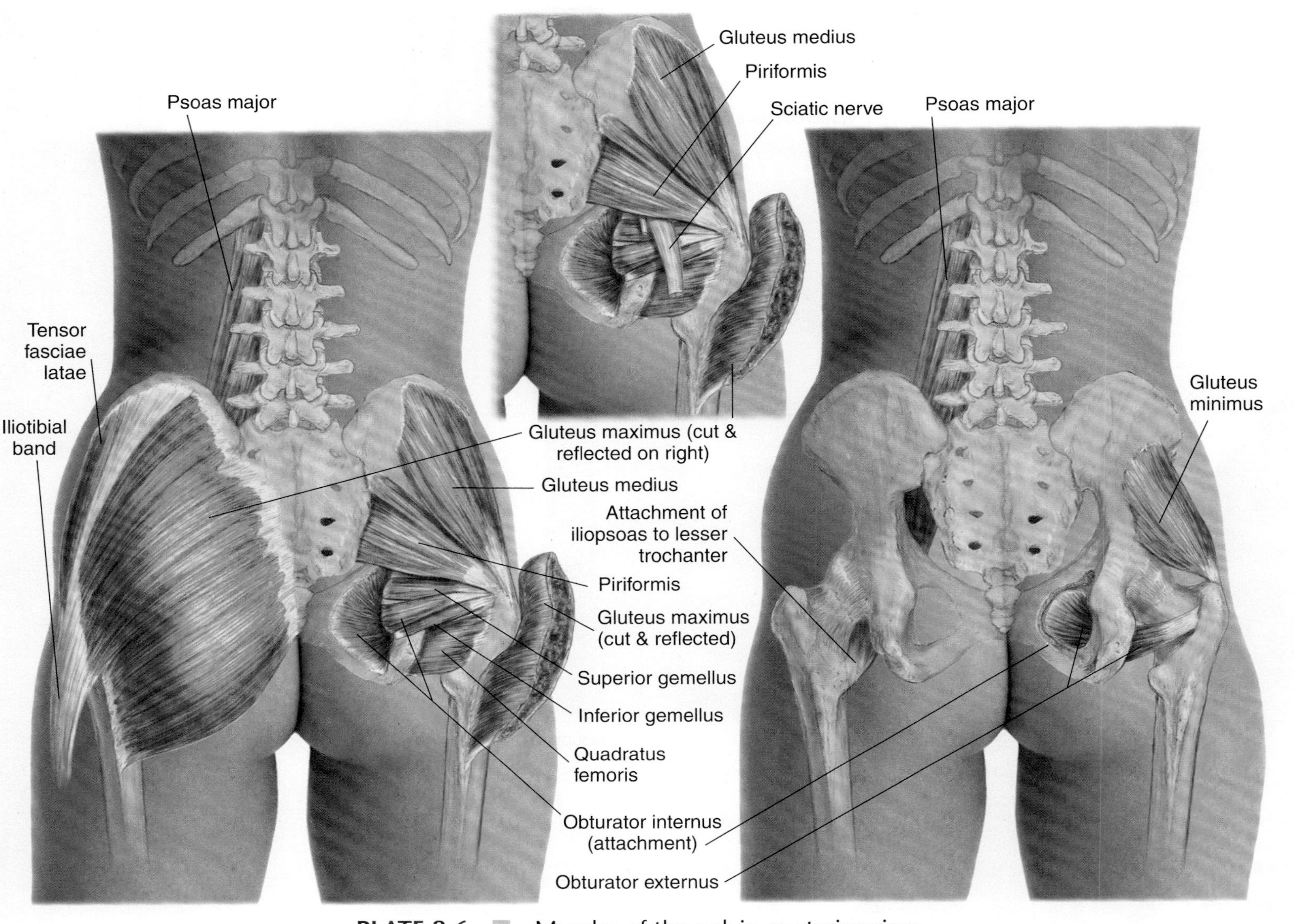

PLATE 8-6 ■ Muscles of the pelvis, posterior view

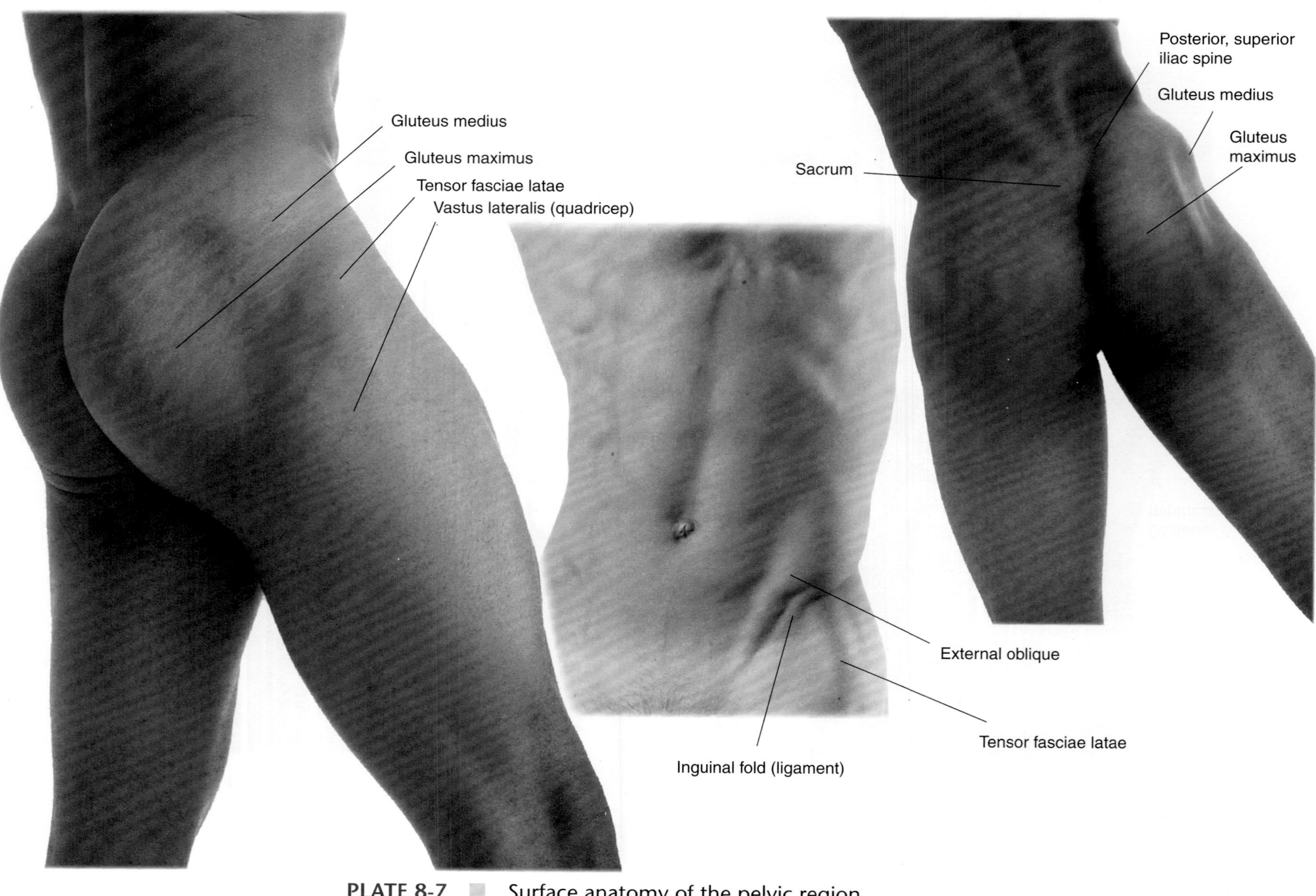

PLATE 8-7 ■ Surface anatomy of the pelvic region

Overview of the Region (Plates 8-1 to 8-7)

The structural, functional, and emotional importance of the human pelvis cannot be overemphasized. The pelvis balances the torso and its appendages on the legs. It is the container, support, and protector of the abdominal and pelvic organs, especially the organs of reproduction and elimination. It is, therefore, a very personal and intimate area. Its position and freedom of movement are of principal importance in postural alignment, and in gait.

Although we tend to think of the pelvis as a single entity, it is actually composed of two halves, or hemipelves, connected posteriorly at the sacroiliac joints and anteriorly at the symphysis pubis. The pelvis as a whole can be rotated forward or backward, or tilted to either side. Each hemipelvis, however, can have a greater or lesser anterior or posterior rotation in relation to the other, resulting in what is called a torqued pelvis. The position of the hemipelvis will affect the position of the hip joint and its corresponding leg because each hemipelvis is the site of one acetabulum, the socket in which the head of the femur rests. The anterior or posterior rotation of the pelvis as a whole will also affect the normal curve of the lumbar spine, which in turn will affect the carriage of the entire upper body.

A lateral tilt in the pelvis, determined by the relative positions of the two posterior, superior iliac spines (PSIS), will result in an uneven distribution of the body weight on the legs and will require a compensatory shifting of the spine, rib cage and its attached structures. Any combination of tilt or rotation in the frontal or sagittal planes and torque of the hemipelves will result in a postural misalignment that is likely to cause a wide variety of myofascial problems in both the lower extremities and the entire upper body. In addition to postural issues, tightness or trigger points in the muscles of the pelvis can interfere with reproductive or eliminatory functions and can refer pain into the viscera.

The muscles of the pelvis should always be considered and addressed in any interview and examination. Because of the intimate nature of the pelvic region, it is necessary to approach examination and treatment with a great deal of sensitivity to the client's feelings and concerns with regard to privacy and modesty. Examination and treatment should be carried out only with specific written informed consent, with particular care paid to draping and to maintaining the client's feelings of safety and security.

ethics **ETHICAL CAUTION**

Remember that a client always has the right of refusal, even if they have already given consent. If the client feels uncomfortable at any time, they are able to withdraw that consent. It's important to be tuned in to the client's body language and nonverbal cues, as some people will hesitate to tell you that they feel uncomfortable.

PSOAS MAJOR (ILIOPSOAS)

SO-az MAY-jer

ETYMOLOGY Greek *psoa*, the muscles of the loins + Latin *major*, larger

Overview

Psoas major (Fig. 8-1), which joins **iliacus** at the groin to form **iliopsoas**, is one of the most important muscles in the body, not only for its primary function as hip flexor, but also for its postural and clinical significance.

In four-legged domestic animals, iliopsoas has little challenging work to do, since it has no real postural function and acts only to swing the hind leg forward in walking. For this reason, it tends to be a tender cut of meat: it is the tenderloin or filet, the source of the filet mignon. In humans, the story is altogether different: since we walk upright, much greater muscular effort is required to flex the hip and lift the leg against the pull of gravity. In addition, psoas plays a major role in determining the positioning of the pelvis and low back in relation to each other.

During gestation, the hips of the fetus remain fully flexed most of the time. If you observe human babies, you will notice that they do not lie flat—the hips tend to stay partially flexed. In fact, a baby does not usually attain full extension of the hips until she begins to walk. This full extension is necessary for a relaxed and comfortable upright posture. Children spend a great deal of time sitting, either in class at school, or at home studying or watching television. Most adults spend even more time in this position at desks or computers or, again, in front of the television. Iliopsoas, therefore, spends a lot of time shortened and very little time stretched.

Psoas attaches to the lumbar vertebrae and passes downward through the abdominal cavity to the groin, where it merges with iliacus and passes over the anterior rim of the ilium, then obliquely in a posterior and inferior direction to attach to the **lesser trochanter** of the femur. In this way, it uses the anterior rim of the ilium as a pulley, exerting an inferior and posterior force against it. Thus, by pulling

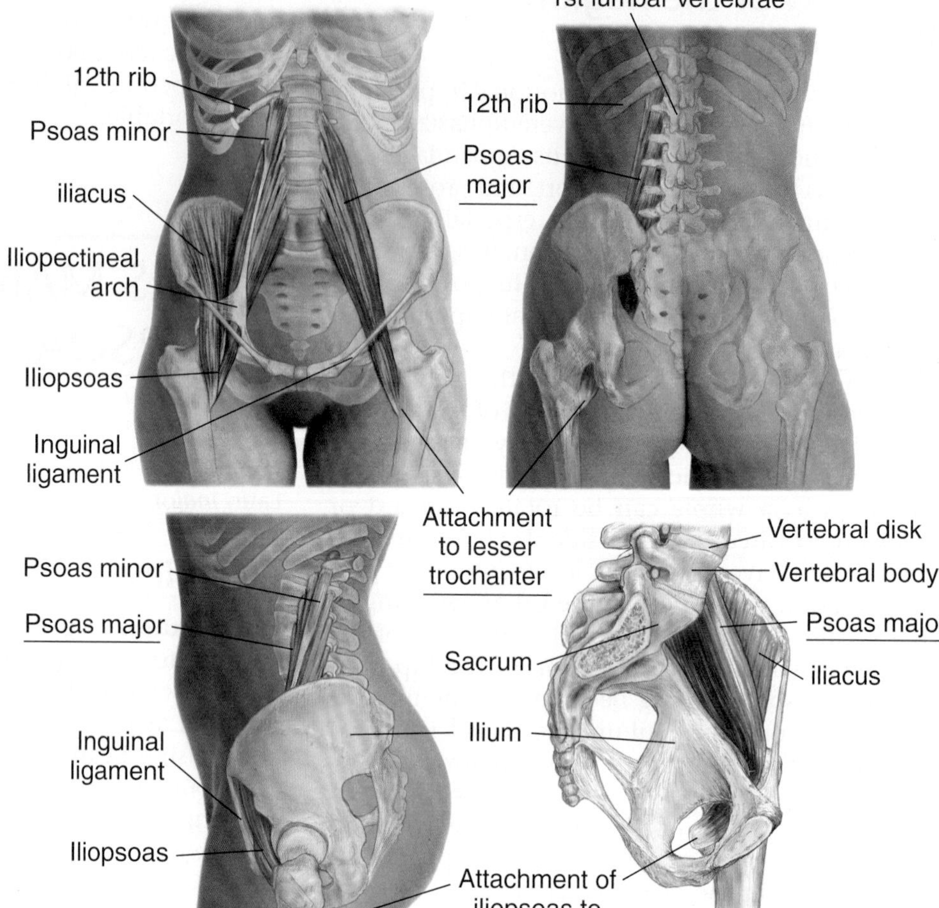

FIGURE 8-1 Anatomy of psoas major

forward on the lumbar spine and pressing downward and backward on the anterior inferior ilium, it rotates the pelvis forward and draws the lumbar curve into lordosis (Fig. 8-2). This effect can easily be seen in children, who tend to have this rotation and lordosis to a pronounced degree, and it is quite common for this postural tendency to persist into adulthood to a lesser, but still measurable, extent. One result of an anterior pelvic rotation is to shift the weight of the contents of the abdominal cavity forward, causing the abdomen to protrude. In addition, this rotation moves the hip joint posteriorly, placing strain on the muscles controlling the knees and ankles. An exaggerated lumbar lordosis requires compensatory positioning of all the structures superior to it.

The clinical significance of psoas is both indirect and direct: indirect, in the postural influences described above, and direct, by referring pain into the low back, abdomen, groin, and upper thigh. The pain referral patterns of psoas can include the viscera. In this way, psoas problems can mimic pain from visceral causes.

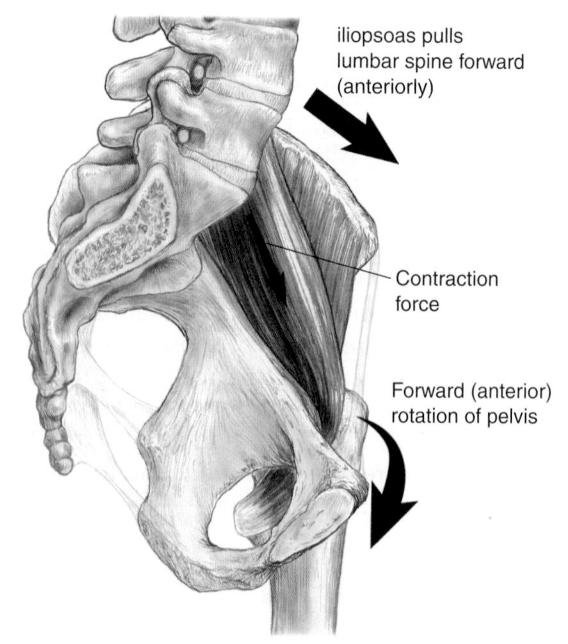

FIGURE 8-2 Influence of psoas major on anterior pelvic rotation

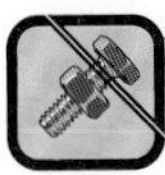

ATTACHMENTS

- Origin: vertebral bodies and intervertebral disks of the twelfth thoracic to the fifth lumbar, and to the transverse processes of the lumbar vertebrae
- Insertion: with the iliacus muscle to the lesser trochanter of the femur

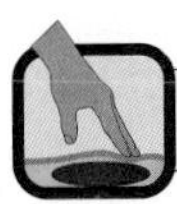

PALPATION

Belly is discernible with the fingertips just below and two to three inches to either side of the umbilicus by having the client raise the corresponding leg. Lower psoas is discernible in the groin below the inguinal ligament just medial to the iliopubic eminence. Architecture is parallel, and fibers run vertically except where they pass over the anterior pelvic brim, where the superior ramus of the pubis joins the anterior ilium.

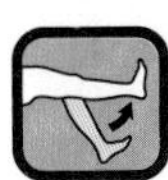

ACTION

Flexes, adducts and laterally rotates the hip; can contribute to flexion and lateral bending of the lumbar spine, is a major postural muscle

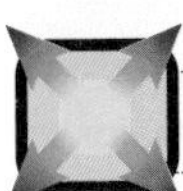

REFERRAL AREAS

- To the medial lumbar region
- To the abdomen from the epigastrium to the groin
- To the anterior thigh from the groin halfway to the knee

OTHER MUSCLES TO EXAMINE

- Iliacus
- Rectus abdominis
- Abdominal obliques
- Diaphragm
- Hip adductors
- Quadratus lumborum
- Lumbar erector spinae muscles

MANUAL THERAPY

Compression

- The client lies supine, with the hip and knee on the side to be treated flexed about 45°.
- The therapist stands beside the client, at the client's hip.
- Place the fingertips of the hand nearest the client on the near side of the abdomen, a few inches inferior and lateral to the navel (Fig. 8-3).
- Press firmly and slowly into the abdomen, moving the fingertips in a circular fashion.
- When you encounter the psoas, press into the muscle searching for tender areas (Fig. 8-4). Hold for release.
- Move the hand caudally so that the fingertips are just inferior to the previous spot.
- Repeat this procedure until you reach the inguinal ligament.
- Repeat at the groin below the inguinal ligament (the circular motion is not necessary here) (Fig. 8-5).
- This work on psoas may also be done from the opposite side of the client, with the client in a sitting position (Fig. 8-6) or standing bent over the table.

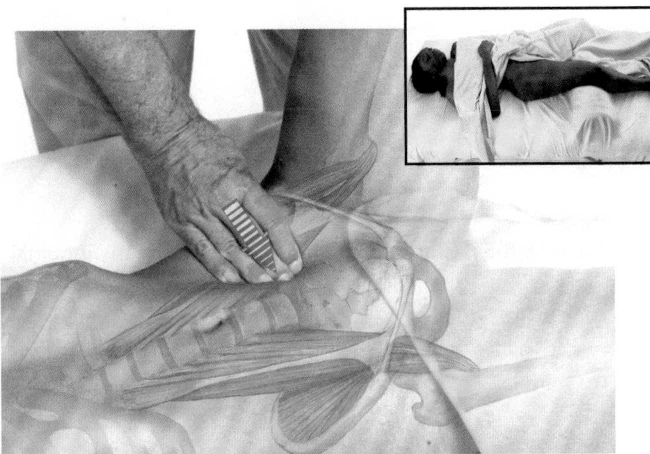

FIGURE 8-3 Position of hand for work on psoas major

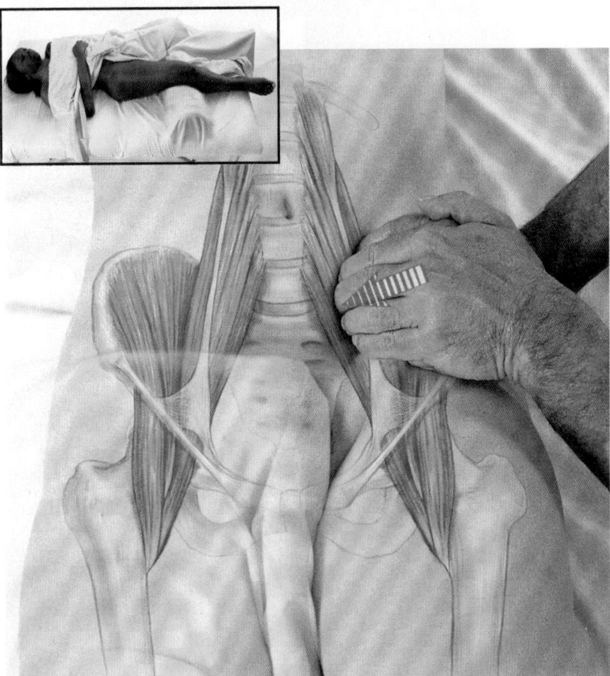

FIGURE 8-4 Compression of psoas major

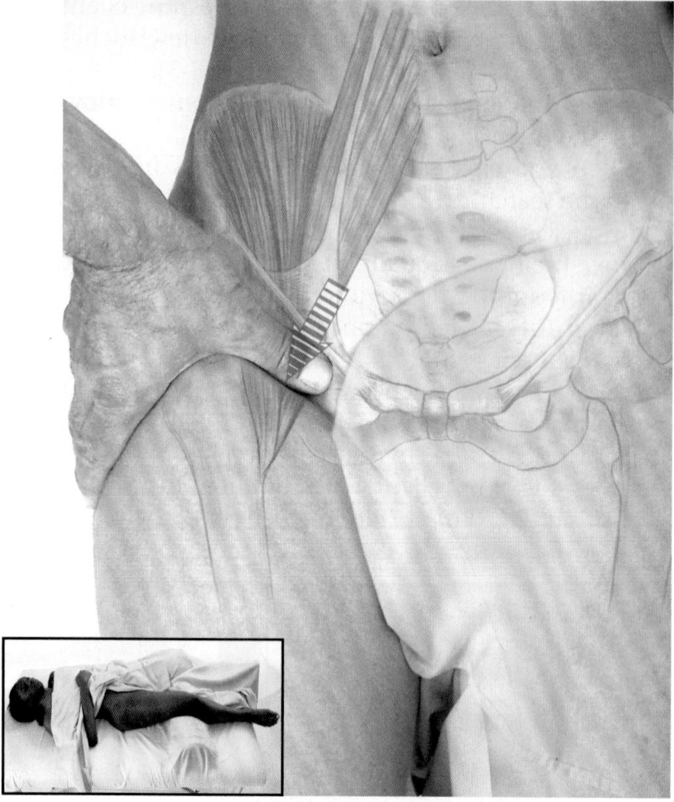

FIGURE 8-5 Compression of iliopsoas below the inguinal ligament

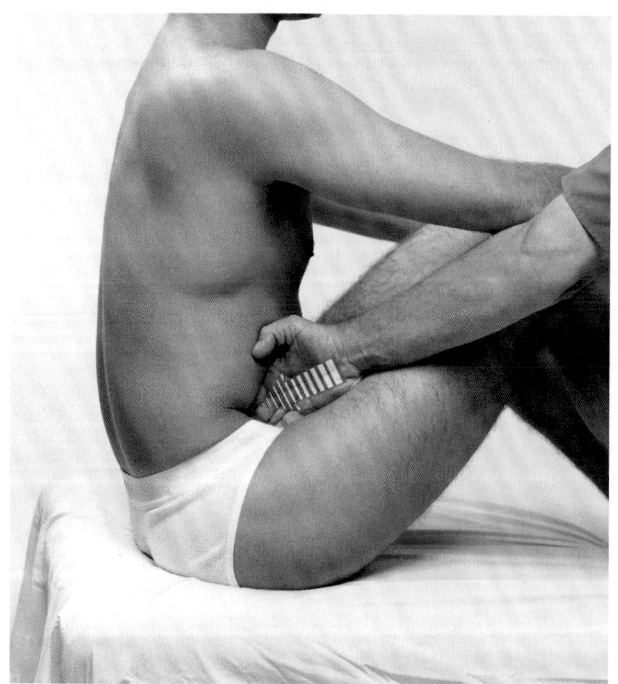

FIGURE 8-6 Compression of psoas major with client in sitting position

Compression of the Inferior Attachment

- The client lies supine.
- The therapist stands beside the client at the client's knees.

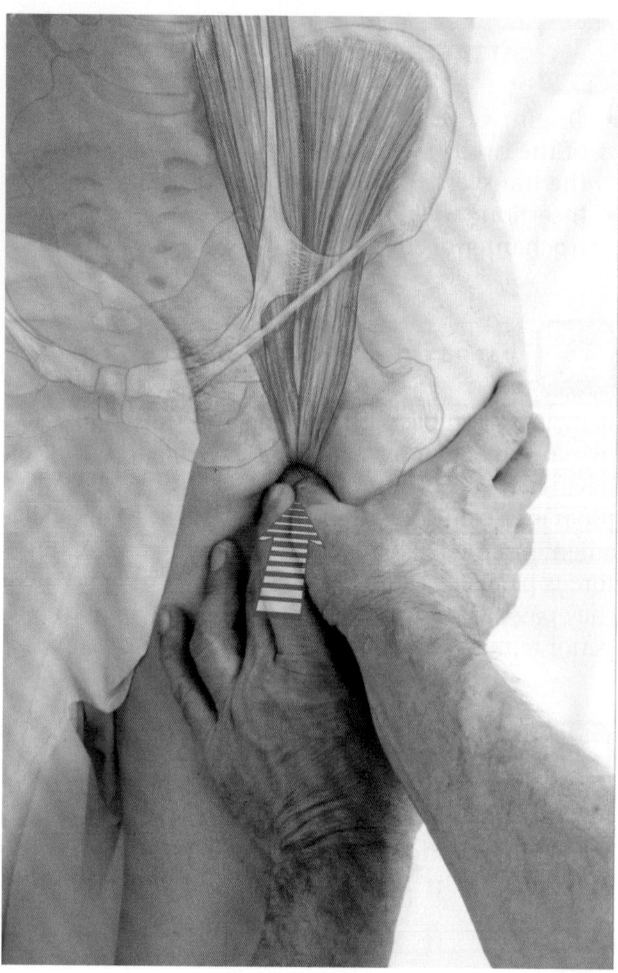

FIGURE 8-7 Compression of attachment of psoas major to lesser trochanter

- Place the supported thumb on the anterior thigh, about two inches below the groin, medial to the rectus femoris.
- Press firmly into the tissue, looking for the attachment to the lesser trochanter (Fig. 8-7). If tender, hold for release.

ILIACUS

il-lee-ACK-us, il-EYE-a-cus

ETYMOLOGY Relating to the ***ilium***: Latin ***ilium***, flank, groin

Overview

See discussion of psoas, above.

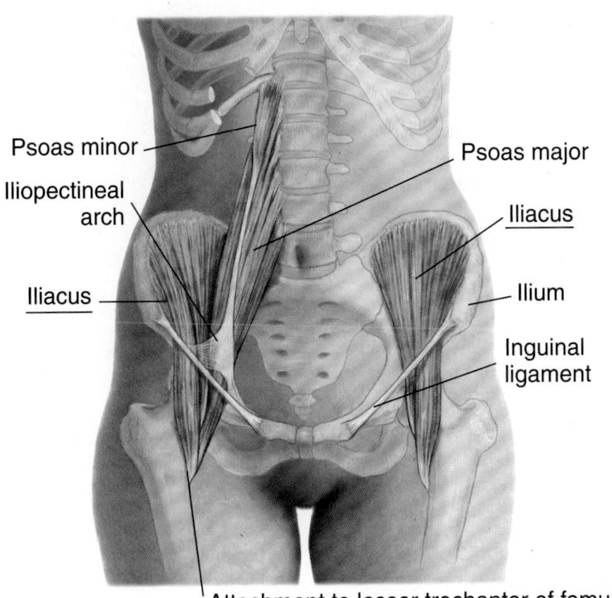

FIGURE 8-8 Anatomy of iliacus

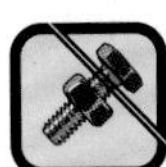

ATTACHMENTS

- Origin: iliac fossa on the interior side of the hip bone, and also from the region medial to the anterior inferior iliac spine (Fig. 8-8)
- Insertion: tendon of psoas, the anterior surface of lesser trochanter, and the capsule of the hip joint

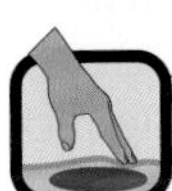

PALPATION

Can be discerned with the fingertips curled over the ilium. The architecture is convergent.

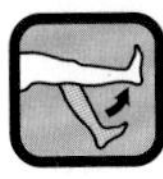

ACTION

Flexes, adducts and laterally rotates the hip along with the psoas major

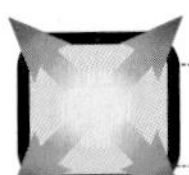

REFERRAL AREA

See psoas, above

OTHER MUSCLES TO EXAMINE

See psoas, above

MANUAL THERAPY

Stripping and Cross-fiber Stroking

- The client lies supine.

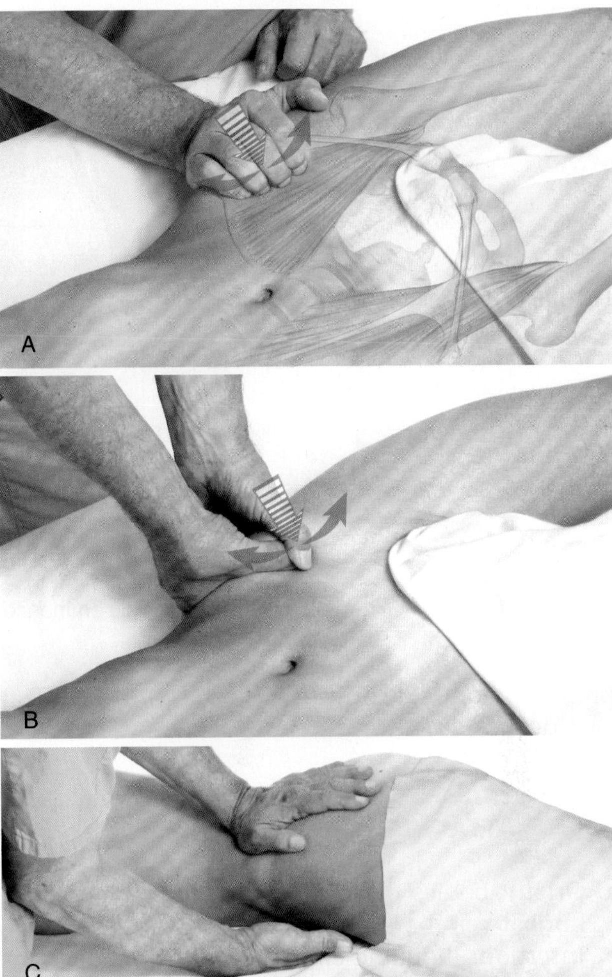

FIGURE 8-9 Stripping and cross-fiber stroking of iliacus with fingertips (A), supported thumb (B), and from underneath the client (C)

- The therapist stands beside the client at the hip.
- Place the fingertips just medial to the ilium.
- Pressing firmly into the tissue, move the fingertips back and forth and rotate the hand from side to side to slide the fingertips across the muscle (Fig. 8-9A).
- This procedure may also be carried out with the supported thumb (Fig. 8-9B), or with the client prone and the hand underneath the pelvis (Fig. 8-9C).

PSOAS MINOR

SO-az MY-ner

ETYMOLOGY Greek ***psoa***, the muscles of the loins + Latin ***minor***, smaller

Overview

Psoas minor (Fig. 8-10) is absent in approximately 50% of the population, and in some people may be

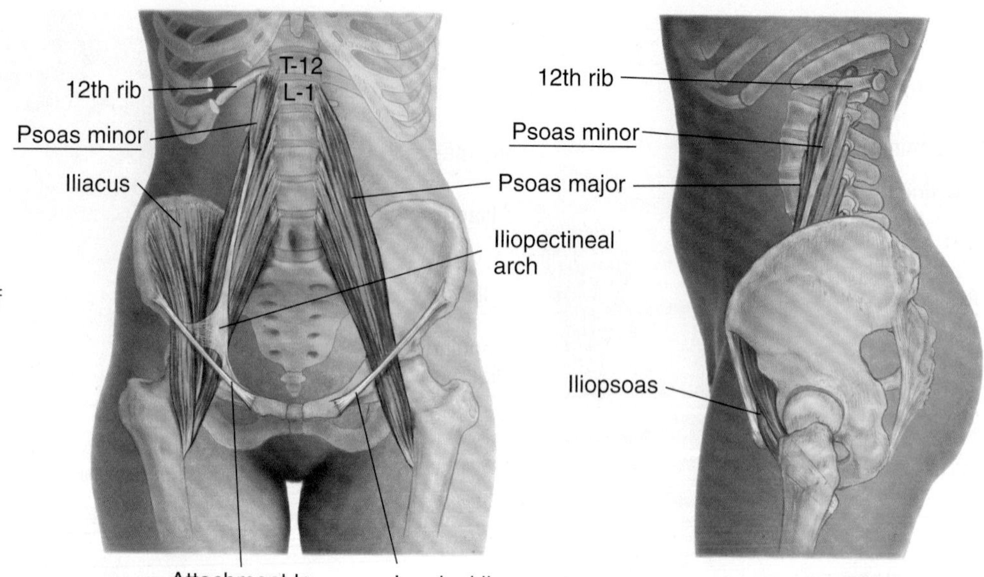

FIGURE 8-10 Anatomy of psoas minor

present on one side only. It has no recorded clinical significance.

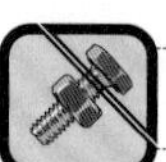

ATTACHMENTS

- Origin: bodies of the twelfth thoracic and first lumbar vertebrae and the disk between them
- Insertion: iliopubic eminence via the iliopectineal arch (iliac fascia)

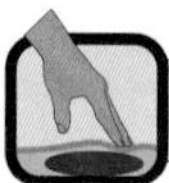

PALPATION

Not palpable

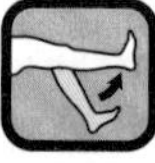

ACTION

Assists in flexion of the lumbar spine

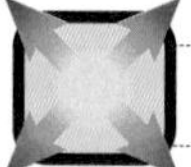

REFERRAL AREA

Not applicable

OTHER MUSCLES TO EXAMINE

Not applicable

MANUAL THERAPY

Not applicable

Overview of the Muscles of the Pelvic Floor

The pelvic floor might more usefully be called the pelvic hammock, both for psychological reasons (a hammock sounds softer than a floor) and descriptive reasons. These muscles form a supportive hammock for the pelvic organs, secured to the coccyx behind, the pubis in front, the ischial tuberosities on either side, as well as to various connective tissue structures in between.

The muscle group has openings to admit the rectum, the vagina, and the urethra, and parts of it serve as sphincters for these passages. It is common for people to hold tension in the pelvic floor muscles along with the buttock muscles, and this tension can affect the pelvic organs and cause discomfort in such activities as bowel movements and sexual intercourse.

Some examination and treatment of these muscles can be carried out externally, working between the buttocks and on the perineum, but a thorough and effective treatment will often require internal work through the rectum. Internal examination and treatment of the pelvic floor muscles is an advanced, specialized technique that is beyond the scope of this book. Very few states in the USA allow massage therapists to perform internal work.

For external work between the buttocks or on the perineum, the client may lie prone, preferably with a pillow or bolster under the hips.

ETHICAL CAUTION

The practice act in some states may prohibit work on pelvic floor muscles, as they may be considered part of the genitals; in some states it is considered the domain of physical therapists, not massage therapists. When pelvic floor work *is* allowed to massage therapists, there should be specific written informed consent and a thorough discussion prior to performing any work in that area on the client. Unfortunately, there are also some clients who will claim having injured their groin or perineum in an attempt to get massage therapists to perform massage that is sexual in nature. Some therapists choose to protect themselves by requiring a doctor's prescription or medical records demonstrating an injury before performing pelvic floor work. Some may also require that a third party be present in the treatment room.

COCCYGEUS

cock-SIDGE-us

ETYMOLOGY Latin, relating to the ***coccyx***, from Greek ***kokkyx***, cuckoo, coccyx

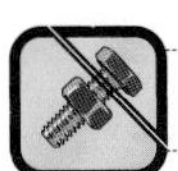

ATTACHMENTS

- Origin: spine of the ischium and the sacrospinous ligament (Fig. 8-11)
- Insertion: sides of the lower part of the sacrum and the upper part of the coccyx

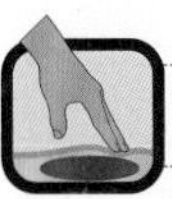

PALPATION

The superior attachments can be palpated externally on either side of the coccyx. Although outside the scope of practice of massage therapists in most states, the muscle can be palpated internally with the index finger from the coccyx moving inferiorly. Its architecture is convergent.

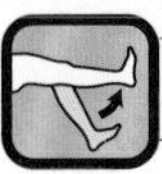

ACTION

Assists in the support of the pelvic floor, especially when intra-abdominal pressures increase; if the human coccyx was mobile it could produce wagging of the "tail" (lateral flexion of coccyx).

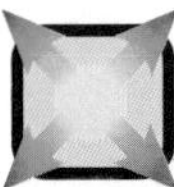

REFERRAL AREA

To the lower sacrum, the coccyx, and the surrounding area (medial aspect of the buttocks)

OTHER MUSCLES TO EXAMINE

- Gluteus maximus
- Obturator internus
- Quadratus lumborum

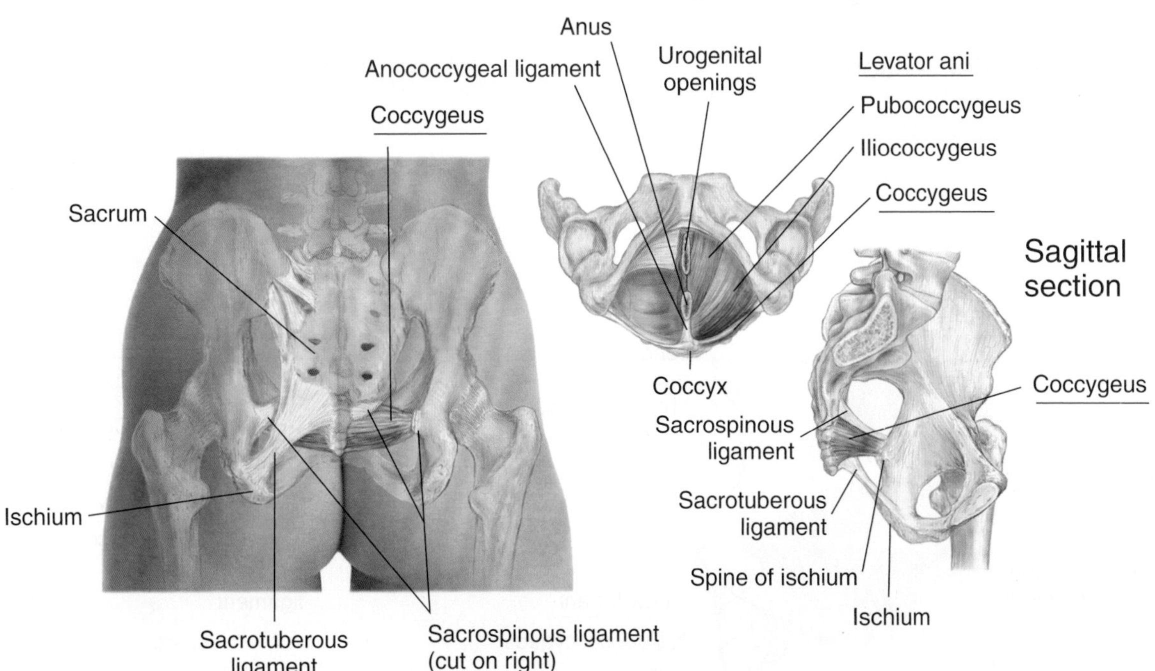

FIGURE 8-11 Anatomy of coccygeus

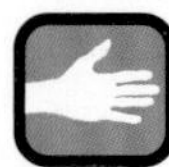

MANUAL THERAPY

See Manual Therapy for the Pelvic Floor Muscles and Obturator Internus, below.

LEVATOR ANI

le-VAY-ter AYN-eye

ETYMOLOGY Latin *levator*, raiser + *ani*, of the anus

Overview

Levator ani comprises the pubococcygeus, iliococcygeus, and puborectalis muscles, forming the pelvic diaphragm (Fig. 8-12).

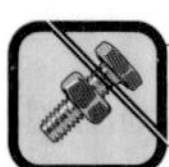

ATTACHMENTS

- Origin: posterior body of the pubis, the tendinous arch of the obturator fascia, and the spine of the ischium
- Insertion: anococcygeal ligament, the sides of the lower part of the sacrum and of the coccyx

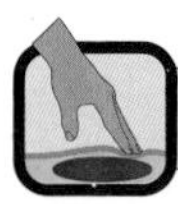

PALPATION

Can only be palpated internally—outside the scope of practice of massage therapists in most states

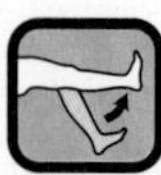

ACTION

Resists prolapsing forces and draws the anus upward following defecation; helps support the pelvic viscera.

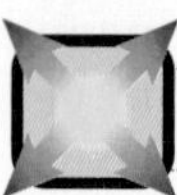

REFERRAL AREA

To the lower sacrum, the coccyx, and the surrounding area (medial aspect of the buttocks)

OTHER MUSCLES TO EXAMINE

- Gluteus maximus
- Obturator internus
- Quadratus lumborum

MANUAL THERAPY

Levator ani cannot be externally treated effectively.

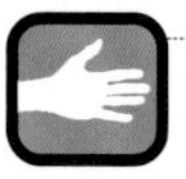

MANUAL THERAPY FOR THE PELVIC FLOOR MUSCLES AND OBTURATOR INTERNUS

Compression

- The client lies prone. A pillow may be placed under the client's pelvis.
- The therapist stands beside the client at the hip.

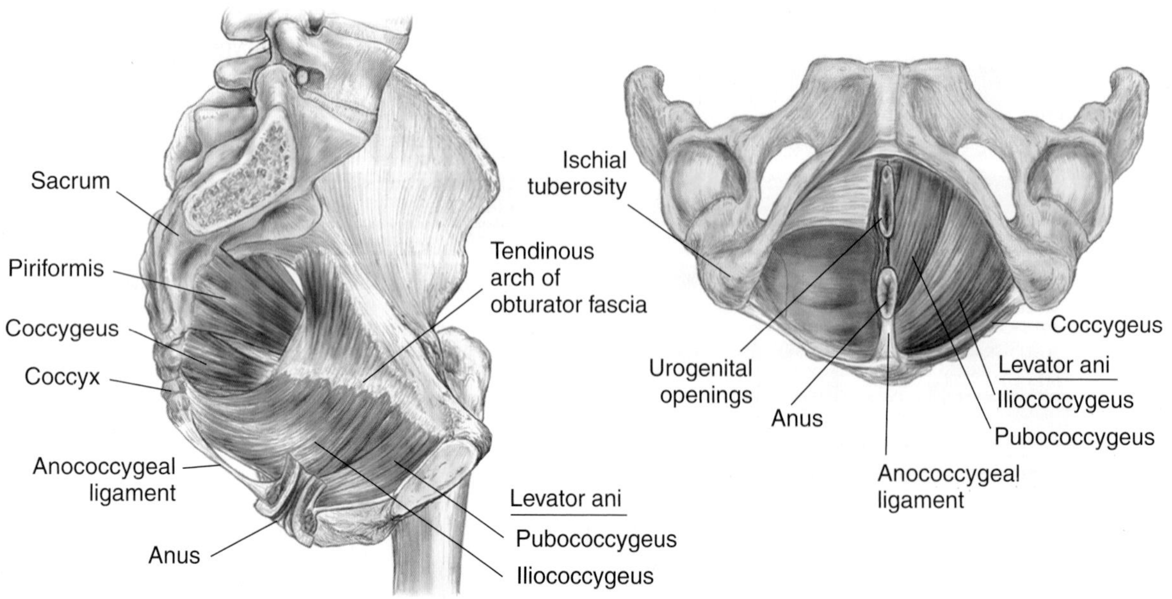

FIGURE 8-12 Anatomy of levator ani

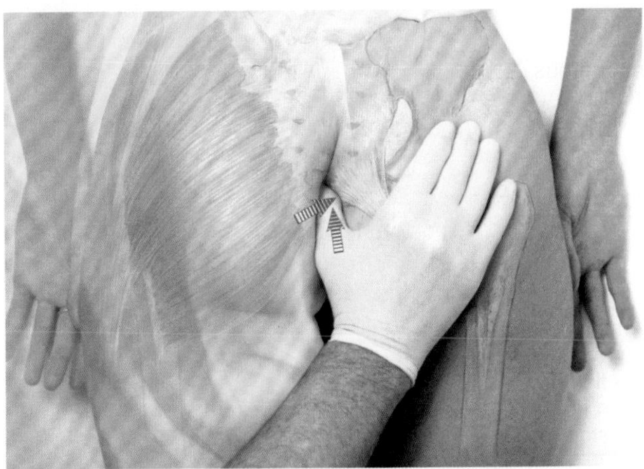

FIGURE 8-13 External examination under the coccyx

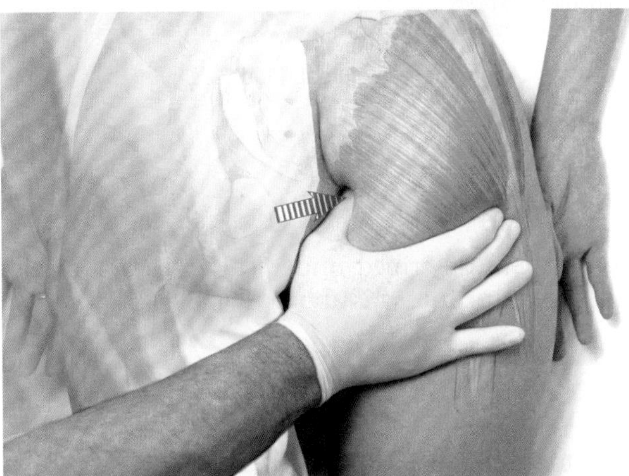

FIGURE 8-14 External examination and treatment between the buttocks

- Place the palm of the gloved hand nearest the client on the opposite buttock, inserting the thumb between the buttocks to rest on the inferior end of the coccyx externally. Avoid touching the anal sphincter.
- Press firmly under the coccyx (Fig. 8-13), then into the tissue on either side of the coccyx, looking for tender spots. Hold for release.
- Repeat this procedure, shifting the thumb in an inferior direction, exploring the pelvic floor muscles and the inner aspect of gluteus maximus (Fig. 8-14).
- At the level of the obturator foramen, press into the foramen to explore obturator internus, holding for release as necessary (Fig. 8-15).

Overview of the Gluteal Muscles

Since gluteus maximus and fascia associated with the iliotibial band cover gluteus medius and much of gluteus minimus, much of the work on the buttock applies to all three muscles, especially over the lateral aspect. The only distinction lies in the intention and depth of the work. Therapy of the gluteal muscles will be found after descriptions of all the individual muscles.

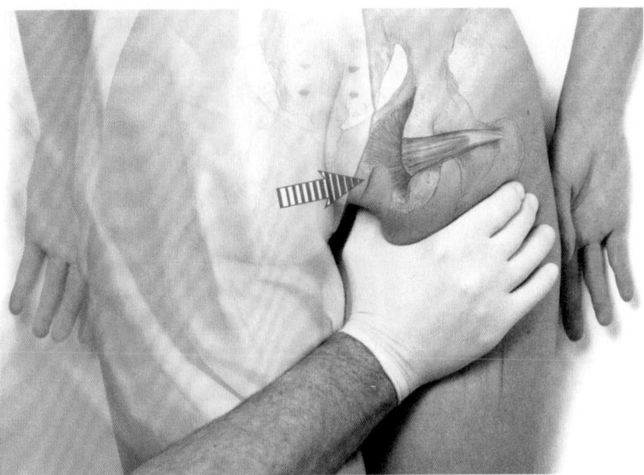

FIGURE 8-15 Compression of obturator internus

ETHICAL CAUTION

Gluteal muscles, though not genitalia, are close enough in proximity that caution should be used and utmost care to safeguarding the comfort and modesty of the client. Discuss the involvement of the gluteals in the client's pain before touching the area. Use proper draping techniques. Check the practice act in your state; some allow for temporary removal of the drape in order to apply treatment, while others may expect that treatment is applied through the drape. Even if removal is allowed, maintain the client's modesty by exposing only one side at a time.

GLUTEUS MAXIMUS

GLUE-tee-us MAX-im-us

ETYMOLOGY Latin ***gluteus***, buttock muscle + ***maximus***, largest

Overview

Gluteus maximus (Fig. 8-16) is the most powerful hip extensor for actions such as climbing. Its size, power, and role in upright posture and locomotion distinguish humans from our ape relatives. It is an antagonist to iliopsoas and very commonly involved in low back pain.

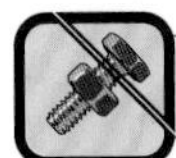

ATTACHMENTS

- Origin: ilium behind the posterior gluteal line, to the posterior surface of the sacrum and coccyx, and to the sacrotuberous ligament
- Insertion: iliotibial band of the fascia lata (superficial three-quarters of the muscle) and to the gluteal tuberosity of the femur (posterolateral proximal one-quarter)

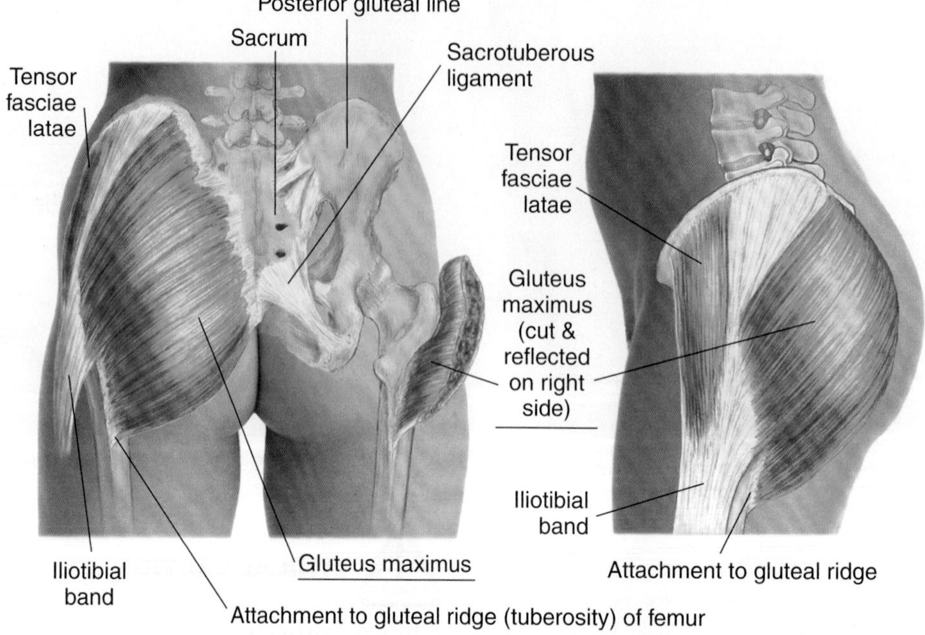

FIGURE 8-16 Anatomy of gluteus maximus

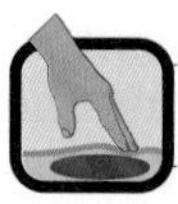

PALPATION

Discernible over most of the buttock, moving downward diagonally to the iliotibial band. Medial edge is discernible between the buttocks. Architecture is convergent, and fibers are primarily diagonal.

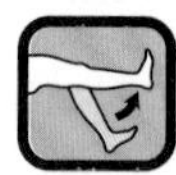

ACTION

Externally rotates and extends the hip, especially from a flexed position, as in climbing stairs or rising from a sitting position

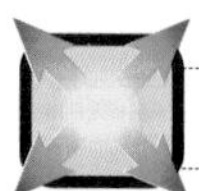

REFERRAL AREA

To the entire buttock and into the upper posterior thigh

OTHER MUSCLES TO EXAMINE

- Other gluteal muscles
- Deep lateral rotators of the hip
- Quadratus lumborum
- Pelvic floor muscle

MANUAL THERAPY

See Manual Therapy for the Gluteal Muscles, below. Note: For working the medial aspect of gluteus maximus, use the technique for external work between the buttocks described under Pelvic Floor Muscles and Obturator Internus above (Fig. 8-14).

GLUTEUS MEDIUS

GLUE-tee-us ME-dee-us

ETYMOLOGY Latin ***gluteus***, buttock muscle + ***medius***, middle

Overview

Gluteus medius (Fig. 8-17), with gluteus minimus, is a powerful abductor of the hip and an important lateral stabilizer while walking, running or any time the body weight is supported on one leg. It is very commonly involved in low back pain.

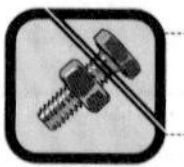

ATTACHMENTS

- Origin: ilium between the anterior and posterior gluteal lines
- Insertion: lateral surface of the greater trochanter

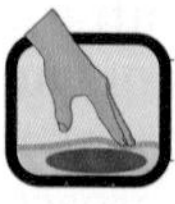

PALPATION

Discernible only on the lateral and superior aspect of the buttock. Architecture is convergent, and fibers are diagonal.

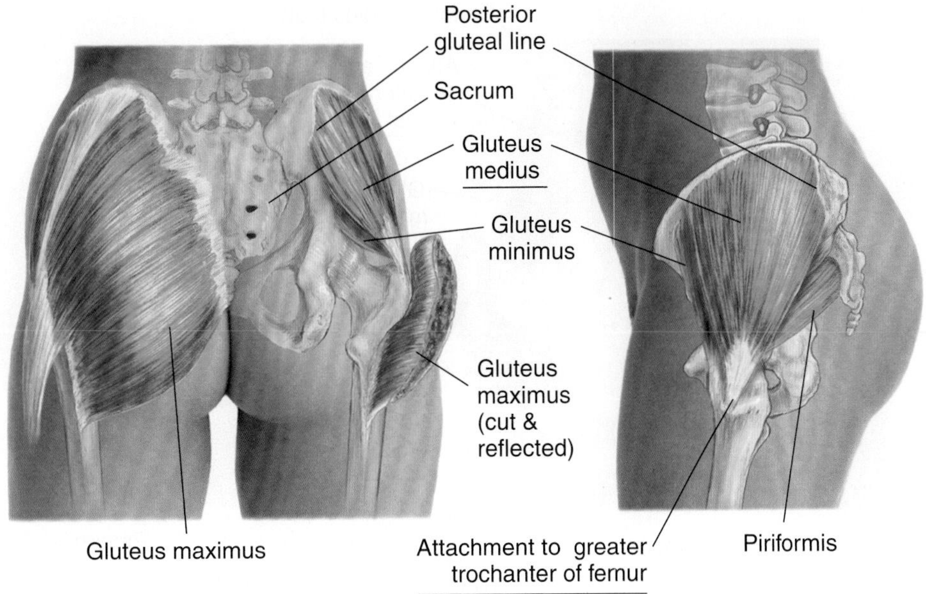

FIGURE 8-17 Anatomy of gluteus medius

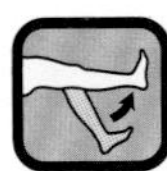

ACTION

Abducts and contributes to flexion, extension, lateral and medial rotation of the hip joint.

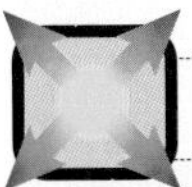

REFERRAL AREAS

- Over the buttock
- Over the sacrum
- Into the medial lumbar region
- Into the upper posterior thigh

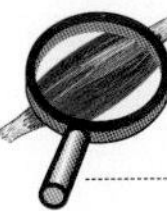

OTHER MUSCLES TO EXAMINE

- Quadratus lumborum
- Lumbar erector spinae muscles
- Other gluteal muscles
- Deep lateral rotators of the hip
- Pelvic floor muscles

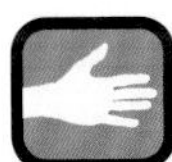

MANUAL THERAPY

See Manual Therapy for the Gluteal Muscles, below.

GLUTEUS MINIMUS

GLUE-tee-us MIN-im-us

ETYMOLOGY Latin ***gluteus***, buttock muscle + ***minimus***, smallest

Overview

Gluteus minimus (Fig. 8-18), with gluteus medius, is a powerful abductor of the hip. It has a pain referral pattern that may mimic sciatica, but is differentiated in that actual sciatica may also include numbness, tingling, and weakness. Gluteus minimus is commonly involved in most hip and leg pain, which sometimes radiates down the lateral leg and other times down the posterior leg.

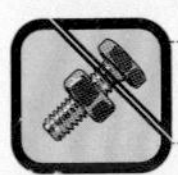

ATTACHMENTS

- Origin: ilium between the anterior and inferior gluteal lines
- Insertion: greater trochanter of the femur

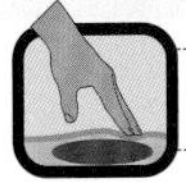

PALPATION

Discernible on the lateral aspect of the buttock between gluteus medius and tensor fasciae latae. Architecture is convergent.

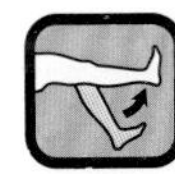

ACTION

Abducts, flexes and medially rotates the hip

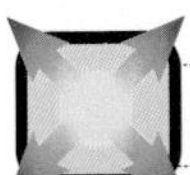

REFERRAL AREAS

- Over the buttock and lateral hip
- Over the posterior thigh
- Over the posterior calf
- Over the lateral thigh
- Over the lateral calf to the ankle

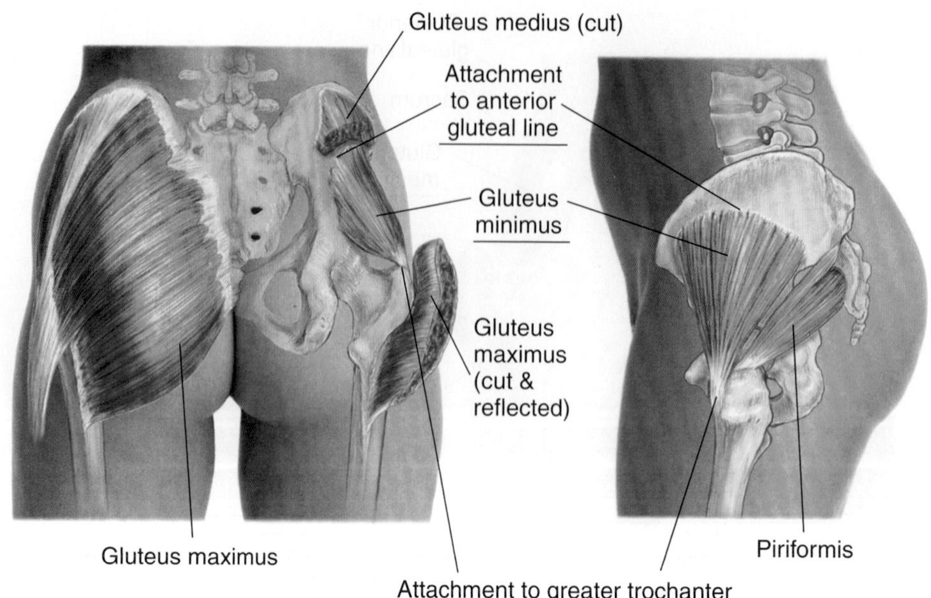

FIGURE 8-18 Anatomy of gluteus minimus

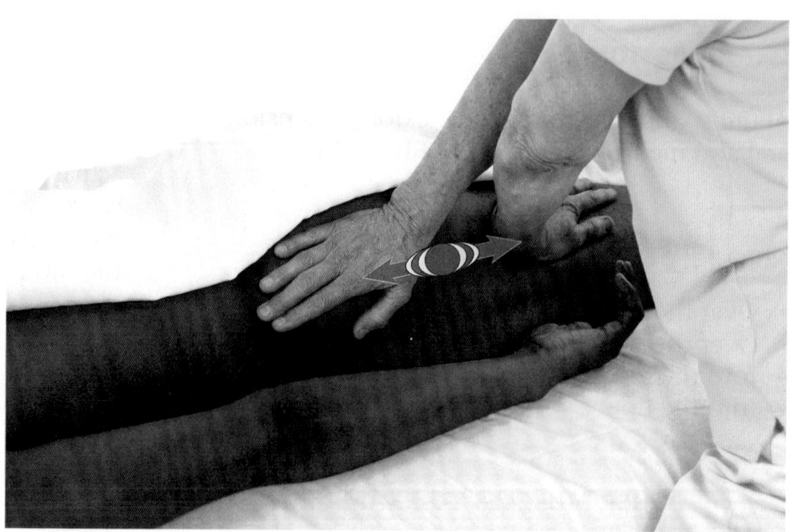

FIGURE 8-19 Myofascial release on gluteal region

OTHER MUSCLES TO EXAMINE

- Other gluteal muscles
- Deep lateral rotators of the hip
- Tensor fascia latae
- Iliotibial band
- Vastus lateralis
- Hamstrings
- Calf muscles

MANUAL THERAPY FOR THE GLUTEAL MUSCLES

Myofascial Stretch

- The client lies prone.
- The therapist stands beside the client at the waist, facing the client.
- Place the palm of your cephalad hand on the upper aspect of the client's near buttock, the fingers pointing inferiorly.
- Cross the caudad hand over, placing it on the client's waist at the iliac crest.
- Lean into the hands to push them apart, pressing firmly into the tissue (Fig. 8-19).
- Hold this stretch until you feel the underlying tissue release.

Stripping

- The client lies prone.
- The therapist stands beside the client at the level of the chest.
- Place the palm of the hand on the buttock just above the iliac crest and lateral to the sacrum, the thumb pointing inferiorly (Fig. 8-20A).

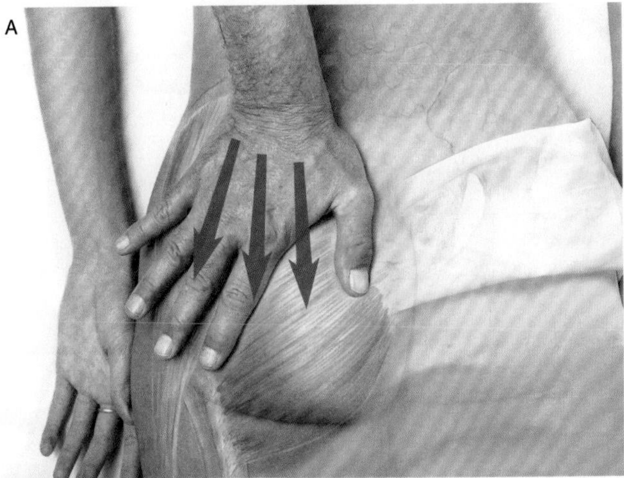

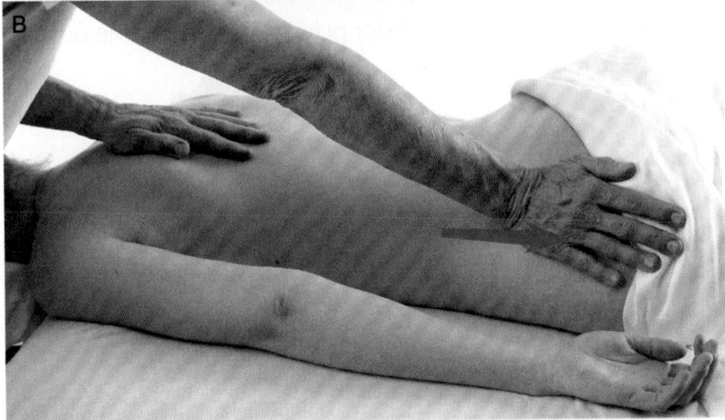

FIGURE 8-20 Stripping of gluteal muscles with the heel of the hand: (A) beginning stroke; (B) ending stroke

- Pressing firmly into the tissue with the heel of the hand, slide the hand along the muscle to its most inferior aspect.
- Beginning just lateral to the previous spot, repeat this procedure until the entire buttock has been covered, including the attachment of gluteus maximus to the iliotibial band, and gluteus minimus along the side of the hip (Fig. 8-20B).
- The same procedure may be carried out with the knuckles (Fig. 8-21), the fingertips (Fig. 8-22), or the supported thumb (Fig. 8-23).

Stripping

- The client lies on her/his side, with the lower leg straight and the upper leg flexed at the hip and knee.
- The therapist stands beside the client at the waist.
- Place the supported thumb on the superior lateral aspect of the buttock at the iliac crest.
- Pressing firmly into the tissue, slide the thumbs inferiorly along the muscle to its attachments on the greater trochanter (Fig. 8-24).

Compressifon

- The client lies prone.
- The therapist stands beside the client at the client's waist.
- Place the supported thumb on the lateral aspect of the buttock just inferior to the iliac crest.

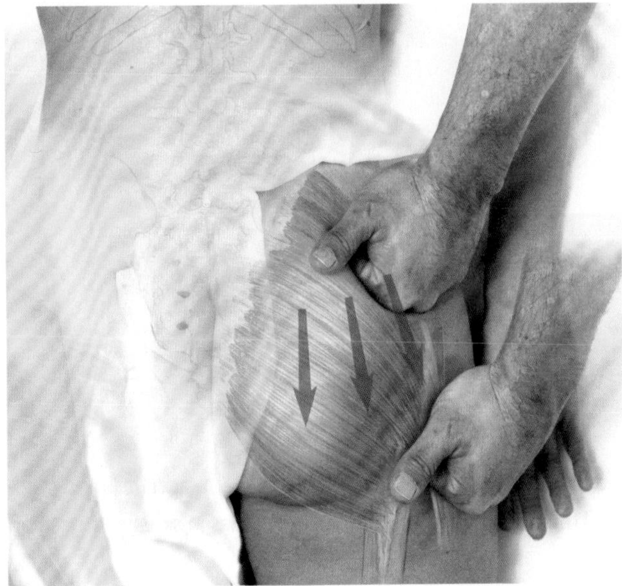

FIGURE 8-21 Stripping of gluteal muscles with the knuckles

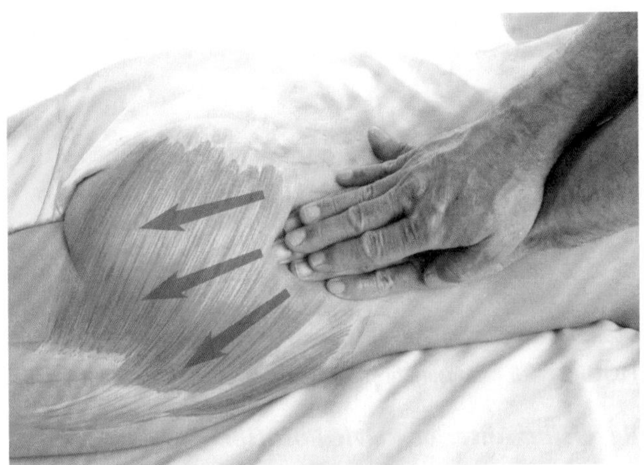

FIGURE 8-22 Stripping of gluteal muscles with the fingertips

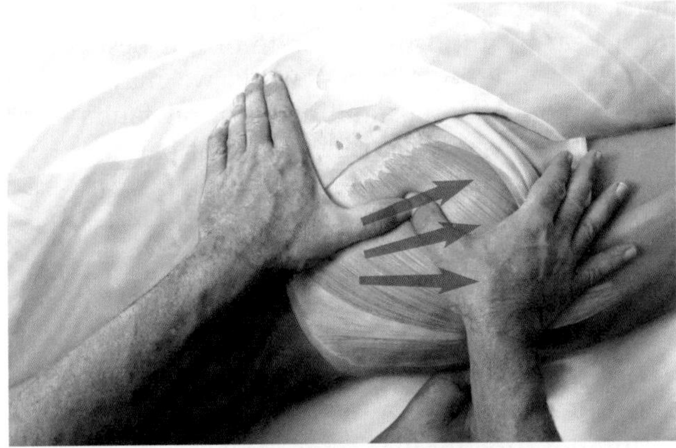

FIGURE 8-23 Stripping of gluteal muscles with the thumb

- Press firmly into the tissue, moving your thumb back and forth, to search for tender areas. Hold for release (Fig. 8-25).
- Explore the gluteal muscles in this way over the entire buttock.

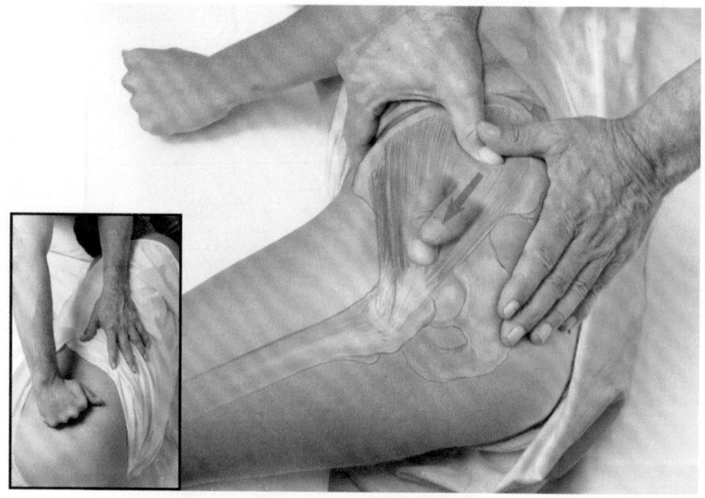

FIGURE 8-24 Stripping of gluteal muscles in side-lying position

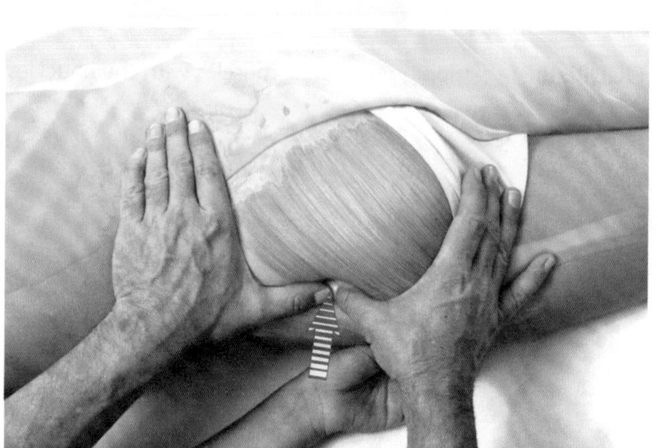

FIGURE 8-25 Examination and compression of gluteal muscles

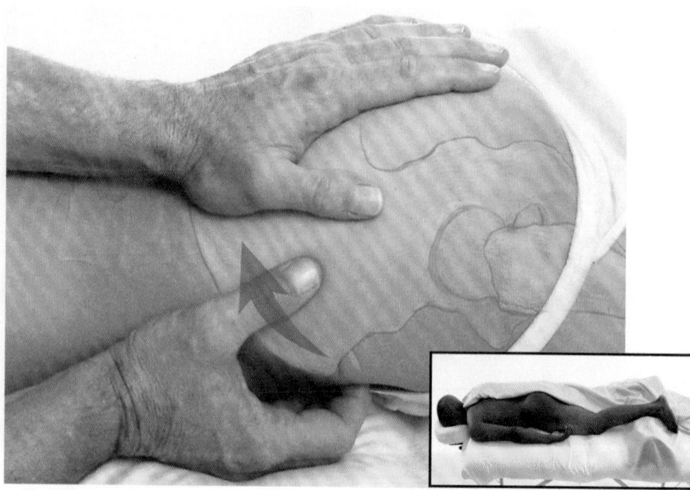

FIGURE 8-26 Reversing anterior pelvic rotation in prone position

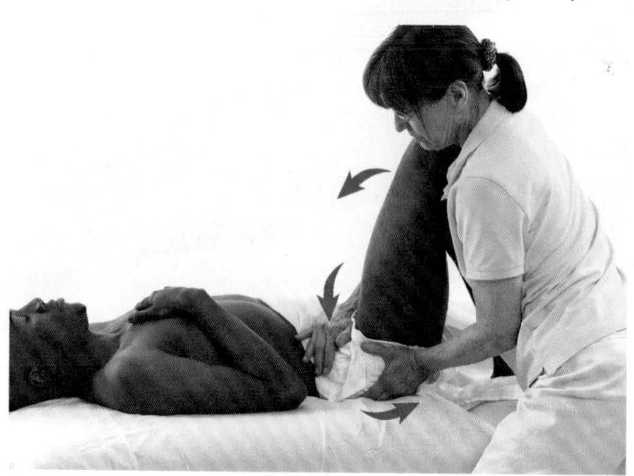

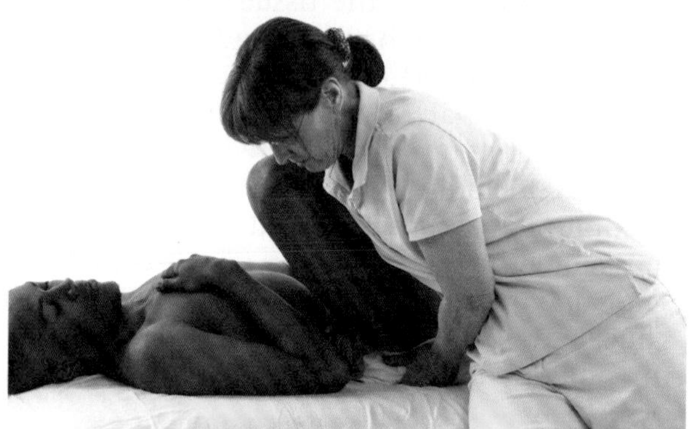

FIGURE 8-27 Reversing anterior pelvic rotation in supine position

Reversing Anterior Pelvic Rotation

These procedures should be performed after working all the muscles affecting anterior pelvic rotation (quadratus lumborum, gluteal muscles, latissimus dorsi, iliopsoas, rectus femoris, hip adductors). We must bear in mind that in spite of our best intentions and offering our best work, we may not be able to correct long-standing postural faults—nor are they necessarily causing the client pain.

Prone Position

- The client lies prone.
- The therapist stands beside the client at the client's waist.
- Place one hand on the buttock at the iliac crest, the fingers pointing inferiorly. Place the other hand under the ilium with the fingertips on the anterior superior iliac spine (ASIS).
- Simultaneously pull the ASIS in a superior direction while pushing the iliac crest in an inferior direction (Fig. 8-26).

Supine Position

- The client lies supine, with the leg flexed at the hip and the knee.
- The therapist stands beside the client's leg, facing the head.
- Wrapping the arm nearest the client around the client's leg, place your shoulder firmly just below the knee and the heel of your hand on the ASIS.
- Place your far hand underneath the client's buttock, with the fingertips resting on the iliac crest.
- Ask the client to resist you with 20% of her/his strength as you simultaneously press the leg to the client's chest, push superiorly against the ASIS, and pull inferiorly on the buttock and iliac crest (Fig. 8-27).

DEEP LATERAL ROTATORS OF THE HIP

PIRIFORMIS

PEER-re-FORM-is

ETYMOLOGY Latin ***pirum***, pear + ***forma***, form

Overview

Piriformis (Fig. 8-28) is a primary lateral rotator of the hip, as well as a principal stabilizer of the hip joint along with the gluteus medius. It has profound clinical significance.

The sciatic nerve may pass under, over, or even through (or partially through) piriformis, depending on the individual. Therefore, a taut piriformis may cause pain not only through its own referral patterns, but also by entrapment of the sciatic nerve. This entrapment is called *piriformis syndrome*. Piriformis problems are common in ballet dancers because of the constant demand for "turnout" (lateral rotation of the hip) in ballet. It is also very common in general because of its role in stabilizing the hip and may be particularly painful for people who sit all day, such as office personnel and truck drivers.

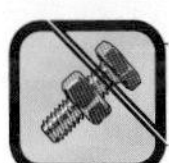

ATTACHMENTS

- Origin: margins of the anterior pelvic sacral foramina, the greater sciatic notch of the ilium, the sacroiliac joint capsule, and the sacrotuberous ligament
- Insertion: upper border of greater trochanter

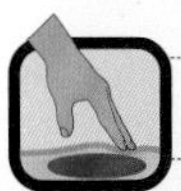

PALPATION

Palpable only if pathologically hypercontracted, through gluteus maximus on a line between the lower sacrum and the greater trochanter. Superior attachment is discernible intra-anally underneath the lower sacrum, outside the scope of practice of most massage therapists. Architecture is convergent.

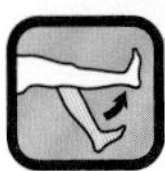

ACTION

Extends, abducts and rotates hip laterally; stabilizes hip joint

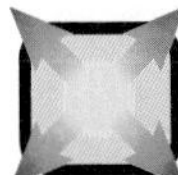

REFERRAL AREAS

- Over the buttock (especially the lateral border of the sacrum and the inferolateral aspect of the buttock)
- Into the posterior thigh
- By entrapment of the sciatic nerve, over the entire posterior leg to the foot, and into the low back, hip, groin, perineum, and rectum

OTHER MUSCLES TO EXAMINE

- Gluteal muscles
- Other deep lateral rotators of the hip
- Quadratus lumborum

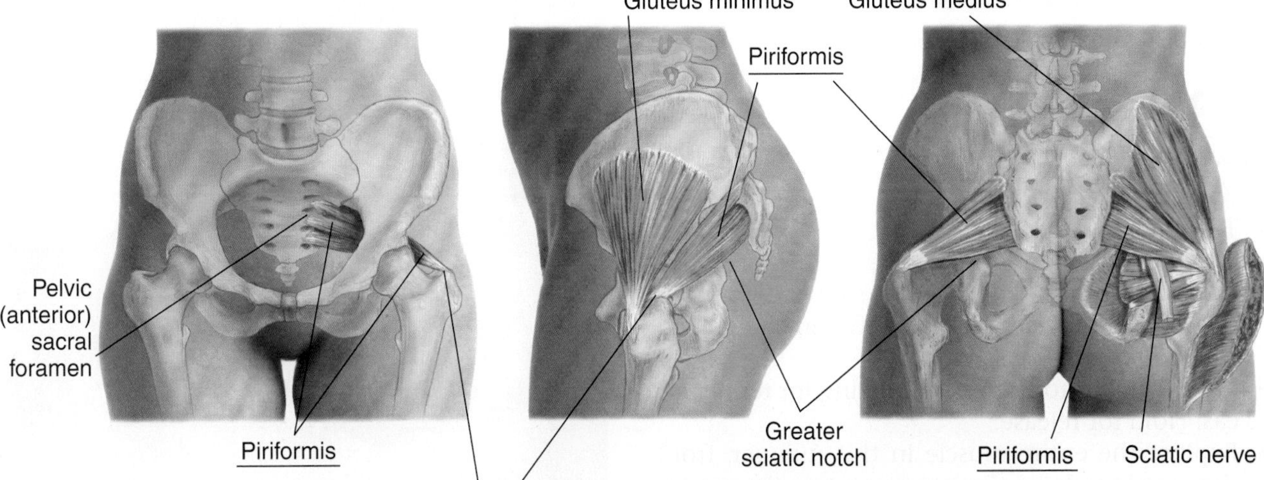

FIGURE 8-28 Anatomy of piriformis

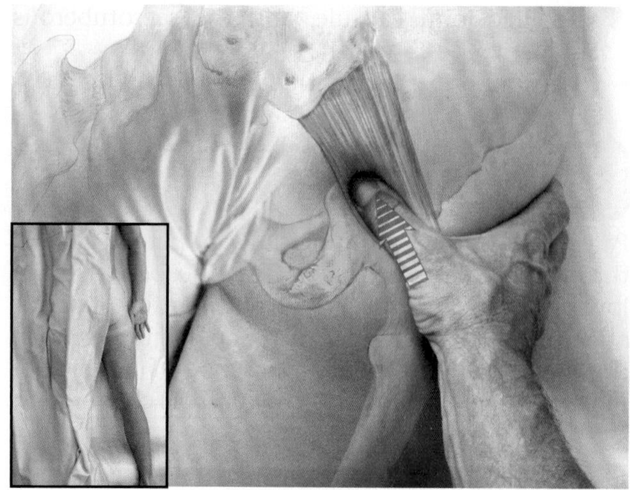

FIGURE 8-29 Compression of piriformis with thumb

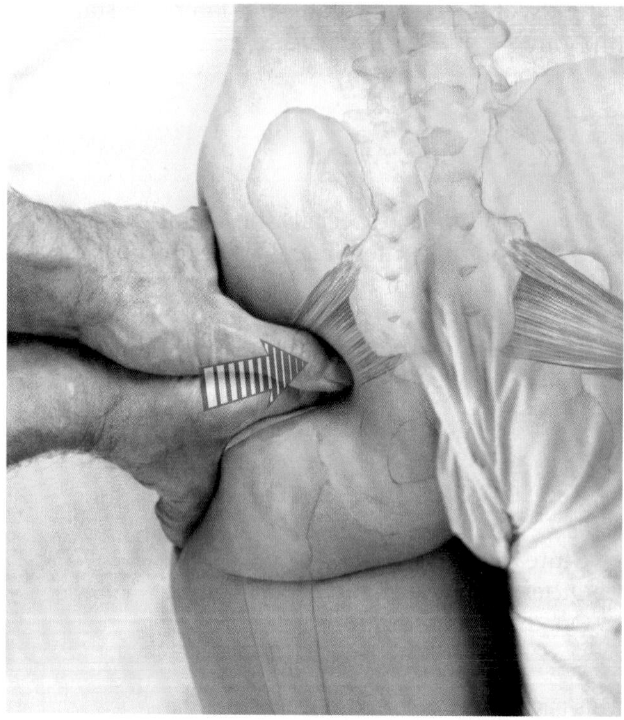

FIGURE 8-30 Compression of piriformis with supported thumb

MANUAL THERAPY

Compression

- The client lies prone.
- The therapist stands beside the client's hip.
- Place the thumb (Fig. 8-29) or supported thumb (Fig. 8-30) on the midpoint between the greater trochanter and the sacrum.
- Press firmly into the tissue, looking for tender areas. Hold for release.
- Explore the entire muscle in this manner, from the sacral border to the attachment on the greater trochanter (Fig. 8-31).

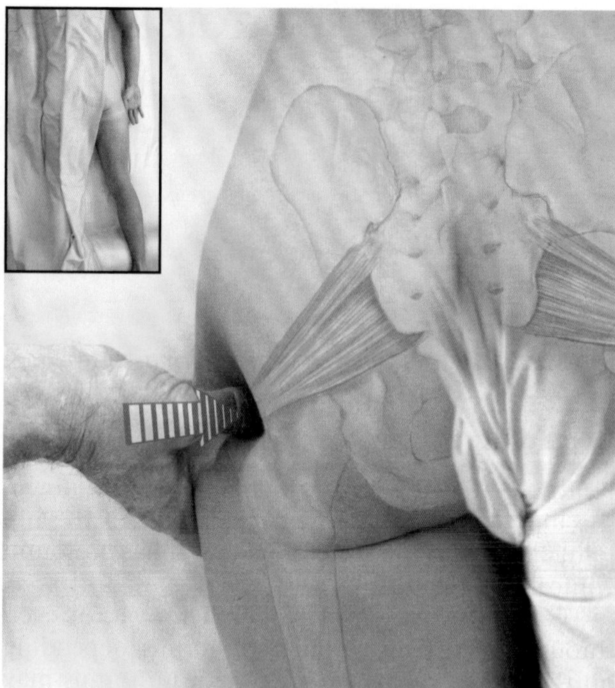

FIGURE 8-31 Compression of piriformis attachment at greater trochanter

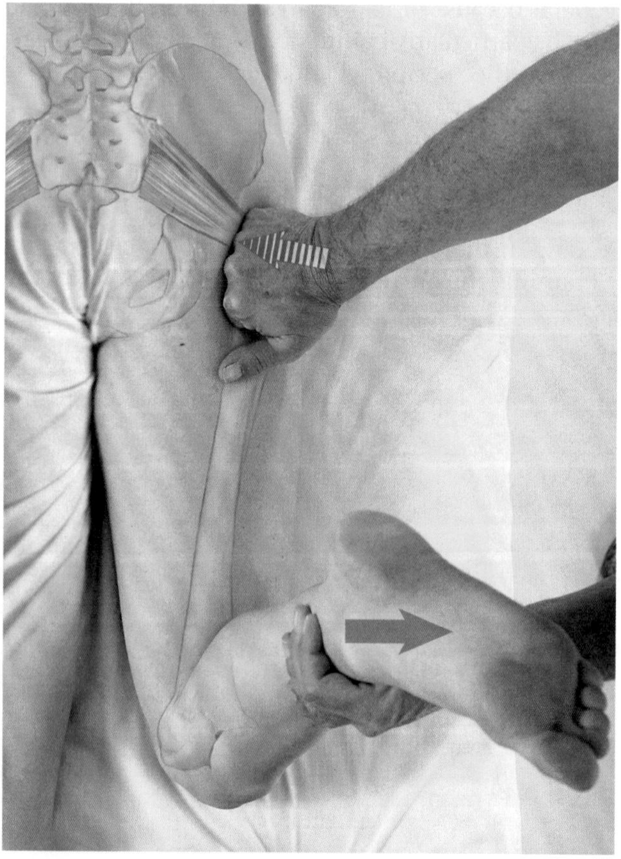

FIGURE 8-32 Passive stretch of piriformis

Compression with Stretch

- The client lies prone.
- The therapist stands at the client's hip.
- Place the knuckles of one hand on the buttock just medial to the greater trochanter, pressing firmly in a medial and anterior direction.
- With the other hand, grasp the client's ankle and flex the knee to 90°.
- Still holding the knuckles firmly against piriformis, pull the client's foot toward yourself, rotating the hip medially (Fig. 8-32).

SUPERIOR GEMELLUS

sue-PEER-ee-or je-MELL-us

ETYMOLOGY Latin ***superior***, higher + ***gemellus***, diminutive of geminus, twin

Overview

Superior gemellus (Fig. 8-33) has no clinical significance separate from piriformis.

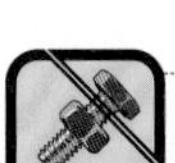

ATTACHMENTS

- Origin: ischial spine and margin of the lesser sciatic notch
- Insertion: medial surface of the greater trochanter via the tendon of obturator internus

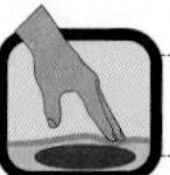

PALPATION

Not palpable

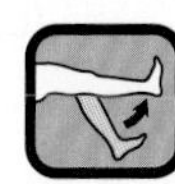

ACTION

Rotates hip laterally; assists extension and abduction; stabilizes the hip joint

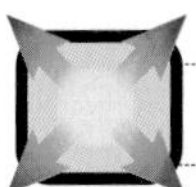

REFERRAL AREA

Not applicable

OTHER MUSCLES TO EXAMINE

Not applicable

MANUAL THERAPY

Not applicable

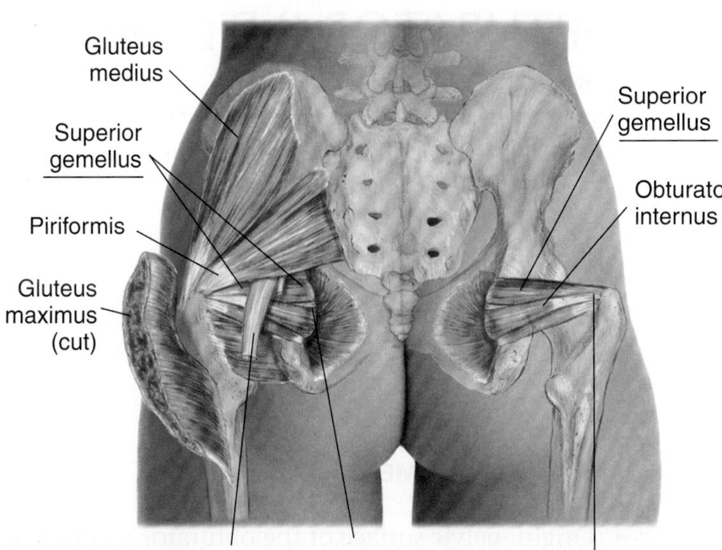

FIGURE 8-33 Anatomy of superior gemellus

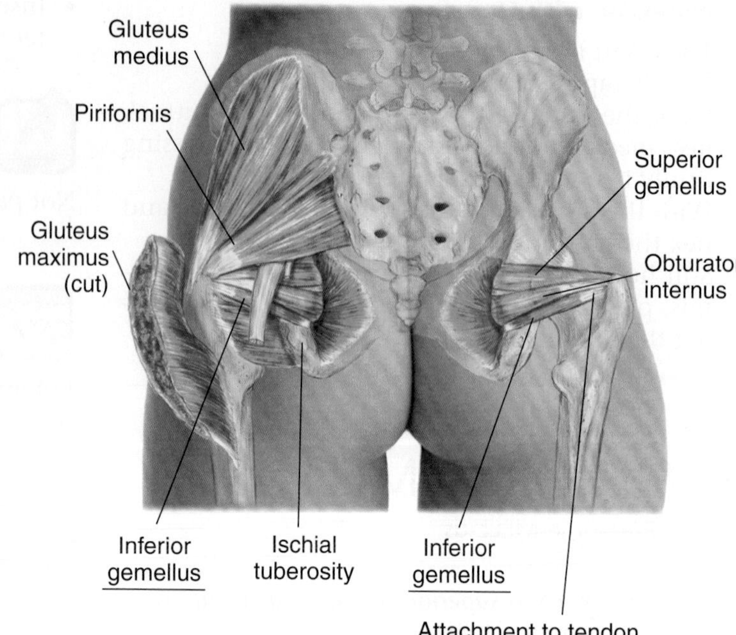

FIGURE 8-34 Anatomy of inferior gemellus

INFERIOR GEMELLUS

in-FEER-ee-or je-MELL-us

ETYMOLOGY Latin ***inferior***, lower + ***gemellus***, diminutive of geminus, twin

Overview

Inferior gemellus (Fig. 8-34) has no clinical significance separate from piriformis.

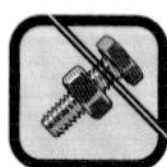

ATTACHMENTS

- Origin: medial ischial tuberosity
- Insertion: medial surface of the greater trochanter via the tendon of obturator internus

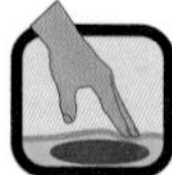

PALPATION

Not palpable

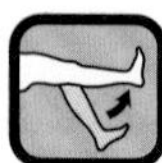

ACTION

Rotates hip laterally; assists extension and adduction

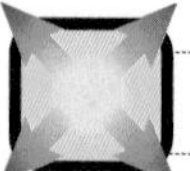

REFERRAL AREA

Not applicable

OTHER MUSCLES TO EXAMINE

Not applicable

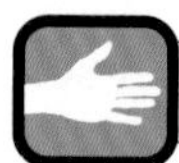

MANUAL THERAPY

Not applicable

OBTURATOR INTERNUS

AHB-tu-ray-ter in-TURN-us

ETYMOLOGY Latin ***obturator***, that which occludes or stops up + ***internus***, internal

Overview

Obturator internus (Fig. 8-35) has much the same referral pattern as levator ani and coccygeus, discussed above.

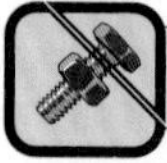

ATTACHMENTS

- Origin: pelvic surface of the obturator membrane and margin of obturator foramen
- Insertion: through the lesser sciatic notch, turning 90° to insert into the medial surface of the greater trochanter

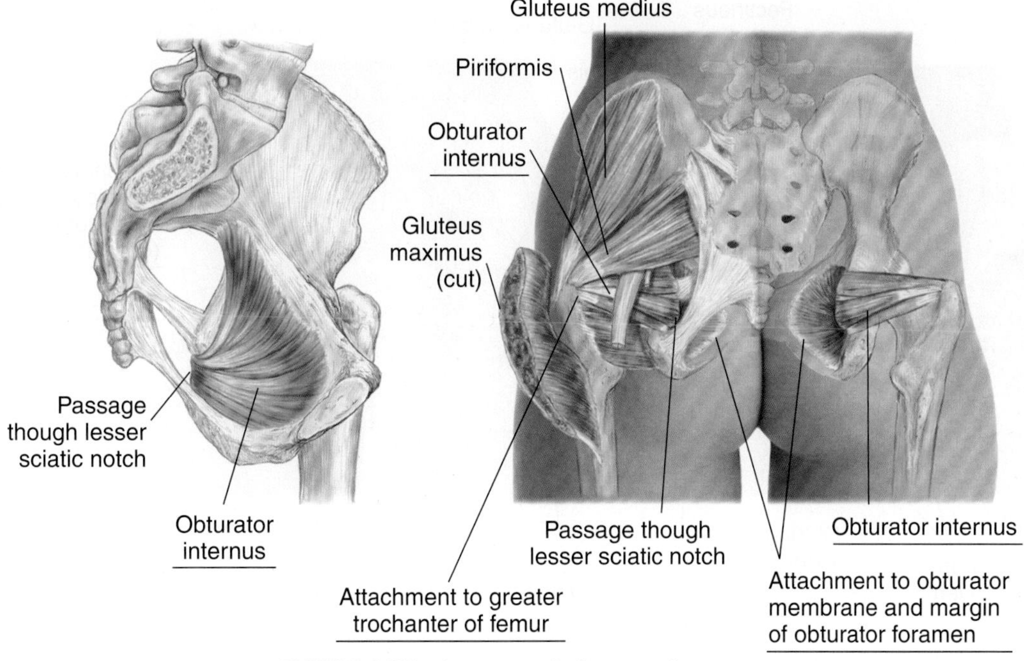

FIGURE 8-35 Anatomy of obturator internus

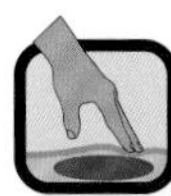

PALPATION

Discernible with the thumb between the buttocks pressing into the obturator foramen. Architecture is convergent as a whole.

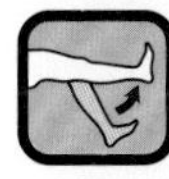

ACTION

Rotates hip laterally; assists extension and abduction; stabilizes the hip joint

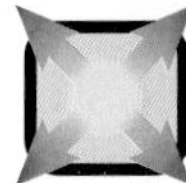

REFERRAL AREAS

- To the lower sacrum and coccyx
- Into the posterior upper thigh

OTHER MUSCLES TO EXAMINE

- Pelvic floor muscles
- Piriformis
- Gluteus maximus

MANUAL THERAPY

See Manual Therapy for the Pelvic Floor Muscles and Obturator Internus, above

OBTURATOR EXTERNUS

AHB-tu-ray-ter ex-TURN-us

ETYMOLOGY Latin ***obturator***, that which occludes or stops up + ***externus***, external

Overview

Obturator externus (Fig. 8-36) may, with quadratus femoris, cause tenderness just medial to the lower aspect of the greater trochanter. This muscle may be palpated deeply in the groin between pectineus and adductor brevis.

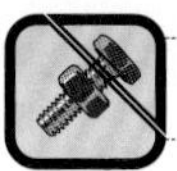

ATTACHMENTS

- Origin: lower half of margin of obturator foramen and adjacent part of external surface of obturator membrane
- Insertion: trochanteric fossa of greater trochanter

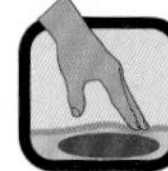

PALPATION

Not palpable

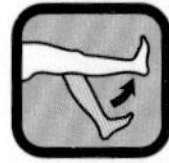

ACTION

Rotates thigh laterally; assists extension and adduction; stabilizes the hip joint

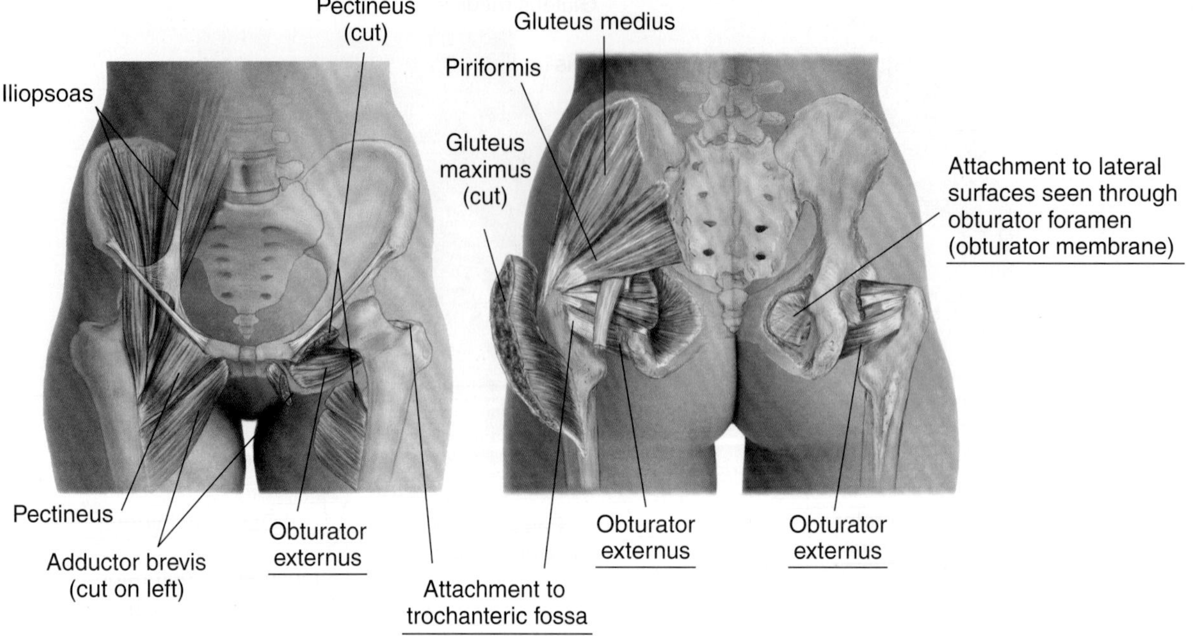

FIGURE 8-36 Anatomy of obturator externus

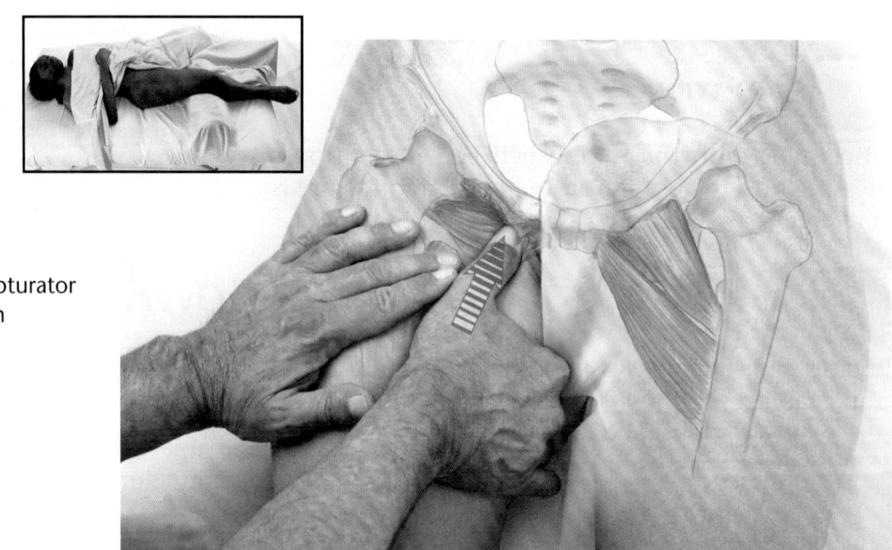

FIGURE 8-37 Compression of obturator externus through the groin

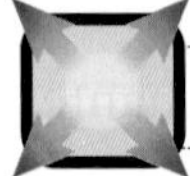

REFERRAL AREA

Just medial to the lower aspect of the greater trochanter

OTHER MUSCLES TO EXAMINE

- Quadratus femoris and other deep lateral rotators of the hip
- Pectineus
- Adductor brevis

MANUAL THERAPY

Compression

- The client lies supine.
- The therapist stands at the client's knee.
- Using the thumb, locate pectineus and adductor brevis.
- Press firmly and deeply into the tissue between pectineus and adductor brevis, exploring for tenderness (Fig. 8-37). Hold for release.

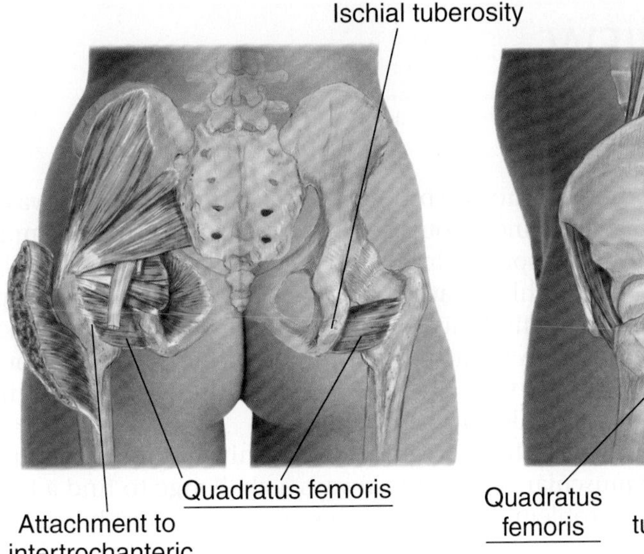

FIGURE 8-38 Anatomy of quadratus femoris

QUADRATUS FEMORIS

kwa-DRAY-tus FEM-or-is

ETYMOLOGY Latin ***quadratus***, four-sided + ***femoris***, of the femur (thigh bone)

Overview

Quadratus femoris (Fig. 8-38) may, with obturator externus, cause tenderness just medial to the lower aspect of the greater trochanter.

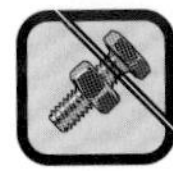

ATTACHMENTS

- Origin: lateral border of tuberosity of ischium
- Insertion: intertrochanteric crest of femur

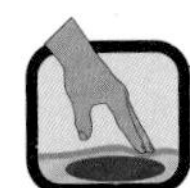

PALPATION

Palpable just posterior and medial to the greater trochanter. Architecture is parallel.

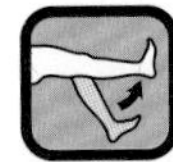

ACTION

Rotates hip laterally; assists extension and adduction

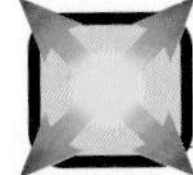

REFERRAL AREA

With obturator externus, just medial to the lower aspect of the greater trochanter

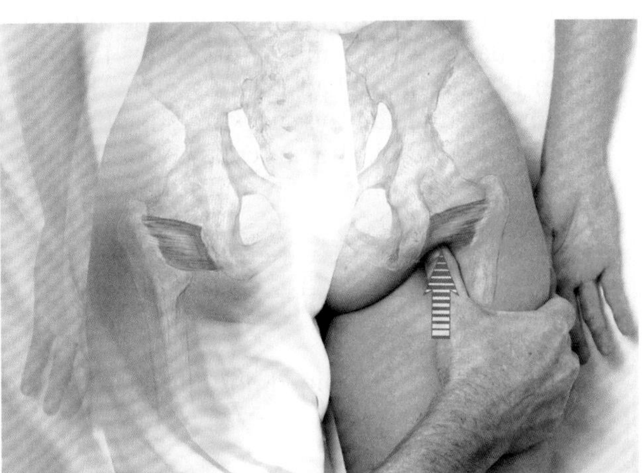

FIGURE 8-39 Compression of quadratus femoris

OTHER MUSCLES TO EXAMINE

- Obturator externus
- Other deep lateral rotators of the hip

MANUAL THERAPY

Compression

- The client lies prone.
- The therapist stands at the client's knee.
- Place the thumb at the crease of the buttock between the ischial tuberosity and the greater trochanter.
- Press firmly in a superior direction, exploring for tender areas (Fig. 8-39). Hold for release.

CHAPTER REVIEW

CASE STUDY

B.F. was 8 years old the first time her mother brought her in for massage. She was a competitive gymnast who had started at the age of 6 and quickly outshone everyone else—true Olympic material. Her mother is a client, and an M.D., but is a hospital administrator who doesn't practice. She viewed massage as a generally good thing for the child athlete, rather than seeking it for any specific problem. Over the next 5 years, B.F. was in training on a daily basis and received massage once a week, and sometimes more frequently if she was recovering from injury—something that happens with young gymnasts more frequently than people realize. Over the years she suffered wrist injuries, ankle injuries, pulled hamstrings, a concussion . . . a lot for a young child to go through.

B.F.'s frequent complaint was in the gluteals and deep hip rotators, not surprising for a gymnast. She was a tiny girl but very muscular, and it was always a challenge to find a balance between working deeply enough to address her problems and not being so deep as to hurt her. Even when she had no specific injuries, her overall body was taut as a guitar string. In addition to her daily hours of practice, she was a straight-A student in school and one who pushed herself to excel at everything she attempted. She would be particularly tense in the days immediately before a big competition. Sometimes her massage was rehabilitative in nature, but many times it was just for stress and general muscle tension.

When B.F. was 13, her mother came in for her own appointment one day, and said "You won't believe it, my daughter has quit gymnastics." I expressed my surprise and she said that her daughter had said, "I'm 13, and I have had 13 MRIs, all for injuries I got during gymnastics." She decided that was enough. Her mother had always supported her, but never pushed her into it, and it was her own decision to quit.

In high school, she ran cross-country and was still a client, though with less frequency than before. She is away at college now and still comes in for a massage whenever she is visiting home.

C.T., LMBT

REVIEW QUESTIONS

1. The ______ are joined posteriorly at the sacroiliac joints.
   a. Puborectales
   b. Hemipelves
   c. Orbiculares
   d. Acetabula

2. A lateral tilt of the pelvis is determined by a misalignment in the relative position of the two ______.
   a. Pubis symphysis
   b. Greater trochanters
   c. Acromion
   d. PSIS

3. Iliopsoas is composed of the _______and the ________.
   a. Psoas minor and iliac crest
   b. Psoas minor and ilium
   c. Psoas major and iliacus
   d. Psoas major and iliac crest

4. The levator ani can be palpated ______.
   a. At the medial border of T-12
   b. On the lateral third of the iliac crest
   c. Superior to the psoas
   d. Only internally.

5. You should never perform pelvic work on a client without _______.
   a. Letting them know it might be ticklish
   b. Telling them it's illegal
   c. Obtaining specific informed consent
   d. Taking their pelvic measurements

6. _______syndrome is an entrapment of the sciatic nerve.
   a. Piriformis
   b. Sacroiliac
   c. ITB
   d. Pectoralis minor

7. The most powerful muscle for climbing is the _______.
   a. Obturator
   b. Levator ani
   c. Gemellus
   d. Gluteus maximus

8. Internal work on pelvic floor muscles is usually _______.
   a. Sexual in nature
   b. Outside the scope of practice of massage therapy
   c. Performed at the beginning of the session
   d. Too painful for the client

9. The position of turning the foot out that ballet dancers often use is known as _______.
   a. Lateral hip rotation
   b. Adduction
   c. Flexion of the hip
   d. Flexion of the femur

10. The condition resulting from one hemipelves having a greater or lesser anterior or posterior rotation in relation to the other results in a ______ pelvis.
    a. Torqued
    b. Fractured
    c. Warped
    d. Dropped

thePoint Additional helpful resources are available at http://thePoint.lww.com.

CHAPTER 9

The Thigh

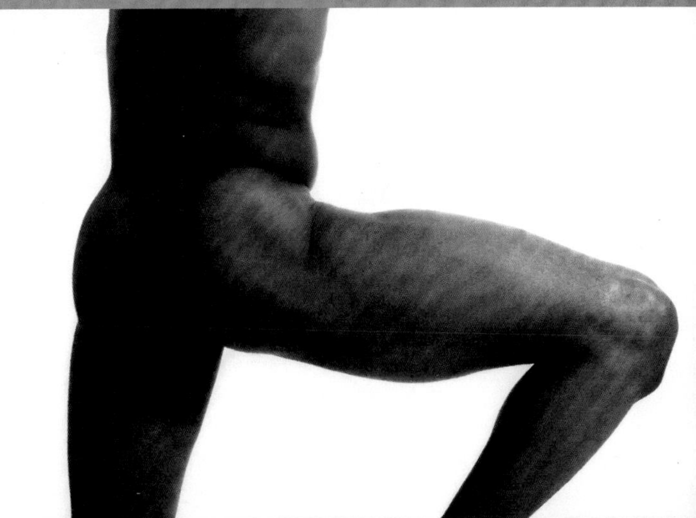

LEARNING OBJECTIVES

At the end of this chapter, the learner will be able to:

- State the correct terminology of the muscles of the thigh.
- Palpate the muscles of the thigh.
- Identify their attachments at the origins and insertions.
- Explain the actions of the muscles.
- Describe their pain referral areas.
- Recall related muscles.
- Recognize any endangerment sites and ethical cautions for massage therapy.
- Demonstrate proficiency in manual therapy techniques for muscles of the thigh.

The Overview of the Region begins on page 284, after the anatomy plates.

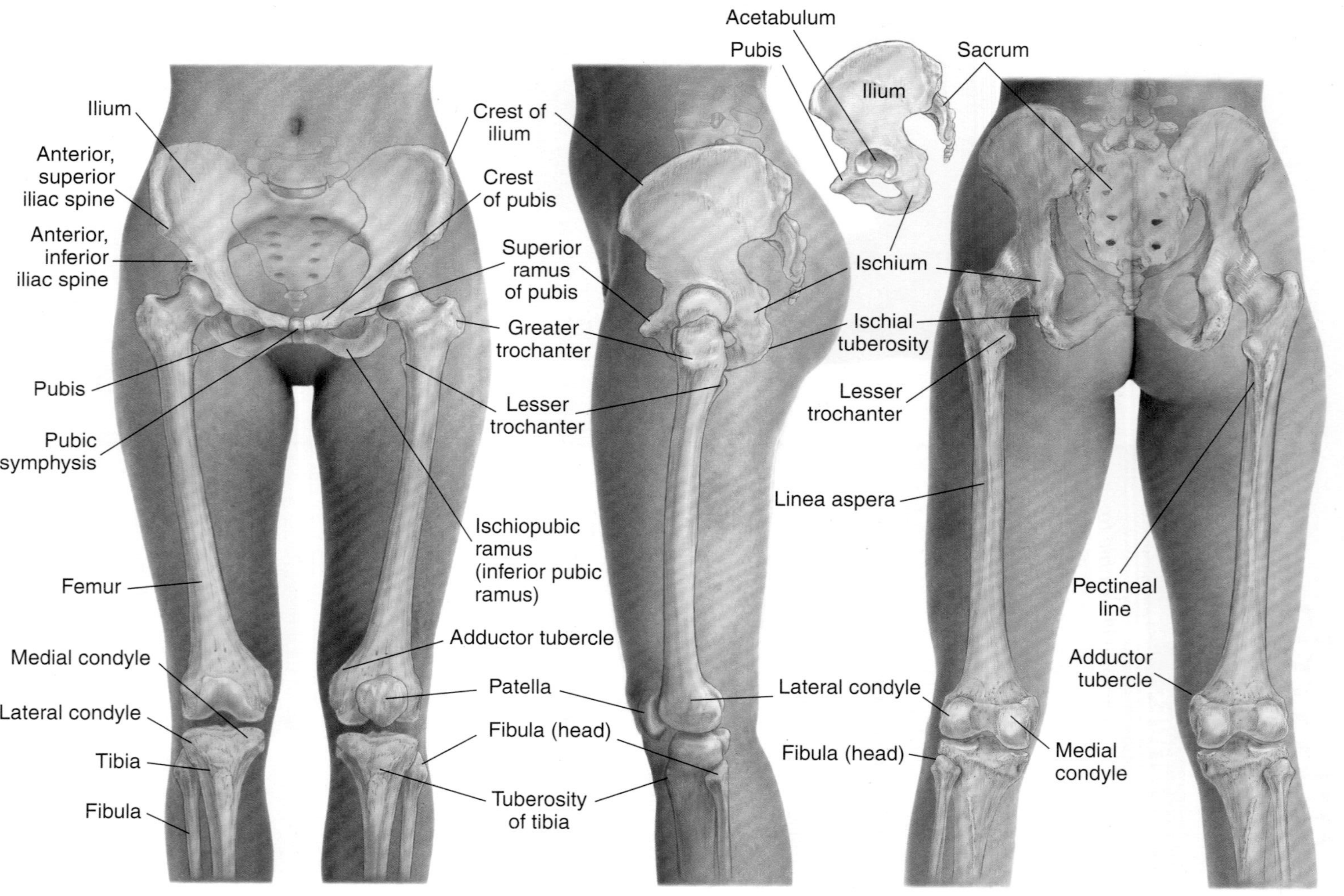

PLATE 9-1 ■ Skeletal features of the thigh

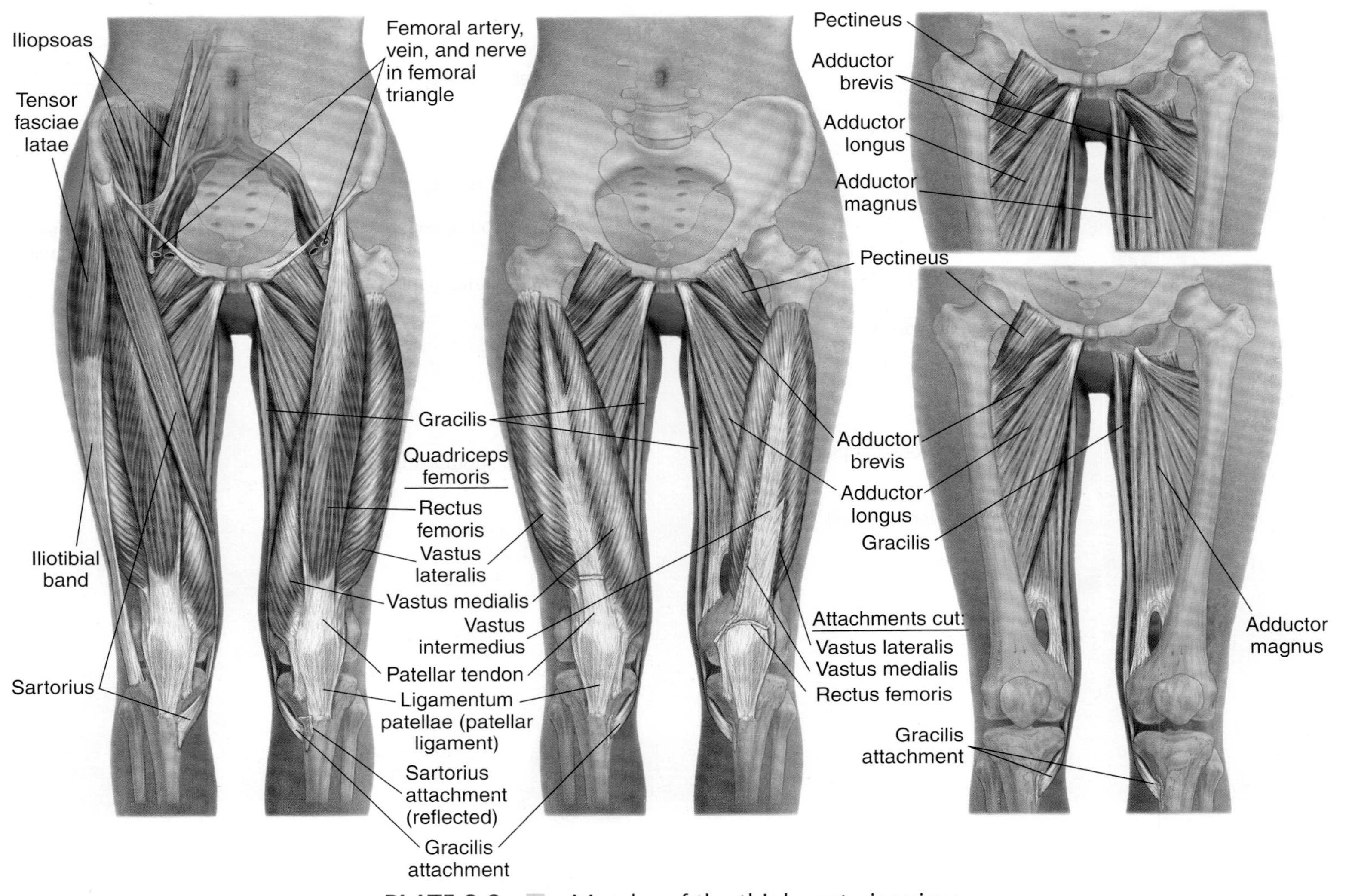

PLATE 9-2 ■ Muscles of the thigh, anterior view

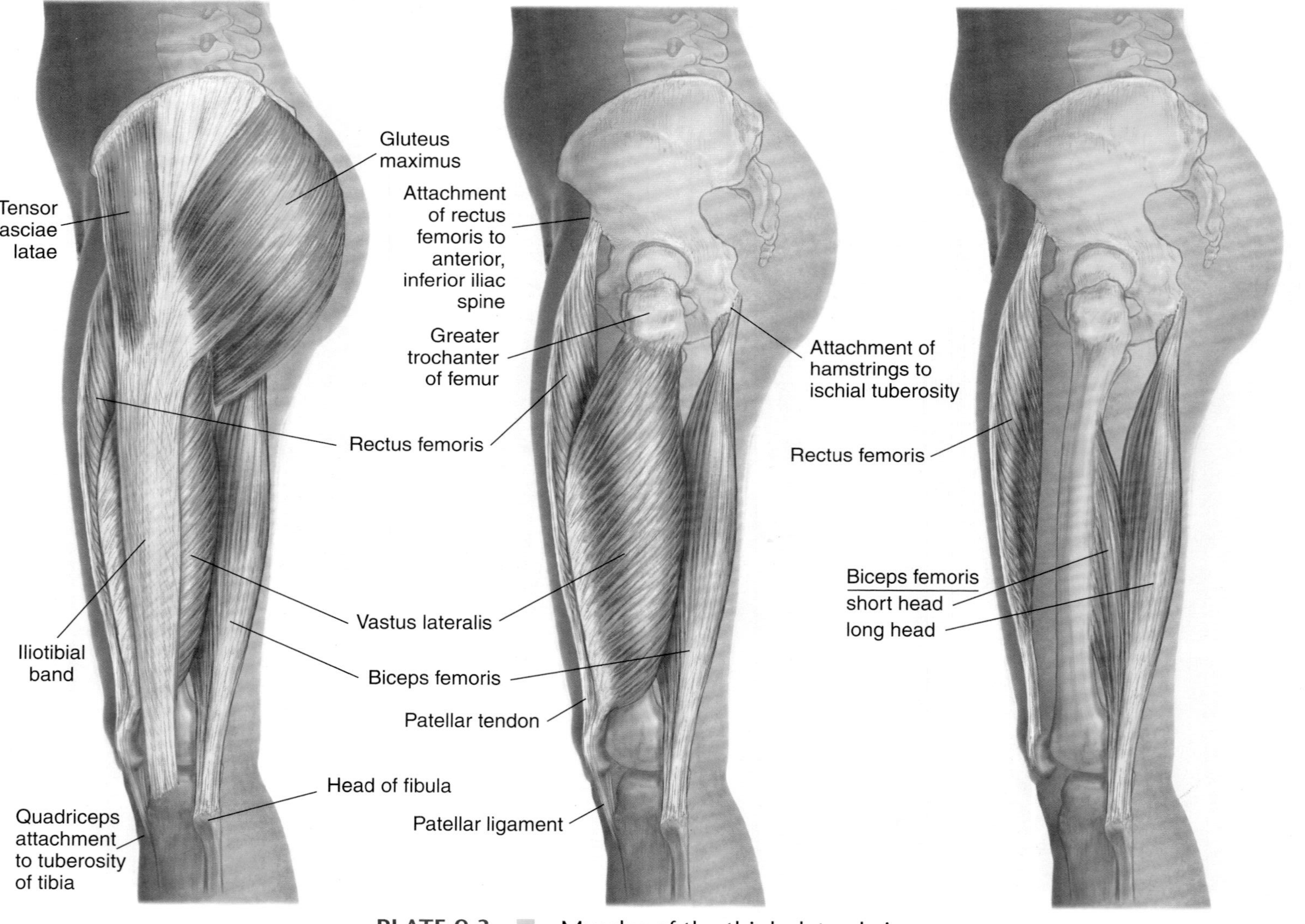

PLATE 9-3 ■ Muscles of the thigh, lateral view

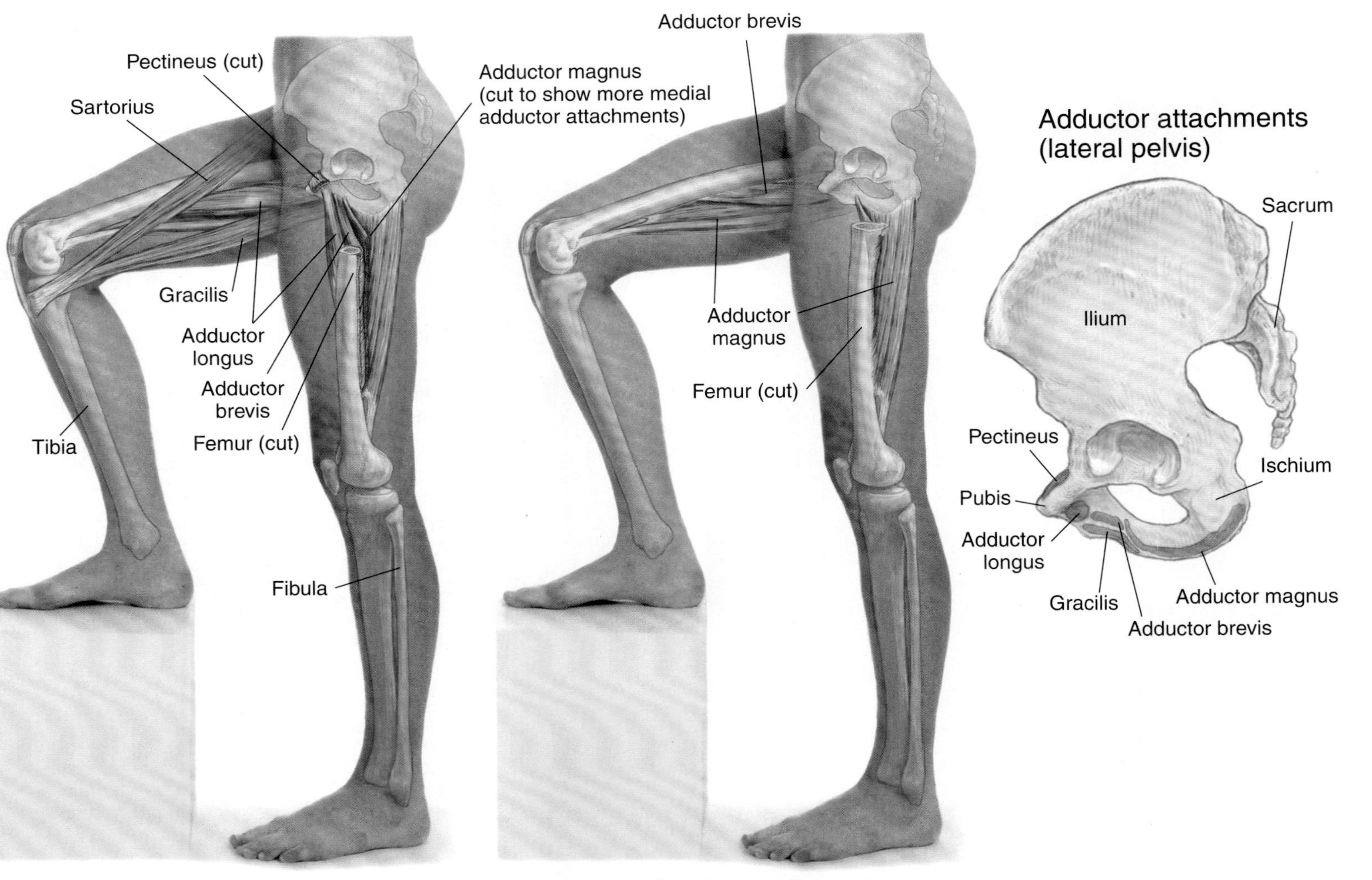

PLATE 9-4 ■ Adductors of the hip, medial and lateral views

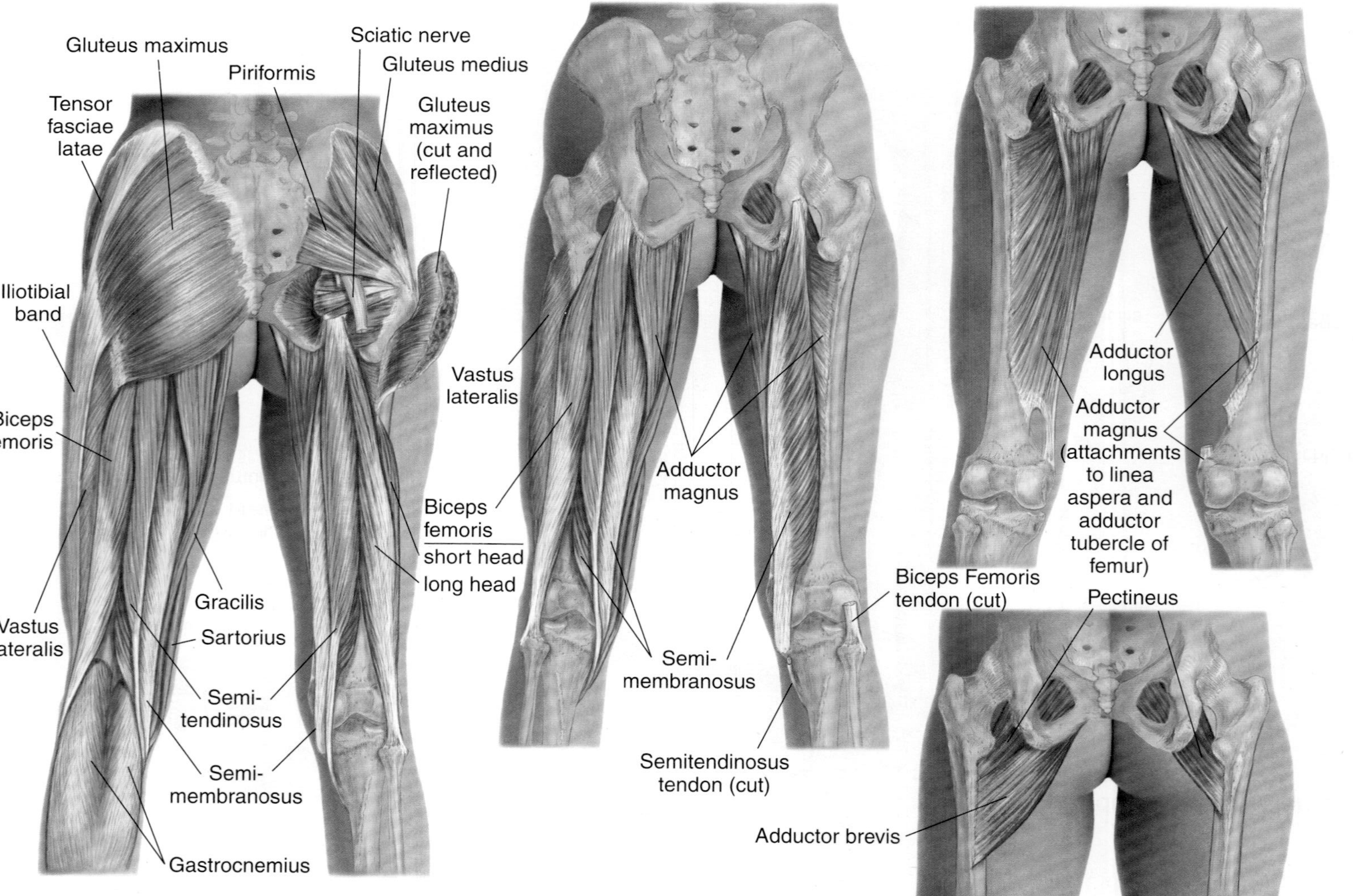

PLATE 9-5 ■ Muscles of the thigh, posterior view

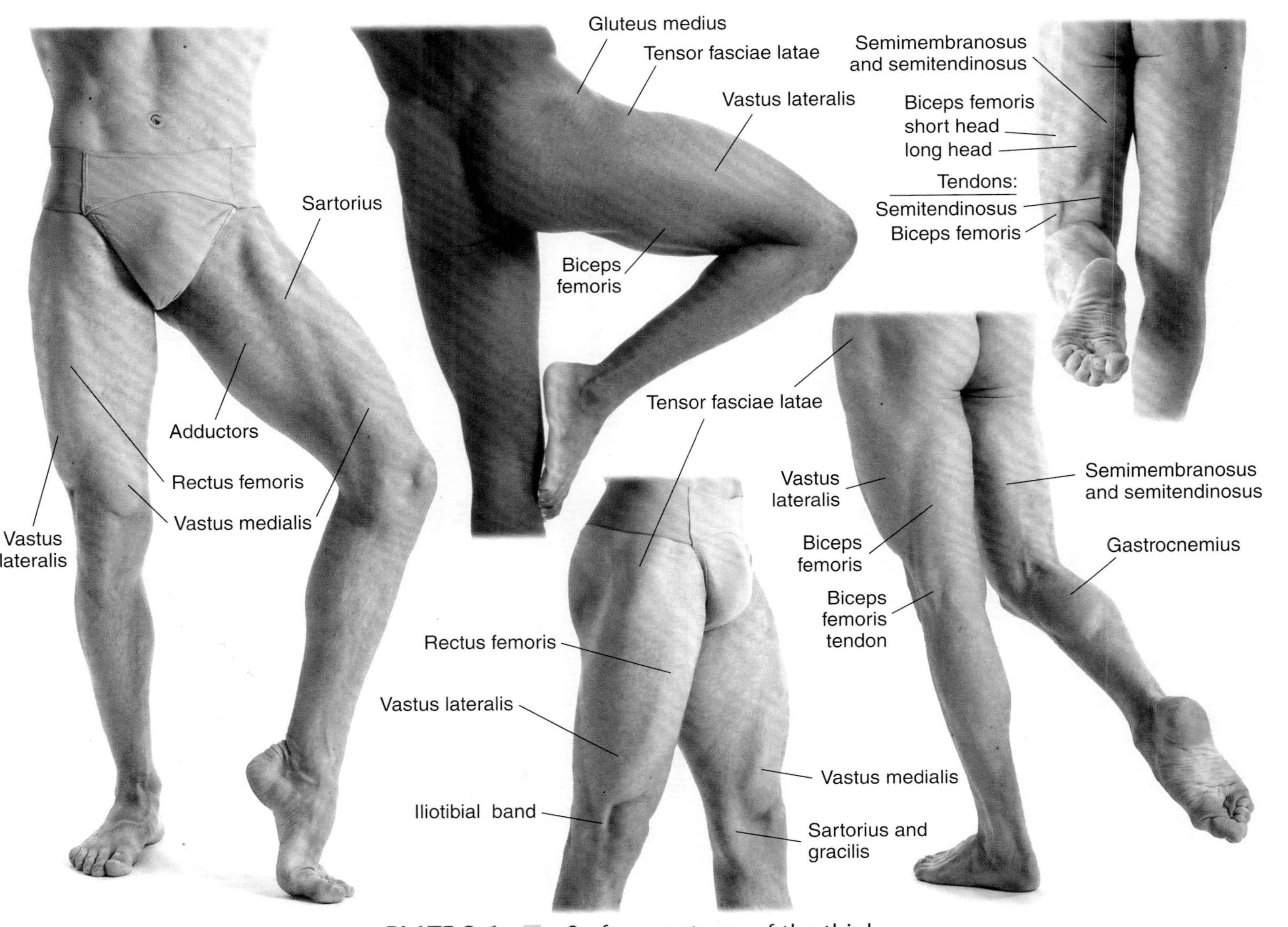

PLATE 9-6 ■ Surface anatomy of the thigh

Overview of the Region (Plates 9-1 to 9-6)

The powerful muscles of the thigh can be divided into four basic groups: anterior **(quadriceps** and **sartorius),** posterior **(hamstrings),** lateral **(tensor fasciae latae** and **iliotibial band),** and medial **(hip adductors).** Although some pain in the thigh is referred from superior muscles in and around the pelvis and from the lower leg, pain may also originate in the thigh muscles themselves.

The muscles of the thigh are one of the principal contributors to knee pain, as their primary function is to move and stabilize the knee joint. Their importance in maintaining posture is considerable, both in their control of the knee and in the influence of **rectus femoris** and the hip adductors on the position of the pelvis. Rectus femoris attaches at the **anterior inferior iliac spine (AIIS),** and **adductor longus, adductor brevis, pectineus,** and **gracilis** all have attachments to various anterior aspects of the **pubis.** Therefore, all these muscles are hip flexors and can contribute to an anterior pelvic rotation. The hamstrings, on the other hand, attach to the ischial tuberosity, are hip extensors, and can pull the pelvis into posterior rotation. When we say that quadriceps and hamstrings are antagonists, we usually think of their opposing functions in extending or flexing the knee, but they are also antagonists in the positioning of the pelvis.

When the quadriceps and hamstrings are shortened, they can cause increased pressure of the patella against the joint surfaces of the femur. This may cause worn, damaged cartilage and knee pain. In addition, since the muscles of the **quadriceps** group attach to the **tibia** via a common tendon enclosing the **patella,** these muscles determine the position of the patella. Together, the quadriceps and hamstrings dictate the position and balance of stress in the knee joint. The knee joint is usually included among the most structurally complex joints in the body. That, combined with the physical forces encountered in bearing body weight during movement, makes it one of the most vulnerable and susceptible to injury.

Careful observation of the gait of the client in the initial examination will reveal much information about the muscles of the thigh, such as relative strength and tension, because they affect the position and movement of the hips and knees throughout the gait cycle.

Note that the connective tissue structure attaching quadriceps to the tibia and enclosing the patella is generally referred to as the *patellar tendon* above the patella (connects muscle to bone) and as the *patellar ligament* below the patella (connects bone to bone).

CAUTION Be familiar with the femoral triangle, a triangular space at the upper part of the thigh, bounded by sartorius laterally, adductor longus medially, and the inguinal ligament superiorly (see Plate 9-2). Deep to these muscles, it is bounded laterally by iliopsoas and medially by pectineus. The femoral triangle contains the femoral vessels and the branches of the femoral nerve. The popliteal triangle, or fossa, at the back of the knee, contains the tibial and common peroneal (fibular) nerve, popliteal artery (a continuation of the femoral artery), popliteal vein, small saphenous vein, popliteal lymph nodes, and vessels. When working on the thigh, take care not to exert pressure on these structures.

ethics **ETHICAL CAUTION**

Working with the attachments of the upper thigh can require contact with the genitals, which is prohibited in most regulated states in the USA. Keep the client draped as securely as possible, and remain in constant communication. It may make the client feel more secure if you suggest that they place their own hand over their genitals while you are working in the area.

Overview of the Muscles of the Anterior Thigh

Most of the muscles of the anterior thigh are extensors of the knee and flexors of the hip joint, but some move only the knee while others may flex both joints. They provide stability while standing and help produce locomotion.

QUADRICEPS FEMORIS

KWAD-ris-seps fe-MOR-is, FEM-or-is

ETYMOLOGY Latin ***quadri***, four + ***caput***, head, therefore, four-headed

Overview

Three of the muscles (the vasti) of the quadriceps group cross and move only the knee joint, while one (rectus femoris) crosses and moves both the hip and the knee joints. All have a common inferior attachment via the patellar tendon and apply their considerable extension force to the anterior tibia (Fig. 9-1).

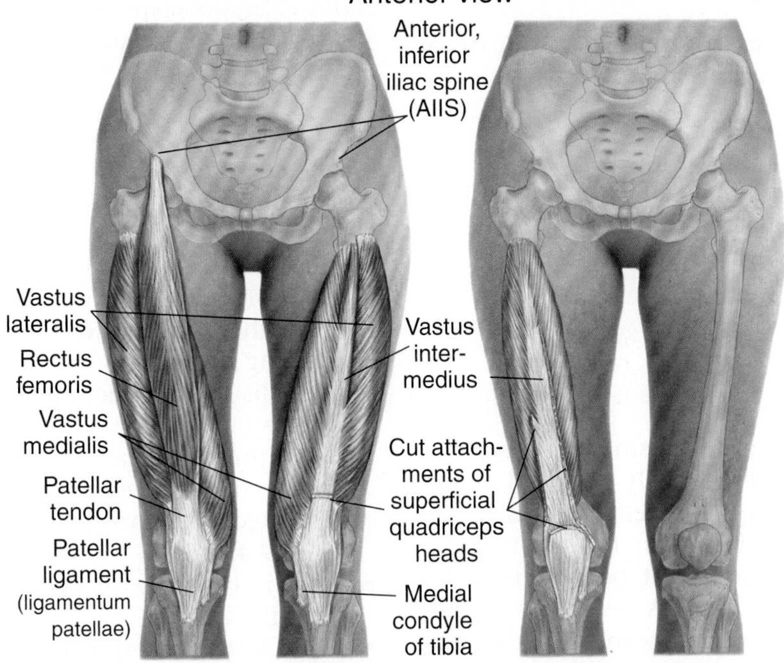

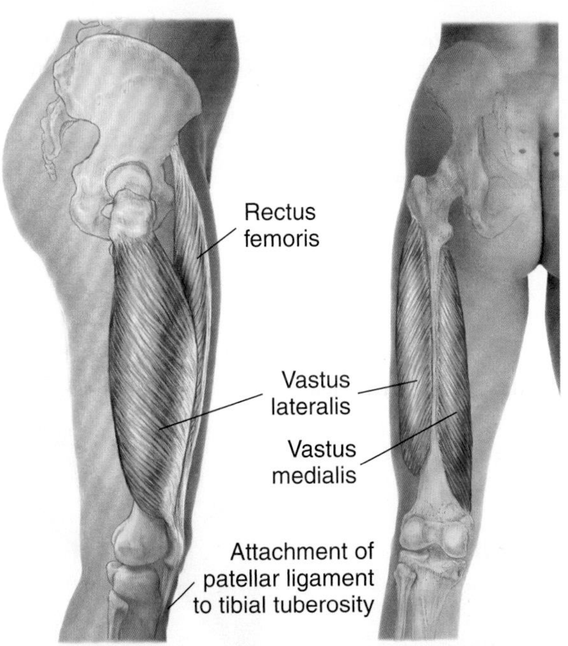

FIGURE 9-1 Anatomy of quadriceps femoris

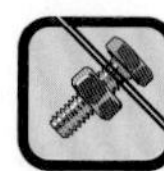

ATTACHMENTS

Origins

- Rectus femoris: to the anterior inferior iliac spine (AIIS) and upper margin of acetabulum
- Vastus lateralis: to the lateral lip of the linea aspera and wrapping from lateral to anterior femur just below the greater trochanter
- Vastus medialis: to the medial lip of the linea aspera
- Vastus intermedius: to the upper three-fourths of the anterior surface of the shaft of the femur

Insertions

- All to the patella, and thence by the patellar ligament (ligamentum patellae) to the tibial tuberosity; vastus medialis also to the medial condyle of the tibia

PALPATION

Palpation is easy, but distinguishing the muscles is very challenging. All are easily palpated at the attachment to the superior patella. Rectus femoris (architecture bipennate) can be followed up to its superior attachment just below the anterior superior iliac spine. Vastus lateralis and medialis (architecture unipennate) can be followed to their superior attachments to the femur laterally and medially. Vastus intermedius is not directly palpable.

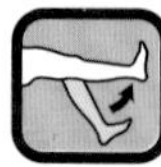

ACTION

All extend the knee; rectus femoris also flexes the hip

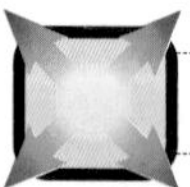

REFERRAL AREA

- Vastus medialis and intermedius: to the anterior thigh and the knee
- Vastus lateralis: to the lateral thigh and the knee

OTHER MUSCLES TO EXAMINE

- Hip adductors
- Tensor fasciae latae and iliotibial band
- Obturator internus (may cause pain in the anterior thigh through entrapment of the obturator nerve)

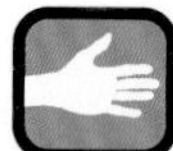

MANUAL THERAPY

CAUTION These procedures should not be performed on a client who has had recent knee surgery, or is scheduled for such surgery. If a client has had knee surgery in the past, or complains of knee pain, question the client thoroughly before proceeding. When in doubt, have the client obtain permission from her or his physician before proceeding.

Stripping

- The client lies supine.
- The therapist stands beside the client at the lower legs.
- Place the heel of the hand, the thumb, or the fingertips (Fig. 9-2) on the quadriceps tendon where it attaches to the patella on the medial side.
- Pressing firmly into the tissue, slide along vastus medialis to its attachment on the upper femur (Fig. 9-3).
- Beginning again at the kneecap in the center, repeat this procedure, continuing the stroke along rectus femoris to its attachment at the ASIS (Figs. 9-4, 9-5).
- Repeat the same procedure laterally on vastus lateralis (Figs. 9-6, 9-7).
- Note: Vastus intermedius lies deep to the other quadriceps muscles and is therefore treated through them.

Cross-fiber Friction for the Patellar Tendon and Ligament

- The client lies supine.
- The therapist stands beside the client at the legs.

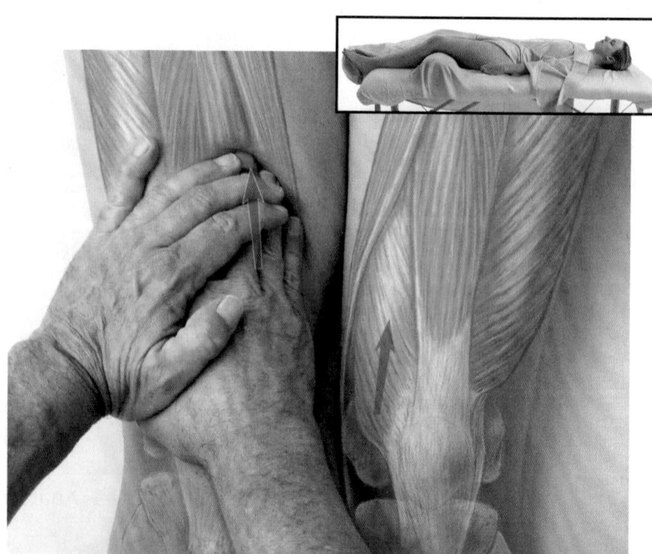

FIGURE 9-2 Stripping of vastus medialis with the fingertips

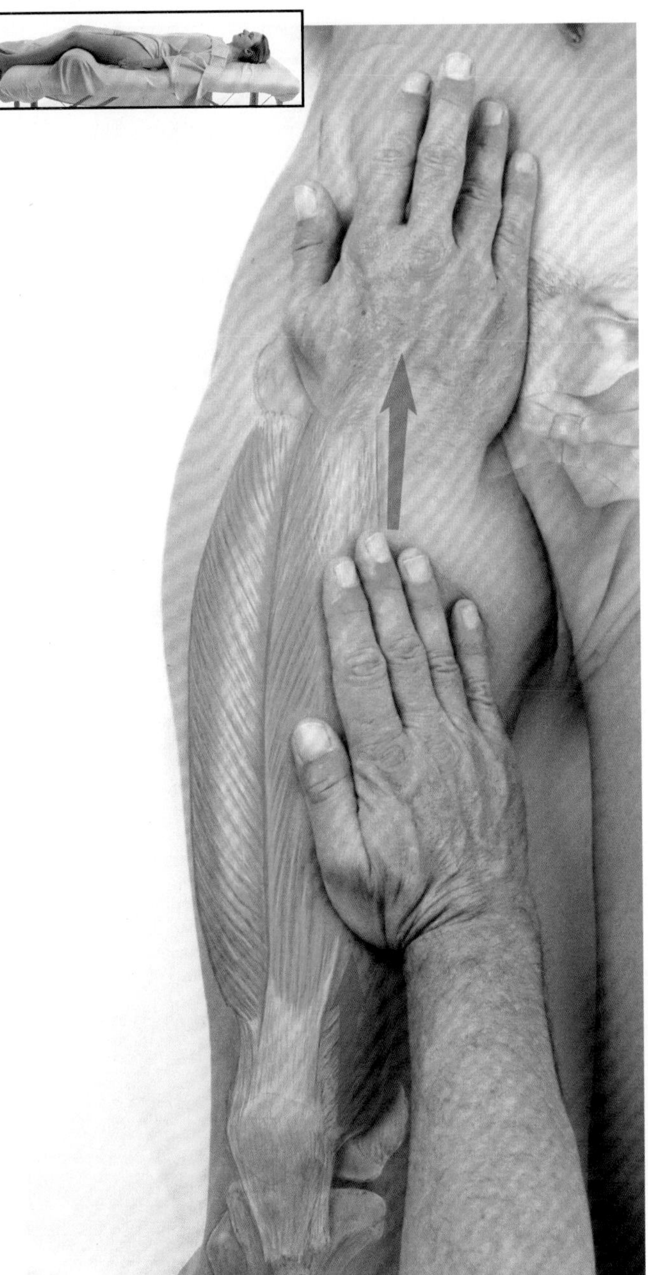

FIGURE 9-3 Stripping of vastus medialis

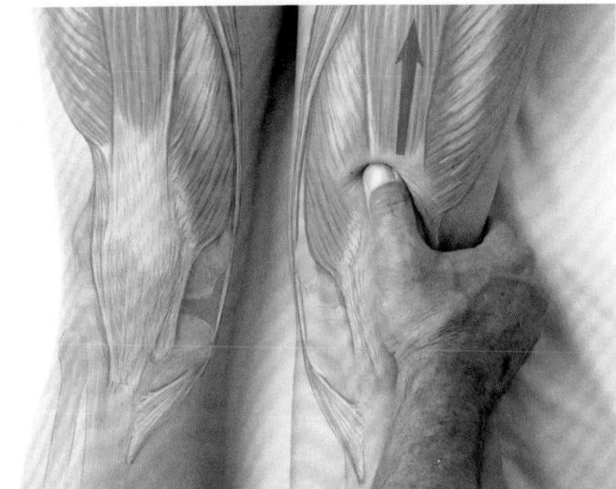

FIGURE 9-4 Stripping of rectus femoris with the thumb

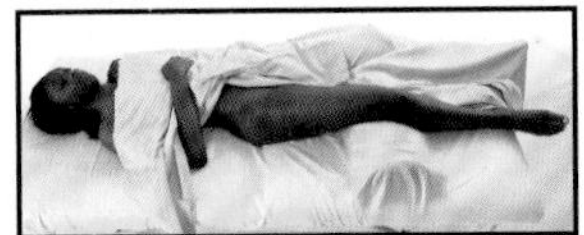

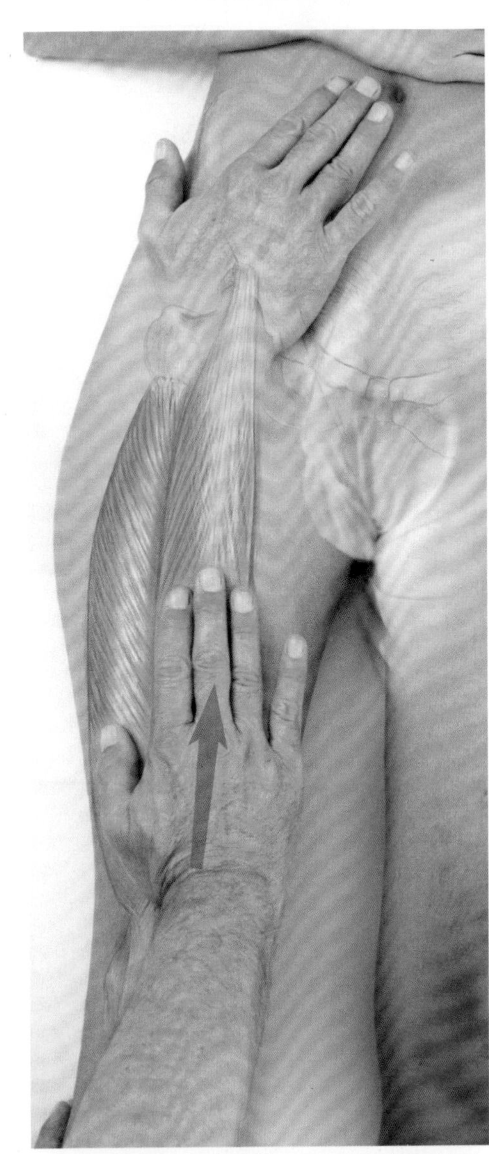

FIGURE 9-5 Stripping of rectus femoris

- Place the thumb on the patellar tendon (superior to the patella).
- Press firmly into the tissue, and move the thumb back and forth across the tendon until you feel a decreased tension in the tendon (Fig. 9-8A).
- Repeat this procedure on the patellar ligament (inferior to the patella) (Fig. 9-8B).

Cross-fiber Friction on Deep Surface of Patella

- With one hand, displace the patella away from yourself.
- Place the fingertips of the other hand under the patella.

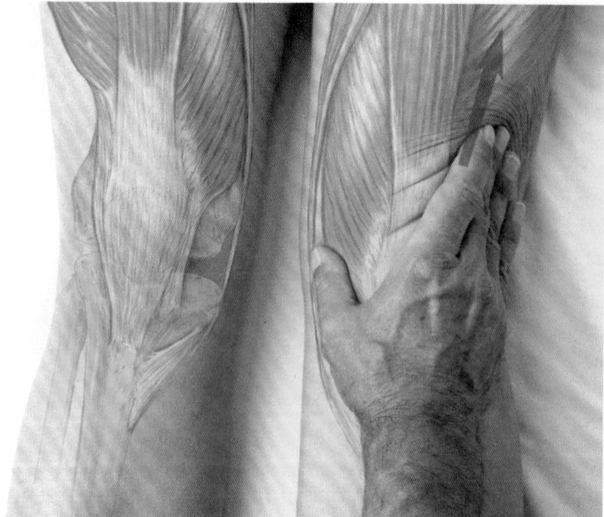

FIGURE 9-6 Stripping of vastus lateralis with the fingertips

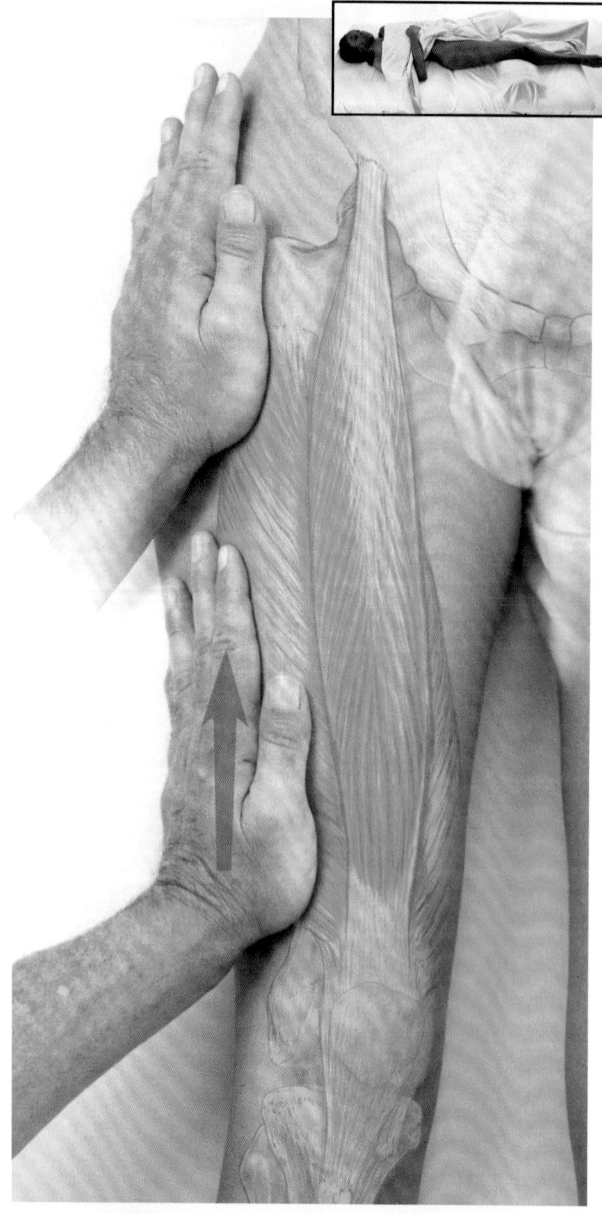

FIGURE 9-7 Stripping of vastus lateralis

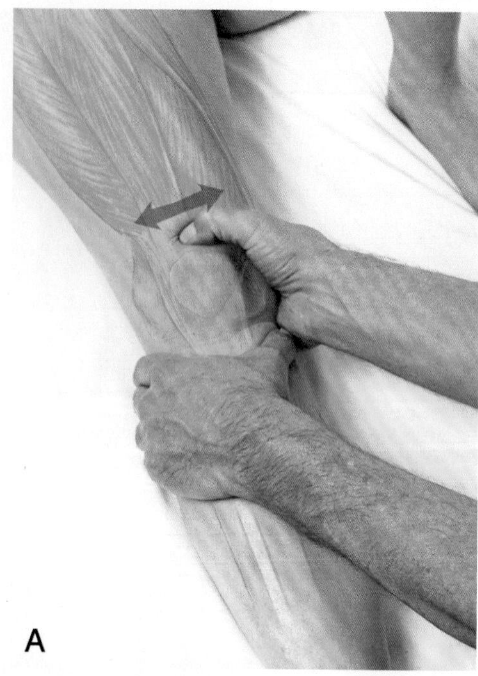

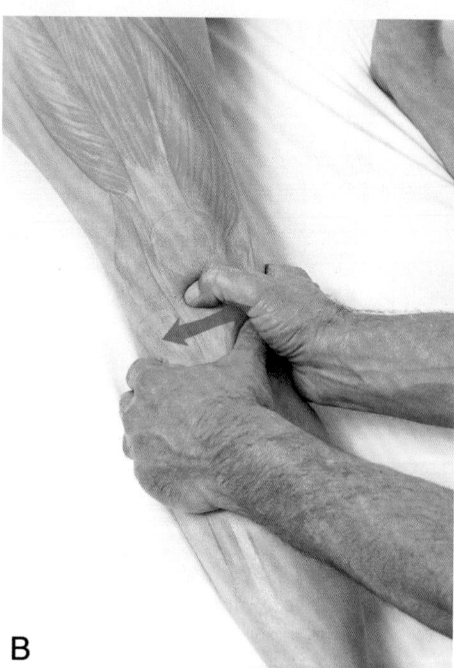

FIGURE 9-8 Cross-fiber friction of the patellar tendon **(A)** and ligament **(B)**

- Pressing upward into the patella, move your fingertips back and forth until you feel a decreased tension in the tendon (Fig. 9-9A).
- Repeat the procedure medially (Fig. 9-9B).

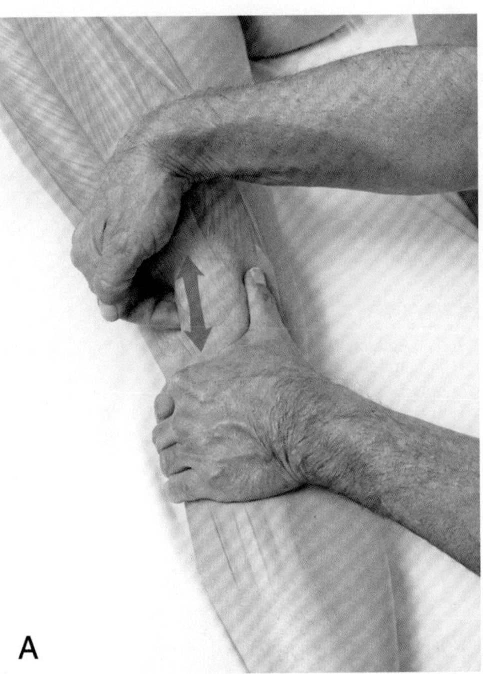

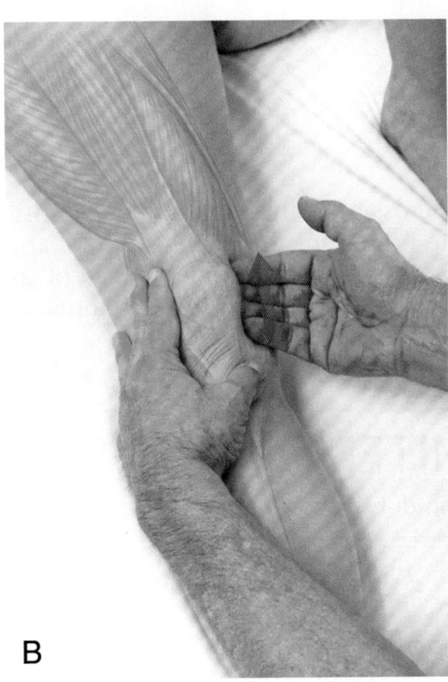

FIGURE 9-9 Cross-fiber friction underneath the patella laterally **(A)** and medially **(B)**

SARTORIUS

sar-TORE-ee-us

ETYMOLOGY Latin *sartor*, tailor (from the cross-legged position in which a tailor sits)

Overview

Sartorius has the distinction of being the longest muscle of the body. It flexes and rotates both the hip and knee. A taut sartorius muscle (Fig. 9-10) will often interfere with the stretching of piriformis. If you attempt to stretch piriformis and the client reports feeling the stretch in the anterior thigh, release sartorius before proceeding.

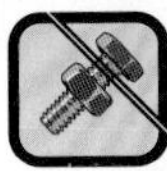

ATTACHMENTS

- Origin: anterior superior iliac spine
- Insertion: medial border of the tuberosity of the tibia after passing behind the knee

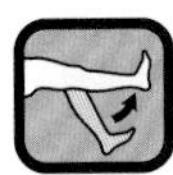

ACTION

Flexes hip and knee, rotates knee medially and hip laterally

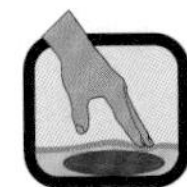

PALPATION

Ask the client to laterally rotate and flex the thigh at the hip joint and feel for the contraction of the sartorius immediately distal and slightly medial to the ASIS. Its architecture is parallel.

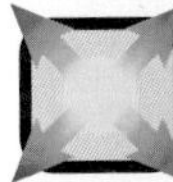

REFERRAL AREA

To the anterior and medial aspects of the thigh

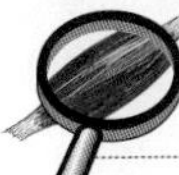

OTHER MUSCLES TO EXAMINE

- Quadriceps
- Hip adductors

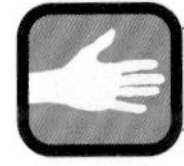

MANUAL THERAPY

Stripping

- The client lies supine.
- The therapist stands beside the client at the legs.
- Place the heel of the hand, thumb, or fingertips on the medial thigh just superior to the patella.
- Pressing firmly into the tissue, slide the fingertips diagonally along the muscle across the quadriceps to its attachment on the ASIS (Fig. 9-11).

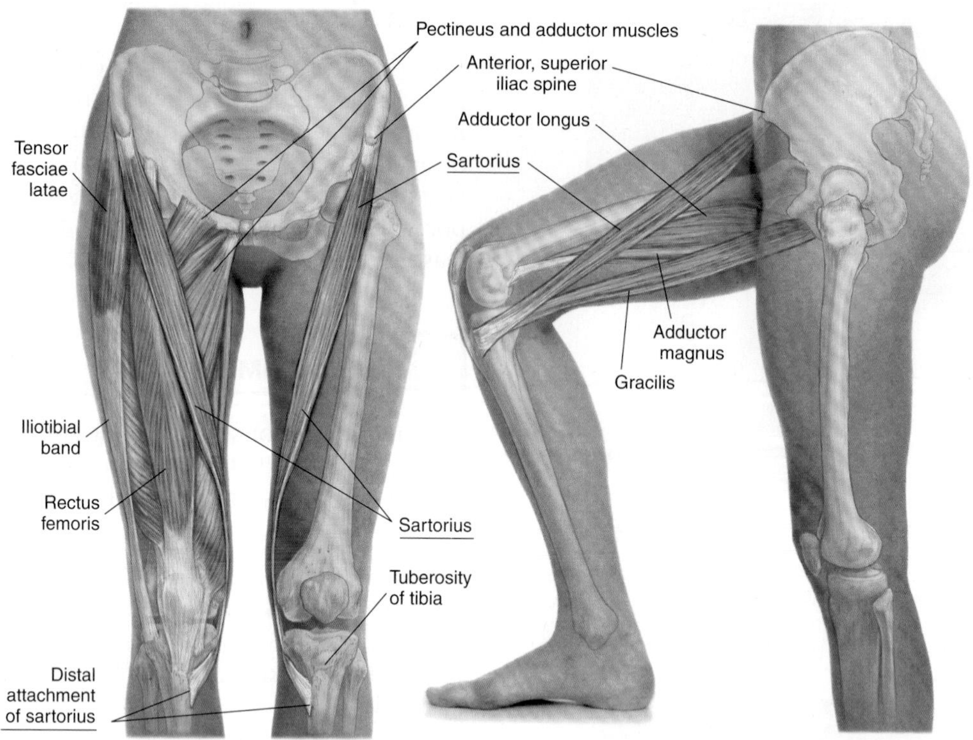

FIGURE 9-10 Anatomy of sartorius

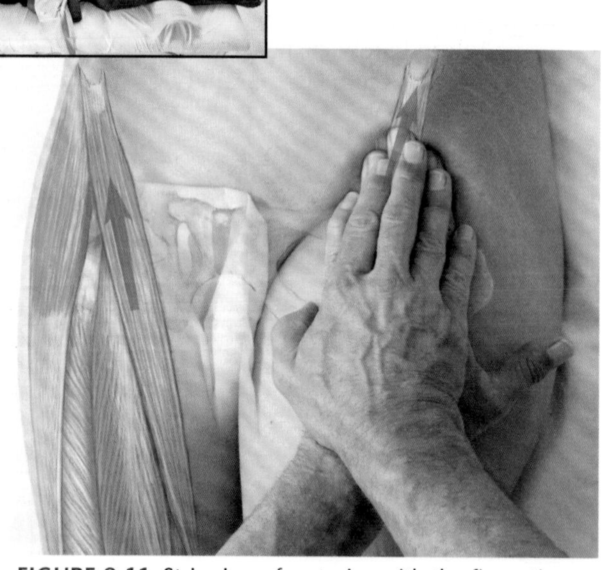

FIGURE 9-11 Stripping of sartorius with the fingertips

Overview of the Muscles of the Posterior Thigh (Hamstrings)

From the word "ham," denoting the buttock and back of the thigh, "hamstrings" is an old term for the muscles of the posterior thigh, comprising the long head of biceps femoris, the semitendinosus, and the semimembranosus muscles. Note that these muscles cross both the hip and knee joints and are therefore important in both movement and stabilization of these joints. The short head of the biceps femoris crosses and moves the knee only.

SEMITENDINOSUS

SEM-i-ten-di-NO-sus

ETYMOLOGY Latin ***semi***, half + ***tendinosus***, tendinous

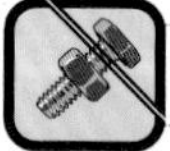

ATTACHMENTS

- Origin: ischial tuberosity (Fig. 9-12)
- Insertion: anterior, medial condyle of the tibia after passing behind the knee with sartorius and gracillis

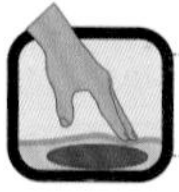

PALPATION

The hamstrings, like quadriceps femoris, are easy to palpate but difficult to distinguish. Biceps femoris can be followed on the lateral side to its attachment to the head of the fibula where its single tendon can be palpated crossing behind the knee. The two tendons

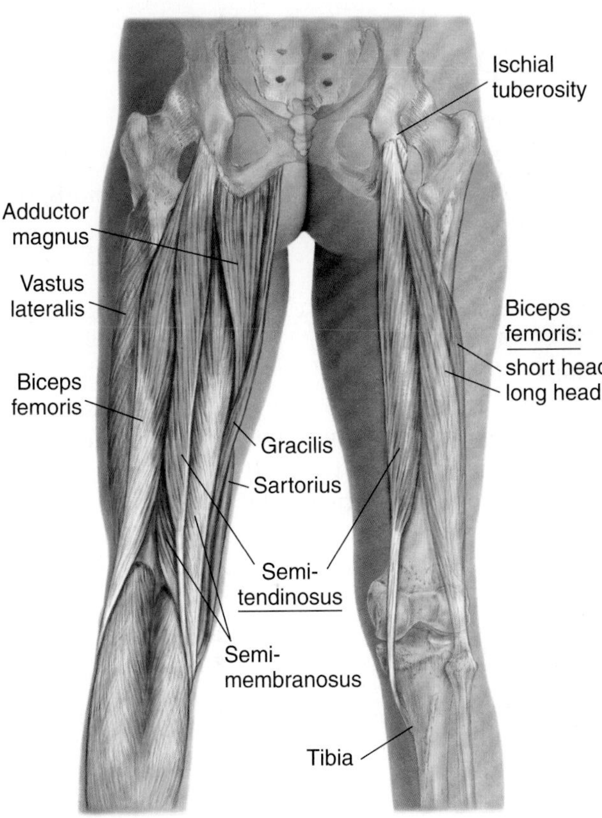

FIGURE 9-12 Anatomy of semitendinosus

belonging to the semitendinosus and semimembranosus can be palpated as they cross medially behind the knee. Semimembranosus can be followed to its attachment to the posterior, medial condyle of the tibia. Semitendinosus is difficult to distinguish at its inferior attachment to the anterior, medial tibia. The superior heads of the hamstrings can be felt underneath the ischial tuberosity. Biceps femoris and semimembranosus are bipennate; semitendinosus is unipennate.

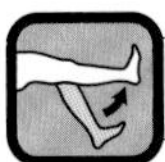

ACTION

Extends and medially rotates the hip; flexes the knee and rotates it medially when the knee is flexed; action is identical to semimembranosus.

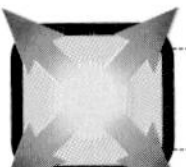

REFERRAL AREA

Over the back of the leg from the buttock to the mid-calf

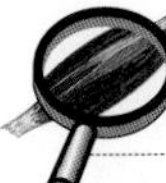

OTHER MUSCLES TO EXAMINE

- Quadratus lumborum
- Piriformis
- Gluteal muscles
- Hip adductors

SEMIMEMBRANOSUS

SEM-i-mem-bra-NO-sus

ETYMOLOGY Latin ***semi***, half + ***membranosus***, membranous

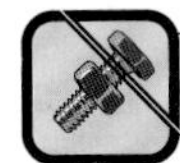

ATTACHMENTS

- Origin: ischial tuberosity (Fig. 9-13)
- Insertion: posterior aspect of the medial condyle of the tibia

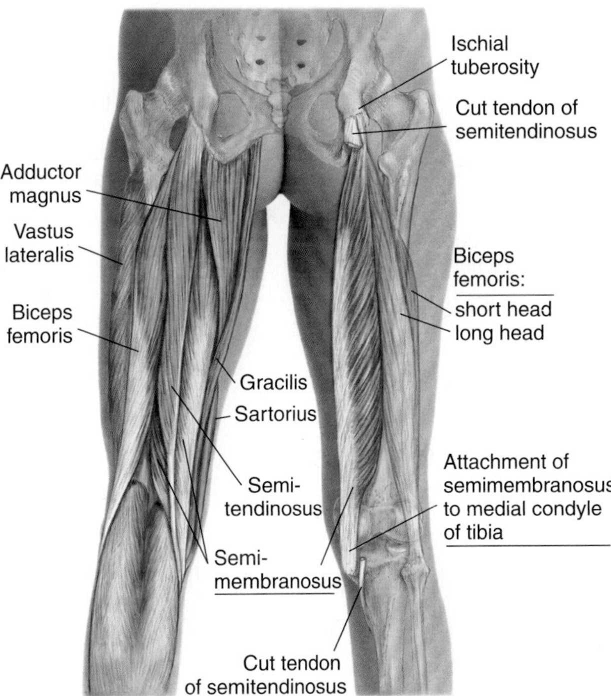

FIGURE 9-13 Anatomy of semimembranosus

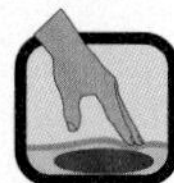

PALPATION

See semitendinosus

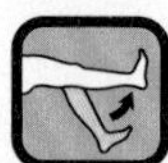

ACTION

Extends and medially rotates the hip; flexes the knee and rotates it medially when the knee is flexed; action is identical to semitendinosus

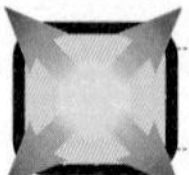

REFERRAL AREA

Over the back of the leg from the buttock to the mid-calf

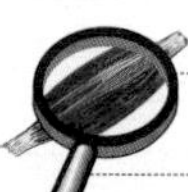

OTHER MUSCLES TO EXAMINE

- Quadratus lumborum
- Piriformis
- Gluteal muscles
- Hip adductors

BICEPS FEMORIS

BUY-seps fe-MORE-is

ETYMOLOGY Latin ***biceps***, two-headed + ***femoris***, of the femur

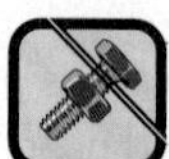

ATTACHMENTS

- Origin: long head to the ischial tuberosity, the short head to the lower two-thirds of the lateral lip of linea aspera (Fig. 9-14)
- Insertion: head of the fibula

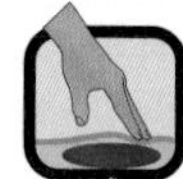

PALPATION

See semitendinosus

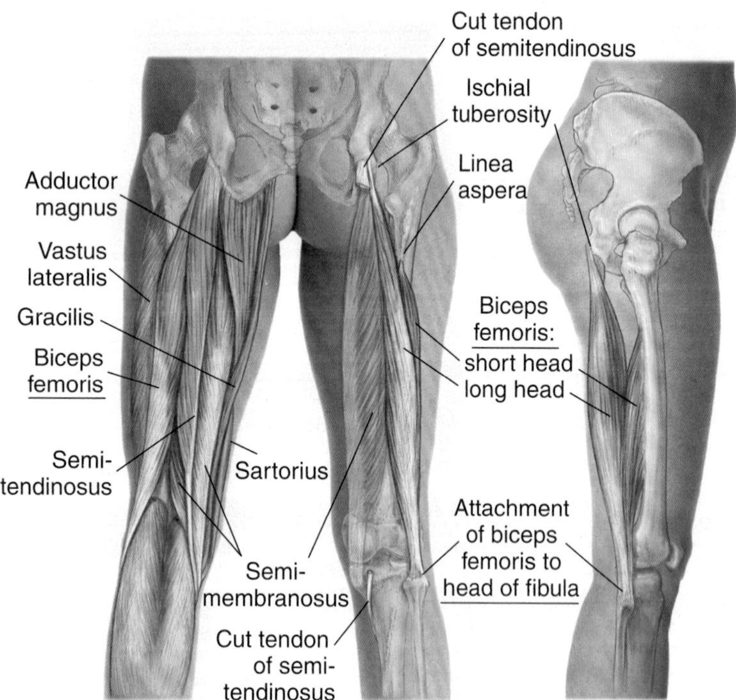

FIGURE 9-14 Anatomy of biceps femoris

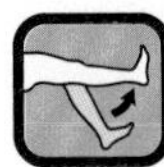

ACTION

Flexes knee and rotates flexed knee laterally; long head extends and laterally rotates the hip.

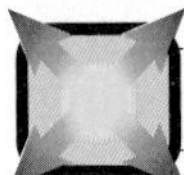

REFERRAL AREA

Over the back of the leg from the buttock to the mid-calf

OTHER MUSCLES TO EXAMINE

- Quadratus lumborum
- Piriformis
- Gluteal muscles
- Hip adductors

MANUAL THERAPY

CAUTION Always avoid applying pressure into the popliteal space behind the knee.

HAMSTRINGS

Stripping

- The client lies prone.
- The therapist stands beside the client at the calves.
- Place the fingertips, heel of the hand, forearm, or knuckles on the medial aspect of the hamstrings just superior to the knee.
- Pressing firmly into the tissue, slide along the muscle to its attachment on the ischial tuberosity (Fig. 9-15).
- Beginning in the center, repeat this procedure (Fig. 9-16).
- Repeat the same procedure on the lateral aspect (Fig. 9-17).

Compression and Cross-fiber Friction

- Place the thumbs on the attachment of the hamstrings to the ischial tuberosity (Fig. 9-18).
- Press superiorly into the tissue and hold for release.
- Alternatively, move the thumbs from side to side until you feel a softening and relaxation in the tissue.

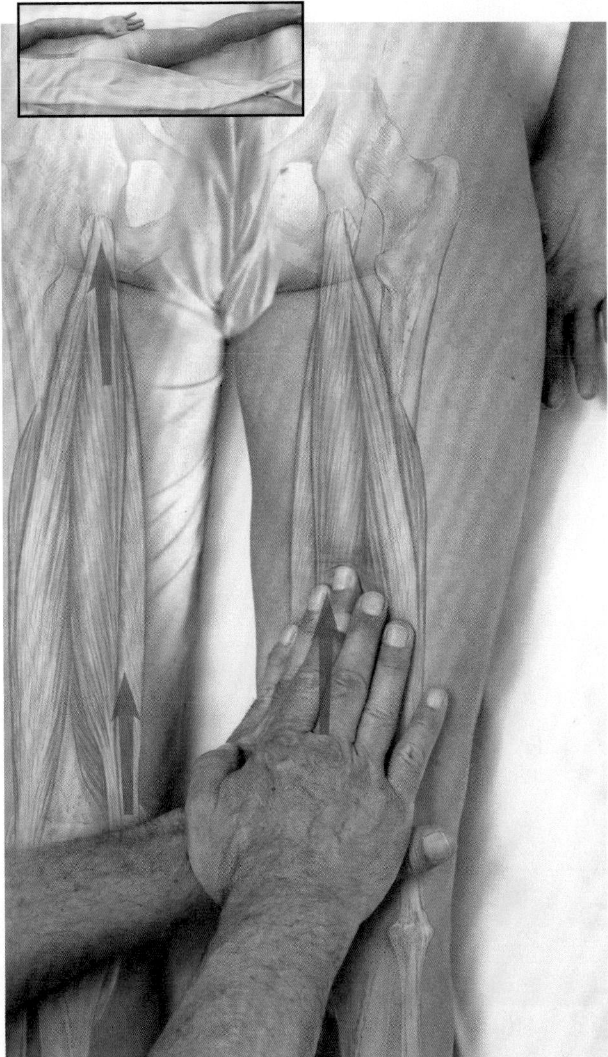

FIGURE 9-15 Stripping of medial hamstrings with the fingertips

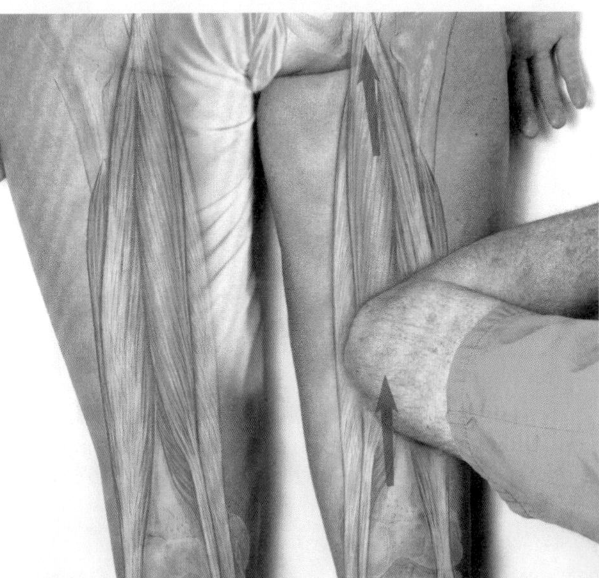

FIGURE 9-16 Stripping of hamstrings with the forearm

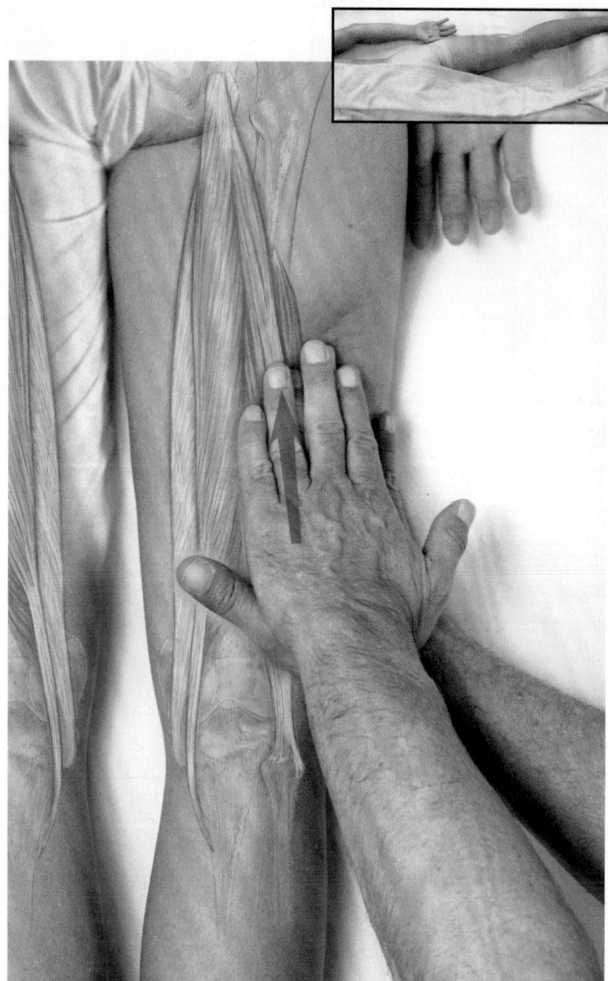

FIGURE 9-17 Stripping of lateral hamstrings with the fingertips

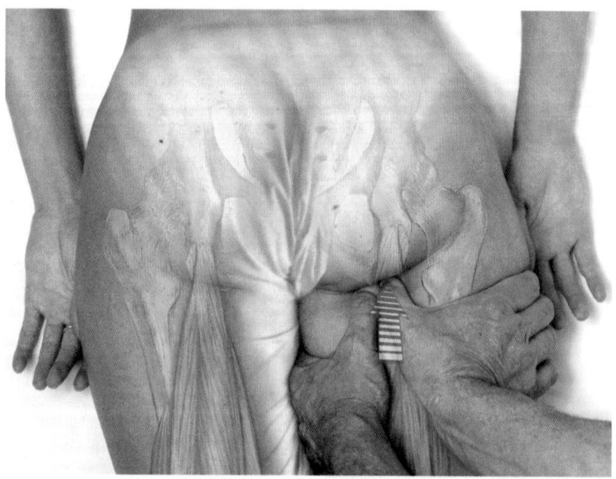

FIGURE 9-18 Compression of hamstring attachments against the ischial tuberosity

Overview of the Lateral Thigh: Tensor Fasciae Latae and the Iliotibial Band (ITB or Iliotibial Tract)

The iliotibial band (ITB) is not strictly a muscle; rather, it is a fibrous reinforcement (thickening) of the fascia lata (the deep fascia of the thigh) on the lateral surface of the thigh, extending from the crest of the ilium to the lateral condyle of the tibia. It helps ligaments stabilize the knee both in extension and in partial flexion and is therefore used constantly during walking and running. In leaning forward with slightly flexed knee, the tract is the main support of knee against gravity. Tensor fasciae latae attaches to the anterior edge of the ITB and part of the gluteus maximus attaches to the posterior edge. Together they tense and control this deep fascia. Tensor fasciae latae pulls on the ITB to serve as a flexor, abductor, and medial rotator of the hip. The force of the gluteus maximus on the ITB produces extension, abduction, and lateral rotation of the hip. Iliotibial band syndrome is a problem that occurs when the tensor fasciae latae, gluteus maximus, and the iliotibial band become taut. This causes the tendon-like ITB to rub against the outside of the knee joint capsule, which results in inflammation and pain. ITB syndrome is a common injury among runners, especially if they do extensive running uphill or downhill or begin exercising after a long layoff period. It is often an "overload"-type injury.

TENSOR FASCIAE LATAE AND THE ILIOTIBIAL BAND

TEN-ser FASH-a LAT-a

ILL-ee-o-TIB-ee-al band

ETYMOLOGY Latin ***tensor,*** tightener + ***fasciae,*** of the bandage + ***latae,*** wide

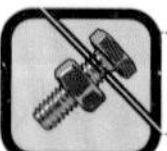

ATTACHMENTS

- Origin: (tensor fasciae latae), anterior superior iliac spine and the adjacent lateral and anterior surface of the ilium (Fig. 9-19)
- Insertion: iliotibial band of fascia lata, which attaches to the lateral condyle of the tibia

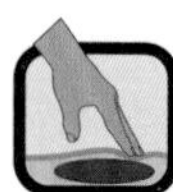

PALPATION

Tensor fasciae latae can be palpated laterally, just below the anterior superior iliac spine, and moving

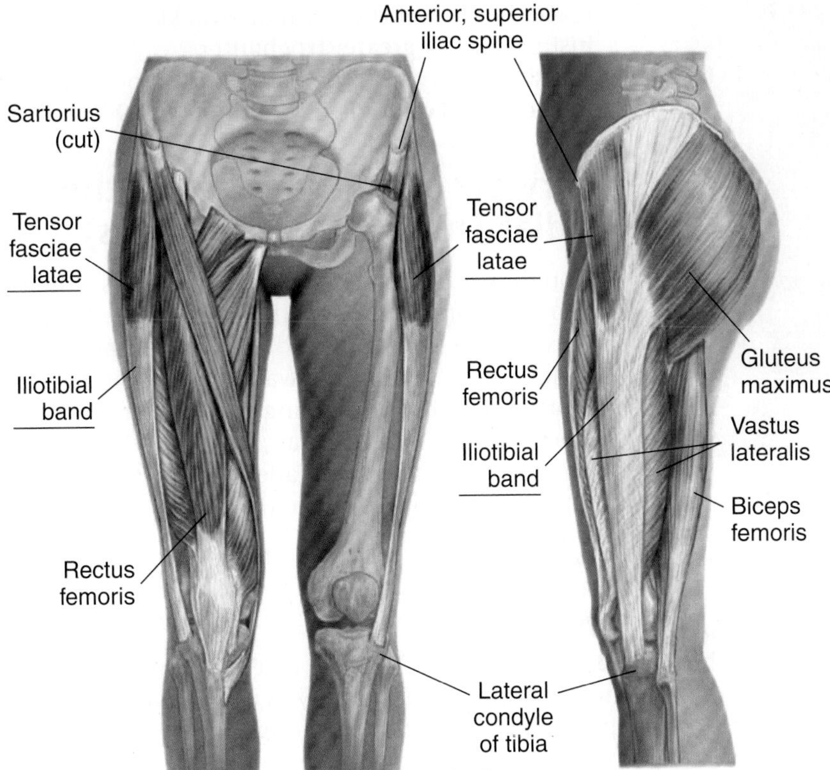

FIGURE 9-19 Anatomy of tensor fasciae latae and the iliotibial band

posteriorly into the iliotibial band (ITB). The ITB can be followed from there, and from gluteus maximus, down the side of the thigh to the lateral condyle of the tibia. The muscle architecture is parallel.

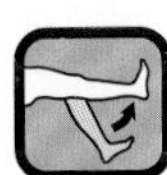

ACTION

Tenses fascia lata; flexes, abducts, and medially rotates hip; also contributes to the lateral stability of the knee

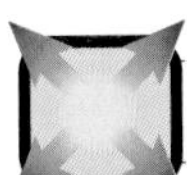

REFERRAL AREA

To the lateral aspect of the thigh

OTHER MUSCLES TO EXAMINE

Vastus lateralis

MANUAL THERAPY

TENSOR FASCIAE LATAE

Compression

- The client lies supine.
- The therapist stands beside the client at the knee.
- Place the fingertips on the tensor fasciae latae between the greater trochanter and the crest of the ilium.
- Press firmly into the tissue, searching for tender areas. Hold for release (Fig. 9-20).

Stripping

- The client lies supine.
- The therapist stands beside the client at the chest.
- Place the fingertips, thumb, or knuckles on the tensor fasciae latae just below the iliac crest.
- Pressing firmly into the tissue, glide along the muscle past the greater trochanter (Fig. 9-21).
- Continue the stroke with the next technique for the ITB.

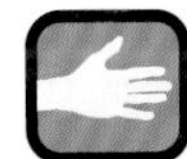

MANUAL THERAPY

THE ILIOTIBIAL BAND (ITB)

Stripping

- The client lies supine.
- The therapist stands beside the client at the waist.
- Place the heel of the hand or knuckles on the ITB just below the greater trochanter.
- Pressing firmly into the tissue, glide along the ITB to the lateral condyle of the tibia (Fig. 9-22).

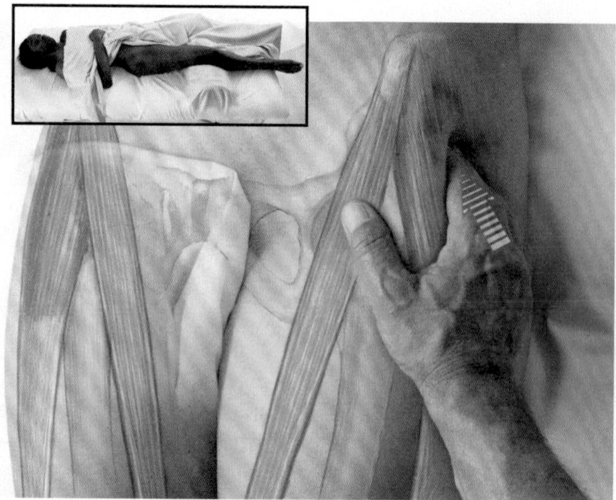

FIGURE 9-20 Compression of tensor fasciae latae with the fingertips

Stripping

- The client lies on her or his side, with the lower leg straight, and the upper leg flexed at the hip and the knee.
- The therapist stands behind the client at the pelvis.
- Place the heel of the hand or knuckles on the ITB just below the greater trochanter.
- Pressing firmly into the tissue, slide along the ITB to the lateral condyle of the tibia (Fig. 9-23).

Overview of the Muscles of the Medial Thigh (Hip Adductors)

Although we associate the hip adductors chiefly with adduction of the hip, they contribute to flexion, extension, rotation, and stability of the hip in complex ways in standing, walking, climbing stairs, and other activities involving the legs. In your assessment of the client's gait, observe the medial thigh closely for any anomalies such as twitches or catches in the motion of the thigh.

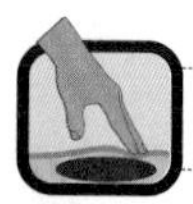

PALPATION

The superior attachments of these muscles follow the pubis from the symphysis all the way to the ischial tuberosity. Adductor longus is the most prominent of the group as it attaches to the anterior,

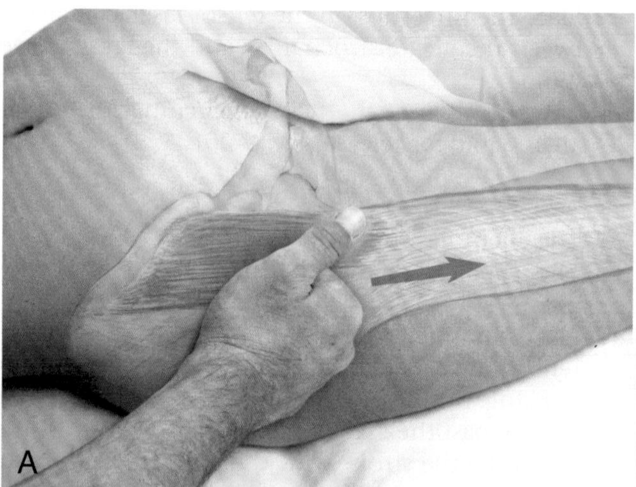

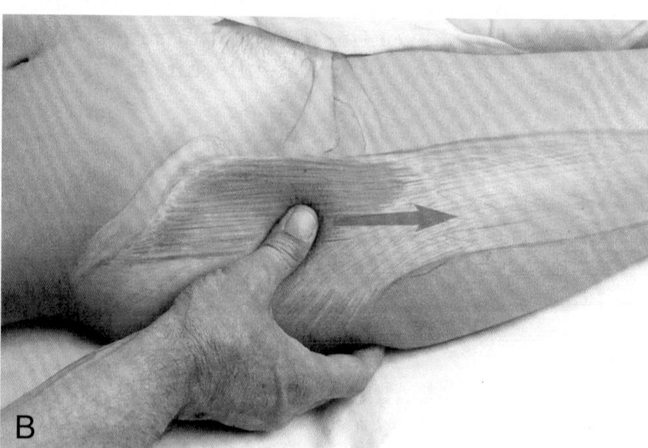

FIGURE 9-21 Stripping of tensor fasciae latae with the knuckles **(A)** and the thumb **(B)**

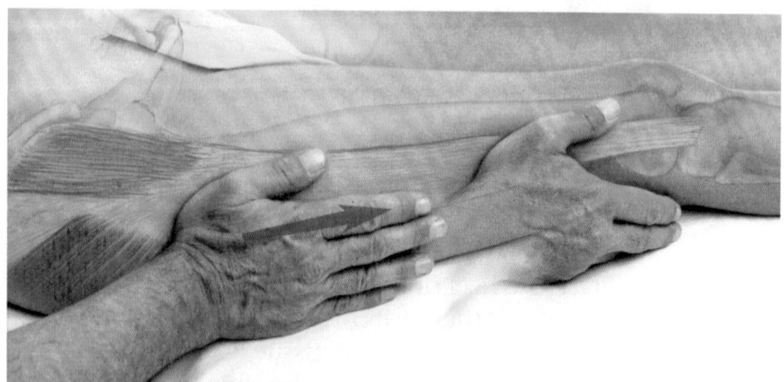

FIGURE 9-22 Stripping of iliotibial band with client supine

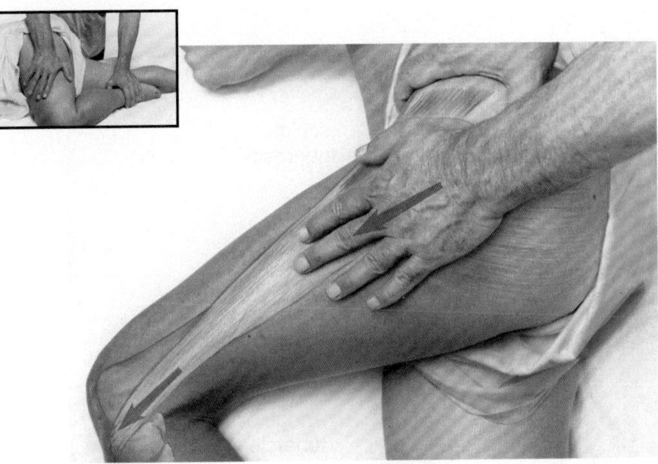
FIGURE 9-23 Stripping of iliotibial band with client side-lying

superior side of the pubic symphysis. Adductor brevis attaches lateral to it, and pectineus to the lateral end of the superior pubic ramus. Behind these are gracilis and then adductor magnus, which attaches to the ischiopubic ramus and the ischial tuberosity. Although it is difficult for the most part to distinguish the attachments, they can be easily palpated and followed from the pubic symphysis to the ischial tuberosity. The attachment of adductor magnus with gracilis to the pubis and ischium forms a distinctively large tendon. The inferior attachments are difficult to palpate except for adductor magnus, which attaches to the adductor tubercle of the femur, and gracilis, which attaches just below the tibial tuberosity. Their architectures are all convergent except gracilis, which is parallel. The area medial to the tibial tuberosity, encompassing the insertions of the semitendinosus, gracilis, and sartorius, is often referred to as the pes anserinus.

ETHICAL CAUTION

Palpation at the pubis may seem invasive; exercise extra care with draping and communication to maintain the client's feelings of safety and security. The client should always be allowed to keep their underwear on, if they prefer. Avoid touching pubic hair, and although you are working in close proximity, make special effort to avoid touching genitalia.

ADDUCTOR MAGNUS

ad-DUCK-ter MAG-nus

ETYMOLOGY Latin ***ad***, toward + ***ducere***, pull + ***magnus***, large

Overview

The adductor magnus is the largest and most powerful hip adductor. It also has the most extensive attachments and produces more types of movement than the others. The anterior, superior lateral part of adductor magnus (Fig. 9-24) is called adductor minimus when it sometimes forms a distinct muscle.

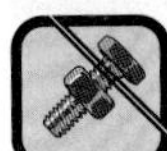

ATTACHMENTS

- Origin: lateral ischial tuberosity and ischiopubic ramus
- Insertion: linea aspera and adductor tubercle of the femur

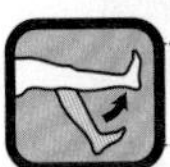

ACTION

Adducts the hip joint; parts of it can flex, extend, laterally and medially rotate the hip

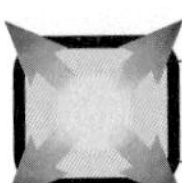

REFERRAL AREA

To the medial aspect of the thigh

OTHER MUSCLES TO EXAMINE

Other hip adductors

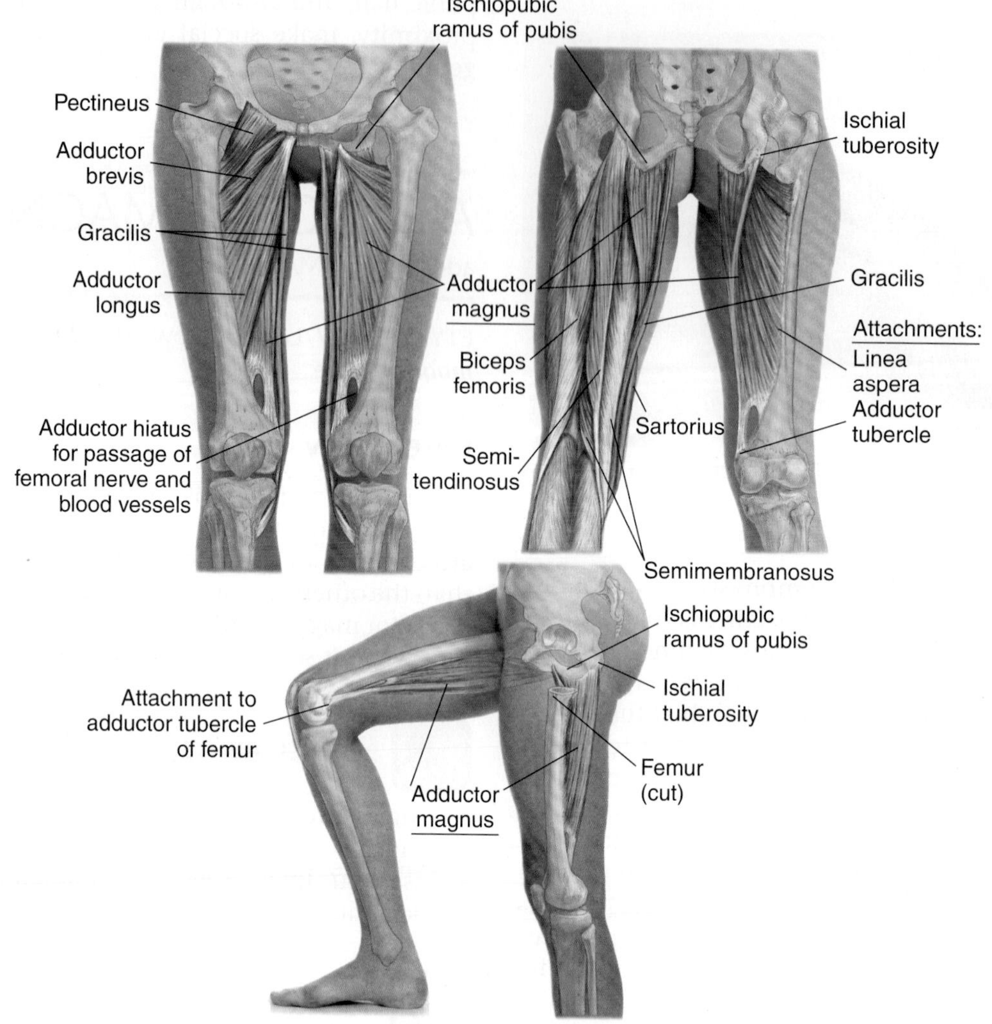

FIGURE 9-24 Anatomy of adductor magnus

ADDUCTOR LONGUS

ad-DUCK-ter LONG-gus

ETYMOLOGY Latin ***ad***, toward + ***ducere***, pull + ***longus***, long

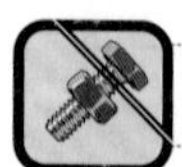

ATTACHMENTS

- Origin: just lateral to the symphysis and below the crest of pubis (Fig. 9-25)
- Insertion: middle third of medial lip of linea aspera of the femur

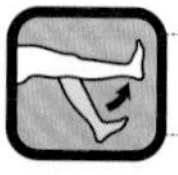

ACTION

Adducts, flexes and laterally rotates the hip

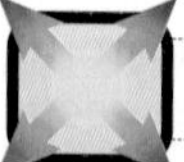

REFERRAL AREA

To the medial aspect of the thigh

OTHER MUSCLES TO EXAMINE

Other hip adductors

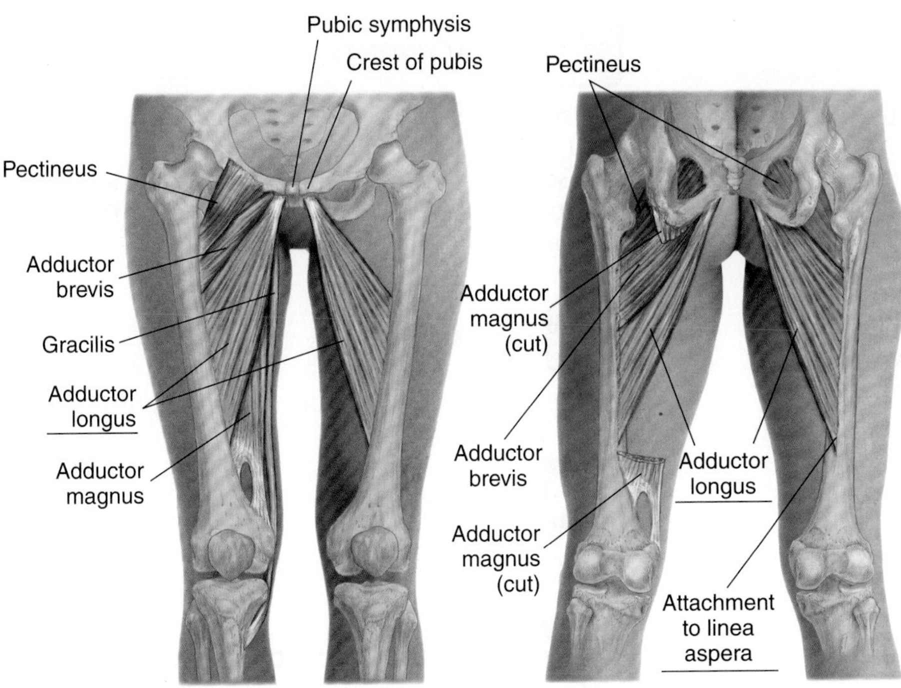

FIGURE 9-25 Anatomy of adductor longus

ADDUCTOR BREVIS

ad-DUCK-ter BREV-is

ETYMOLOGY Latin ***ad***, toward + ***ducere***, pull + ***brevis***, short

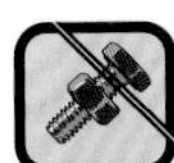

ATTACHMENTS

- Origin: inferior ramus of the pubis (Fig. 9-26)
- Insertion: upper third of medial lip of linea aspera

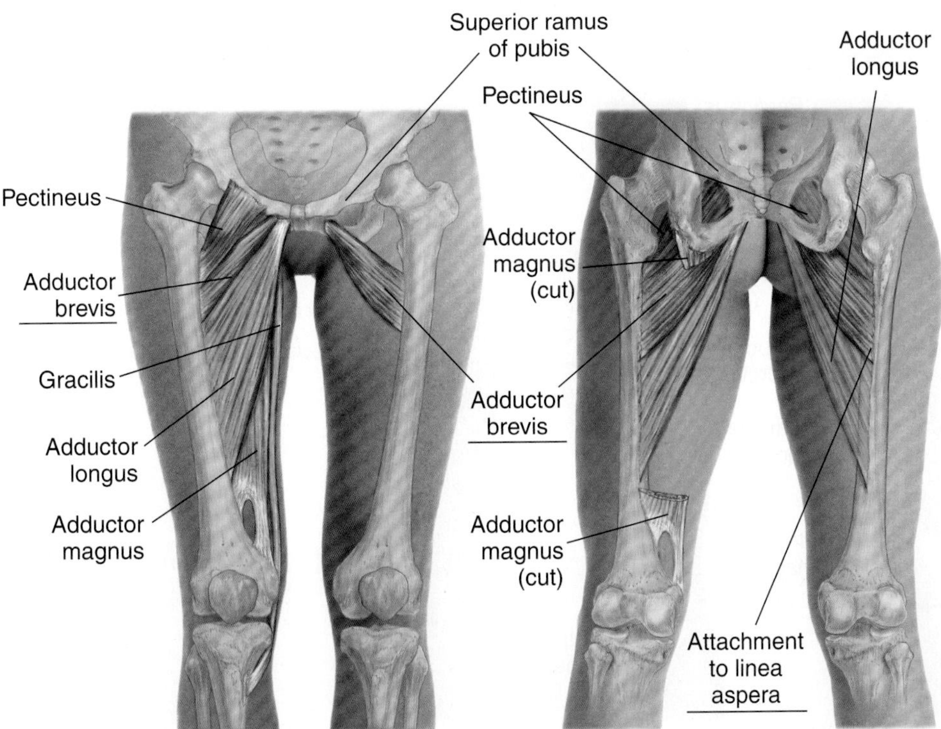

FIGURE 9-26 Anatomy of adductor brevis

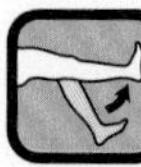

ACTION

Adducts, flexes and laterally rotates the hip

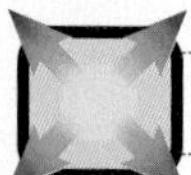

REFERRAL AREA

To the medial aspect of the thigh

OTHER MUSCLES TO EXAMINE

Other hip adductors

PECTINEUS

peck-TIN-ee-us

ETYMOLOGY Latin ***pecten***, comb

Overview

Pectineus (Fig. 9-27) is named for its attachment to the pecten, a sharp ridge on the superior pubic ramus.

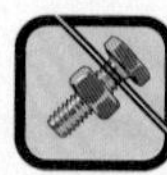

ATTACHMENTS

- Origin: crest of the pubis and laterally along the superior pubic ramus (the pecten)
- Insertion: pectineal line of the posterior femur between the lesser trochanter and the linea aspera

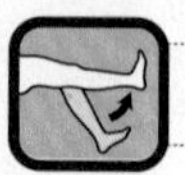

ACTION

Adducts, flexes and laterally rotates the hip

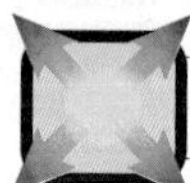

REFERRAL AREA

To the medial aspect of the thigh

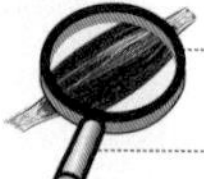

OTHER MUSCLES TO EXAMINE

Other hip adductors

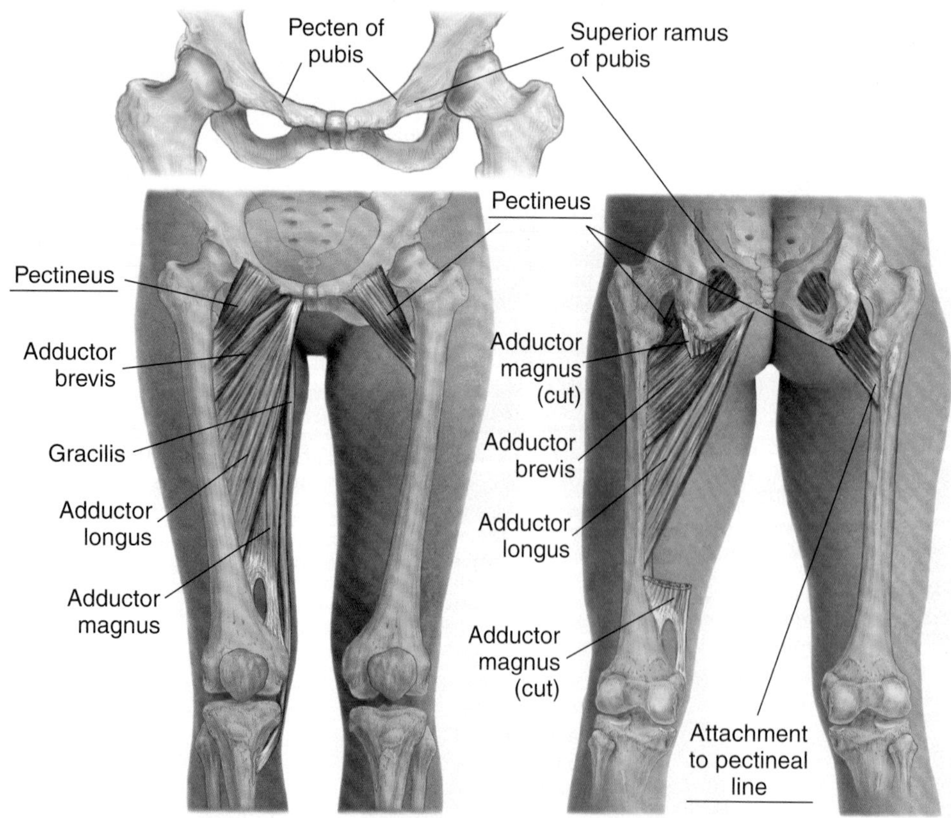

FIGURE 9-27 Anatomy of pectineus

GRACILIS

GRASS-ill-iss, gra-SILL-iss

ETYMOLOGY Latin ***gracilis***, slender

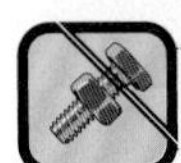

ATTACHMENTS

- Origin: body and inferior ramus of the pubis near the symphysis (Fig. 9-28)
- Insertion: anterior, medial condyle of the tibia after passing behind the knee with sartorius and semitendinosus

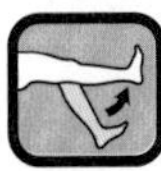

ACTION

Adducts the hip, flexes the knee, rotates the flexed knee medially

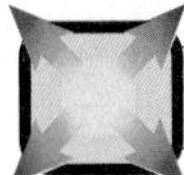

REFERRAL AREA

To the medial aspect of the thigh

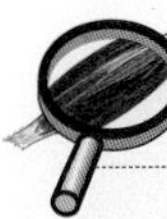

OTHER MUSCLES TO EXAMINE

Other hip adductors

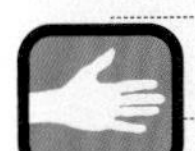

MANUAL THERAPY

THE HIP ADDUCTORS

Compression of the Adductor Attachments

- The client lies supine.
- The therapist stands beside the client at the knee.
- Place your thumb on the lateral edge of the pubic crest on the attachment of pectineus (Fig. 9-29).
- Press firmly into the tissue, looking for tender spots. Hold for release.
- Shift the thumb inferiorly and posteriorly along the pubic crest, compressing each adductor attachment (Fig. 9-30).
- Repeat this procedure until you reach the attachment of adductor magnus (Fig. 9-31).
- This technique may also be performed with the hip abducted and externally rotated and the knee partially flexed and may also be performed with the fingertips (Fig. 9-32).

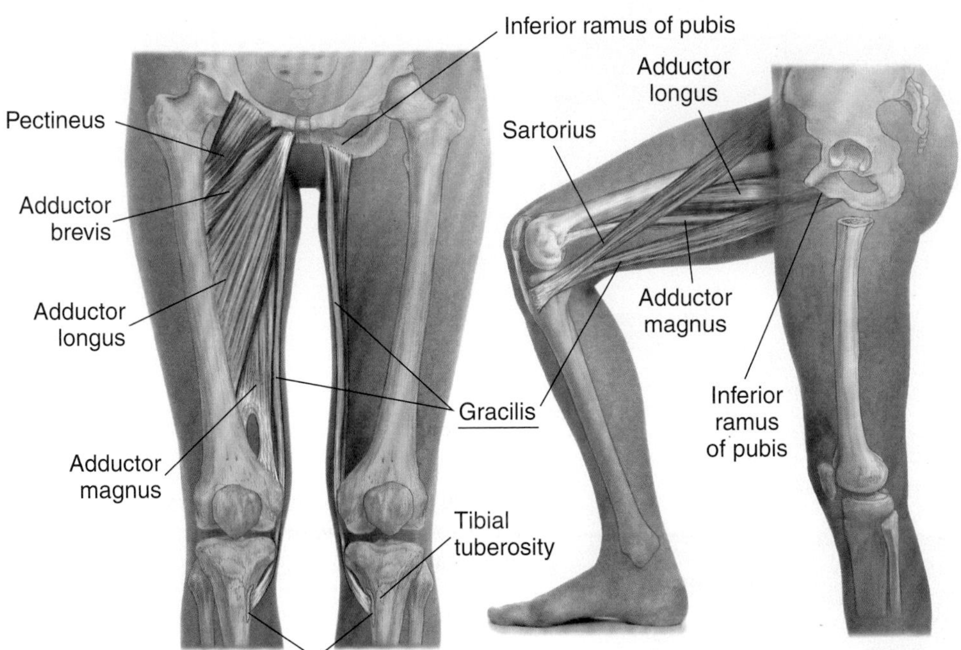

FIGURE 9-28 Anatomy of gracilis

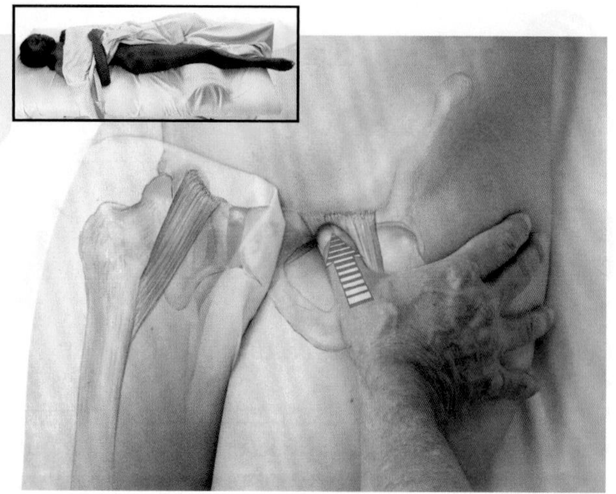

FIGURE 9-29 Compression of attachment of pectineus

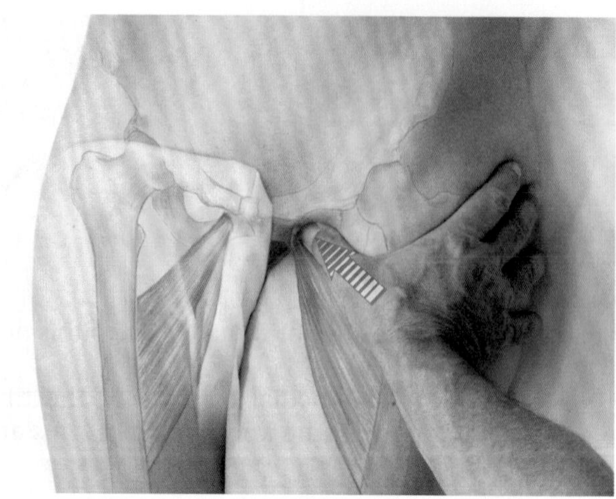

FIGURE 9-30 Compression of attachment of adductor brevis

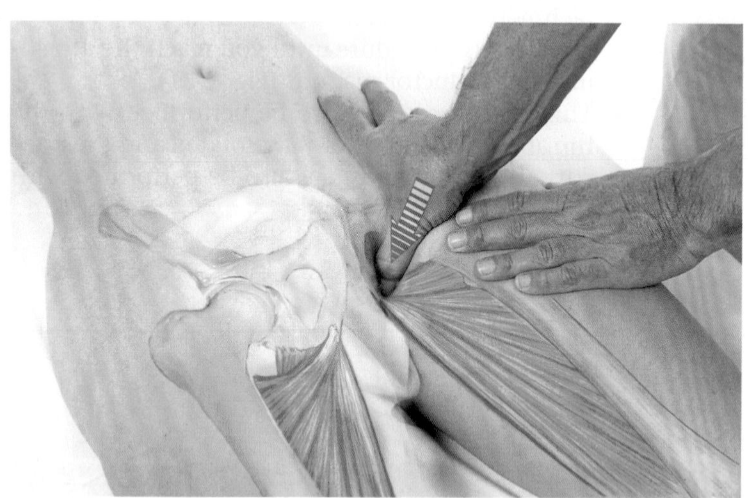

FIGURE 9-31 Compression of attachment of adductor magnus with thumb

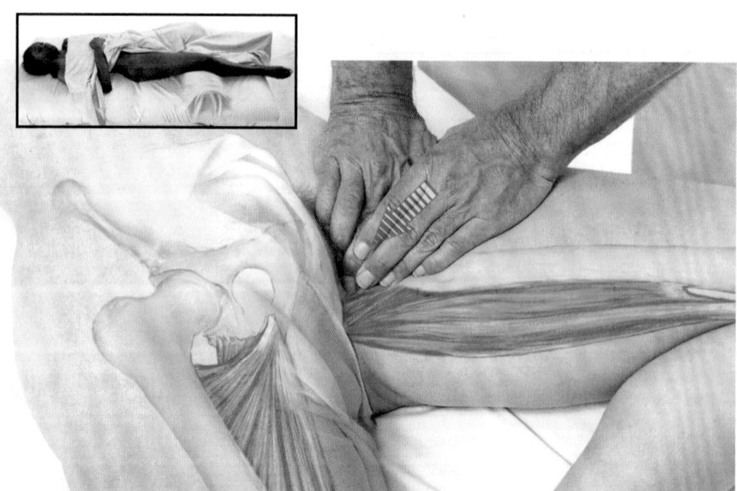

FIGURE 9-32 Compression of attachment of adductor magnus with fingertips, hip abducted and rotated

Stripping and Compression of the Hip Adductors

- The client lies supine, either with the leg straight and the hip slightly abducted, or with the hip abducted and externally rotated and the knee partially flexed.
- The therapist stands beside the client at the knees.
- Place the fingertips or thumb(s) just above the medial epicondyle of the femur.
- Pressing firmly into the tissue, glide the fingertips along the adductors to the anterior aspect of the pubic arch.
- Beginning at the same spot, repeat this procedure, ending each time more posteriorly along the pubis (Fig. 9-33, Fig. 9-34, Fig. 9-35).

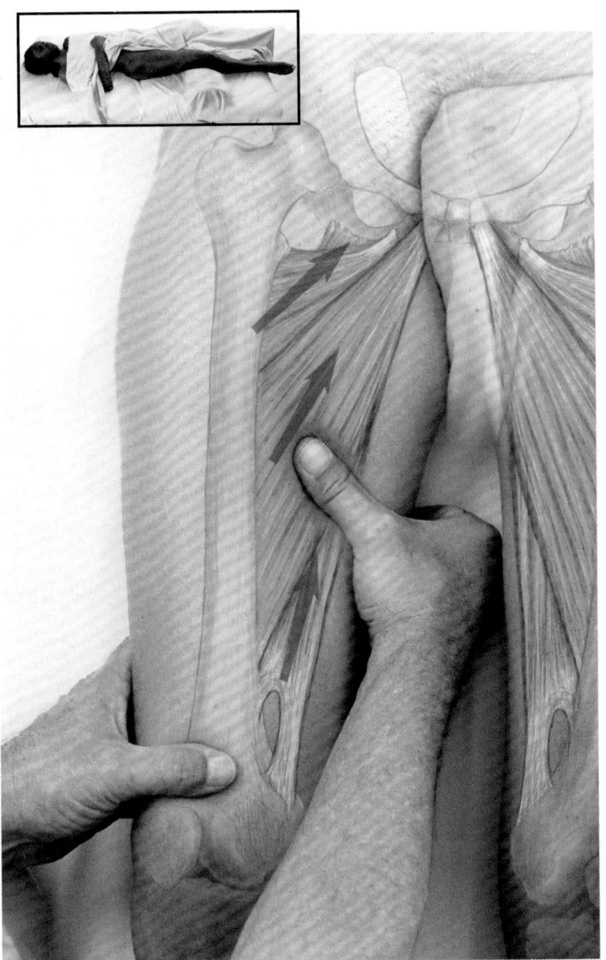

FIGURE 9-33 Stripping of adductor magnus and longus with thumb, client supine, leg straight, hip slightly abducted

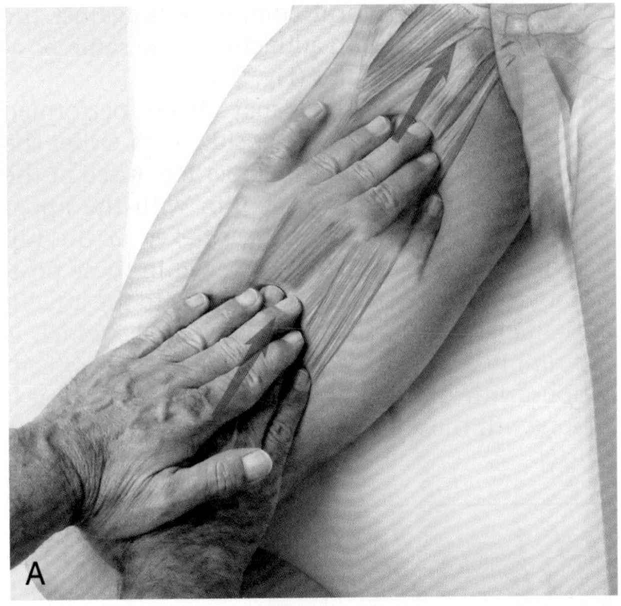

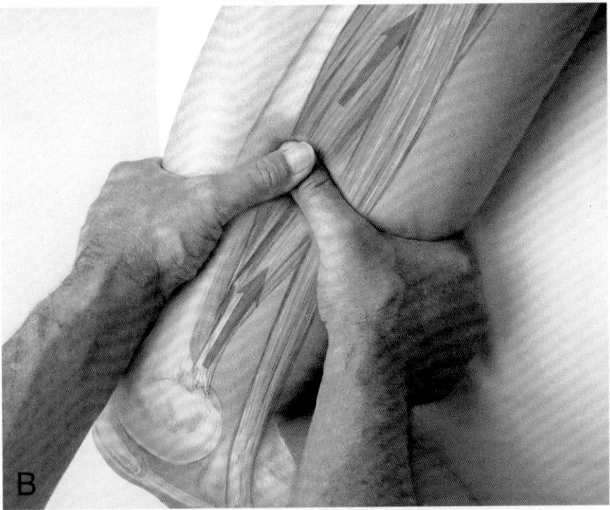

FIGURE 9-34 Stripping of adductor magnus and gracilis, client supine, hip abducted and externally rotated, hip and knee flexed: with fingertips **(A)** and with thumb **(B)**

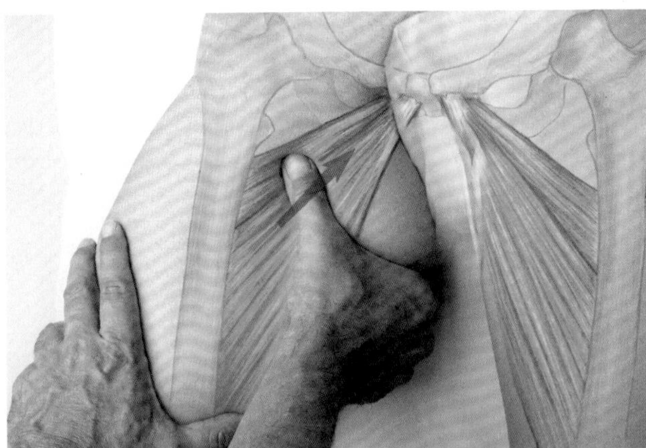

FIGURE 9-35 Stripping of adductor brevis and longus with thumb, client supine, hip abducted and externally rotated, hip and knee flexed.

- You may also perform compression against the femur along each hip adductor in the same position, using the thumbs (Fig. 9-36).
- Both of these procedures may also be performed with the client lying on her side, with either the lower leg straight and the upper leg flexed at the hip and the knee (Fig. 9-37), or with the upper leg straight and the lower leg flexed at the hip and the knee (Fig. 9-38). However, in these positions it is not possible to work close to the attachments without contacting the genitals, which is prohibited in most regulated states. Be very cautious with draping and keep open communication with the client so there is no discomfort.

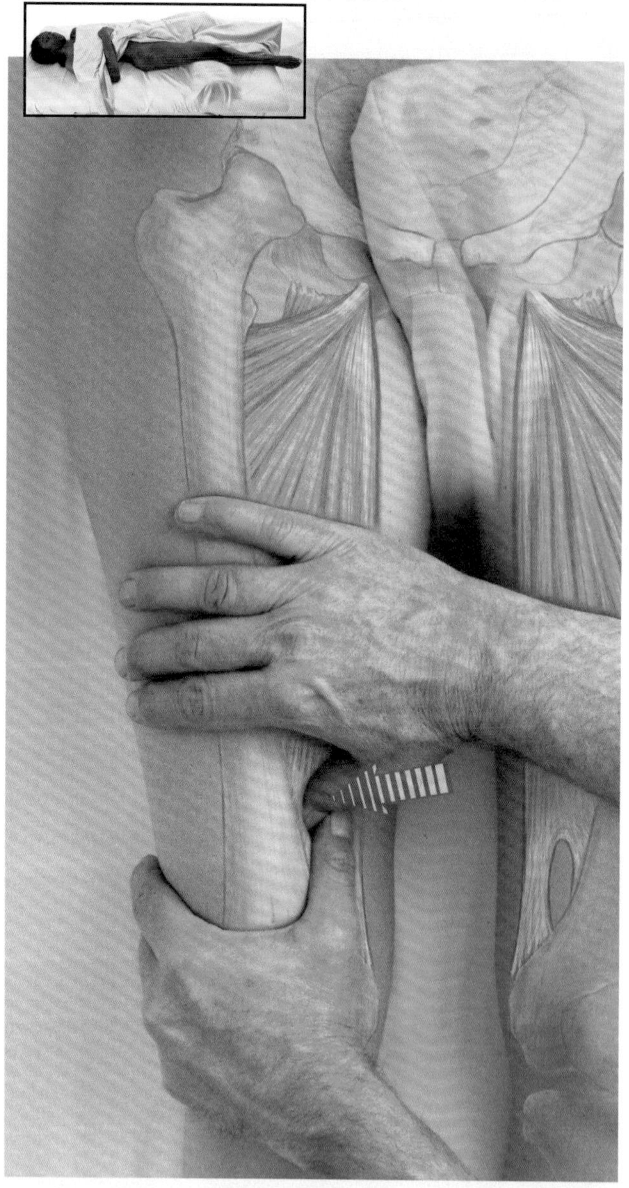

FIGURE 9-36 Compression of adductor magnus with thumb, leg straight

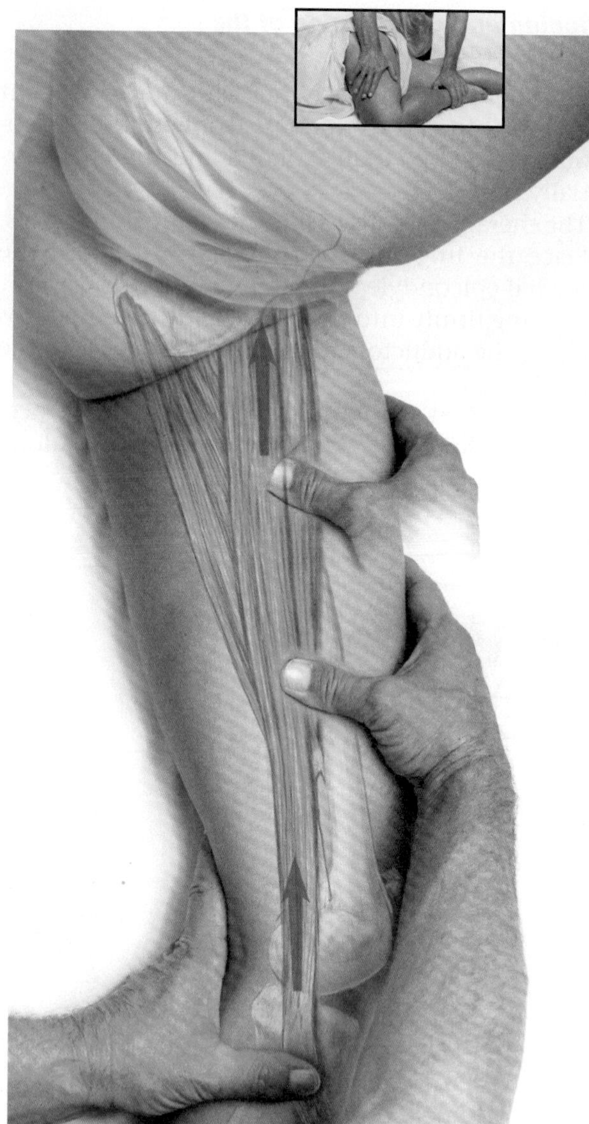

FIGURE 9-37 Stripping of adductors with client side-lying, lower leg straight

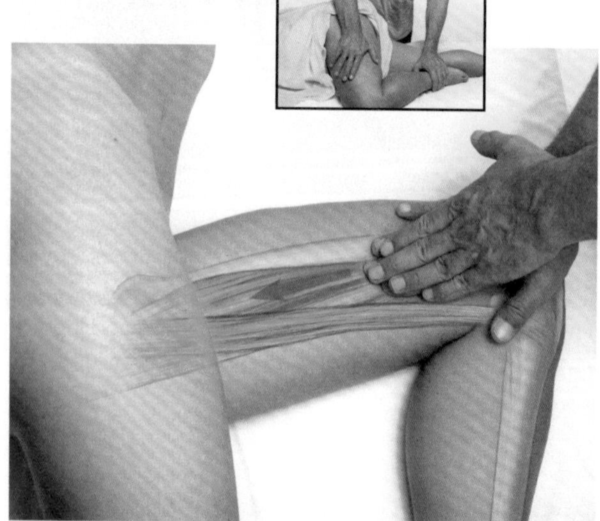

FIGURE 9-38 Stripping of adductors with client side-lying, upper leg straight

CHAPTER REVIEW

CASE STUDY

C.G. is a 64-year-old woman who is taking care of her elderly mother full-time. She stated that her life-long hobby was ballroom dancing until about two years ago, when she underwent a hip replacement. She felt that something went wrong during the surgery; when she came out of anesthesia she said her leg didn't feel "quite right," and as the weeks progressed, she stated that her knee was turning out to the side when it had not done that prior to the surgery. After receiving physical therapy for several weeks with no improvement, the doctor decided to operate again and discovered that a muscle had not been properly reattached; she could not recall which one but thought it was a gluteal muscle. She did not feel that the second surgery, or the subsequent physical therapy, had really improved the situation.

C.G. had seen by chance on the Internet that I was traveling to her country to teach massage classes and contacted me to ask for a consultation. When I saw her she was in obvious distress; the right thigh and knee were rotated laterally. Gait assessment showed awkwardness—like a waddling gait, but not quite, because of the turnout. She stated that it was not painful except some residual pain around the surgery site itself—she was most upset about not being able to dance; she stated that although she had practiced some in the privacy of her home she was embarrassed to dance in public because of the turned leg and awkwardness. Palpation revealed that her thigh and gluteal muscles felt almost flaccid. Assessment demonstrated substantially less strength in the right leg than the left.

As I was only in her town for the day, I could not personally treat C.G. I promised to find an orthopedic massage therapist to help her and was able to locate one near her to refer her to. C.G. emailed me about three months after our consult to say that she had been receiving massage frequently since our meeting and that the therapist was using techniques to strengthen her leg. She stated that while it was not 100% restored, her leg and knee looked almost in their normal position and that she was out walking every day for exercise without feeling self-conscious about her walk. She stated that she intended to start attending dances again soon. With her permission, I spoke to her therapist, who stated that she had been using massage therapy and muscle energy techniques with good success. She had also persuaded C.G. to seek some help in caring for her mother, due to the amount of stress it was putting on her, and stated that her physical condition seemed to start improving as her stress improved.

L.A., LMBT

REVIEW QUESTIONS

1. _______ crosses both the hip joint and the knee joint.
   a. Adductor brevis
   b. Adductor magnus
   c. Pectineus
   d. Rectus femoris

2. Although they are involved in other movements, the medial muscles of the thigh primarily perform _______.
   a. Extension
   b. Adduction
   c. Abduction
   d. Dorsiflexion

3. The muscles of the **quadriceps** group attach to the ______ via a common tendon enclosing the patella.
   a. Fibula
   b. Femur
   c. Tibia
   d. ASIS

4. A taut sartorius can interfere with the stretching of the ______.
   a. Piriformis
   b. Gluteus maximus
   c. Tibialis anterior
   d. Vastus lateralis

5. Two endangerment sites to be aware of when working the thigh muscles are the _______ and _______ triangles.
   a. Temporal and obturator
   b. Femur and lateralis
   c. Gracilis and vasus medialis
   d. Femoral and popliteal

6. The longest muscle of the body is the _______.
   a. Gracilis
   b. Sartorius
   c. Biceps femoris
   d. Iliotibial band

7. The superior part of adductor magnus is the adductor _______.
   a. Inferior
   b. Posterior
   c. Minimus
   d. Lateralis

8. The _______ is a sharp ridge on the superior pubic ramus.
   a. Pecten
   b. Symphysis
   c. Pectineous
   d. Gracilis

9. The muscle that is grouped with vastus lateralis, vastus medialis, and vastus intermedius is the _______.
   a. Hamstring
   b. Iliotibial band
   c. Rectus femoris
   d. Adductor brevis

10. The massage therapist should be sensitive to invasiveness, using careful draping and clear client communication, when working the anterior thigh because many of the muscles attach on the ______.
    a. Tibial tuberosity
    b. ASIS
    c. PSIS
    d. PubisFIGURE 9-1 Anatomy of quadriceps femoris

thePoint Additional helpful resources are available at http://thePoint.lww.com.

CHAPTER 10

The Leg, Ankle, and Foot

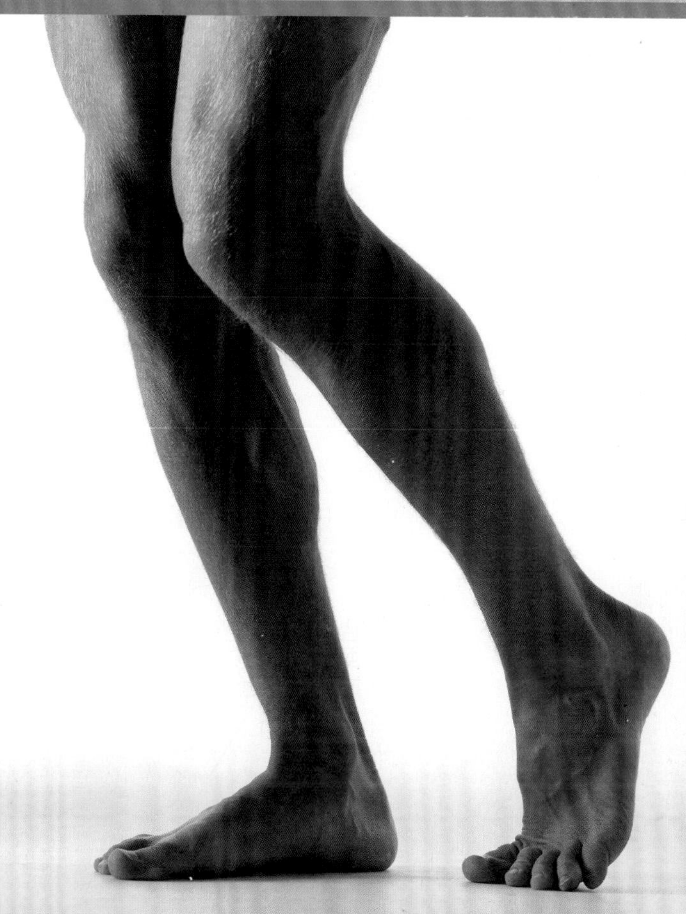

LEARNING OBJECTIVES

At the end of this chapter, the learner will be able to:

- State the correct terminology of the muscles of the leg, ankle, and foot.
- Palpate the muscles of the leg, ankle, and foot.
- Identify their attachments at the origins and insertions.
- Explain the actions of the muscles.
- Describe their pain referral areas.
- Recall related muscles.
- Recognize any endangerment sites and ethical cautions for massage therapy.
- Demonstrate proficiency in manual therapy techniques for muscles of the leg, ankle, and foot.

The Overview of the Region begins on page 316, after the anatomy plates.

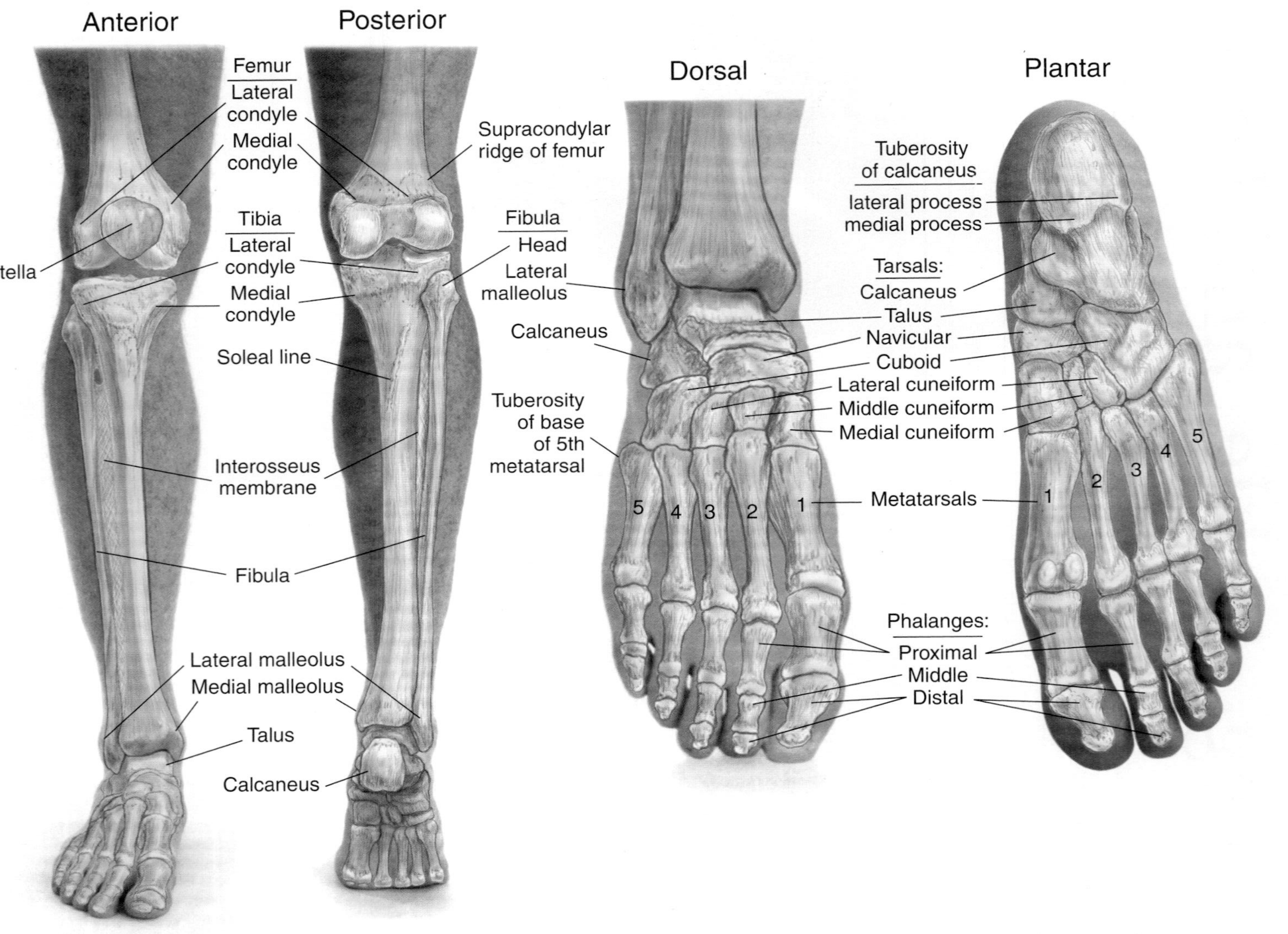

PLATE 10-1 ■ Skeletal features of the leg and foot

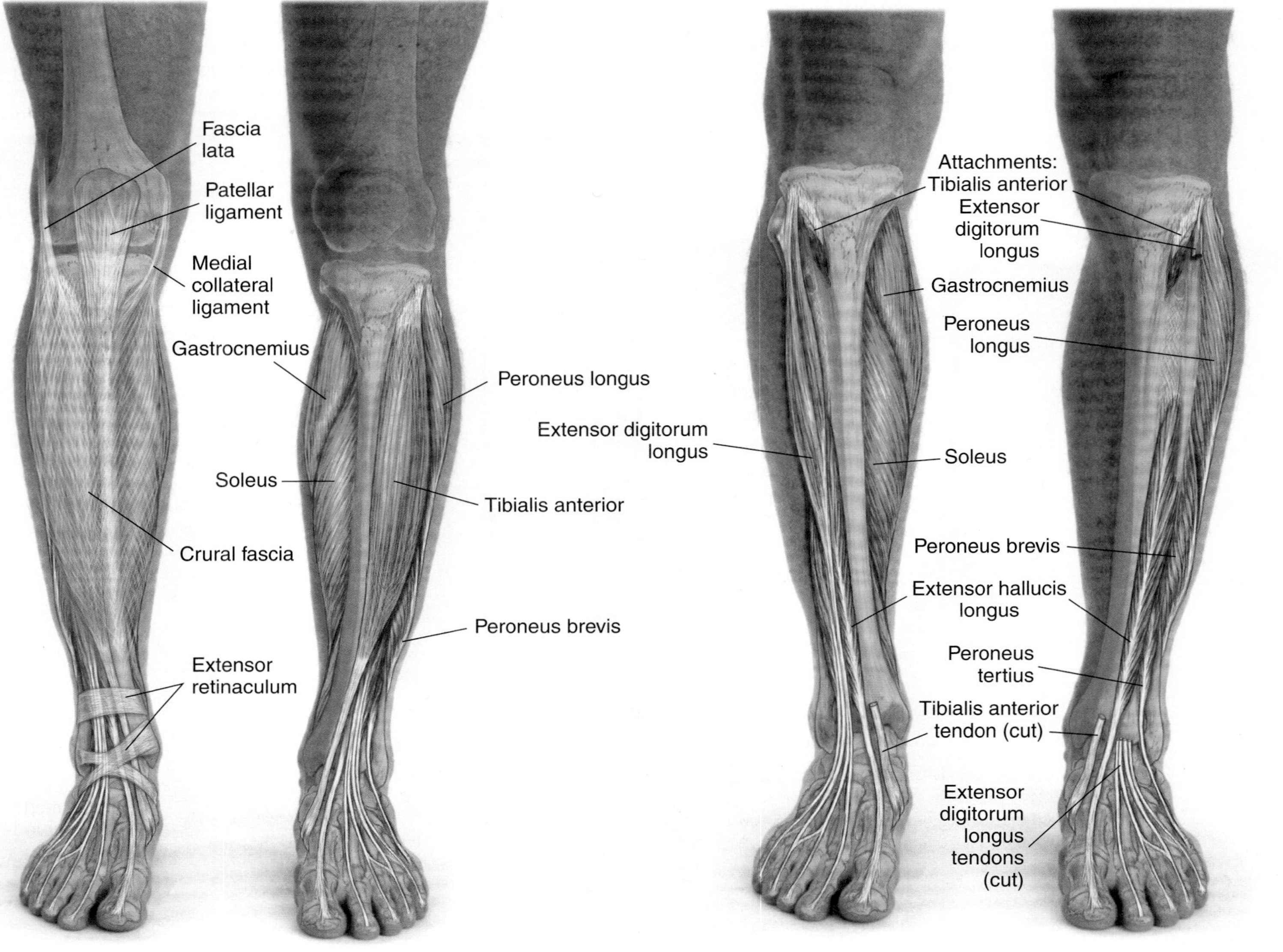

PLATE 10-2 ■ Muscles of the leg, anterior view

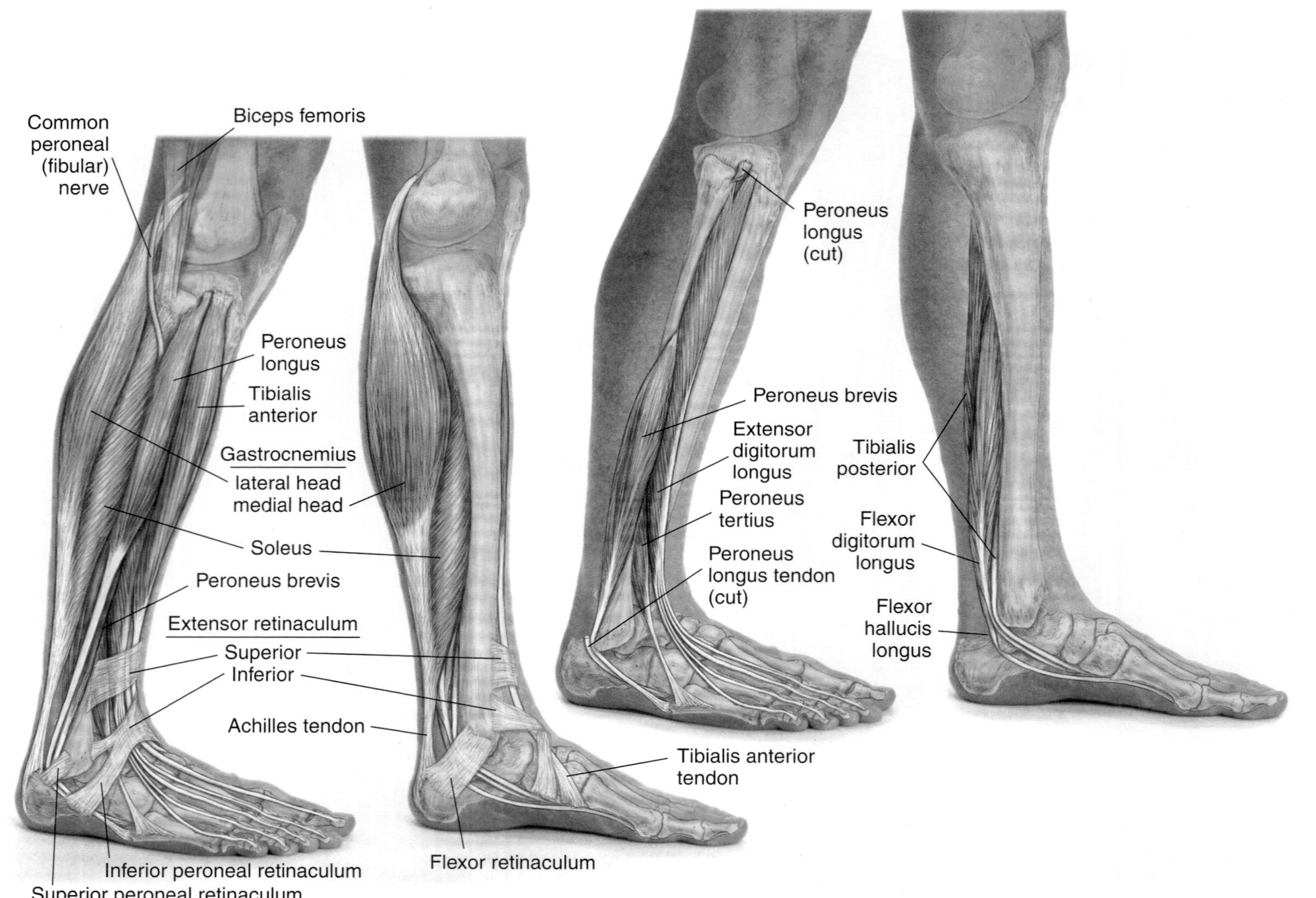

PLATE 10-3 ■ Muscles of the leg, lateral and medial views

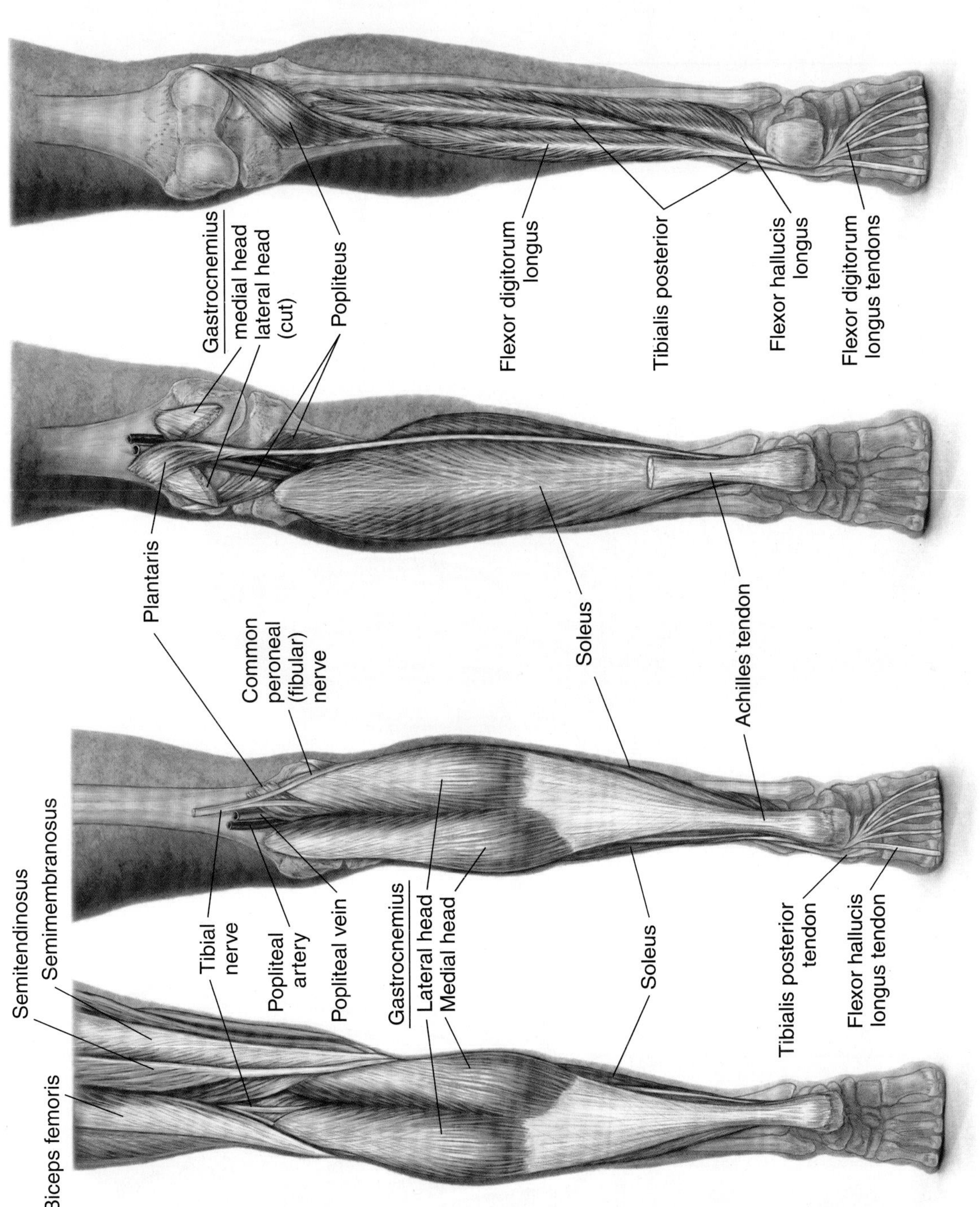

PLATE 10-4 ■ Muscles of the leg, posterior view

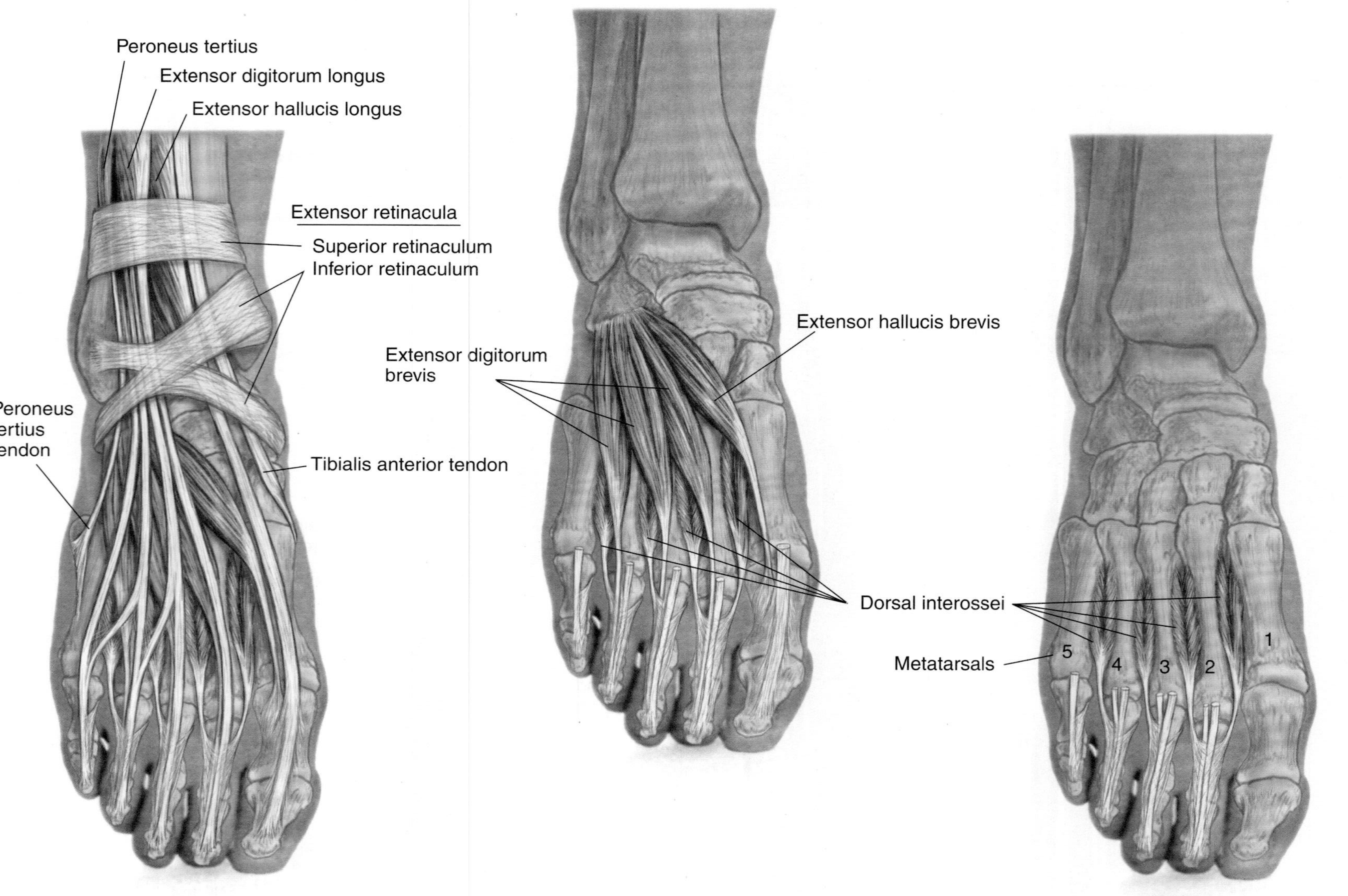

PLATE 10-5 ■ Intrinsic muscles of the foot, dorsal view

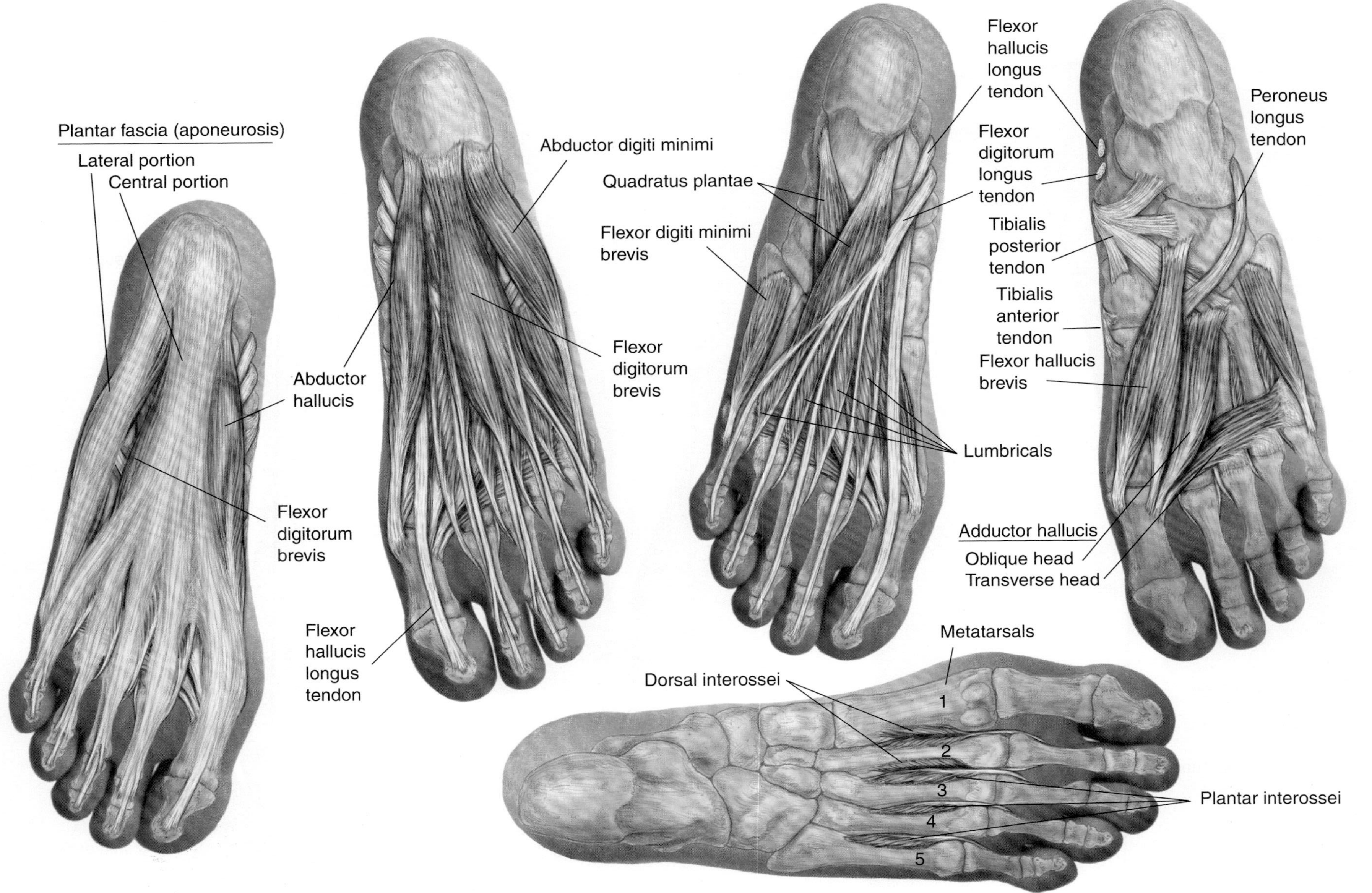

PLATE 10-6 ■ Intrinsic muscles of the foot, plantar view

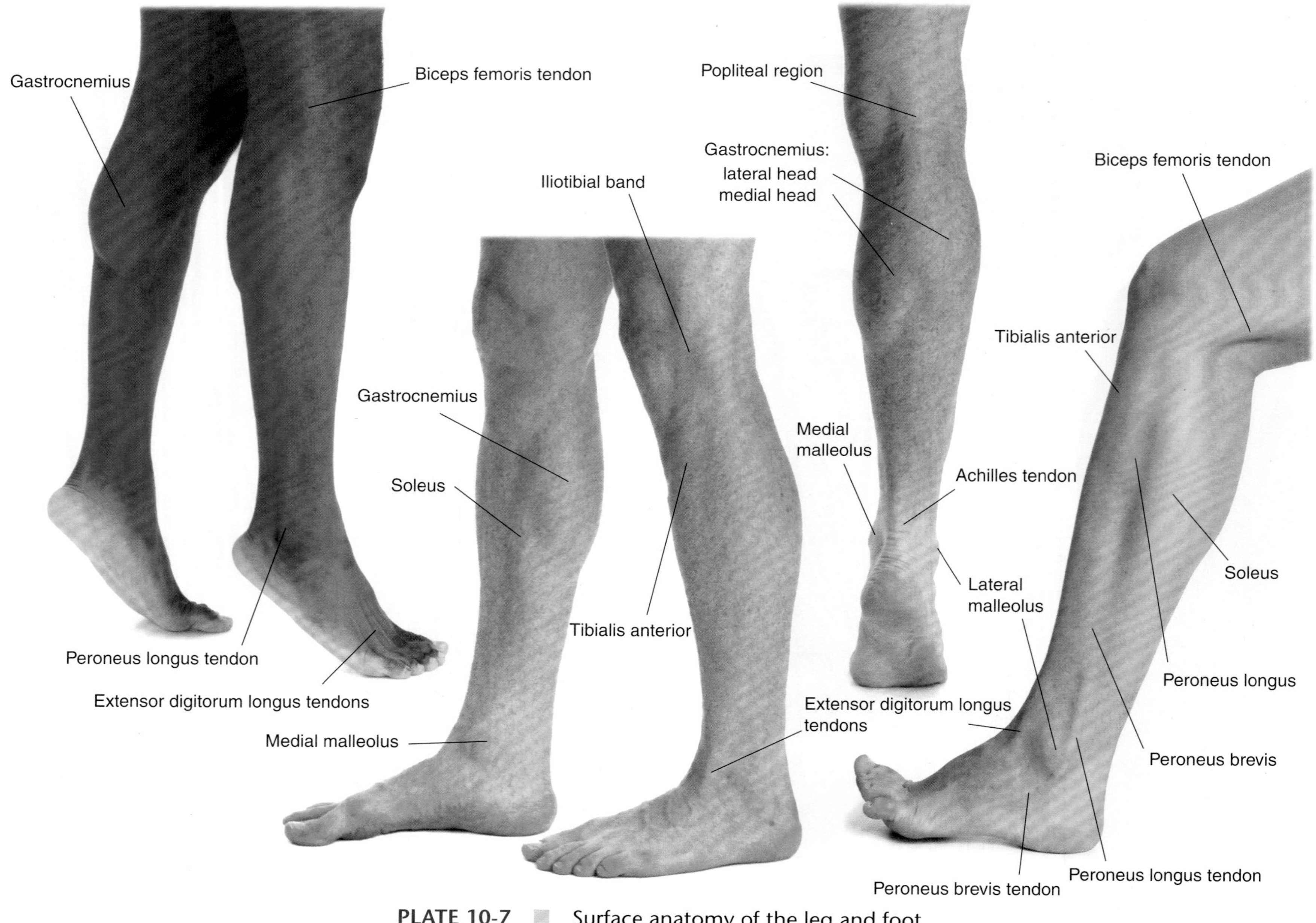

PLATE 10-7 ■ Surface anatomy of the leg and foot

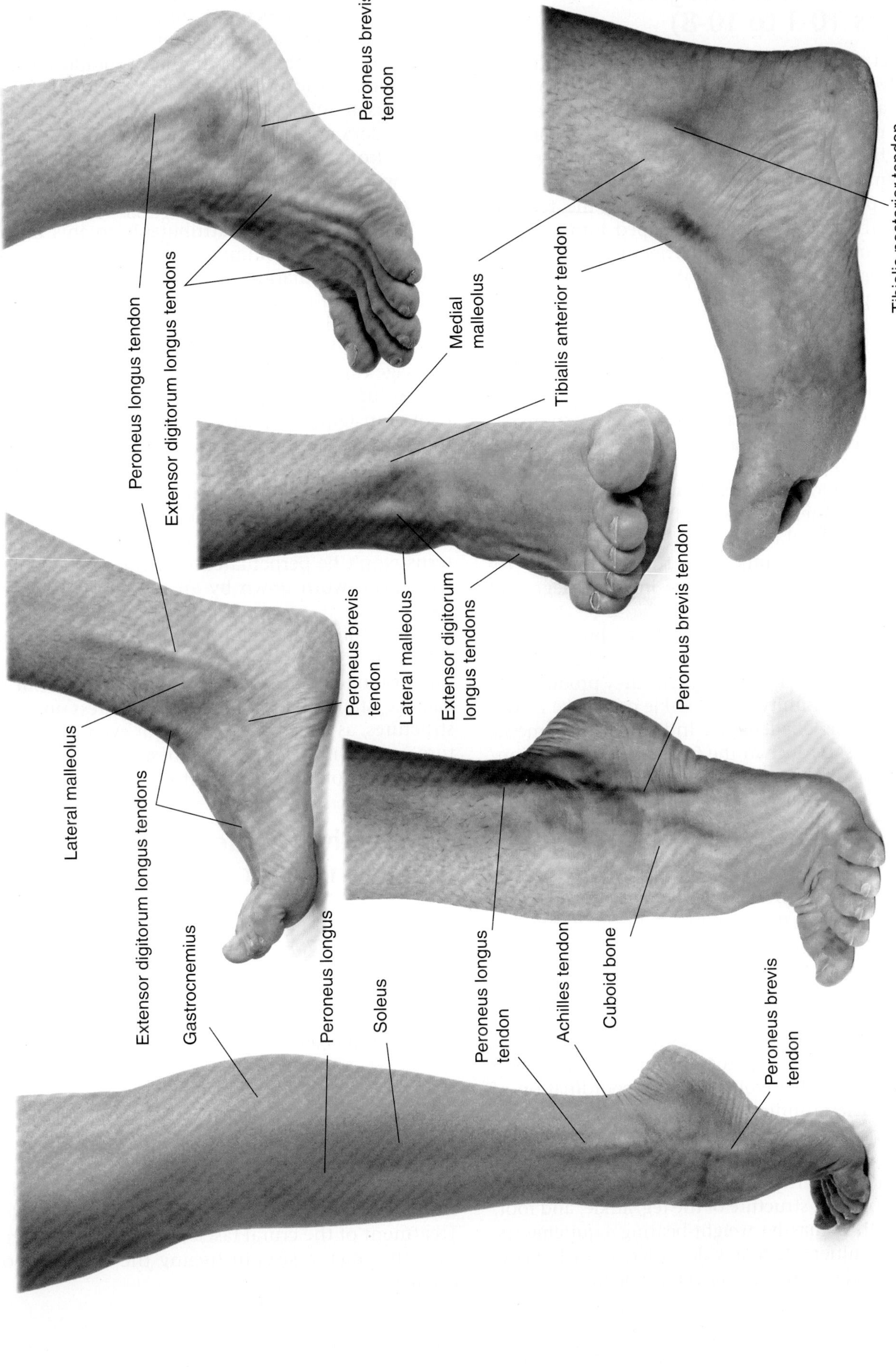

Lateral malleolus
Extensor digitorum longus tendons
Peroneus longus tendon
Extensor digitorum longus tendons
Peroneus brevis tendon
Peroneus brevis tendon
Extensor digitorum longus tendons
Gastrocnemius
Peroneus longus
Soleus
Peroneus longus tendon
Achilles tendon
Cuboid bone
Peroneus brevis tendon
Peroneus brevis tendon
Lateral malleolus
Extensor digitorum longus tendons
Medial malleolus
Tibialis anterior tendon
Tibialis posterior tendon

PLATE 10-8 ■ Surface anatomy of the leg and foot

Overview of the Region (Plates 10-1 to 10-8)

The feet are the foundation of the human body and the pivot points for its locomotion. Note that the bones and joints in the leg, ankle, and foot are similar in number to those in the forearm, wrist, and hand, but their functions and the demands placed on them are quite different.

The principal muscles controlling the feet are found in the leg. They are grouped into anterior, lateral, and posterior compartments separated by fascial partitions. Tendons of these muscles reach various points in the foot via the ankle, usually making right-angle turns and covering long distances to do so. Smaller muscles, referred to as the intrinsic muscles of the foot, are wholly contained within its structure. They assist movements of the larger leg muscles and some are solely responsible for abduction and adduction of the metatarsophalangeal (MP) joints.

The ankle joint allows for virtually no lateral or medial movement; it plantar flexes and dorsiflexes the foot. External and internal rotation of the feet is accomplished primarily at the hip or from rotation of the knee joint while in some degree of flexion.

The movements of the foot are produced by combined movements of the tarsal and metatarsal joints. The number of movements they produce and their close proximity to the ankle can make movement analysis challenging. Individual movements these joints produce in the foot include adduction/abduction, and inversion/eversion. These movements can further combine to produce supination and pronation. The MP and interphalangeal (IP) joints of the toes flex, extend (and hyperextend). The MP joints also abduct, and adduct.

Ankle plantar and dorsal flexion (dorsiflexion) are the primary movements of locomotion, and they are accompanied by complex activity in both the muscles of the foot that reside on the leg and the intrinsic muscles of the foot. In locomotion, weight is transferred successively from the back to the front as the action proceeds from the heel strike to the function of the toes in pushing off. Many other movements involve intricate coordination of these muscles: running, climbing, diving, and dancing, to name but a few. The healthy foot and leg are well equipped to carry out these activities with impressive dexterity.

The complex structure of the leg, ankle, and foot, along with its massive weight-bearing requirements, makes it vulnerable to a wide variety of orthopedic injuries and chronic myofascial problems.

Because they serve as the foundation, the feet, ankles, and legs affect and are profoundly affected by posture. For balanced posture, the center of gravity (balanced weight) of the body should balance at a point just forward of the ankle. The body will compensate in a variety of ways to ensure that the weight does not fall behind this point. If the weight falls in front of this point, the calf and foot muscles must work constantly to keep the body from falling forward. Chronic tautness and trigger points in the calf muscle are usually attributable to this imbalance and are very common.

Chronic supination or pronation of the foot is a dysfunction requiring correction appropriate to its cause and may necessitate surgery, corrective orthotics or boots, and/or physical therapy. While massage can help in many cases, it may not be the only solution or the primary solution. You can gain a lot of insight into postural problems just by looking at your client's shoes and noting the wear patterns. Therapists who specialize in Rolfing or other structural work often recommend that their clients discontinue wearing old shoes after postural corrections have taken place, so old imbalance patterns won't be perpetuated by wearing shoes that have been worn down by an inverted or everted foot.

Aside from traumatic injuries, the most stressful activity for the legs, ankles, and feet is simply standing for long periods of time. If the posture is out of balance, standing places tremendous stress on these structures, as already described. But even if the posture is good, muscles function best either in motion or at rest—not under constant stress.

Connective Tissue of the Leg, Ankle, and Foot

CRURAL FASCIA

KROO-rul FAHSH-uh

ETYMOLOGY Latin *cruralis,* belonging to the legs + *fasciae,* of the bandage

Overview

The crural fascia (Fig. 10-1) is the deep fascia of the entire lower limb. It is continuous with the fascia lata, attaches to the ligaments of the patella, and thickens at the ankle to form the retinacula. Treatment of the crural fascia, including the fascia over the tibia, assists in freeing the structures of the leg.

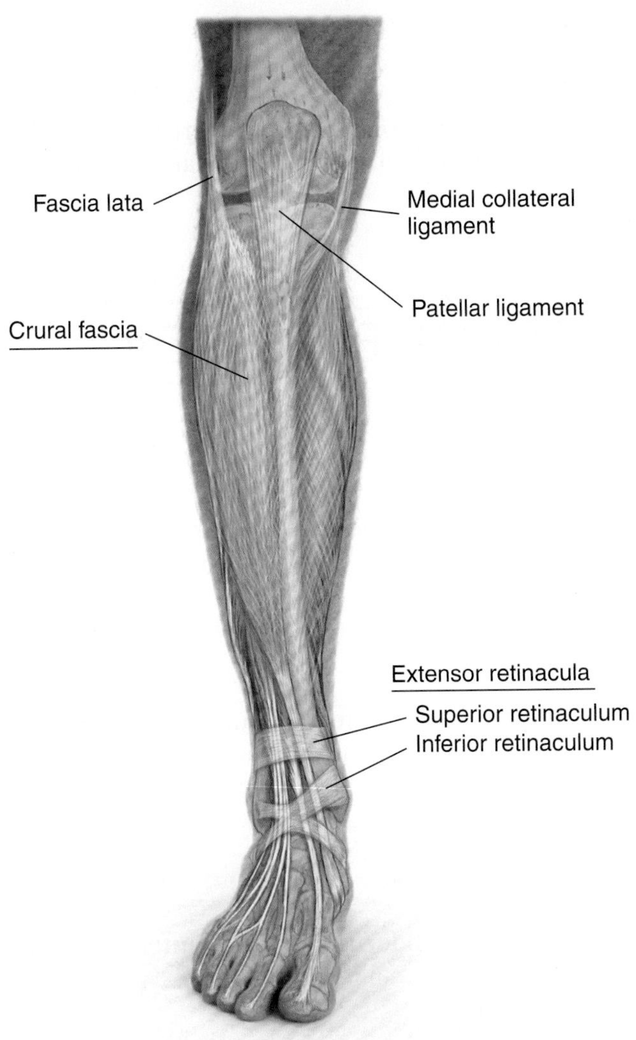

FIGURE 10-1 Anatomy of the crural fascia

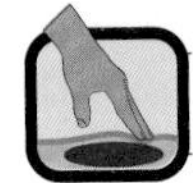

PALPATION

Not separately discernable from the muscle.

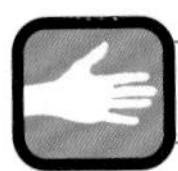

MANUAL THERAPY

Fascial Stripping

- The client lies supine.
- The therapist stands at the client's feet.
- Place the heel of the hand on the medial side of the leg just superior to the ankle.
- Pressing firmly into the tissue, slide the heel of the hand in a cephalad and posterior direction (Fig. 10-2A).

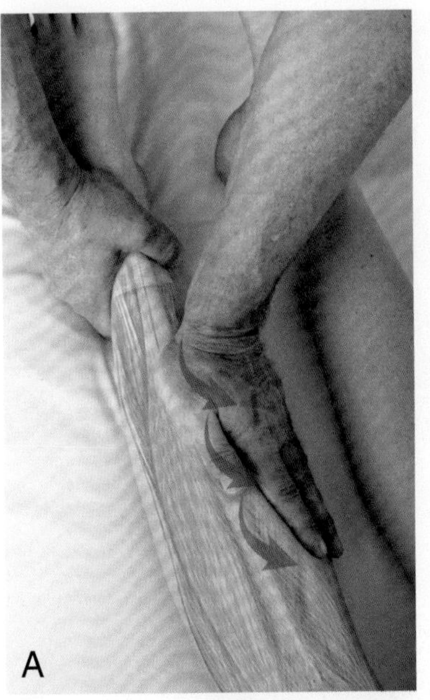

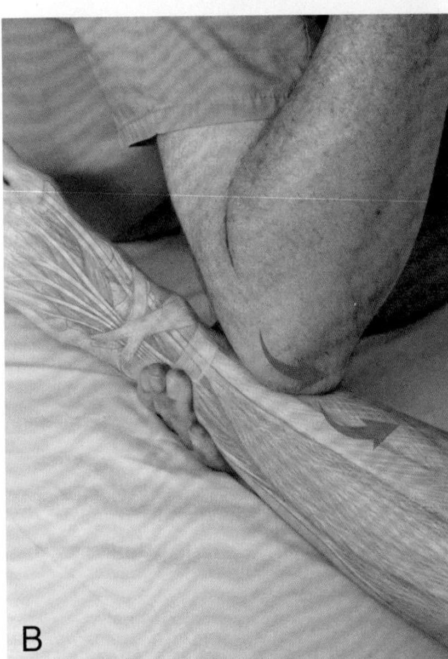

FIGURE 10-2 Deep stroking of the crural fascia with the heel of the hand **(A)** and the elbow **(B)**

- Repeat this procedure, with the hand just above the previous starting position.
- Repeat the same procedure, proceeding up the leg as far as the medial condyle.
- You may also use the elbow (Fig. 10-2B) or supported thumb (Fig. 10-3) for this procedure.

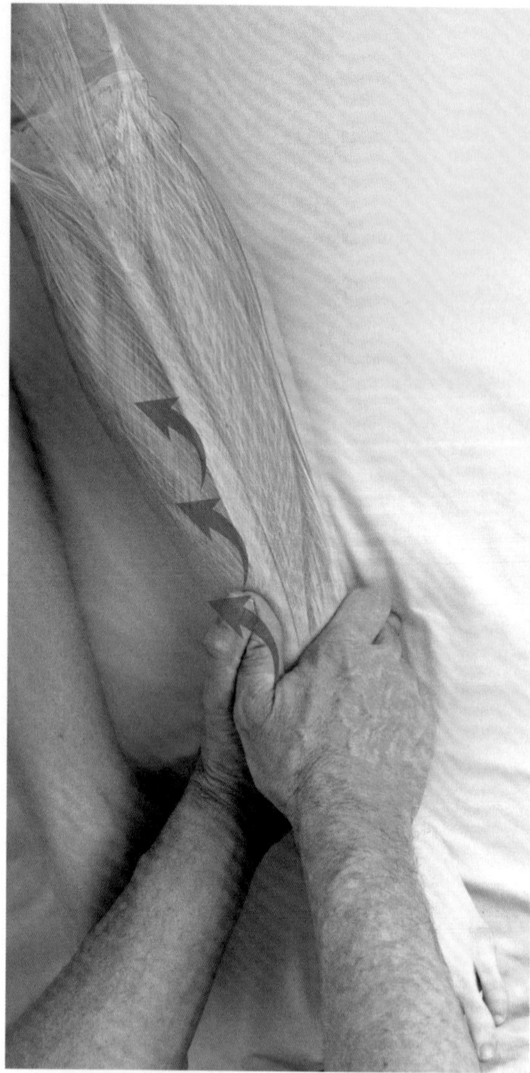

FIGURE 10-3 Deep stroking of the crural fascia with supported thumb

Flexor, Extensor, and Peroneal Retinacula

FLEXOR RETINACULUM

FLEX-er reh-tin-AK-yu-lum

ETYMOLOGY Latin ***flexor***, bender + ***retinaculum***, band or halter (from ***retinere***, to hold back)

Overview

The flexor retinaculum (Fig. 10-4) is a wide ligamentous band passing from the medial malleolus to the medial and upper border of the calcaneus and to the plantar surface as far as the navicular bone. It holds in place the tendons of the tibialis posterior, flexor digitorum longus, and flexor hallucis longus.

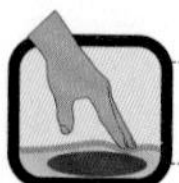

PALPATION

Ask the client to dorsiflex and invert the foot. Palpate between the medial malleolus and medial side of calcaneus.

INFERIOR EXTENSOR RETINACULUM

In-FEER-ee-or ex-TEN-sor reh-tin-AK-yu-lum

ETYMOLOGY Latin ***inferior***, lower + ***extensor***, extender + ***retinaculum***, band or halter (from ***retinere***, to hold back)

Overview

The inferior extensor retinaculum (Fig. 10-4) is a Y-shaped ligament restraining the extensor (and dorsiflexor) tendons of the foot distal to the ankle joint.

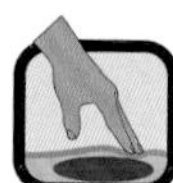

PALPATION

Palpate on either side on the tibialis anterior tendon at the level of the malleoli.

SUPERIOR EXTENSOR RETINACULUM

Su-PEER-ee-or ex-TEN-sor reh-tin-AK-yu-lum

ETYMOLOGY Latin ***superior***, higher + ***extensor***, extender + ***retinaculum***, band or halter (from ***retinere***, to hold back)

Overview

The superior extensor retinaculum (Fig. 10-4) is a ligament that binds the extensor (and dorsiflexor) tendons proximal to the ankle joint; it is continuous with (a thickening of) the deep fascia of the leg.

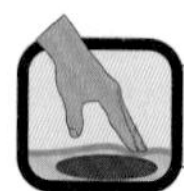

PALPATION

With the client supine, ask them to dorsiflex ankle and extend toes. Retinacula can be palpated one inch proximal to medial malleolus.

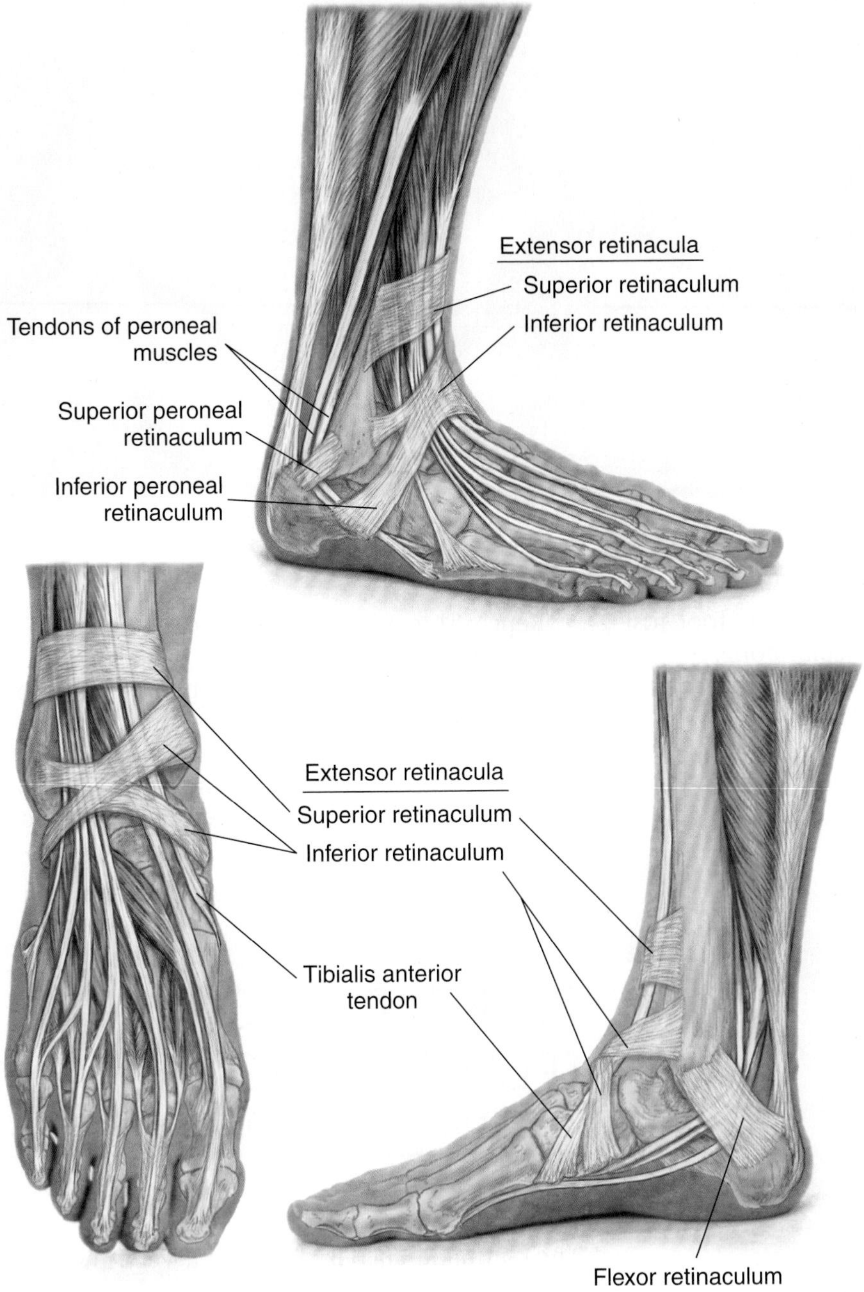

FIGURE 10-4 Anatomy of the flexor, extensor, and peroneal retinacula

PERONEAL RETINACULUM

pur-uh-NEE-ul reh-tin-AK-yu-lum

ETYMOLOGY Latin ***peroneus*** from Greek ***perone***, fibula + Latin ***retinaculum***, band or halter (from ***retinere***, to hold back)

Overview

The peroneal retinaculum (Fig. 10-4) consists of superior and inferior fibrous bands that retain the tendons of the peroneus longus and brevis in position as they cross the lateral side of the ankle behind the lateral malleolus and along the lateral foot.

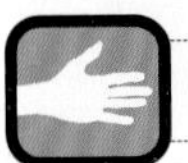

MANUAL THERAPY

RETINACULA

Overview

Although there are distinct retinacula of the ankle, they are treated together.

Cross-fiber Stroking

- The client lies supine.
- The therapist stands at the client's feet.

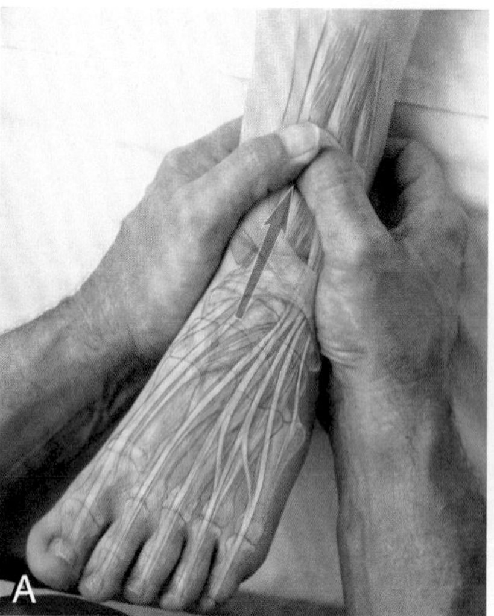

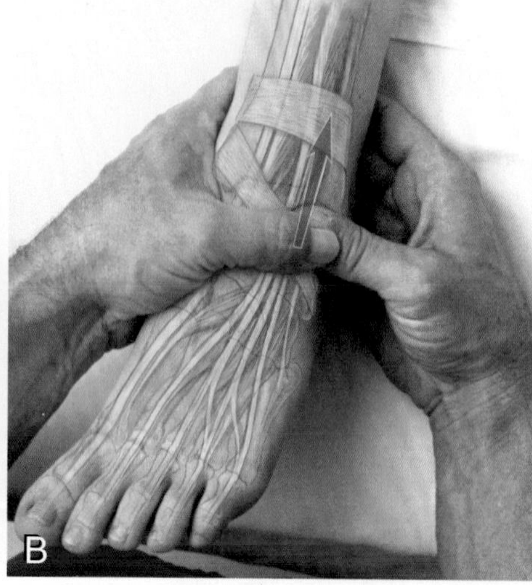

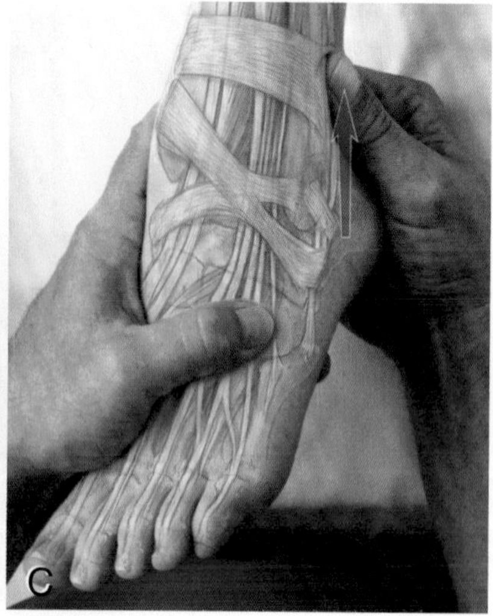

FIGURE 10-5 Deep stroking of the ankle retinacula, moving medial to lateral

- Place the thumb on the dorsum of the foot just below the ankle, over the navicular bone.
- Pressing firmly into the tissue, slide the thumb up the ankle about 3 inches (Fig. 10-5A).
- Repeat this procedure (Fig. 10-5B), moving laterally around the ankle all the way to the Achilles tendon (Fig. 10-5C). Note that the inferior peroneal retinaculum lies more distal on the foot than the retinaculum on the medial side.
- Repeat this procedure, moving around the ankle medially (Fig. 10-6A) all the way to the Achilles tendon (Fig. 10-6B).

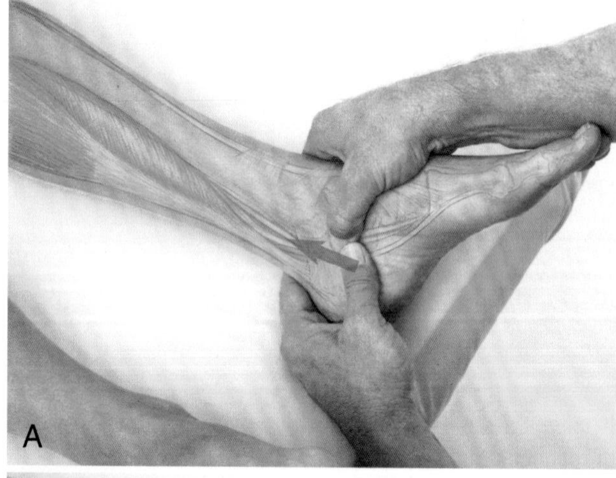

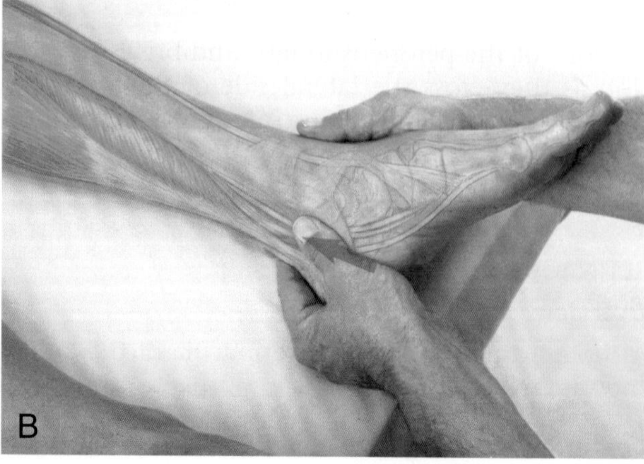

FIGURE 10-6 Deep stroking of the flexor retinaculum: supported thumb **(A)** and unsupported thumb **(B)**

PLANTAR FASCIA (PLANTAR APONEUROSIS)

PLAN-tar FAHSH-uh (PLAN-tar APP-o-nu-RO-sis)

Overview

The plantar fascia (Fig. 10-7) is the very thick, central portion of the fascia investing the plantar muscles; it radiates toward the toes from the medial process of the calcaneal tuberosity and provides attachment to the short flexor muscles of the toes.

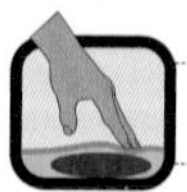

PALPATION

Not separately discernible from the muscle.

MANUAL THERAPY

- The client lies prone, the feet on a pillow or bolster.
- The therapist stands or sits at the client's feet.

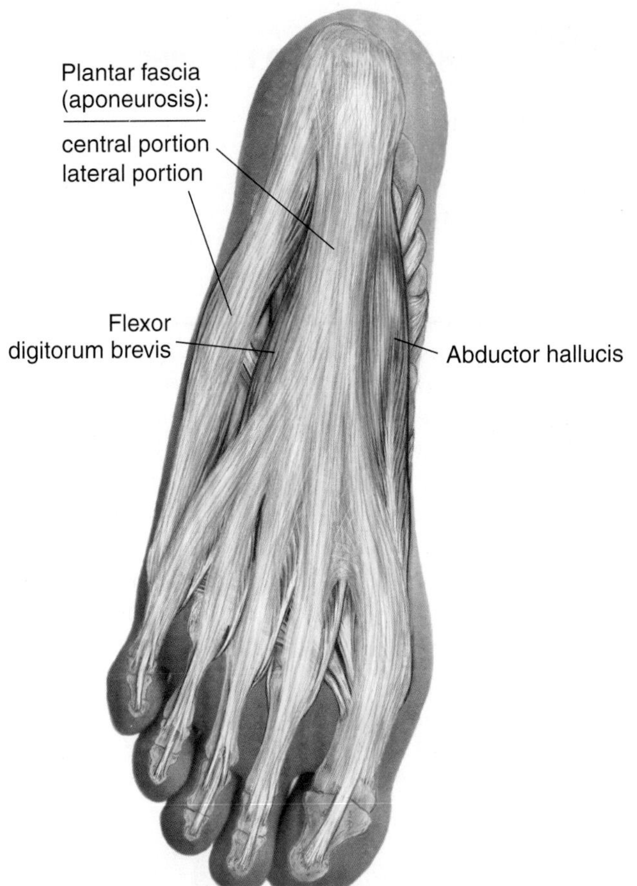

FIGURE 10-7 Anatomy of the plantar fascia

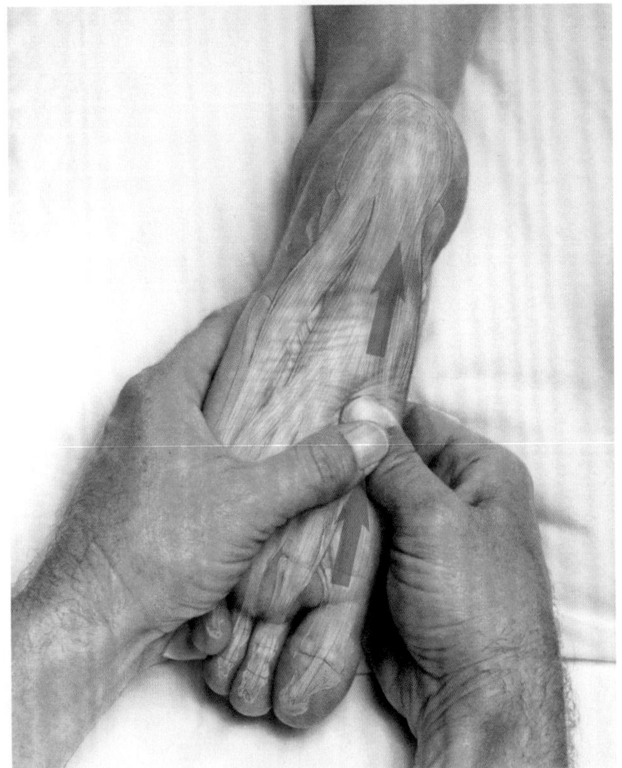

FIGURE 10-8 Deep stroking of the plantar fascia with the thumbs

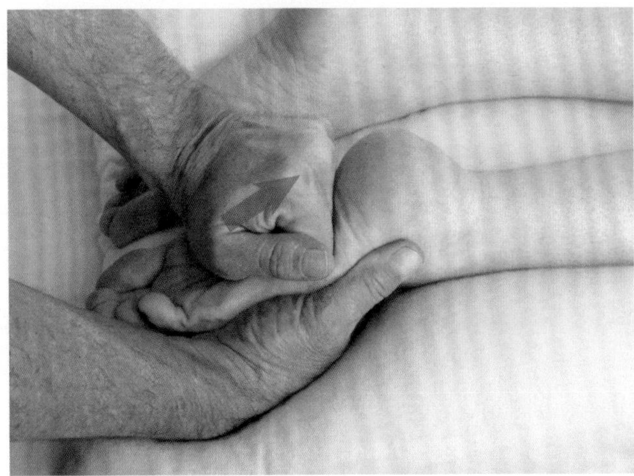

FIGURE 10-9 Deep stroking of the plantar fascia with the knuckles

- Place the thumb or supported thumb on the plantar aspect of the foot on the medial side, just proximal to the base of the big toe.
- Pressing firmly into the tissue, glide the thumb to the heel (Fig. 10-8).
- Repeat this procedure, starting just lateral to the previous starting position.
- Repeat the same procedure until the entire plantar surface has been treated.
- This procedure can be carried out for the entire plantar surface with the knuckles (Fig. 10-9).

Anterior Muscles of the Leg

TIBIALIS ANTERIOR

tib-ee-AL-is an-TEER-ee-or

ETYMOLOGY Latin ***tibialis***, of the tibia + ***anterior***, front

Overview

Be aware that tibialis anterior crosses from the anterolateral side of the leg to the medial side of the foot (Fig. 10-10).

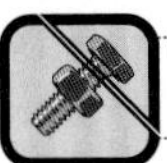

ATTACHMENTS

- Origin: lateral condyle and superior two-thirds of the anterior, lateral surface of tibia and to the interosseous membrane
- Insertion: medial cuneiform and the base of the 1st metatarsal

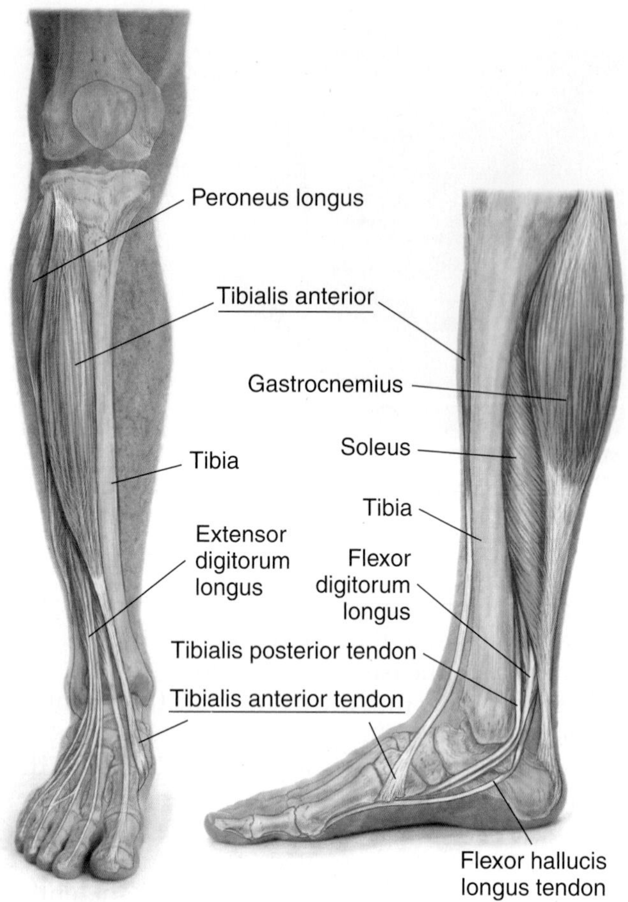

FIGURE 10-10 Anatomy of tibialis anterior

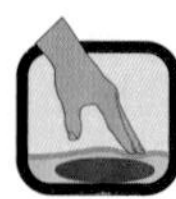

PALPATION

Discernible just lateral to the shin from below the knee to just above the ankle; its tendon can be seen clearly and palpated when the ankle is dorsiflexed and the foot inverted. Architecture is parallel; fibers are essentially vertical until the tendon crosses the ankle.

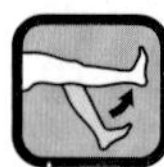

ACTION

Dorsiflexion of the foot at the ankle joint and inversion (supination) of the foot at the intertarsal joints.

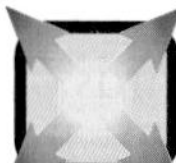

REFERRAL AREAS

- To the anterior aspect of the ankle
- Over the dorsal aspect of the phalanx of the great toe

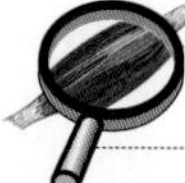

OTHER MUSCLES TO EXAMINE

Extensor hallucis longus

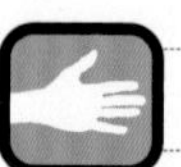

MANUAL THERAPY

Stripping

- The client lies supine.
- The therapist stands at the client's feet.
- Stabilize the foot with the nontreating hand.
- Place the fingertips on the distal end of the tibialis anterior, just proximal to the ankle.
- Pressing firmly into the tissue, slide the fingertips along the muscle to its attachments on the proximal tibia (Fig. 10-11).
- This procedure may also be carried out with the supported thumb (Fig. 10-12) or the heel of the hand (Fig. 10-13).

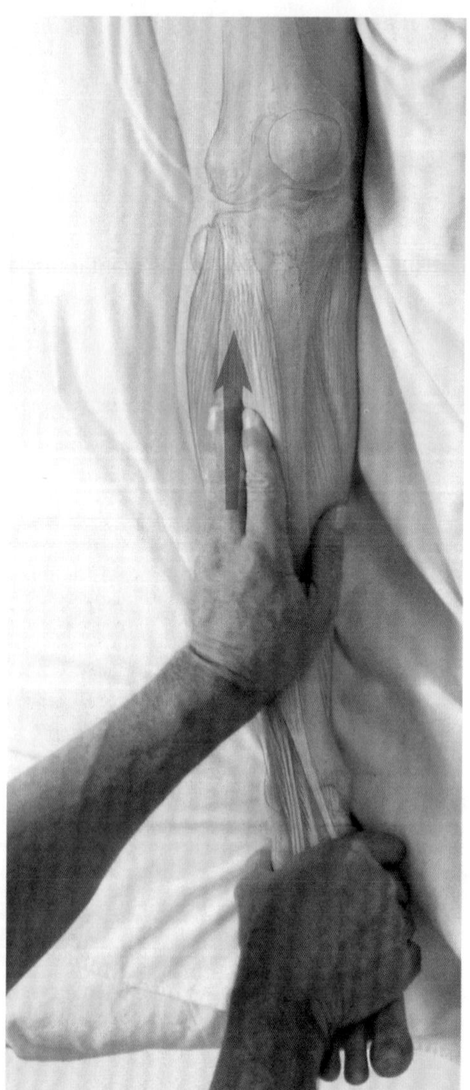

FIGURE 10-11 Stripping of tibialis anterior with the fingertips

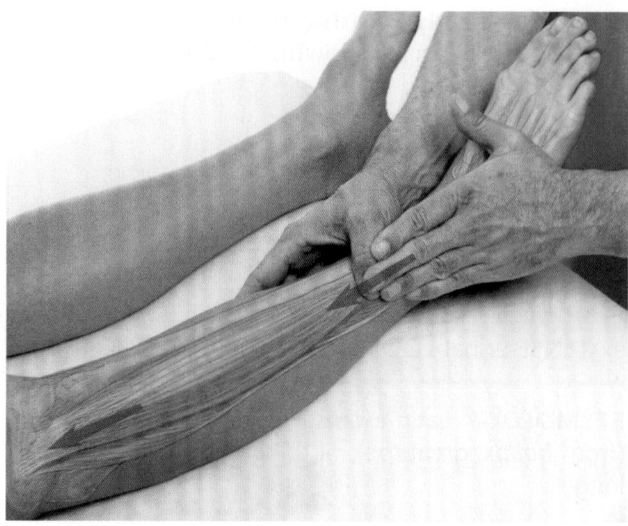

FIGURE 10-12 Stripping of tibialis anterior with supported thumb

FIGURE 10-13 Stripping of tibialis anterior with the heel of the hand

EXTENSOR DIGITORUM LONGUS

ex-TENSE-er didge-i-TORE-um LONG-us

ETYMOLOGY Latin ***extensor***, extender + ***digitorum***, of the digits + ***longus***, long

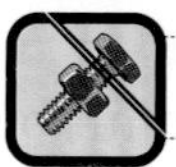

ATTACHMENTS

- Origin: lateral condyle of the tibia, superior two-thirds of the anterior margin of the fibula, upper part of interosseous membrane, and anterior intermuscular septum (Fig. 10-14)
- Insertion: by four tendons to the dorsal surfaces of the bases of the proximal, middle, and distal phalanges of the 2nd to 5th toes

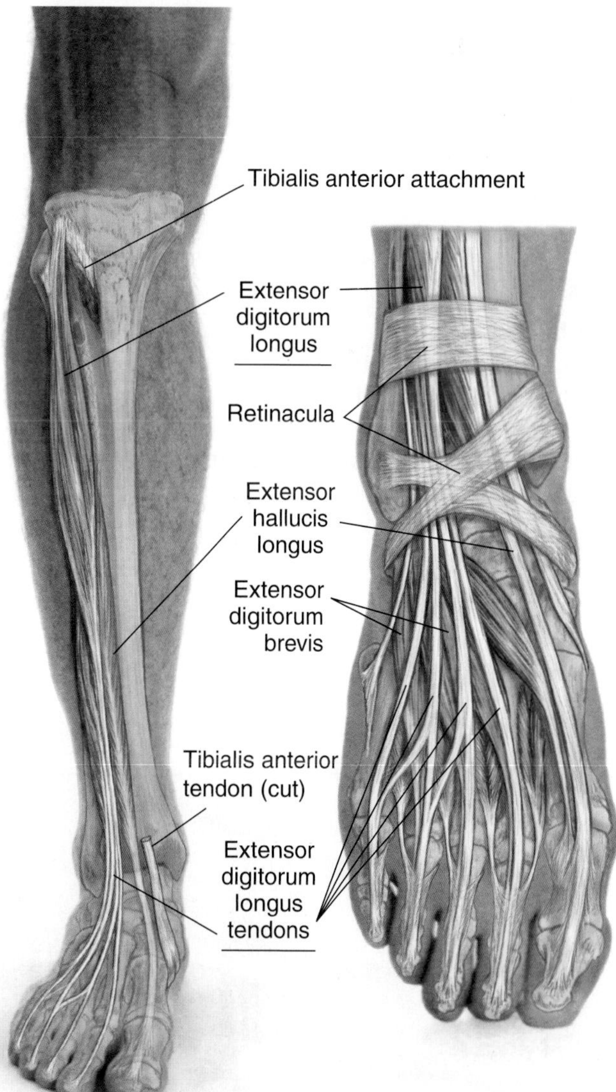

FIGURE 10-14 Anatomy of extensor digitorum longus

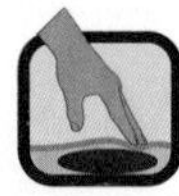

PALPATION

Discernible posterior to tibialis anterior. Architecture is unipennate. The tendons can be seen and palpated as they cross the anterior ankle and dorsum of the foot.

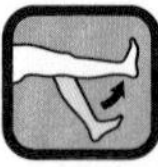

ACTION

Extends (and hyperextends) the MP and IP joints of the four lateral toes; dorsiflexes the ankle and assists pronation of intertarsal joints

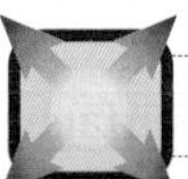

REFERRAL AREA

Over the dorsal aspect of the 2nd, 3rd, and 4th digits of the foot

OTHER MUSCLES TO EXAMINE

Extensor digitorum brevis

MANUAL THERAPY

Stripping

- The client lies supine.
- The therapist stands beside the client at the feet.
- Place the thumb on extensor digitorum longus at its distal end, just anterior and superior to the lateral malleolus.
- Pressing firmly into the tissue, slide the thumb along the muscle following the fibula to its head (Fig. 10-15).

EXTENSOR HALLUCIS LONGUS

ex-TENSE-er hal-LOOSE-is, HAL-loose-is LONG-us

ETYMOLOGY Latin ***extensor***, extender + ***hallucis*** (from ***hallux***, great toe), of the great toe + ***longus***, long

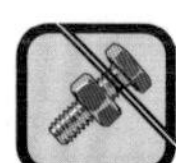

ATTACHMENTS

- Origin: anteromedial surface of the fibula and the interosseous membrane (Fig. 10-16)
- Insertion: base of the distal phalanx of the great toe

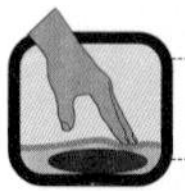

PALPATION

Obvious tendon; palpate at the base of the great toe across dorsum of foot by extending the great toe.

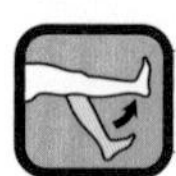

ACTION

Extends (and hyperextends) the MP and IP joints of the great toe; dorsiflexes the ankle assists supination of intertarsal joints

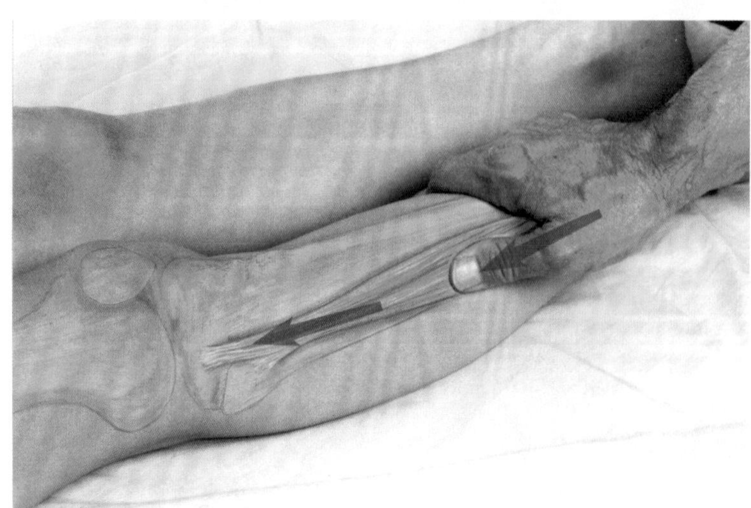

FIGURE 10-15 Stripping of extensor digitorum longus with thumb

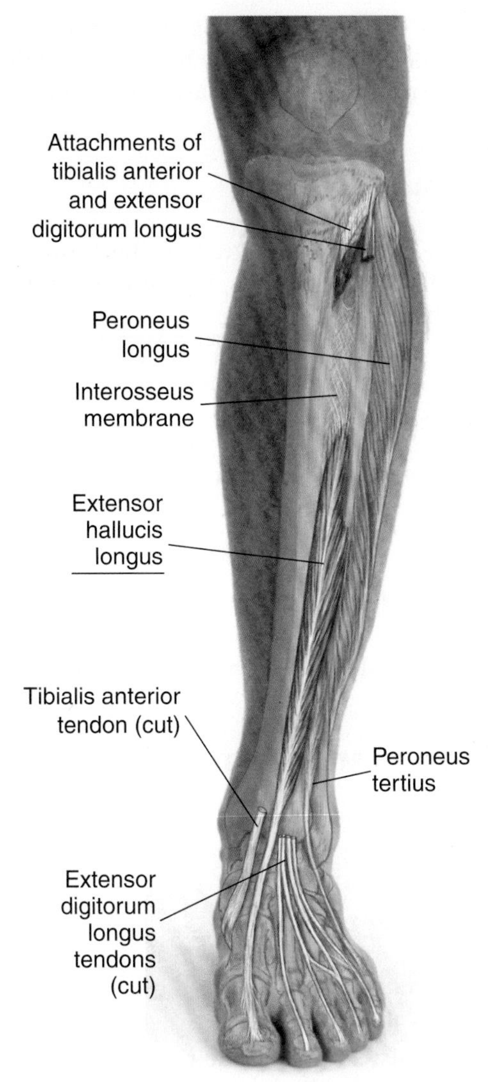

FIGURE 10-16 Anatomy of extensor hallucis longus

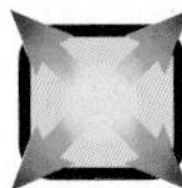

REFERRAL AREA

Over the dorsal aspect of the phalanx of the great toe

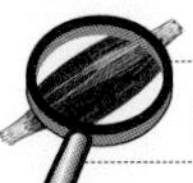

OTHER MUSCLES TO EXAMINE

Tibialis anterior

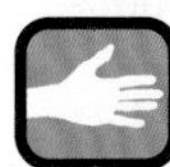

MANUAL THERAPY

EXTENSORS OF THE FOOT

Stretch

- Client may lie prone or supine.
- Holding the leg in one hand, take the foot in the other hand and slowly plantarflex it (Fig. 10-17).

Lateral Muscles of the Leg

PERONEUS LONGUS

pe-ROE-nee-us LONG-us

ETYMOLOGY Latin ***peroneus*** from Greek ***perone***, fibula + ***longus***, long. The name "fibularis" is sometimes used in place of "peroneus."

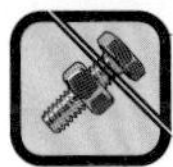

ATTACHMENTS

- Origin: superior two-thirds of the outer surface of the fibula and to the lateral condyle of tibia (Fig. 10-18)

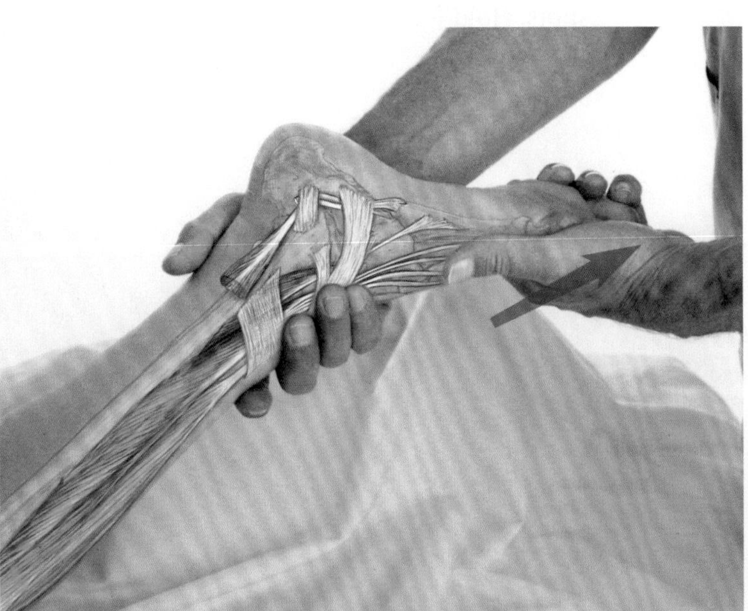

FIGURE 10-17 Stretch of the extensors (dorsiflexors) of the foot

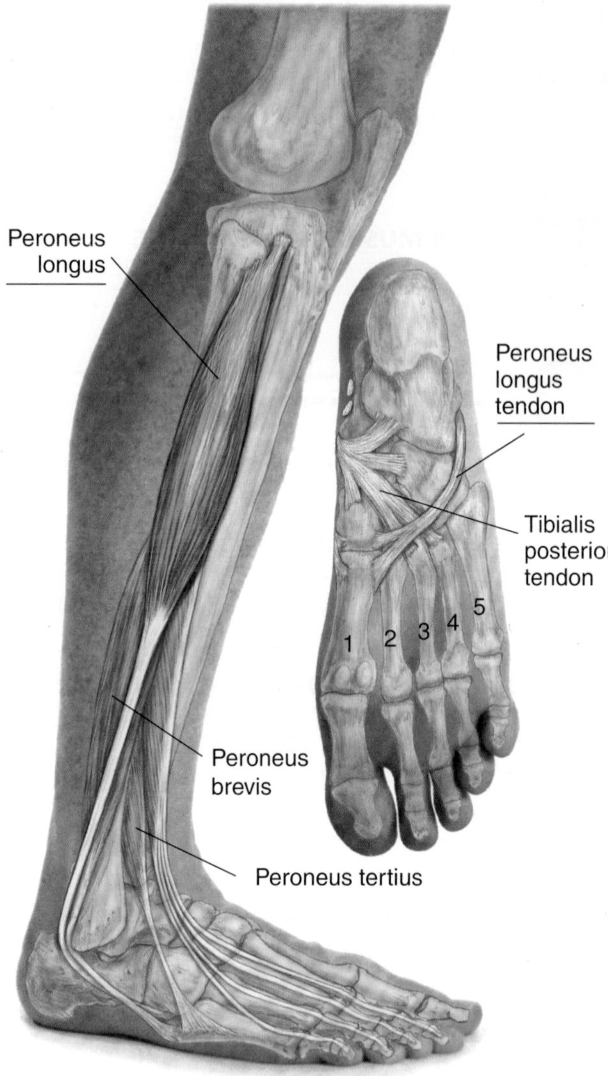

FIGURE 10-18 Anatomy of peroneus longus

- Insertion: by the tendon passing posterior to the lateral malleolus and across the sole of the foot to the medial cuneiform and base of the 1st metatarsal

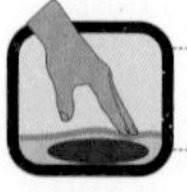

PALPATION

Discernible posterior to extensor digitorum longus in the upper half of the leg, but not beyond. Architecture is bipennate.

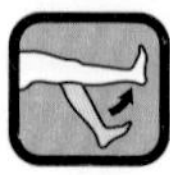

ACTION

Plantar flexes the ankle and everts (pronates) the foot (intertarsal joints)

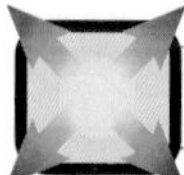

REFERRAL AREA

To the lateral calf and around the lateral malleolus

OTHER MUSCLES TO EXAMINE

Peroneus brevis

MANUAL THERAPY

Compression

- The client lies prone.
- The therapist stands beside the client at the leg.
- Place a hand on the lateral aspect of the leg over the fibula, with the thumb pressing into the tissue a few inches below the knee.
- Press firmly into the tissue, searching for tender spots. Hold for release (Fig. 10-19).

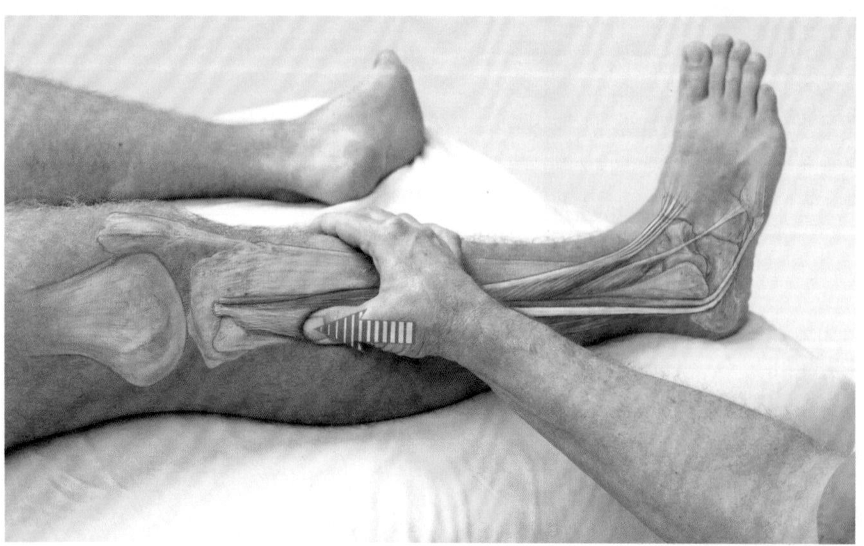

FIGURE 10-19 Compression of peroneus longus trigger point

PERONEUS BREVIS

pe-ROE-nee-us BREV-is

ETYMOLOGY Latin ***peroneus*** from Greek ***perone,*** fibula + ***brevis,*** short. The name "fibularis" is sometimes used in place of "peroneus."

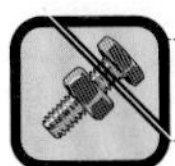

ATTACHMENTS

- Origin: lower two-thirds of the lateral surface of the fibula (Fig. 10-20)
- Insertion: base of the 5th metatarsal bone

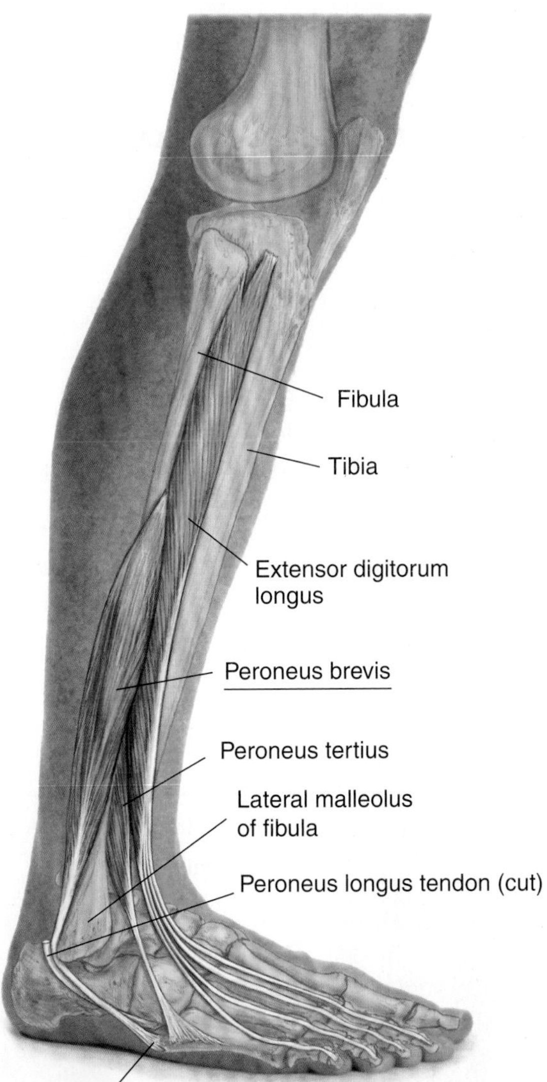

FIGURE 10-20 Anatomy of peroneus brevis

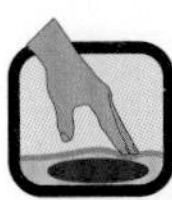

PALPATION

Discernible posterior to tibialis anterior in the lower, lateral half of the leg. Architecture is bipennate.

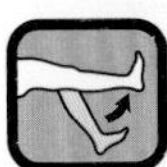

ACTION

Plantar flexes the ankle and everts (pronates) the foot (intertarsal joints)

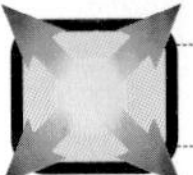

REFERRAL AREA

Around the lateral malleolus

OTHER MUSCLES TO EXAMINE

Peroneus longus

MANUAL THERAPY

Muscle Stripping

- The client lies prone.
- The therapist stands beside the client at the leg.
- Place a hand on the lateral aspect of the leg over the fibula, with the thumb pressing into the tissue about one-third of the way below the knee.
- Press firmly into the tissue, searching for tender spots. Hold for release.

PERONEUS TERTIUS

pe-ROE-nee-us TER-shus

ETYMOLOGY Latin ***peroneus*** from Greek ***perone,*** fibula + ***tertius,*** third. The name "fibularis" is sometimes used in place of "peroneus."

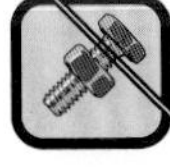

ATTACHMENTS

- Origin: distal third of the anterior fibula and interosseus membrane (Fig. 10-21)
- Insertion: dorsum of base of 5th metatarsal bone near peroneus brevis

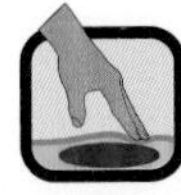

PALPATION

Palpate just anterior and superior to the lateral malleolus.

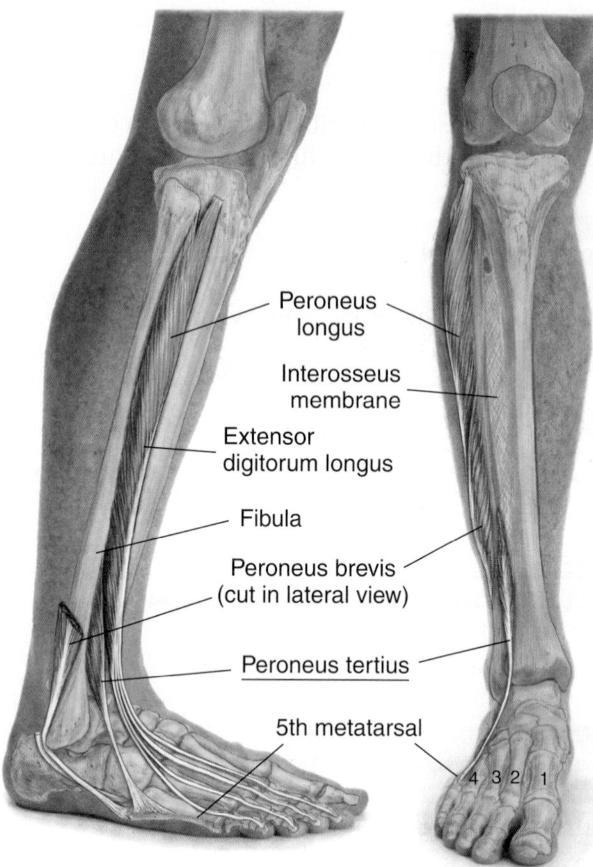

FIGURE 10-21 Anatomy of peroneus tertius

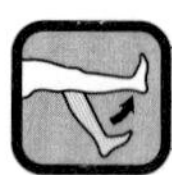

ACTION

Assists in dorsiflexion of the ankle and eversion (pronation) the foot (intertarsal joints)

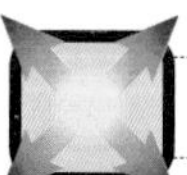

REFERRAL AREA

- Over the anterior lateral ankle and proximal dorsal foot
- Over the lateral aspect of the heel

OTHER MUSCLES TO EXAMINE

Extensor digitorum longus

Posterior Muscles of the Leg

POPLITEUS

pop-LIT-ee-us

ETYMOLOGY Latin ***poples, poplit-***, the ham of the knee

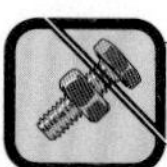

ATTACHMENTS

- Origin: lateral condyle of the femur (Fig. 10-22)
- Insertion: posterior surface of the tibia above the soleal line

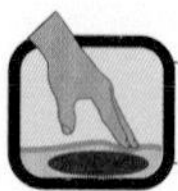

PALPATION

Not discernible

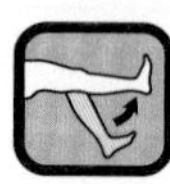

ACTION

Unlocks the knee to begin flexion; assists medial rotation of the knee

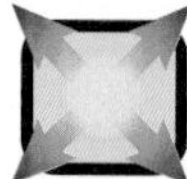

REFERRAL AREA

To the posterior knee, toward the medial side.

OTHER MUSCLES TO EXAMINE

Gastrocnemius

MANUAL THERAPY

Compression

- The client lies on the unaffected side, with the knee to be treated flexed slightly.
- The therapist stands at the client's knees.

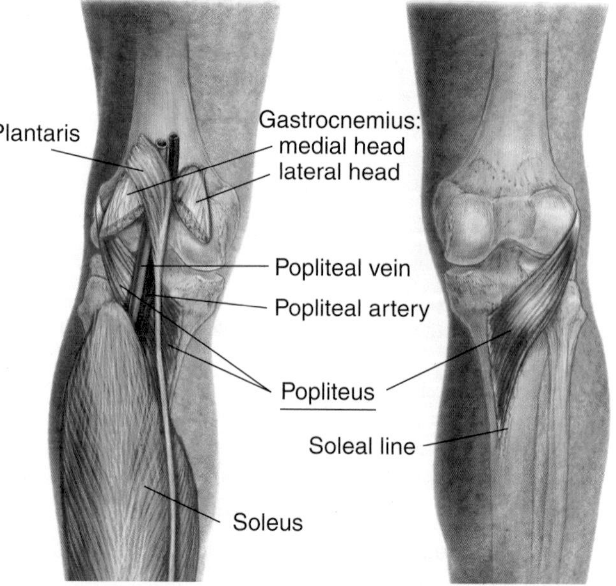

FIGURE 10-22 Anatomy of popliteus

- Place the hand nearest the client on the posterior aspect of the knee, the thumb placed distal to the knee toward the medial side, pressing the gastrocnemius laterally to gain access to popliteus.
- Press firmly into the tissue, searching for tender spots. Hold for release (Fig. 10-23).

CAUTION Avoid pressure on the popliteal artery and tibial nerve, which run along the midline of the posterior knee and overlie this muscle.

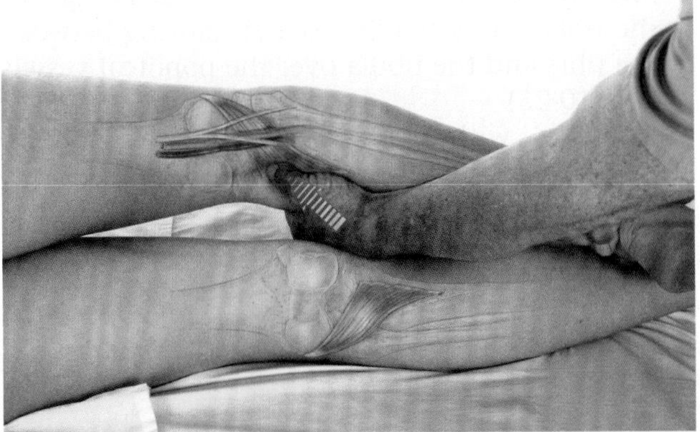

FIGURE 10-23 Compression of popliteus trigger point

GASTROCNEMIUS

GAS-trock-NEEM-ee-us

ETYMOLOGY Greek ***gastroknemia***, calf of the leg, from ***gaster (gastr-)***, belly, + ***kneme***, leg

Overview

Note that gastrocnemius (Fig. 10-24) crosses both the knee and ankle joints, while soleus crosses only the ankle joint. Therefore, while soleus can be stretched with the knee flexed, gastrocnemius can only be stretched with the knee straight.

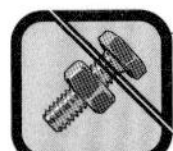

ATTACHMENTS

- Origin: by two heads (lateral and medial) from the lateral and medial epicondyles on the posterior femur
- Insertion: with soleus by the Achilles tendon into the inferior half of the posterior surface of the calcaneus

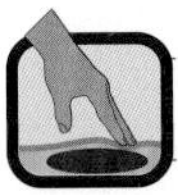

PALPATION

Easily palpable from Achilles tendon up to the division high on the calf, then on either side of the calf across the knee joint inside the hamstring tendons. Architecture as a whole is bipennate.

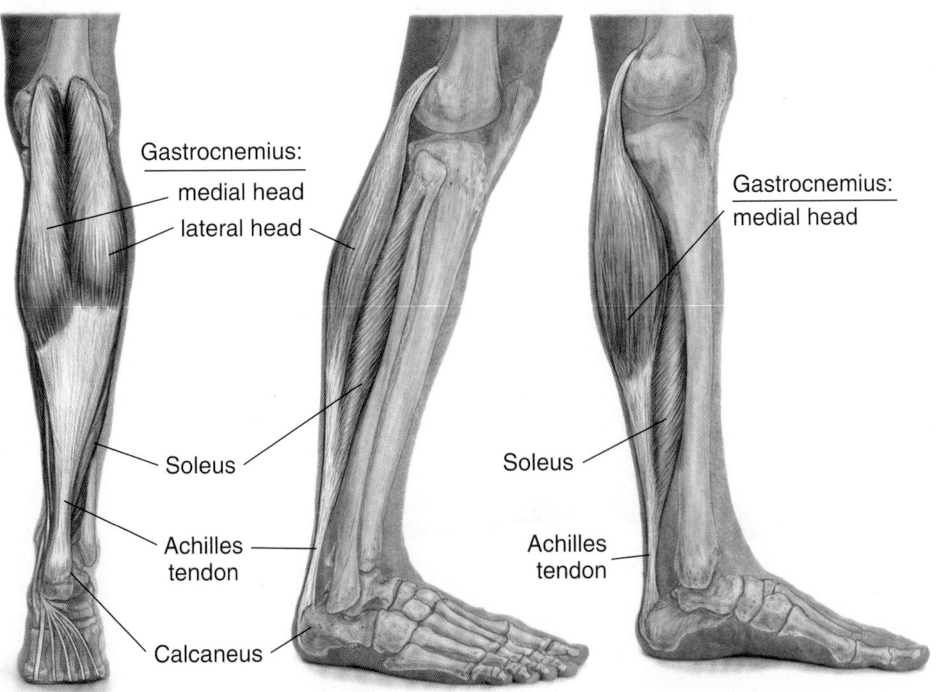

FIGURE 10-24 Anatomy of gastrocnemius

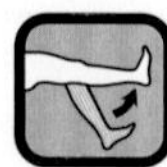

ACTION

Plantar flexion of the ankle; assists knee flexion

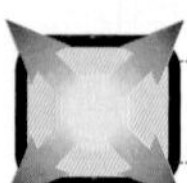

REFERRAL AREA

- Over the bellies of the muscle
- To the medial surface of the ankle
- To the longitudinal arch (medial surface of the plantar foot)

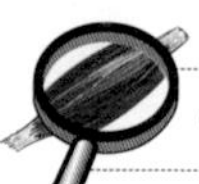

OTHER MUSCLES TO EXAMINE

- All other muscles of the calf
- Piriformis

MANUAL THERAPY

See Manual Therapy of the Calf Muscles, below.

SOLEUS

SO-lee-us

ETYMOLOGY Latin ***solea***, a sandal, sole of the foot (of animals), from ***solum***, bottom, floor, ground

Overview

A soleus trigger point is one of the most common causes of pain in the heel due to its insertion on the calcaneus

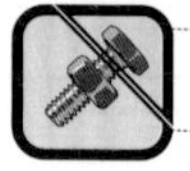

ATTACHMENTS

- Origin: posterior surface of the head and superior third of the shaft of the fibula, the soleal line and middle third of the medial margin of the tibia, and a tendinous arch passing between the tibia and the fibula over the popliteal vessels (Fig. 10-25)
- Insertion: with gastrocnemius by the Achilles tendon into the tuberosity of the calcaneus

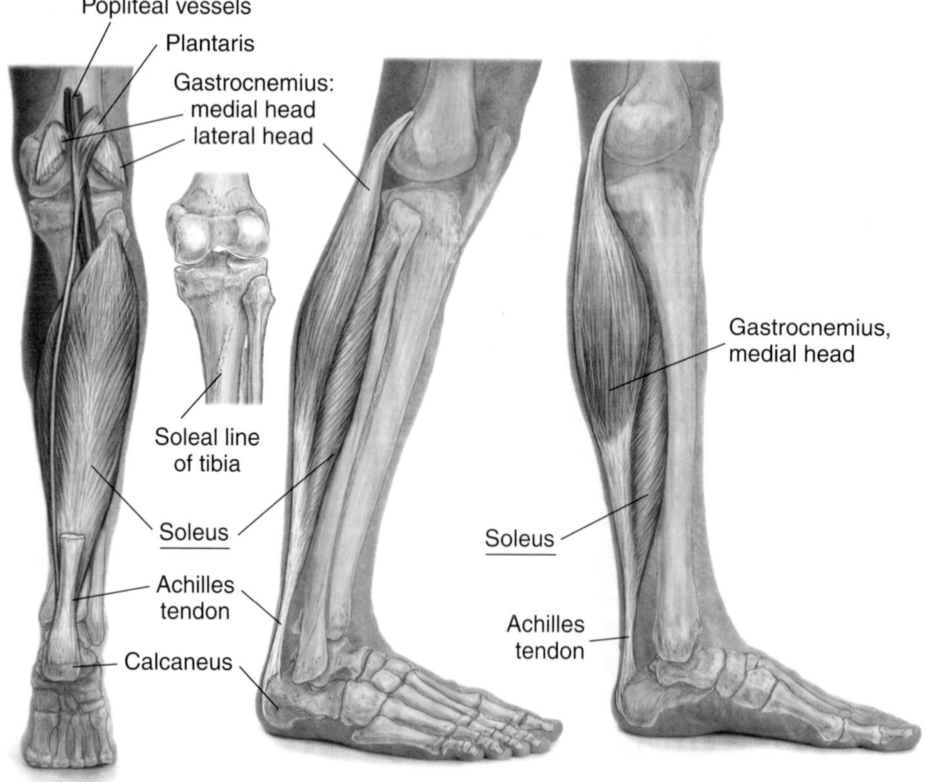

FIGURE 10-25 Anatomy of soleus

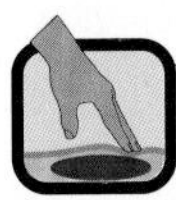

PALPATION

The fibers of the soleus bulge from under the gastrocnemius along both sides of the leg and extend further distal than the heads of the gastrocnemius. Asking the client to stand on tiptoes or to alternatively dorsiflex and plantar flex the ankle as you palpate on the medial or lateral side of the leg will make it prominent.

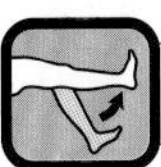

ACTION

Plantar flexion of ankle

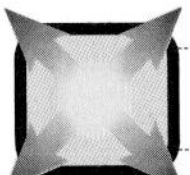

REFERRAL AREA

Over the Achilles tendon to the plantar surface of the heel

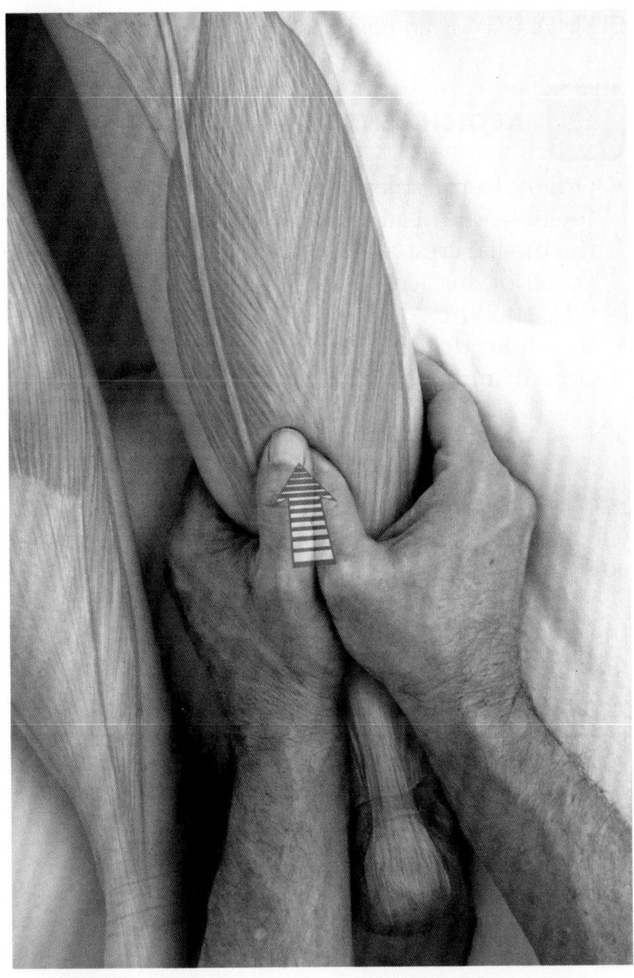

FIGURE 10-26 Compression of soleus trigger point

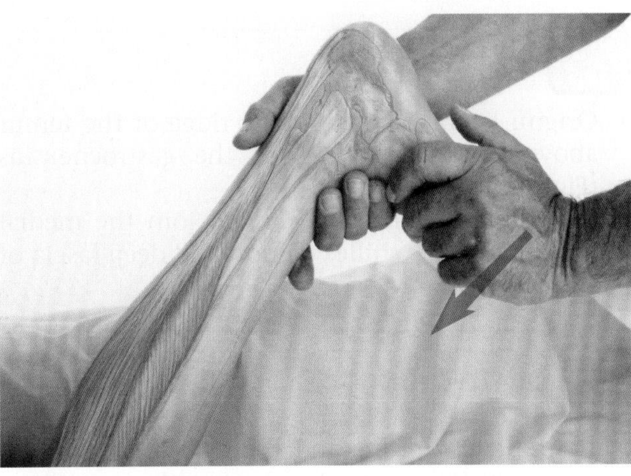

FIGURE 10-27 Stretch of soleus

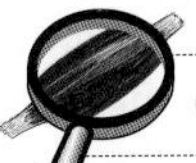

OTHER MUSCLES TO EXAMINE

Quadratus plantae

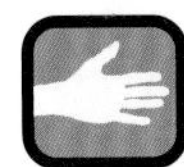

MANUAL THERAPY

Compression

- The client lies prone.
- The therapist stands at the client's feet.
- Place the hand on the soleus, the thumb pressing into the muscle proximal to the ankle about a third of the way to the knee (Fig. 10-26).
- Press firmly into the tissue, searching for tender spots. Hold for release.

Stretch of Soleus

- Holding the client's leg in one hand with the knee partly flexed, grasp the foot with the other hand and slowly dorsiflex it (Fig. 10-27).

See also Manual Therapy of the Calf Muscles, below.

PLANTARIS

plan-TARE-is

ETYMOLOGY Latin ***plantaris***, plantar (relating to the sole of the foot)

Overview

The structure of plantaris varies. It is a long, slender muscle that may have one belly high up in the calf, or two smaller bellies separated by a tendon.

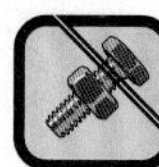

ATTACHMENTS

- Origin: lateral supracondylar ridge of the femur above the lateral head of the gastrocnemius (Fig. 10-28)
- Insertion: by a long tendon to join the medial margin of the Achilles tendon and deep fascia of the ankle

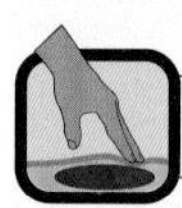

PALPATION

With the client prone and the knee flexed to approximately 90°, cover the heel with your distal hand while your forearm is applied against the plantar aspect of the foot, allowing a simultaneous resistance to plantar flexion of the foot and flexion of the knee.

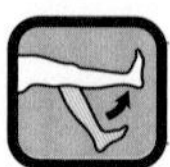

ACTION

Weakly assists in plantar flexion of the ankle

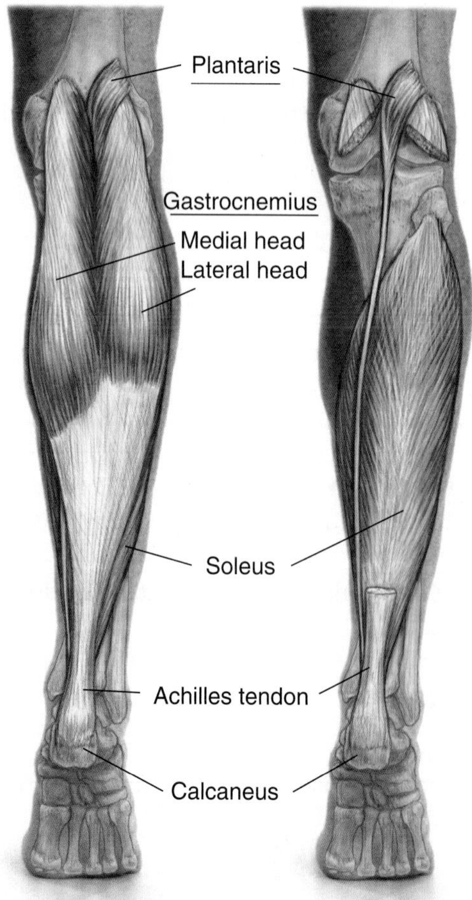

FIGURE 10-28 Anatomy of plantaris

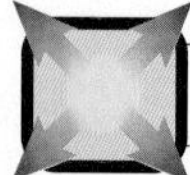

REFERRAL AREA

To the posterior knee and the upper calf

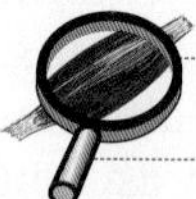

OTHER MUSCLES TO EXAMINE

- Soleus
- Piriformis

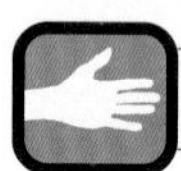

MANUAL THERAPY

See Manual Therapy of the Calf Muscles, below.

TIBIALIS POSTERIOR

tib-ee-AL-is pos-TEER-ee-or

ETYMOLOGY Latin ***tibialis***, of the tibia + ***posterior***, back

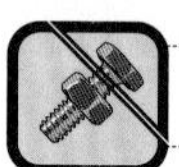

ATTACHMENTS

- Origin: to the soleal line and posterior surface of the tibia, the head and shaft of the fibula between the medial crest and interosseous border, and the posterior surface of the interosseous membrane (Fig. 10-29)
- Insertion: to the navicular; three cuneiform; cuboid; and 2nd, 3rd, and 4th metatarsal bones

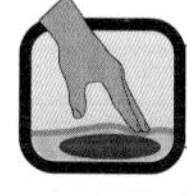

PALPATION

Client prone with knee flexed; locate the medial edge of the tibia with your fingertips.

Slide your fingers posteriorly and hook around the edge of the tibia onto the fibers of tibialis posterior, deep in the posterior leg between the tibia and fibula.

Asking the client to resist plantar flexion and inversion will assist in palpation.

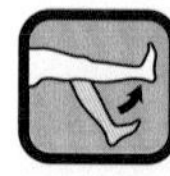

ACTION

Plantar flexion of the ankle and inversion (supination) of foot (intertarsal joints)

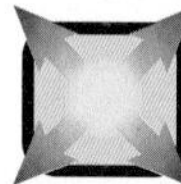

REFERRAL AREA

- Primarily, to the Achilles tendon

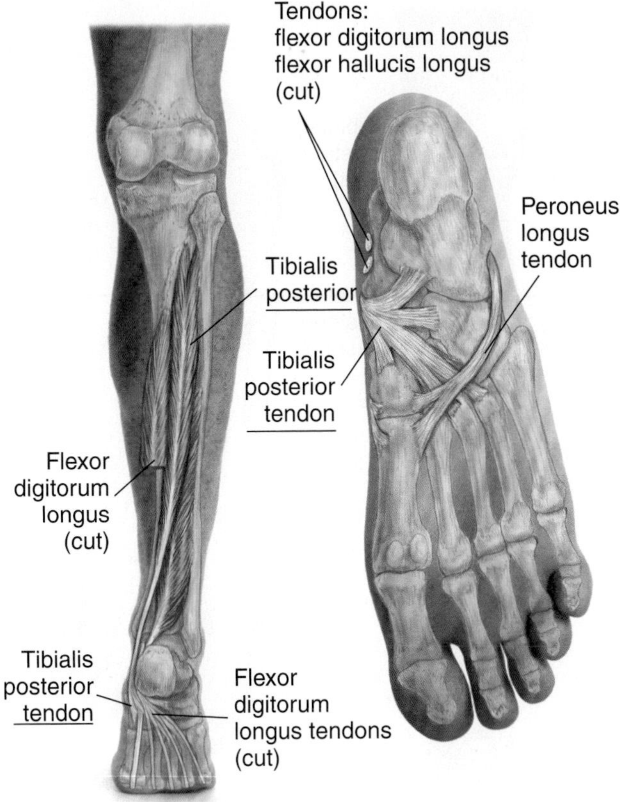

FIGURE 10-29 Anatomy of tibialis posterior

- Secondarily, to the surface of the calf, and the plantar surface of the heel and foot

OTHER MUSCLES TO EXAMINE

- Soleus
- Gastrocnemius
- Peroneal muscles

MANUAL THERAPY

See Manual Therapy of the Calf Muscles, below.

FLEXOR DIGITORUM LONGUS

FLEX-er DIDGE-i-TORE-um LONG-us

ETYMOLOGY Latin ***flexor***, flexor + ***digitorum***, of the digits + ***longus***, long

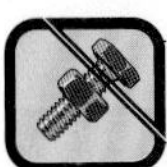

ATTACHMENTS

- Origin: middle third of the posterior surface of the tibia (Fig. 10-30)
- Insertion: by four tendons, perforating those of the flexor brevis, into the bases of the distal phalanges of the four lateral toes

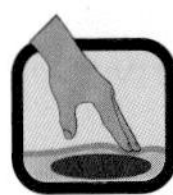

PALPATION

With the client supine and the foot in neutral position, place your hand on the plantar surface of the toes and ask them to plantar flex the toes as you offer resistance to them on the plantar surface.

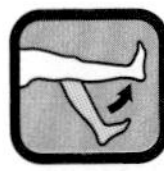

ACTION

Flexes MP and IP joints of 2nd to 5th toes; plantar flexes the ankle and inverts (supinates) the foot (intertarsal joints)

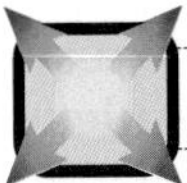

REFERRAL AREA

- To the medial surface of the calf
- To the central plantar surface of the foot

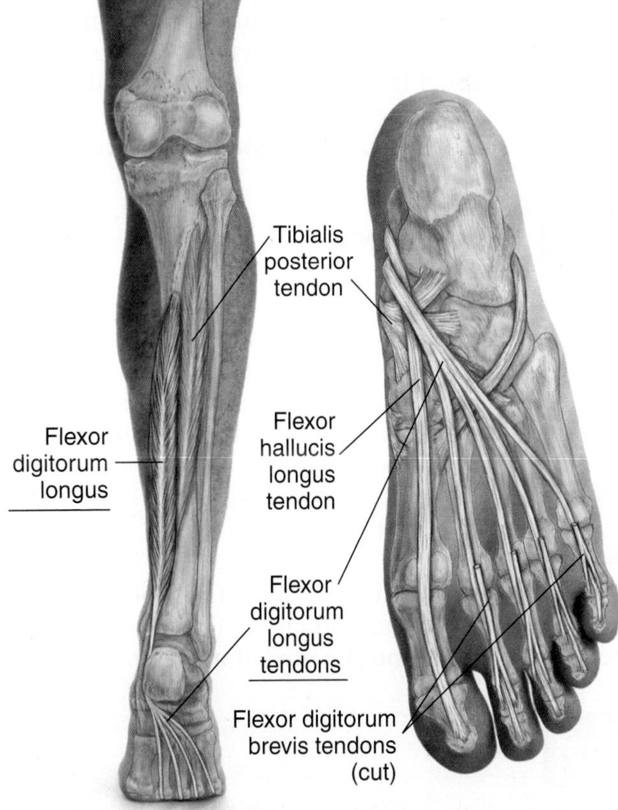

FIGURE 10-30 Anatomy of flexor digitorum longus

OTHER MUSCLES TO EXAMINE

- Other calf muscles
- Other muscles of the plantar foot

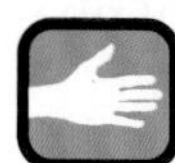

MANUAL THERAPY

See Manual Therapy of the Calf Muscles, below.

FLEXOR HALLUCIS LONGUS

FLEX-er hal-LOOSE-is, HALL-loose-is LONG-us

ETYMOLOGY Latin ***flexor***, flexor + ***hallucis*** (from ***hallux***, great toe), of the great toe + ***longus***, long

Overview

This muscle is particularly vulnerable to tenosynovitis in classical ballet dancers and in athletes who require forefoot push-off and extreme plantar flexion, such as runners, gymnasts, ice skaters, and swimmers. Tenosynovitis is an inflammation of the protective sheath covering the tendon (most commonly occurring at the ankle and wrist joints). This muscle is also vulnerable at the point where its tendon passes under the 1st metatarsal at the ball of the foot. The cause may be due to infection or disease, but is frequently the result of strain or overuse.

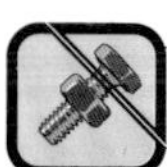

ATTACHMENTS

- Origin: lower two-thirds of the posterior surface of the fibula, and at its lowest part, from the lower part of the interosseous membrane, and from fascia covering the tibialis posterior (Fig. 10-31)
- Insertion: base of the distal phalanx of the great toe

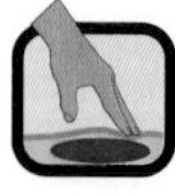

PALPATION

Ask the supine client to dorsiflex the foot while you palpate just posterior and lateral to the tibialis posterior tendon behind the medial malleolus.

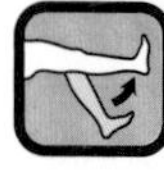

ACTION

Flexes the MP and IP joint of the great toe; plantar flexes the ankle

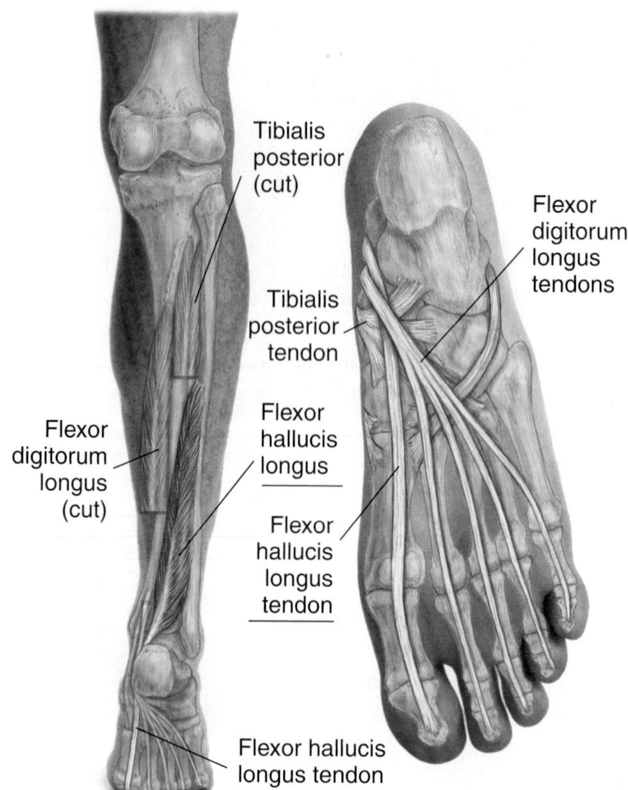

FIGURE 10-31 Anatomy of flexor hallucis longus

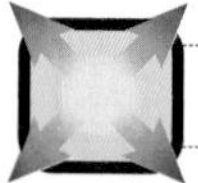

REFERRAL AREA

To the ball of the foot and the great toe

OTHER MUSCLES TO EXAMINE

Flexor hallucis brevis

MANUAL THERAPY

See Manual Therapy of the Calf Muscles, below.

Manual Therapy of the Calf Muscles

When treating the calf muscles with the client prone, avoid excessive plantar flexion of the ankle by placing the ankles on a pillow or bolster or having the client lie with the feet off the end of the table.

Stripping

- The client lies prone.
- The therapist stands at the client's feet.

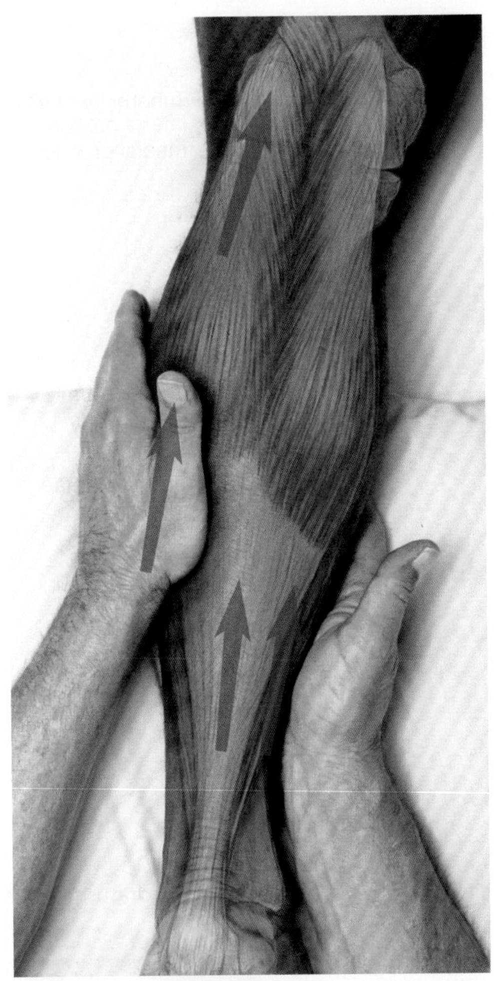

FIGURE 10-32 Stripping of calf muscles with the heel of the hand

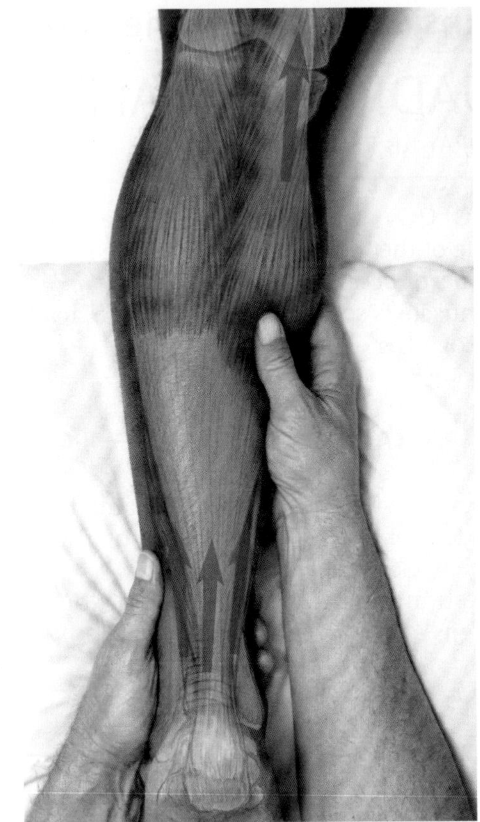

FIGURE 10-33 Stripping of calf muscles with the thumb

- Place the heel of the hand on the calf at the proximal end of the Achilles tendon, starting on the lateral side.
- Pressing firmly into the tissue (Fig. 10-32), slide the heel of the hand along the muscle to the knee.
- Repeat this procedure on the posterior calf.
- Repeat this procedure on the medial calf.
- This procedure may also be carried out using the fingertips, thumbs (Fig. 10-33), or supported thumb (Fig. 10-34).

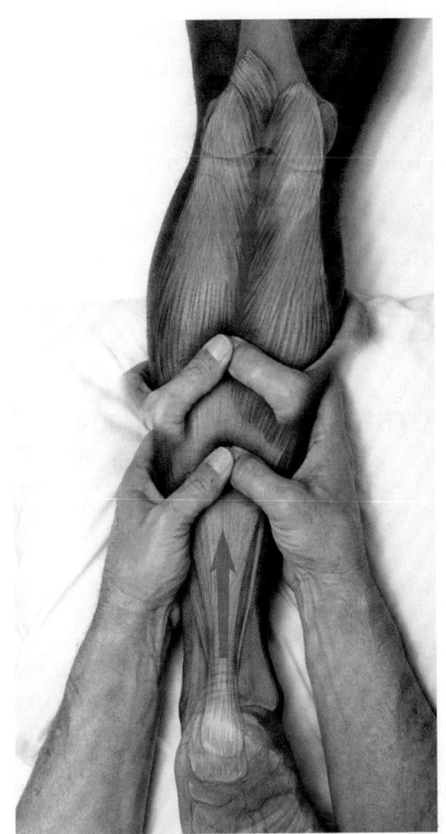

FIGURE 10-34 Stripping of calf muscles with the supported thumb

Intrinsic Muscles of the Foot

QUADRATUS PLANTAE

kwa-DRAY-tus PLAN-tay

ETYMOLOGY Latin ***quadratus***, square + ***plantae***, of the sole of the foot. Quadratus plantae is sometimes called ***flexor accessorius.***

This muscle is sometimes lacking one head or missing altogether.

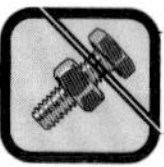

ATTACHMENTS

- Origin: by two heads from the lateral and medial borders of the inferior surface of the calcaneus (Fig. 10-35)
- Insertion: to the tendons of flexor digitorum longus

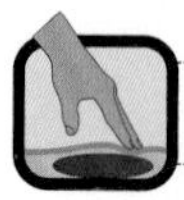

PALPATION

Client supine, foot in the neutral position, stabilize the metatarsals with one hand, and ask the client to flex the four toes as you offer resistance to them on the plantar surface.

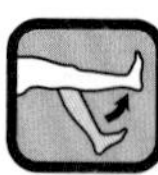

ACTION

Assists flexor digitorum longus in flexion of the MP and IP joints of toes 2 through 5

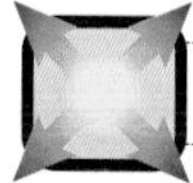

REFERRAL AREA

To the plantar aspect of the heel

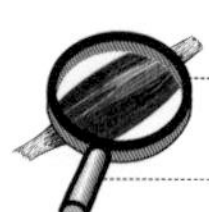

OTHER MUSCLES TO EXAMINE

Soleus

MANUAL THERAPY

Compression

- The client lies prone.
- The therapist stands at the client's feet.
- Hold the foot with both hands, the thumb resting on the plantar surface in the center, just distal to the heel (Fig. 10-36).
- Press firmly into the tissue, searching for tender spots. Hold for release.

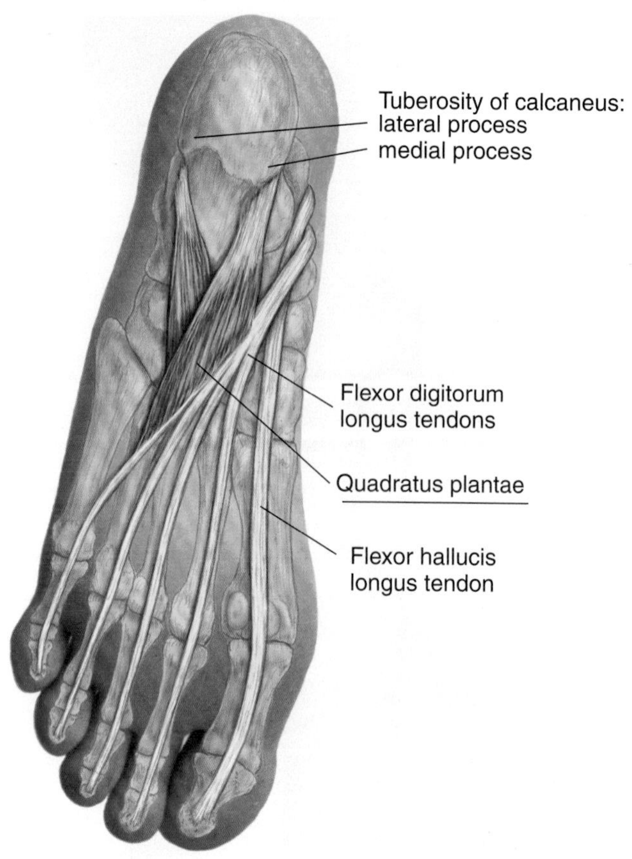

FIGURE 10-35 Anatomy of quadratus plantae

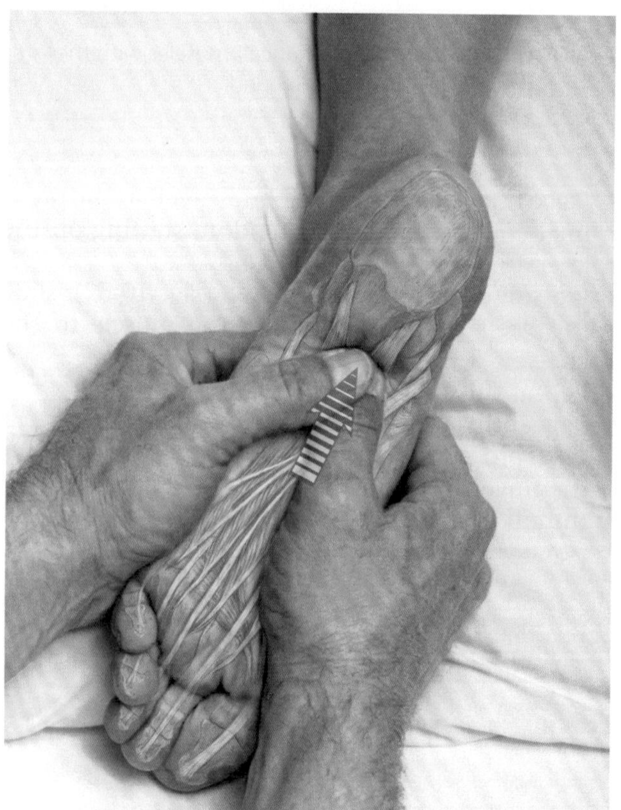

FIGURE 10-36 Compression of quadratus plantae trigger point

FLEXOR DIGITI MINIMI BREVIS

FLEX-er DIDGE-I-tee MIN-I-mee BREV-is

ETYMOLOGY Latin ***flexor***, flexor + ***digiti***, of the digit + ***minimi***, smallest + ***brevis***, short

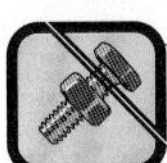

ATTACHMENTS

- Origin: base of the 5th metatarsal bone and the sheath of peroneus longus tendon (Fig. 10-37)
- Insertion: lateral surface of the base of the proximal phalanx of the little toe

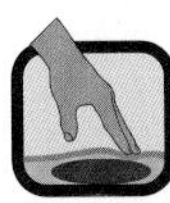

PALPATION

Palpable, but not distinguishable, on the dorsum and side of the foot. Architecture is parallel.

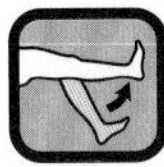

ACTION

Flexes the MP joint of the little toe

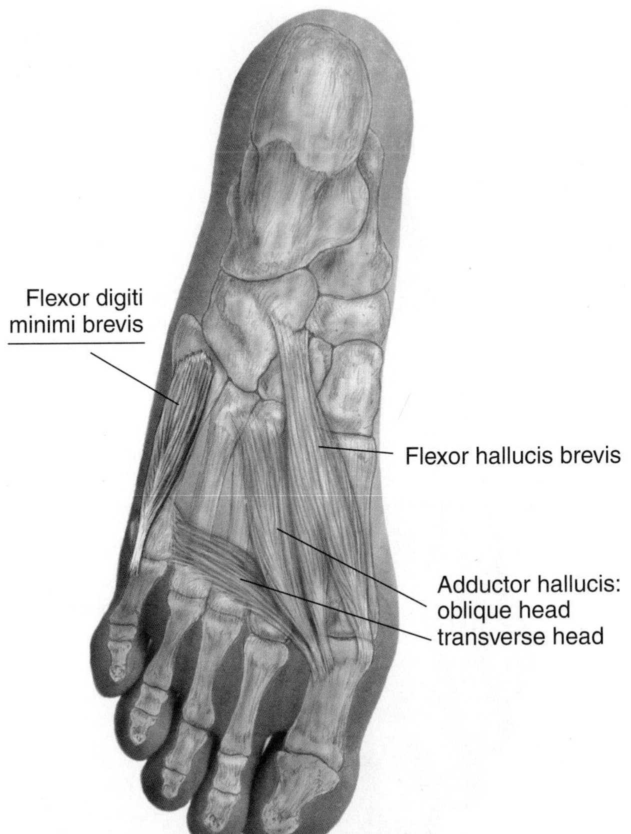

FIGURE 10-37 Anatomy of flexor digiti minimi brevis

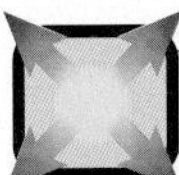

REFERRAL AREA

No isolated pain pattern

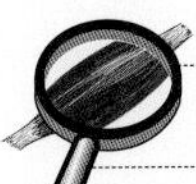

OTHER MUSCLES TO EXAMINE

Not applicable

MANUAL THERAPY

See Manual Therapy of Toe Flexors.

FLEXOR DIGITORUM BREVIS

FLEX-er DIDGE-i-TORE-um BREV-is

ETYMOLOGY Latin ***flexor***, flexor + ***digitorum***, of the digits + ***brevis***, short

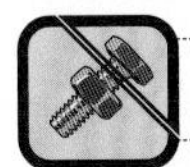

ATTACHMENTS

- Origin: medial process of the tuberosity of the calcaneus and the central portion of the plantar fascia (Fig. 10-38)
- Insertion: middle phalanges of the four lateral toes by tendons perforated by those of flexor digitorum longus

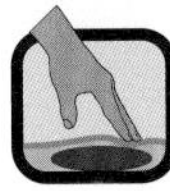

PALPATION

Not directly palpable

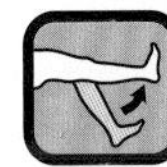

ACTION

Flexes the MP and proximal IP joints of the lateral four toes

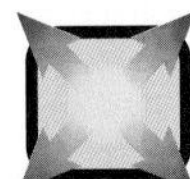

REFERRAL AREA

Across the plantar foot just proximal to the toes

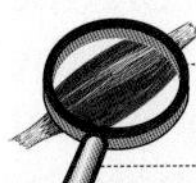

OTHER MUSCLES TO EXAMINE

Other intrinsic muscles of the foot

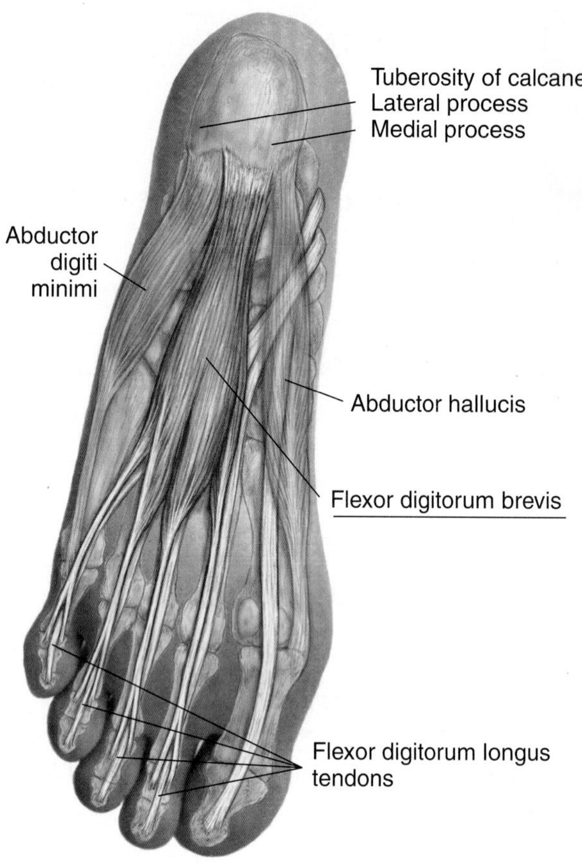

FIGURE 10-38 Anatomy of flexor digitorum brevis

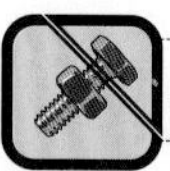

ATTACHMENTS

- Origin: medial surface of cuboid and middle and lateral cuneiform bones (Fig. 10-39)
- Insertion: by two tendons, embracing that of the flexor longus hallucis, into the sides of the base of the proximal phalanx of the great toe

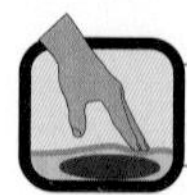

PALPATION

Not separately discernable. May feel the action by asking the client to flex the great toe against resistance.

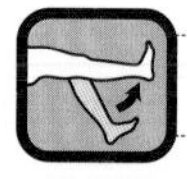

ACTION

Flexes the MP joint of the great toe

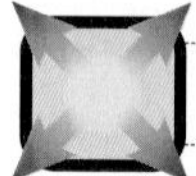

REFERRAL AREA

To the ball of the foot and the great toe on both plantar and dorsal aspects

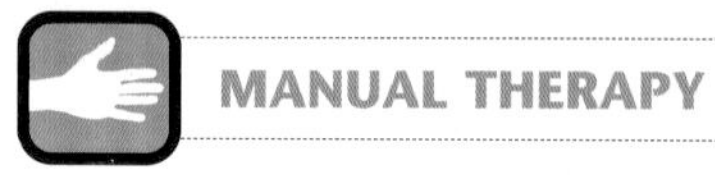

MANUAL THERAPY

See Manual Therapy for Toe Flexors, below.

FLEXOR HALLUCIS BREVIS

FLEX-er hal-LOOSE-is, HALL-loose-is BREV-is

ETYMOLOGY Latin ***flexor***, flexor + ***hallucis*** (from ***hallux***, great toe), of the great toe + ***brevis***, short

Overview

Pain in the ball of the foot extending to the big toe and difficulty in walking is a sign of strain in the flexor hallucis brevis. Like flexor hallucis longus, it is often injured by walking or running on hard or uneven surfaces and by wearing high heels.

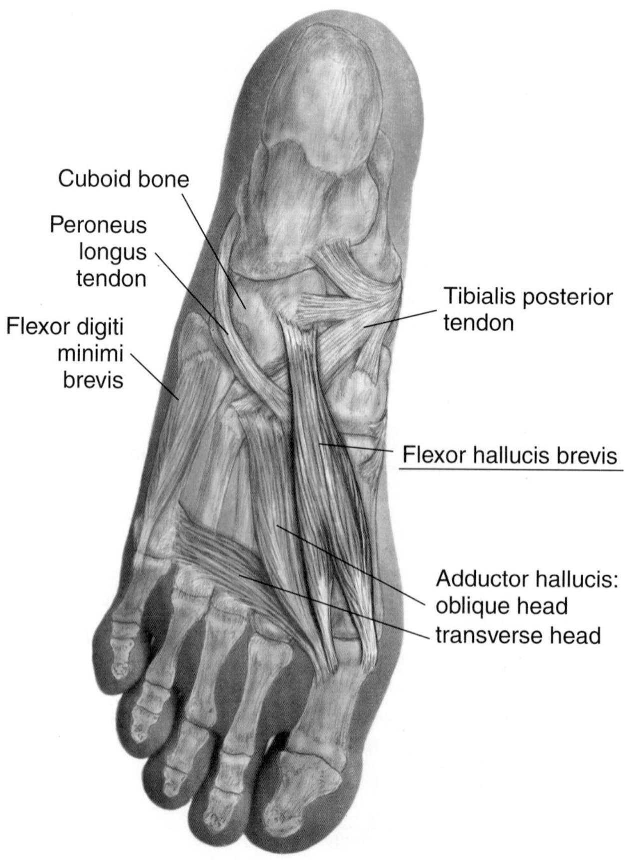

FIGURE 10-39 Anatomy of flexor hallucis brevis

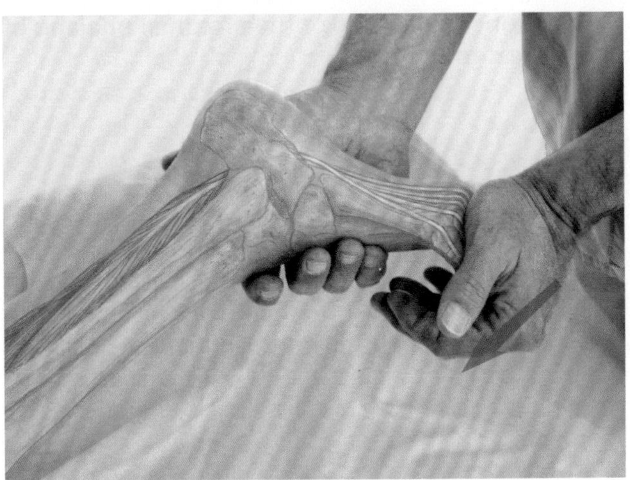

FIGURE 10-40 Stretch of the toe flexors

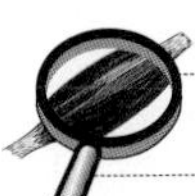

OTHER MUSCLES TO EXAMINE

Flexor hallucis longus

Manual Therapy for Toe Flexors

Stretch

- The client may lie either supine or prone.
- Holding the foot in one hand, place the heel of the other hand on the plantar surface of the toes, and slowly and gently press them into hyperextension (Fig. 10-40).

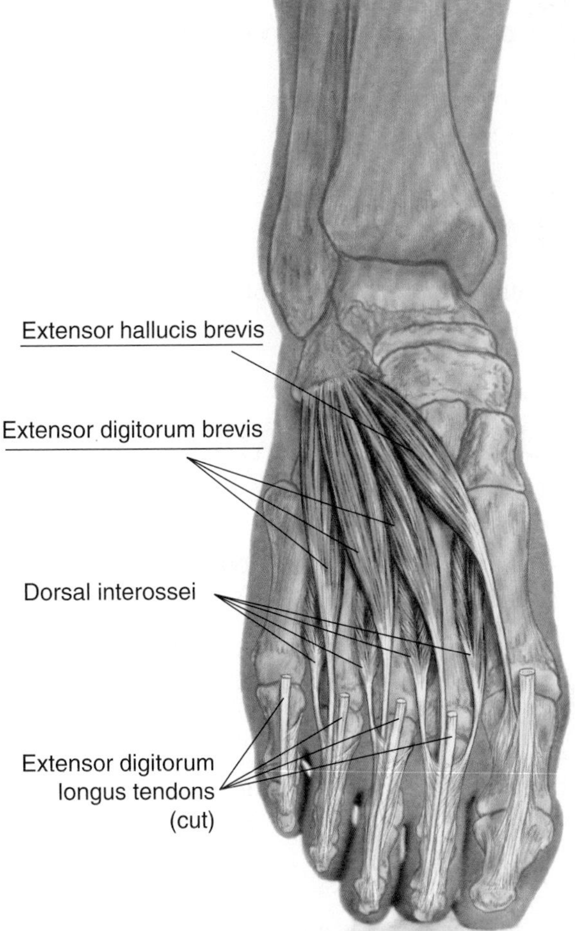

FIGURE 10-41 Anatomy of extensor digitorum brevis

EXTENSOR DIGITORUM BREVIS

ex-TENSE-er didge-i-TORE-um BREV-is

ETYMOLOGY Latin ***extensor***, extender + ***digitorum***, of the digits + ***brevis***, short

Overview

For the purposes of this book, the extensor hallucis brevis is considered to be the medial belly of extensor digitorum brevis, the tendon of which is inserted into the base of the proximal phalanx of the great toe (Fig. 10-41).

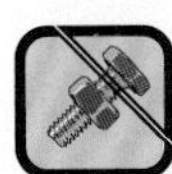

ATTACHMENTS

- Origin: dorsal surface of the lateral calcaneus
- Insertion: by four tendons fusing with those of extensor digitorum longus of the 2nd, 3rd, and 4th toes, and by a slip attached independently to the base of the proximal phalanx of the great toe

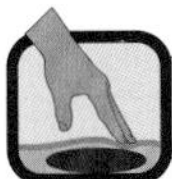

PALPATION

Asking the client to extend the toes while supine with the leg straight (keeping the heel on the table), will make the muscle prominent at the cuboid.

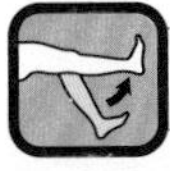

ACTION

Extends the MP joint of toes 1 to 4

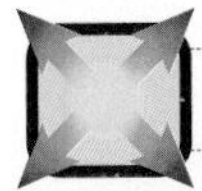

REFERRAL AREA

Over the dorsal aspect of the foot near the ankle

OTHER MUSCLES TO EXAMINE

- Extensor digitorum longus
- Extensor hallucis brevis

MANUAL THERAPY

See General Manual Therapy of the Foot, below.

ABDUCTOR HALLUCIS

ab-DUCK-ter hal-LOOSE-is, HALL-loose-is

ETYMOLOGY Latin ***abductor*** (from ***ab***, away from + ***ducere***, to lead or draw) + ***hallucis*** (from ***hallux***, great toe), of the great toe

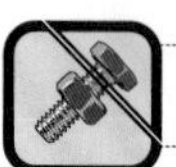

ATTACHMENTS

- Origin: medial process of the calcaneal tuberosity, the flexor retinaculum, and the plantar aponeurosis (Fig. 10-42)

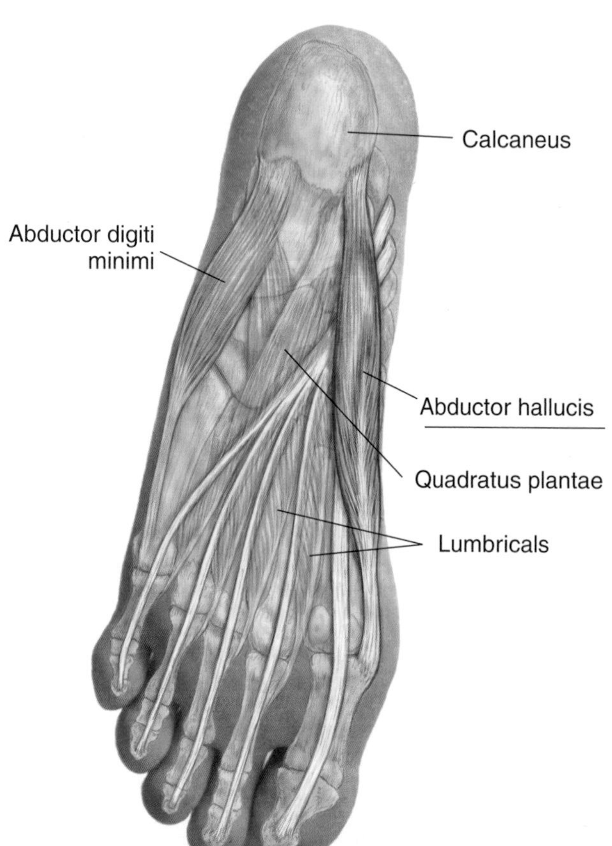

FIGURE 10-42 Anatomy of abductor hallucis

- Insertion: medial side of the proximal phalanx of the great toe

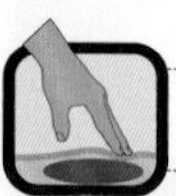

PALPATION

Client supine, legs straight, place fingertips of one hand on dorsal surface of the base of the great toe and the thumb on the planter surface at the base of the great toe. Place the other hand on the lateral side of the foot and ask the client to abduct the great toe.

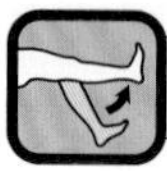

ACTION

Abducts the MP joint of the great toe

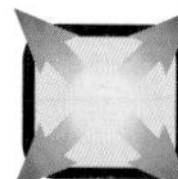

REFERRAL AREA

Medial aspect of heel and foot (arch)

OTHER MUSCLES TO EXAMINE

Gastrocnemius

MANUAL THERAPY

Stripping

- The client lies supine.
- The therapist stands at the client's feet.
- Holding the foot in both hands, place the supported thumb on abductor hallucis at its distal end, just proximal to the base of the big toe.
- Pressing firmly into the tissue, slide the thumb along the muscle as far as the heel (Fig. 10-43).

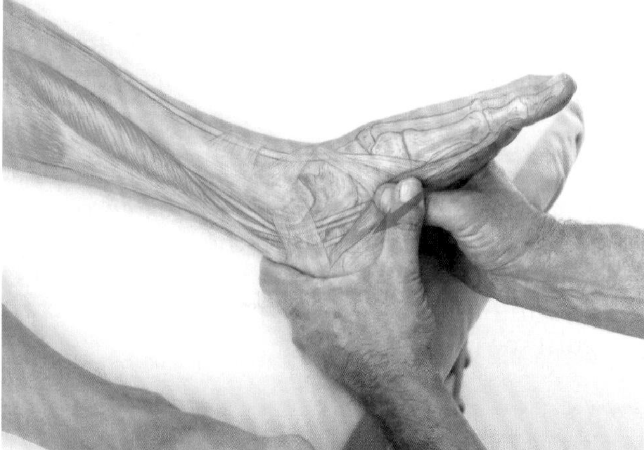

FIGURE 10-43 Stripping of abductor hallucis with supported thumb

ADDUCTOR HALLUCIS

ad-DUCK-ter hal-LOOSE-is, HALL-loose-is

ETYMOLOGY Latin ***adductor*** (from ***ad***, to or toward + ***ducere***, to lead or draw) + ***hallucis*** (from ***hallux***, great toe), of the great toe

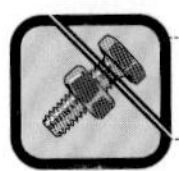

ATTACHMENTS

- Origin: by two heads, the transverse head from the capsules of the lateral four MP joints and the oblique head from the lateral cuneiform and bases of the 3rd and 4th metatarsal bones (Fig. 10-44)
- Insertion: lateral side of the base of the proximal phalanx of the great toe

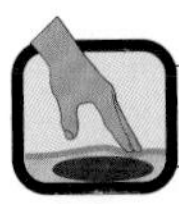

PALPATION

Place your fingertips on the medial side of the foot close to the plantar surface. Asking the client to adduct the 1st phalanx of the great toe will allow you to feel the muscle contraction.

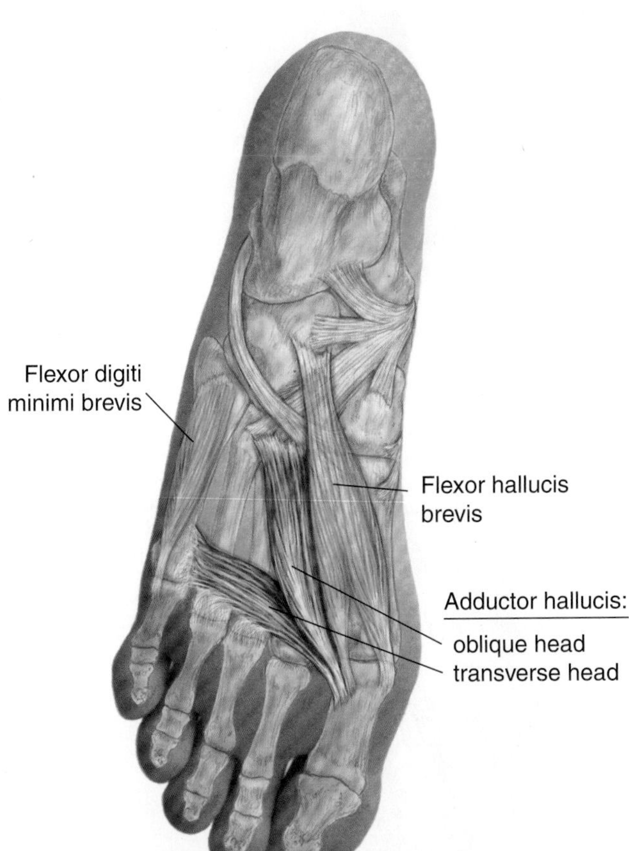

FIGURE 10-44 Anatomy of adductor hallucis

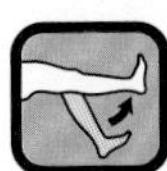

ACTION

Adducts the MP joint of the great toe

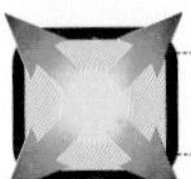

REFERRAL AREA

To the distal plantar aspect of the foot just proximal to the toes, flexor digitorum brevis and flexor hallucis brevis

OTHER MUSCLES TO EXAMINE

Flexor digitorum brevis

MANUAL THERAPY

See General Manual Therapy of the Foot, below.

ABDUCTOR DIGITI MINIMI

ab-DUCK-ter DIJ-I-tee MIN-I-mee

ETYMOLOGY Latin ***abductor*** (***ab***, away from + ***ducere***, to lead), that which draws away + ***digiti***, of the digit + ***minimi***, smallest

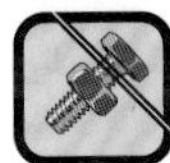

ATTACHMENTS

- Origin: lateral and medial processes of calcaneal tuberosity (Fig. 10-45)
- Insertion: lateral side of proximal phalanx of the 5th toe

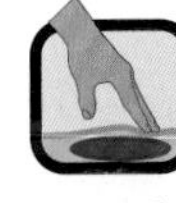

PALPATION

Not directly palpable

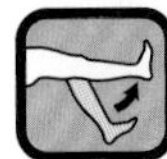

ACTION

Abducts and flexes the MP joint of the little toe

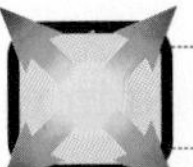

REFERRAL AREA

To the outer edge of the distal aspect of the plantar foot

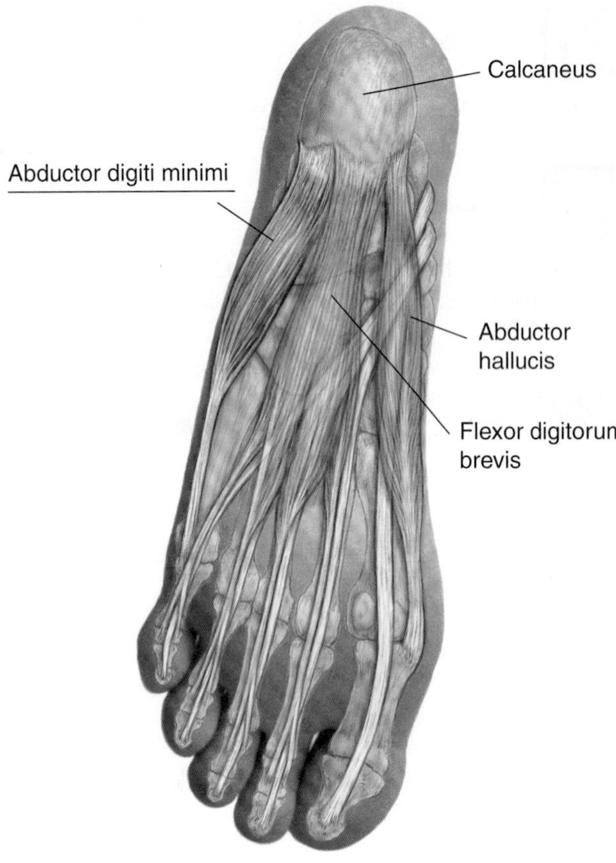

FIGURE 10-45 Anatomy of abductor digiti minimi

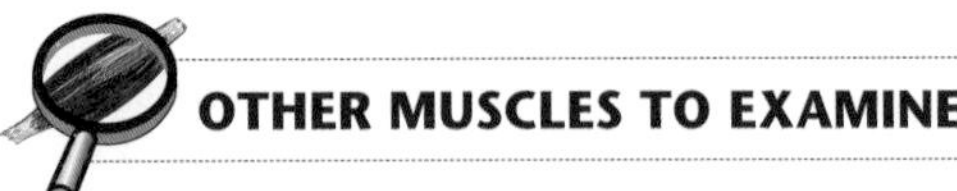

Interossei

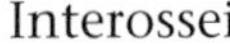

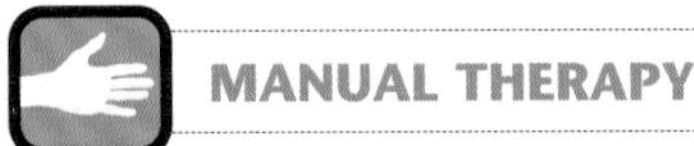

See General Manual Therapy of the Foot, below.

LUMBRICAL MUSCLES OF THE FOOT

LUM-brick-al

ETYMOLOGY Latin ***lumbricus***, earthworm

Overview

One or more of the lumbricals is sometimes missing—or sometimes doubled.

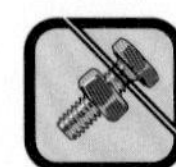

ATTACHMENTS

Origin

- First: from the medial side of the flexor digitorum longus tendon to the 2nd toe (Fig. 10-46)
- Second, third, and fourth: from adjacent sides of the lateral three tendons of flexor digitorum longus (to toes 3-5)

Insertion

- To the tibial side of the extensor tendon on the dorsum of each of the four lateral toes

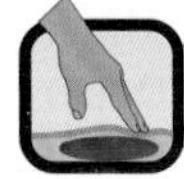

PALPATION

Not directly palpable

ACTION

Flex the MP joint and extend the proximal IP joints of the lateral four toes

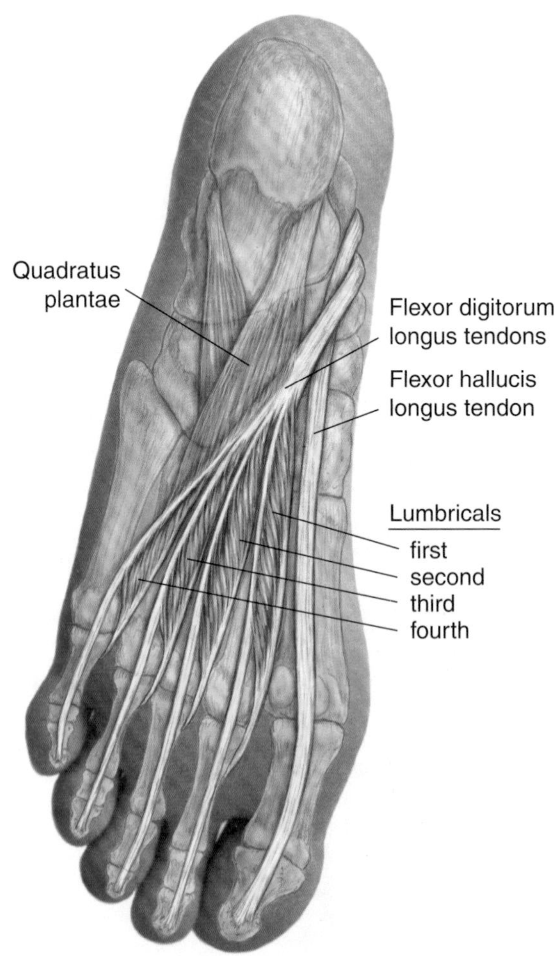

FIGURE 10-46 Anatomy of lumbrical muscles

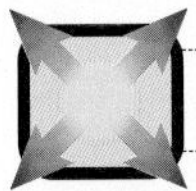

REFERRAL AREA

No isolated pain patterns identified

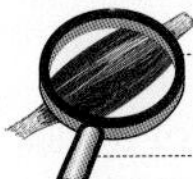

OTHER MUSCLES TO EXAMINE

Not applicable

MANUAL THERAPY

See General Manual Therapy of the Foot, below.

INTEROSSEUS MUSCLES OF THE FOOT (INTEROSSEI)

IN-ter-OSS-ee-us (IN-ter-OSS-eh-ee)

ETYMOLOGY Latin *inter*, between + *os*, bone

Overview

Therapy is restricted to the dorsal interossei, as the plantar interossei cannot be accessed through the plantar fascia and overlying muscles (Fig. 10-47). Interesting to note that if a physician is going to treat the plantar interosseous muscles by injection, they are accessed from the dorsal side of the foot.

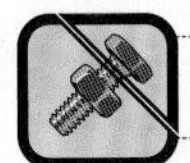

ATTACHMENTS

Dorsal

- Origin: from the sides of adjacent metatarsal bones
- Insertion: first into the medial, second into the lateral side of the proximal phalanx of the 2nd toe, the third and fourth into the lateral side of the proximal phalanx of the 3rd and 4th toes

Plantar

- Origin: medial side of the 3rd, 4th, and 5th metatarsal bones
- Insertion: corresponding side of the proximal phalanx of the same toes

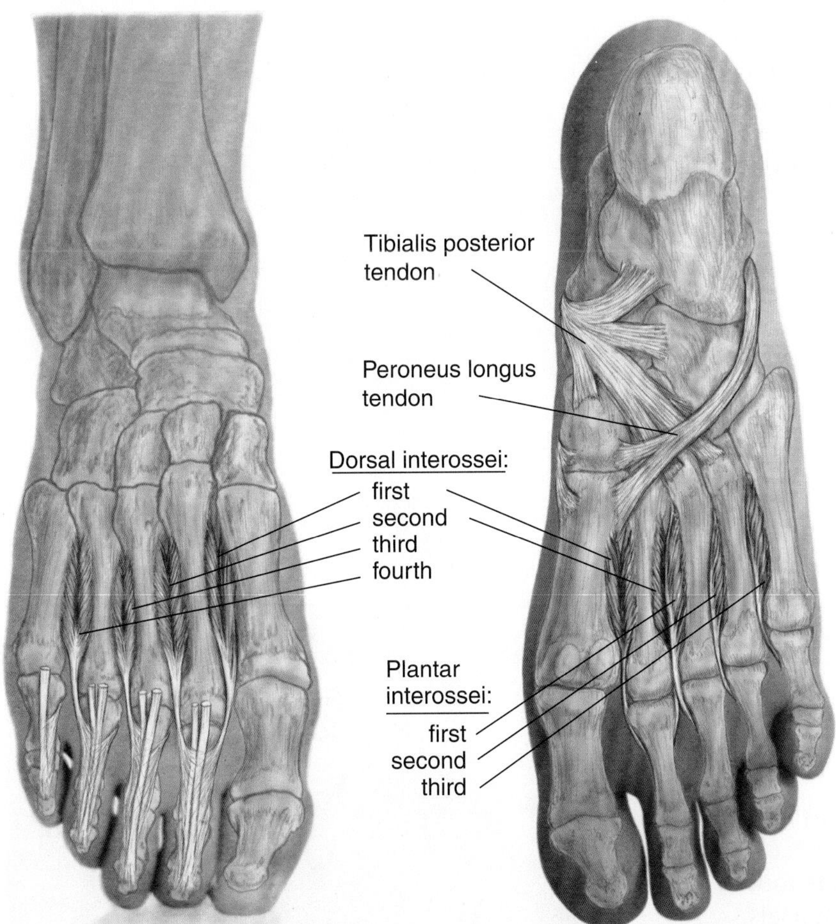

FIGURE 10-47 Anatomy of interosseus muscles (interossei)

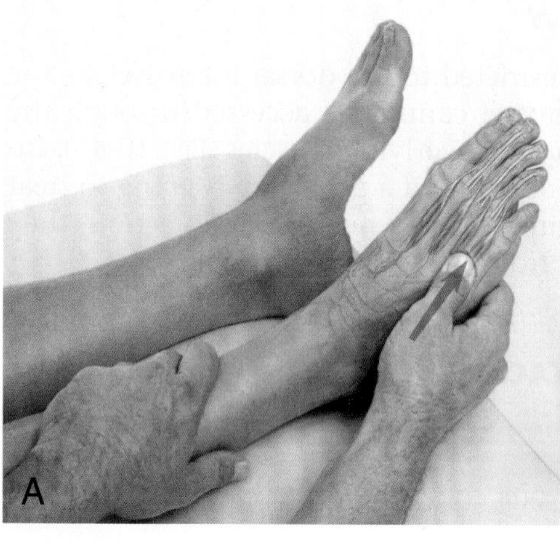

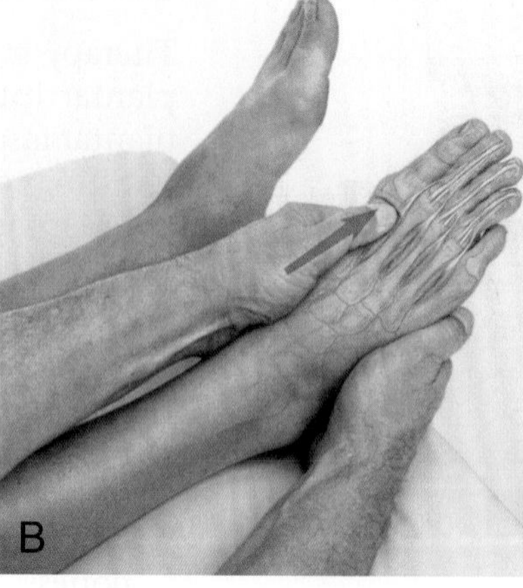

FIGURE 10-48 Stripping of dorsal interossei (therapist at client's legs)

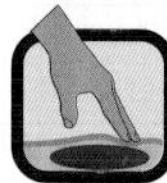

PALPATION

Client supine on the table, knees bent, feet flat on the table. Asking the client to keep the heel on the table and slightly raise the feet will allow you to palpate the interosseous muscles dorsally between the metatarsal bones.

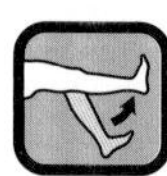

ACTION

- Dorsal: abduct the MP joint of toes 2 to 4 from an axis through the 2nd toe; the first can adduct the MP joint of the 2nd toe
- Plantar: adducts the MP joint of the 3rd through 5th toes

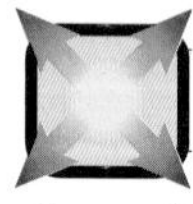

REFERRAL AREA

Over the dorsal or plantar aspects of the corresponding metatarsals

OTHER MUSCLES TO EXAMINE

Flexor and extensor muscles of the toes

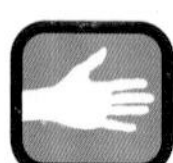

MANUAL THERAPY

DORSAL INTEROSSEOUS MUSCLES

Stripping

- The client lies supine.
- The therapist stands beside the client's legs, facing the feet.
- Place the thumb on the dorsum of the foot in the space between the most lateral metatarsals.
- Pressing firmly into the tissue, slide the thumb along this space to the toes (Fig. 10-48A).
- Repeat this procedure between each pair of metatarsals until the whole foot has been treated (Fig. 10-48B).
- This same procedure can be carried out standing at the client's feet and either pushing the thumb from distal to proximal or pulling the thumb from proximal to distal (Fig. 10-49).

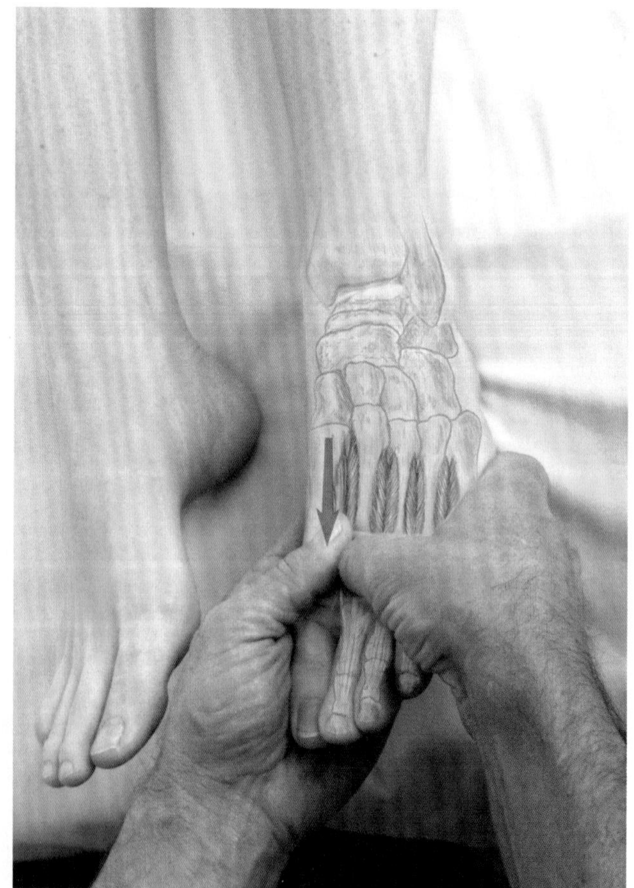

FIGURE 10-49 Stripping of dorsal interossei (therapist standing at client's feet)

General Manual Therapy of the Foot

These are general techniques for loosening the intrinsic muscles of the foot.

Shuckling

- Hold the foot in your lap with both hands grasping it on both sides, and move the hands back and forth (up and down) in opposite directions.
- Do this over the entire breadth of the foot (Fig. 10-50).

Squeezing

- Hold the foot in your lap with both hands and squeeze it, letting your hands slide gradually away from you until they slide off the toes (Fig. 10-51).

Toe-pulling

- Standing at the client's feet, hold the foot with one hand and pull each toe firmly toward yourself (Fig. 10-52).

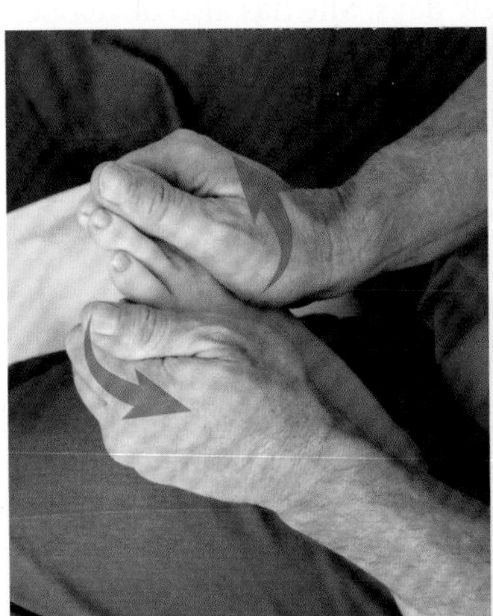
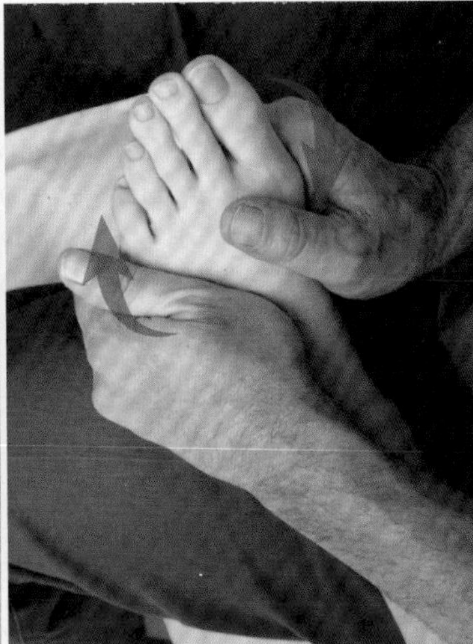

FIGURE 10-50 Shuckling the foot

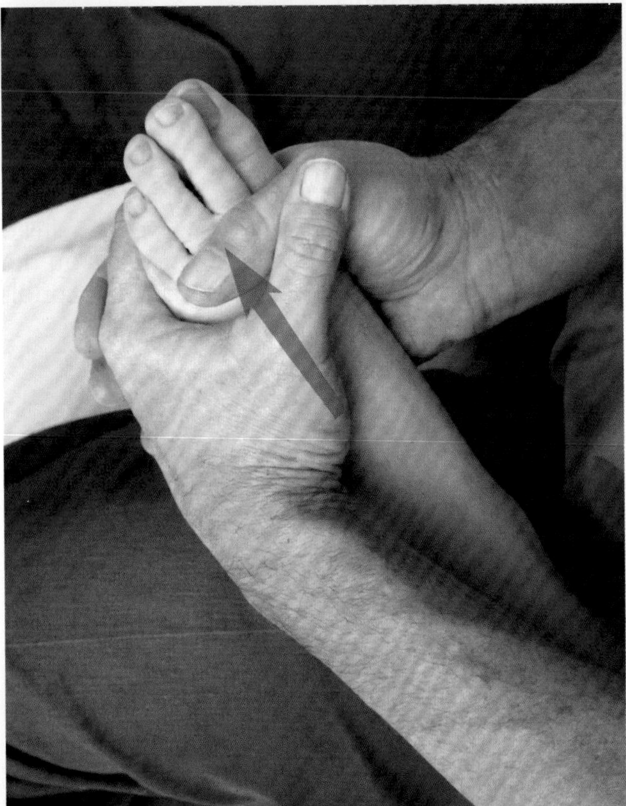

FIGURE 10-51 Squeezing the foot

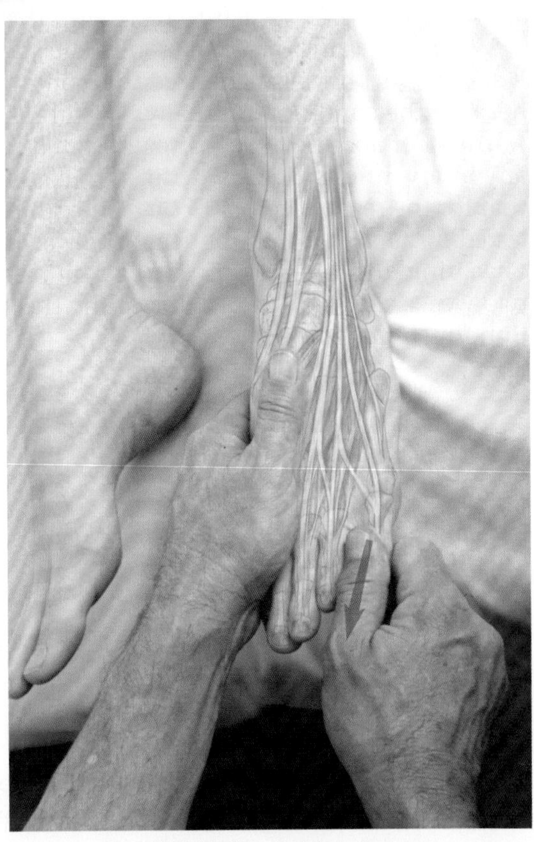

FIGURE 10-52 Pulling the toes

CHAPTER REVIEW

CASE STUDY

L.K. is a 42-year-old woman who has been diagnosed with plantar fasciitis in her left foot. She is a nurse in the psychiatric unit and is on her feet most of the day. She stated that she had been diagnosed by an orthopedist about four months ago and that the doctor had injected her foot with cortisone at that time, fitted her with orthotics, and given her a boot to wear at night that holds the foot in dorsiflexion. He has also given her daily stretches to do, and she reports being diligent about doing them. She stated that the doctor told her at the time she received the injection that for some people it was very effective at stopping the pain and that for some people it may not last long at all. She stated that the shot itself was very painful—and expensive—and that it only brought her relief for a few days. She has also developed a heel spur in response to the plantar fasciitis. She stated that her doctor had informed her that while surgery used to be a common cure for plantar fasciitis, most orthopedists no longer perform it for that purpose. She decided to see if massage therapy would help because she has had success with massage in the past for other muscle ailments. She is also taking NSAIDS and has pain medication that she prefers not to take, but stated that she had to at times, particularly at the end of the day.

L.K. was limping and in obvious pain when she came in. She had worked a double shift the day before and said that the massage was the only reason she was coming out today and that she planned to spend the rest of the day resting. She wears good shoes with good support (in addition to the orthotics). She appears to have no other postural issues. We started the session with her prone, giving Swedish massage for relaxation and warming the muscle, before getting into MFR followed by deep muscle stripping from the ankles to the lower back. The Achilles tendon was sore to the touch; she had a lot of soreness in the gastrocnemius, soleus, ITB, hamstrings, and gluteus. The second half of the session focused on the foot. It was so tender to the touch that an ice cup was applied to the plantar surface for about 5 minutes, followed by palmar effleurage, before beginning any stripping. Passive dorsiflexion was done frequently and held for several seconds each time to give a stretch to the muscle. At the end of the session, I rubbed some peppermint oil into her feet and wrapped them in a warm towel as a feel-good measure more than anything else. She was left to relax with the hot towel for about 10 minutes.

When L.K. came out of the room, she stated that was the best her foot had felt in the 4 months since it started. As I have experienced this condition myself, and had a number of other clients with it, I told her that the condition is usually painful for the better part of a year, which she said her doctor had also warned her about. He had actually stated to her that it usually resolves itself in a year with or without any interventions. She rescheduled to come back in 2 weeks and stated that she was going to budget for that for the rest of the year. When she came in for her second session, she stated that her pain relief had lasted for almost a week but that she was in pain and decided to come weekly for a few weeks instead of waiting until she was already back in pain. After four weekly sessions, she has now gone back on the two-week schedule. She is still wearing the boot at night but says that the massage has made her condition much more bearable.

J.M., LMT

REVIEW QUESTIONS

1. For balanced posture, the weight of the body should rest at a point just _______ of the ankle.
   a. Lateral
   b. Medial
   c. Forward
   d. Backward

2. The _______ fascia is the deep fascia of the lower limb.
   a. Crural
   b. Caudal
   c. Hamstring
   d. Patellar

3. The flexor ______ is a wide band that holds in place the tendons of the tibialis posterior, flexor digitorum longus, and flexor hallucis longus.
   a. Posterior
   b. Hallux
   c. Digitorum
   d. Retinaculum

4. The tibialis anterior crosses from the anterolateral side of the leg to the medial side of the ______.
   a. ASIS
   b. Shin
   c. Soleus
   d. Foot

5. This muscle that is particularly vulnerable to tenosynovitis in classical ballet dancers and in athletes who require forefoot push-off and extreme plantar flexion, such as runners, gymnasts, ice skaters, and swimmers is the ______.
   a. Flexor hallucis longus
   b. Flexor hallucis brevis
   c. Flexor digitorum longus
   d. Flexor digitorum brevis

6. *Quadratus* is descriptive of a muscle that is basically ______.
   a. Trapezoid
   b. Long
   c. Square
   d. Serrated

7. The joints, bones, and musculature of the ankle are comparable to those of the ______.
   a. Foot
   b. Forearm
   c. Hand
   d. Wrist

8. The only one of these muscles that is not considered an "intrinsic" muscle of the foot is the ______.
   a. Quadratus plantae
   b. Extensor digitorum longus
   c. Flexor digitorum brevis
   d. Flexor digiti minimi brevis

9. The ______ cannot be palpated.
   a. Tibialis anterior
   b. Adductor hallucis
   c. Plantar interossei
   d. Gastrocnemius

10. Plantar fasciitis may also be the cause of developing ______.
   a. Heel spurs
   b. Bunions
   c. Corns
   d. Hammertoes

APPENDIX A

Anatomical Prefixes and Suffixes

Greek and Latin Prefixes

Prefix	Meaning
a-	not, without
ab-	away from
abdomen(o)-	of or relating to the abdomen
acr(o)-	extremity; topmost
ad-	to, toward
adip(o)-	relating to fatty tissue
al-	pertaining to
ambi-	both
an-	not, without
ante-	before, in front
anti-	against
arthr(o)-	pertaining to joints, limbs
articul(o)-	joint
bi-	two, both
brady-	slow
burs(o)-	bursa
capit-	pertaining to the head, as a whole
carcin(o)-	relating to cancer
cardi(o)-	relating to the heart
cephal(o)-	relating to the head
cervic-	of or pertaining to the neck
circum-	around
con-	together, with
contra-	against
cost(o)-	of or pertaining to the ribs
cox-	of or relating to the hip, hip joint, or haunch
crani(o)-	belonging or related to the cranium
cyt(o)-	relating to cells
de-	from, down, or not
dextr(o)-	relating to the right side
di-	apart, separation
dia-	through, across
digit-	of or pertaining to the finger
dis-	apart, separate
dys-	painful, faulty
e-	out or away from
ec-	out or away from
ecto-	outside
en-	inside
endo-	inside, within
epi-	over
erythr(o)-	red
eu-	good or normal
ex-	out or away from
exo-	outside
extra-	outside
fibr(o)-	relating to fiber
fore-	before, ahead
gastr(o)-	relating to the stomach
genu-	of or pertaining to the knee
gloss(o)-, glott(o)-	of or pertaining to the tongue
hem(o)-	relating to blood
hemat(o)-	relating to blood
hemi-	half
hist(o)-, histio-	tissue
humer(o)-	pertaining to the upper arm
hydr(o)-	relating to water
hyper-	excessive
hypo-	deficient
ileo-	ilium
ipsi-	same
infra-	below
inter-	between or among
intra-	inside
isch-	restriction
kin(e)-, kin(o)-, kinesi(o)-	movement
latero-	lateral
lip(o)-	relating to fat
lith(o)-	relating to stone
macr(o)-	large
mamm(o)-	of or pertaining to the breast
manu-	of or pertaining to the hand
melan(o)-	black
meso-	middle
meta-	beyond, after, or changed
micro-	small
mono-	one
morph(o)-	form
multi-	many
myel(o)-	of or relating to bone marrow or the spinal cord
necr(o)-	relating to death
neo-	new
neur(i)-, neur(o)-	of or pertaining to the nervous system
ocul(o)-	of or pertaining to the eye
olig(o)-	few
or(o)-	relating to the mouth
orth(o)-	straight
pachy-	thick
pan-	all
para-	beside or abnormal
path(o)-	relating to disease
ped(o)-	relating to children (or sometimes feet)
pelv(i)-, pelv(o)-	hip bone
peri-	position around or surrounding another structure
phob(o)-	relating to excessive fear
phon(o)-	relating to speech
pleur(a)-, pleur(o)-	of or pertaining to the ribs
pod(o)-	relating to feet

poly-	many
post-	after or behind another
pre-	before
pro-	before
psych(o)-	relating to mental function
py(o)-	relating to pus
re-	again or back
reticul(o)-	net
retro-	back or behind
scler(o)-	hard
sarco-	muscular, fleshlike
scoli(o)-	twisted
sigmoid(o)-	S-shaped curvature
sinistr(o)-	relating to the left side
semi-	half
son(o)-	relating to sound
spondyl(o)-	pertaining to the spine
sten(o)-	narrow
sub-	under
super-	above
supra-	above
sym-	with or together
syn-	with or together
tachy-	fast
thorac(i)-, thorac(o)-	pertaining to the thorax
tox(o)-	relating to poison
trans-	situated or moving across or through
tri-	three
troph(o)-	relating to nourishment
ultra-	beyond or excessive
uni-	one
ur(o)-	relating to urine
vas(o)-	relating to vessels
viscer(o)-	of or pertaining to the internal organs

Greek and Latin Suffixes

ac-, acal	pertaining to
-algia	pain
-cele	pouch or hernia
-centesis	puncture
-desis	binding
-dynia	pain
-eal	pertaining to
-ectasis	expansion
-ectomy	removal
-emia	blood
-genesis	origin
-genic	originating
-gram	record
-graph	instrument for recording
-ia	condition
-iasis	presence or formation
-iatric(s), iatry	treatment
-icle	diminutive form
-ism	condition
-ismus	spasm, contraction
-itis	inflammation
-ium	tissue or structure
-logy, logist	study, one who studies
-lysis	dissolution, separation
-malacia	softening
-megaly	enlargement
-meter, metry	measuring device, measurement
-oid	resembling
-ole	diminutive form
-oma	tumor
-osis	condition
-pes	pertaining to the foot
-penia	abnormal reduction
-pexy	fixation
-phil	attraction
-philia	attraction
-plasia	formation
-plasty	surgical repair
-poiesis	formation
-ptosis	falling
-rrhage	burst out
-rrhagia	burst out
-rrhaphy	suture
-rrhea	flow
-rrhexis	rupture
-scope, scopy	instrument for examination, examination
-spasm	involuntary contraction
-stasis	stop
-stomy	creation of an opening
-tension, -tensive	pressure
-tic	pertaining to
-tomy	incision
-tony	tension
-tripsy	crushing
-ula	diminutive form
-ule	diminutive form

Latin Noun Endings

If the nominative singular is –a, then the possessive and the plural are –ae.

Examples:
spina (spine), spinae
scapula, scapulae
fascia (bandage), fasciae
vertebra, vertebrae
Others: tibia, fibula, ulna, fossa, axilla, patella

If the nominative singular is –us, then the possessive and the plural are usually –i.

Examples:
digitus (digit), digiti
humerus, humeri
radius, radii
Others: tarsus, carpus, peroneus, ramus

If the nominative singular is –um, then the possessive is –i and the plural is –a.

Examples:
sacrum, sacri, sacra
sternum, sterni, sterna
cranium, cranii, crania
Others: infundibulum, acetabulum, tectum, cerebrum, pericardium

Some nouns and adjectives are in a different category, where the nominative singular is unpredictable.

Examples:
pectus (chest), pectoris (of the chest), pectora
femur (thigh), femoris, femores
pelvis, pelvis, pelves
pubis, pubis, pubes
nates (buttock), natis, nates
corpus (body), corporis, corpora
latus (side), lateris, latera (not to be confused with the adjective latus = wide)
foramen, foraminis, foramina (aperture)
larynx, laryngis, larynges
coccyx, coccygis, coccyges
mater (mother), matris, matres

Note that adjectives based on these nouns are based not on the nominative, but on the possessive.

Examples:
coccygeal
lateral
pectoral
laryngeal
femoral

APPENDIX B

Directional and Kinetic Terminology

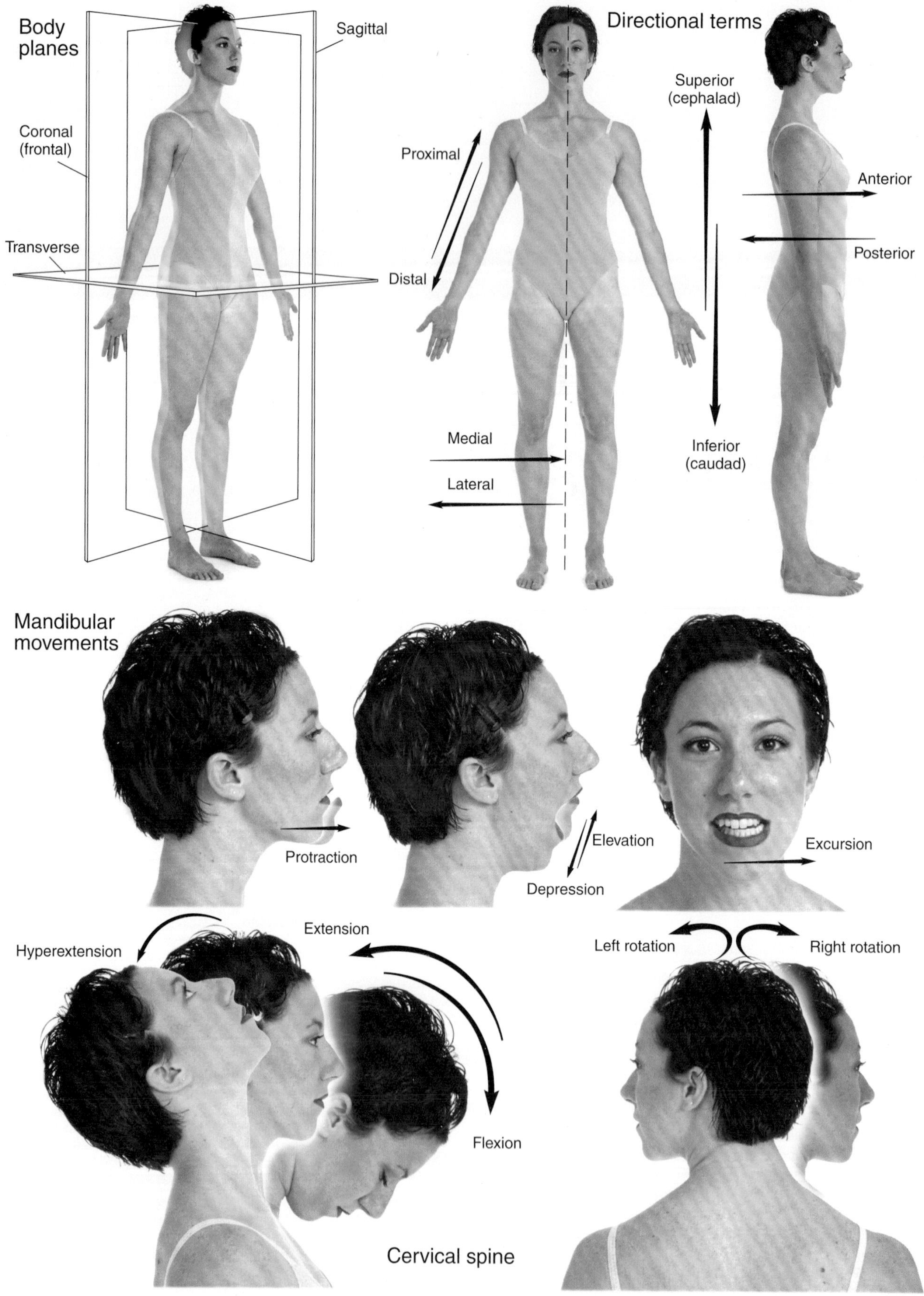
Body planes
Sagittal
Coronal (frontal)
Transverse
Directional terms
Superior (cephalad)
Proximal
Distal
Anterior
Posterior
Medial
Lateral
Inferior (caudad)
Mandibular movements
Protraction
Elevation
Depression
Excursion
Hyperextension
Extension
Flexion
Left rotation
Right rotation
Cervical spine

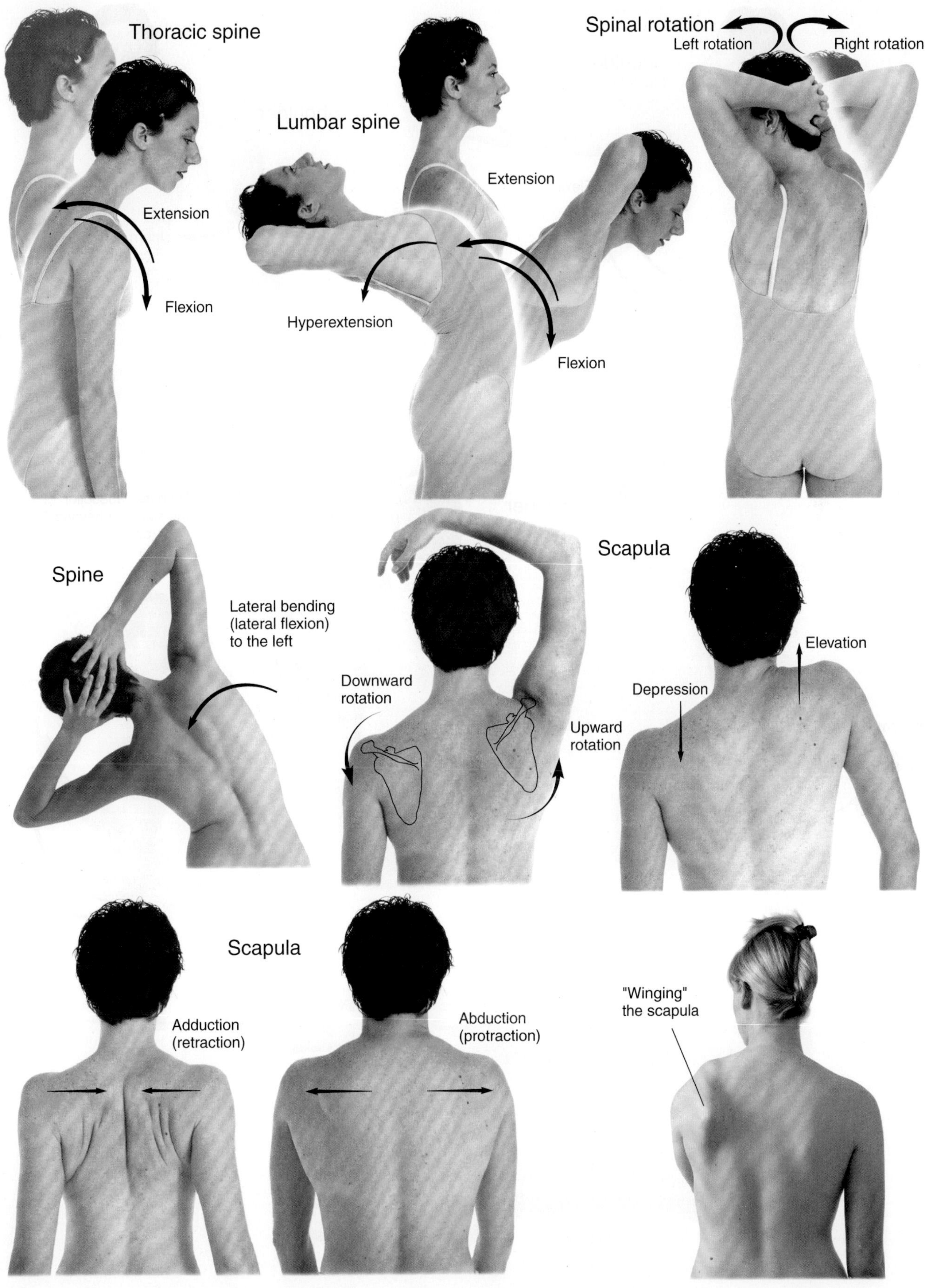
Thoracic spine
Extension
Flexion
Lumbar spine
Extension
Hyperextension
Flexion
Spinal rotation
Left rotation
Right rotation
Spine
Lateral bending
(lateral flexion)
to the left
Scapula
Downward
rotation
Upward
rotation
Elevation
Depression
Scapula
Adduction
(retraction)
Abduction
(protraction)
"Winging"
the scapula

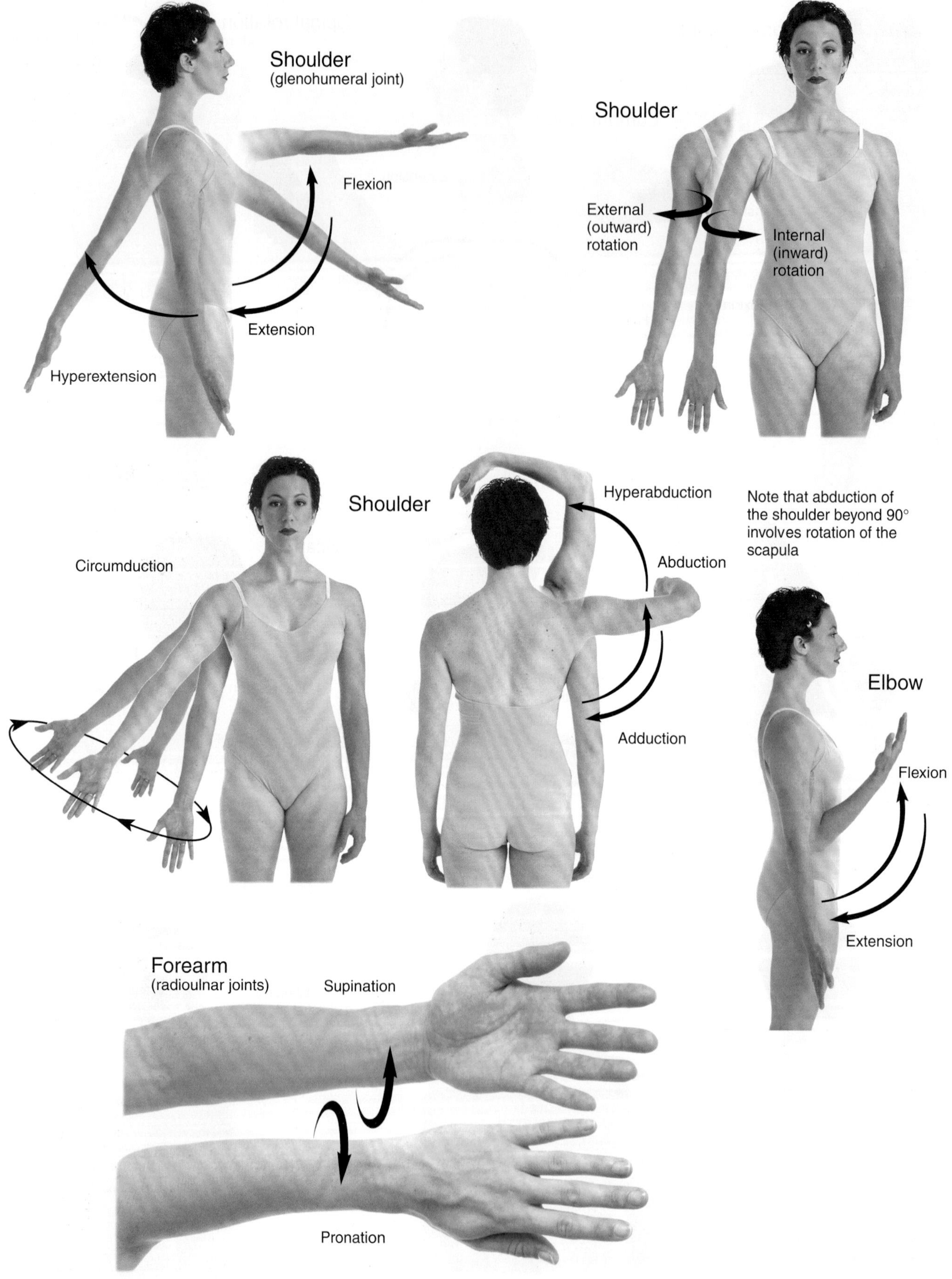
Shoulder
(glenohumeral joint)
Flexion
Extension
Hyperextension
Shoulder
External
(outward)
rotation
Internal
(inward)
rotation
Shoulder
Circumduction
Hyperabduction
Abduction
Adduction
Note that abduction of the shoulder beyond 90° involves rotation of the scapula
Elbow
Flexion
Extension
Forearm
(radioulnar joints)
Supination
Pronation

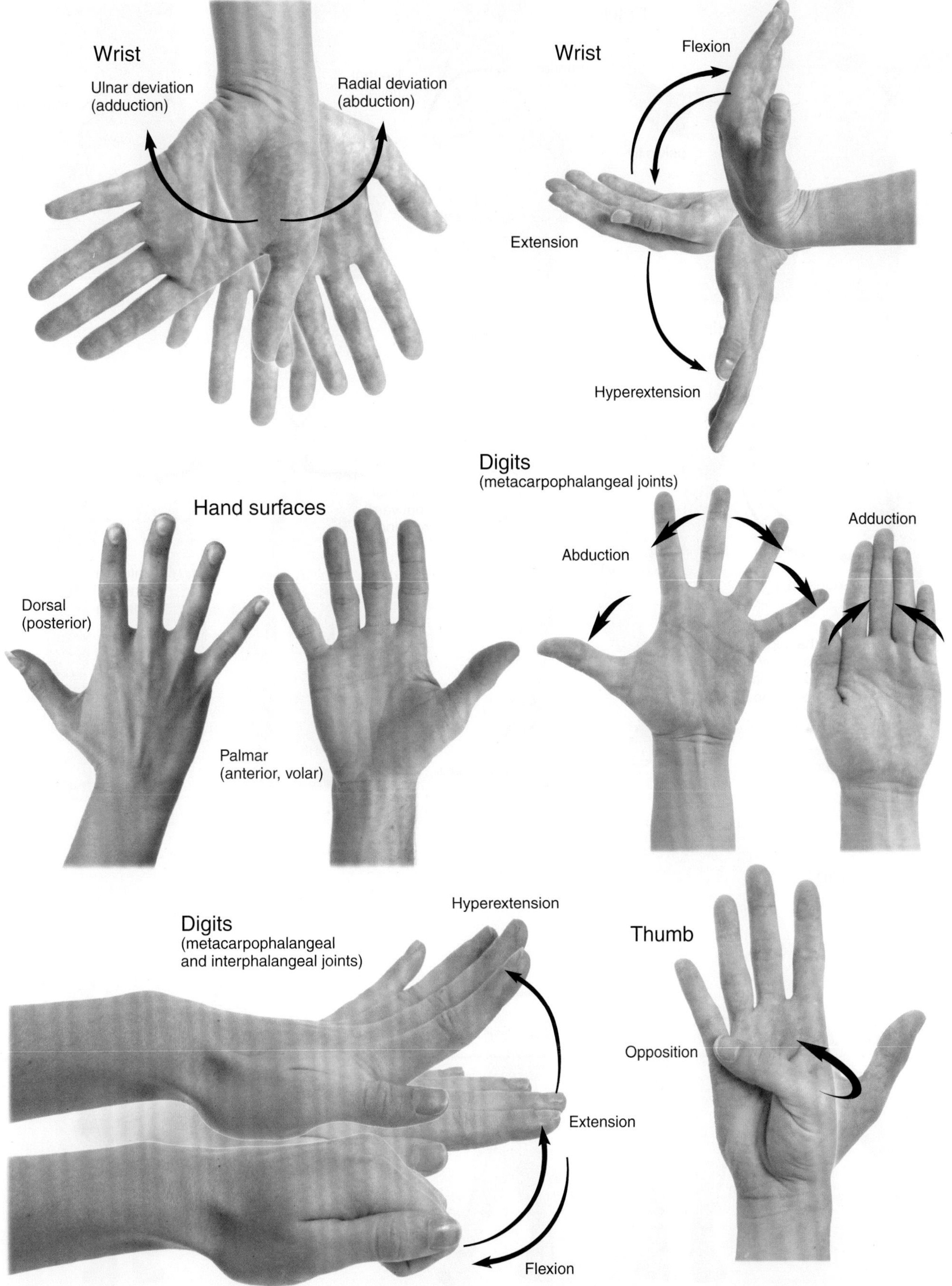
Wrist
Ulnar deviation
(adduction)
Radial deviation
(abduction)
Wrist
Flexion
Extension
Hyperextension
Digits
(metacarpophalangeal joints)
Hand surfaces
Dorsal
(posterior)
Palmar
(anterior, volar)
Abduction
Adduction
Digits
(metacarpophalangeal
and interphalangeal joints)
Hyperextension
Extension
Flexion
Thumb
Opposition

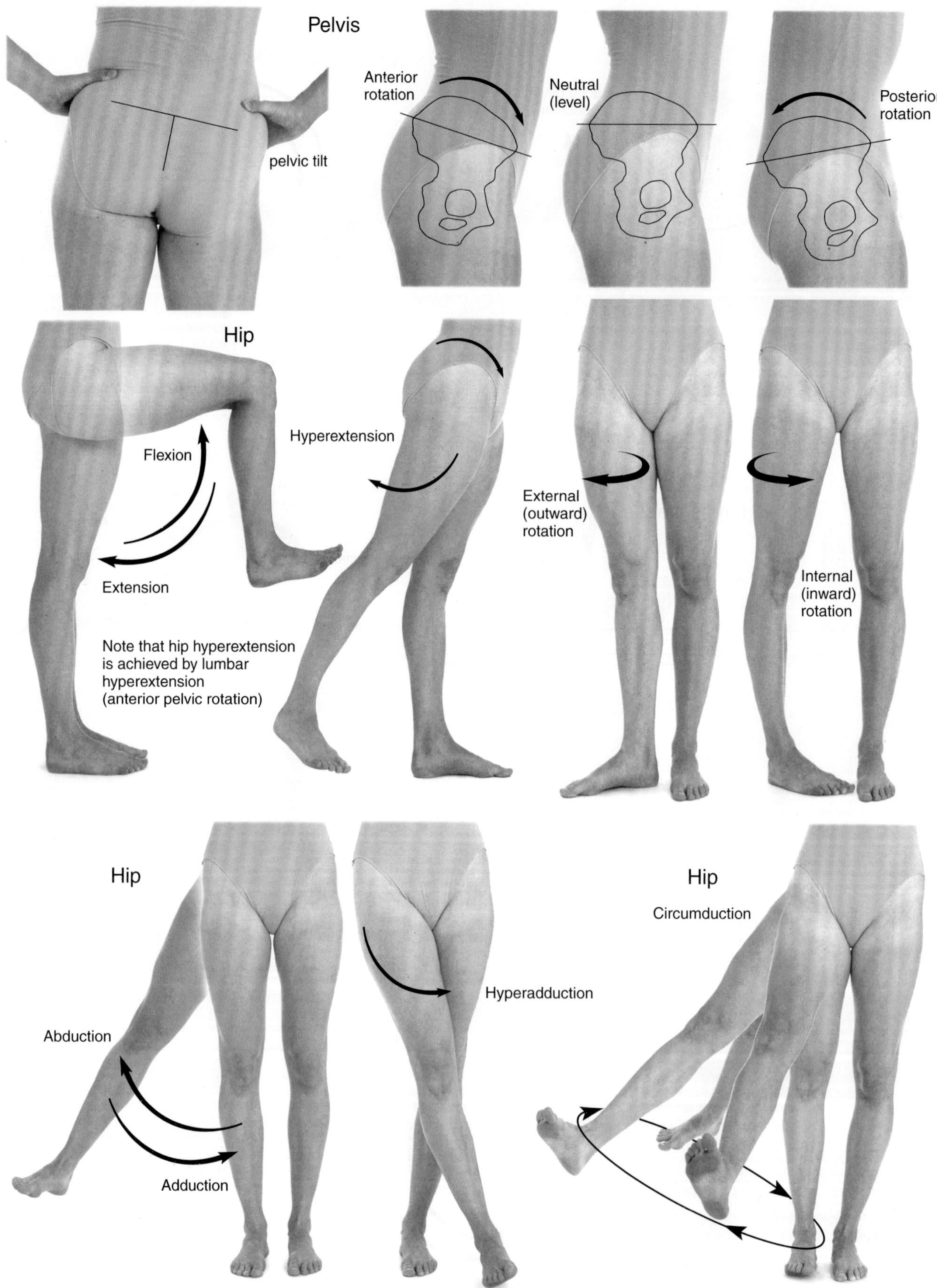
Pelvis
pelvic tilt
Anterior rotation
Neutral (level)
Posterior rotation
Hip
Flexion
Extension
Hyperextension
Note that hip hyperextension is achieved by lumbar hyperextension (anterior pelvic rotation)
External (outward) rotation
Internal (inward) rotation
Hip
Abduction
Adduction
Hyperadduction
Hip
Circumduction

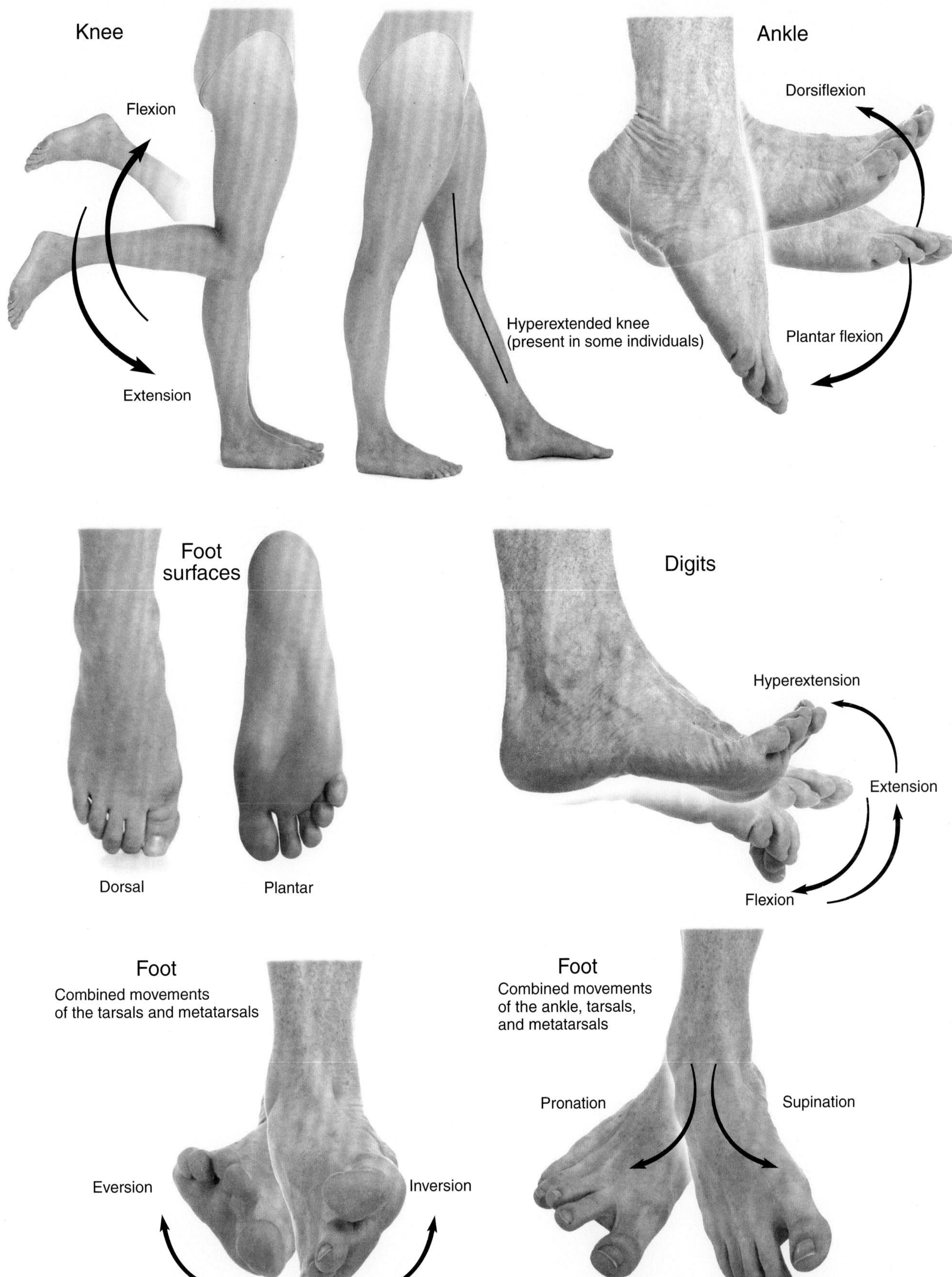
Knee
Flexion
Extension
Hyperextended knee
(present in some individuals)
Ankle
Dorsiflexion
Plantar flexion
Foot
surfaces
Dorsal
Plantar
Digits
Hyperextension
Extension
Flexion
Foot
Combined movements
of the tarsals and metatarsals
Eversion
Inversion
Foot
Combined movements
of the ankle, tarsals,
and metatarsals
Pronation
Supination

APPENDIX C

Muscles by Pain Referral Zone

This is an outline of muscles organized by pain referral zones. Each heading indicates an area in which pain might be experienced; under it is a list of muscles that typically refer pain to that area.

- Head and neck
  - Head
    - Top of head (vertex)
      - Sternocleidomastoid
      - Splenius capitis
    - Back of head
      - Locally, to the back and top of head and can radiate to the ipsilateral eye
      - Trapezius
      - Sternocleidomastoid
      - Semispinalis capitis
      - Semispinalis cervicis
      - Splenius cervicis
      - Suboccipital group
      - Occipitalis
      - Digastric
      - Temporalis
    - Temporal (side of head)
      - Locally, to all or part of temporal region, eyebrow region, cheek, and incisor and molar teeth
      - Trapezius
      - Sternocleidomastoid
      - Temporalis
      - Splenius cervicis
      - Suboccipital group
      - Semispinalis capitis
    - Frontal (forehead)
      - Locally, with pain radiating over the forehead
      - Sternocleidomastoid
      - Semispinalis capitis
      - Frontalis
      - Zygomaticus major
    - Ear and temporomandibular joint (TMJ)
      - Locally, to upper and lower jaw, side of face, ear, and superior to eyebrow
      - Medial and lateral pterygoids
      - Masseter
      - Sternocleidomastoid (clavicular)
    - Eye and eyebrow
      - Locally, superior to the eye and down the side of the nose
      - Sternocleidomastoid (sternal)
      - Temporalis
      - Splenius cervicis
      - Masseter
      - Suboccipital group
      - Occipitalis
      - Orbicularis oculi
      - Trapezius
    - Cheek and jaw
      - Locally, up the cheek and alongside of the nose, and in front of the ear
      - Sternocleidomastoid (sternal)
      - Masseter
      - Lateral pterygoid
      - Trapezius
      - Digastric
      - Medial pterygoid
      - Platysma
      - Orbicularis oculi
      - Zygomaticus major
    - Toothache
      - Temporalis
      - Masseter
      - Digastric
  - Neck
    - Back of neck
      - Trapezius
      - Multifidi
      - Levator scapulae
      - Splenius cervicis
      - Infraspinatus
    - Throat and front of neck
      - Locally, over the anterior neck, and may radiate to upper chest
      - Sternocleidomastoid
      - Digastric
      - Medial pterygoid
- Upper back, shoulder, and arm
  - Upper back and shoulder
    - Upper thoracic back
      - Scalenes
      - Levator scapulae
      - Supraspinatus
      - Trapezius
      - Multifidi
      - Rhomboids
      - Splenius cervicis
      - Triceps brachii
      - Biceps brachii
    - Back of shoulder
      - Deltoids
      - Levator scapulae
      - Scalenes
      - Supraspinatus
      - Teres major
      - Teres minor
      - Subscapularis
      - Serratus posterior superior
      - Latissimus dorsi
      - Triceps brachii
      - Trapezius
      - Iliocostalis thoracis

Front of shoulder
Locally, laterally along the clavicle, over the front of the shoulder and upper arm, along the radial side of the forearm and into the thumb and first two fingers
Infraspinatus
Deltoids
Scalenes
Supraspinatus
Pectoralis major
Pectoralis minor
Biceps brachii
Coracobrachialis

Arm, forearm, wrist, and hand
Back of arm
Scalenes
Triceps
Brachii
Deltoid
Subscapularis
Supraspinatus
Teres major
Teres minor
Latissimus dorsi
Serratus posterior superior
Coracobrachialis
Scalenus minimus

Front of arm
Scalenes
Infraspinatus
Biceps brachii
Brachialis
Triceps brachii
Supraspinatus
Deltoids
Sternalis
Scalenus minimus
Subclavius

Elbow to finger
Outside of the elbow (lateral epicondyle)
Supinator
Brachioradialis
Extensor carpi radialis longus
Triceps brachii
Supraspinatus
Fourth and fifth finger extensors
Anconeus

Inside of the elbow (medial epicondyle)
Triceps brachii
Pectoralis major
Pectoralis minor

Front, or inner (antecubital) surface, of the elbow
Brachialis
Biceps brachii

Back of (dorsal) forearm
Triceps brachii
Teres major
Extensors carpi radialis longus and brevis

Point of the elbow (olecranon)
Triceps brachii
Serratus posterior superior

Radial forearm
Infraspinatus
Scalenes
Brachioradialis
Supraspinatus
Subclavius

Inner (volar) forearm
Palmaris longus
Pronator teres
Serratus anterior
Triceps brachii

Ulnar forearm
Latissimus dorsi
Pectoralis major
Pectoralis minor
Serratus posterior superior

Inner (volar) wrist and palmar
Flexor carpi radialis
Flexor carpi ulnaris
Opponens pollicis
Pectoralis major
Pectoralis minor
Latissimus dorsi
Palmaris longus
Pronator teres
Serratus anterior

Back of (dorsal) wrist and hand
Extensor carpi radialis brevis
Extensor carpi radialis longus
Index to little finger extensors
Extensor indicis
Extensor carpi ulnaris
Subscapularis
Coracobrachialis
Scalenus minimus
Latissimus dorsi
Serratus posterior superior
First dorsal interosseous

Base of thumb and radial hand
Supinator
Scalenes
Brachialis
Infraspinatus
Extensor carpi radialis longus
Brachioradialis
Opponens pollicis
Adductor pollicis
First dorsal interosseous
Flexor pollicis longus

Volar finger (palm side)
Flexors digitorum sublimis and profundus
Interossei
Latissimus dorsi
Serratus anterior
Abductor digiti minimi
Subclavius
Back of (dorsal) finger
Extensor digitorum
Interossei
Scalenes
Abductor digiti minimi
Pectoralis major
Pectoralis minor
Latissimus dorsi
Subclavius
Torso
Upper torso
In the ipsilateral (on the same side) breast and anterior chest, over the anterior shoulder, down the volar (referring to the palm of the hand) surface of the upper arm, over the volar surface of the forearm just below the elbow, and into the middle and ring fingers
Side of chest
Locally, the axilla and across the chest
Serratus anterior
Latissimus dorsi
Front of chest
Pectoralis major
Pectoralis minor
Scalenes
Sternocleidomastoid (sternal)
Sternalis
Iliocostalis cervicis
Subclavius
External abdominal oblique
Mid-thoracic (middle of the back)
Locally, at the side of the back and around the inferior scapula, across the scapula, and the posterior arm
Scalenes
Latissimus dorsi
Levator scapulae
Iliocostalis thoracis
Multifidi
Rhomboids
Serratus posterior superior
Infraspinatus
Trapezius
Serratus anterior
Lower torso
Low thoracic back
Diaphragm
Iliocostalis thoracis
Multifidi
Serratus posterior inferior
Rectus abdominis
Latissimus dorsi
Lumbar (lower back)
Longissimus thoracis
Iliocostalis lumborum
Iliocostalis thoracis
Multifidi
Rectus abdominis
Gluteus medius
Iliopsoas
Buttock
Gluteus medius
Quadratus lumborum
Gluteus maximus
Semitendinosus
Semimembranosus
Piriformis
Gluteus minimus
Rectus abdominis
Soleus
Iliocostalis lumborum
Longissimus thoracis
Iliosacral (base of spine and upper edge of pelvis)
Gluteus medius
Quadratus lumborum
Gluteus maximus
Levator ani
Coccygeus
Rectus abdominis
Soleus
Multifidi
Pelvis
Locally, may mimic visceral pain
Levator ani
Coccygeus
Obturator internus
Adductor magnus
Piriformis
Internal abdominal oblique
Abdomen
Locally, may mimic visceral pain
Rectus abdominis
Abdominal obliques
Iliocostalis thoracis
Multifidi
Quadratus lumborum
Pyramidalis
Transversus abdominis
Hip, leg, and foot
Hip and thigh
Side of (lateral) hip and thigh
Gluteus minimus
Vastus lateralis
Piriformis
Quadratus lumborum

- Tensor fasciae latae
- Iliotibial band
- Vastus intermedius
- Gluteus maximus
- Rectus femoris

Front of (anterior) thigh
- Adductor longus
- Adductor brevis
- Iliopsoas
- Adductor magnus
- Vastus intermedius
- Pectineus
- Sartorius
- Quadratus lumborum
- Rectus femoris

Mid-front of (medial) thigh
- Pectineus
- Vastus medialis
- Gracilis
- Adductor magnus
- Sartorius

Back of (posterior) thigh
- Gluteus minimus
- Semitendinosus
- Semimembranosus
- Biceps femoris
- Piriformis
- Obturator internus

Knee

Front of (anterior) knee
- Rectus femoris
- Vastus medialis
- Adductor longus
- Adductor brevis

Inner surface, toward the front of (anteromedial) knee
- Vastus medialis
- Gracilis
- Rectus femoris
- Sartorius
- Adductor longus
- Adductor brevis

Side of (lateral) knee
- Vastus lateralis

Back of (posterior) knee
- Gastrocnemius
- Biceps femoris
- Popliteus
- Semitendinosus
- Semimembranosus
- Soleus
- Plantaris

Leg, ankle, and foot

Front of calf (anterior leg)
- Tibialis anterior
- Adductor longus
- Adductor brevis

Outside of calf (lateral leg)
- Iliotibial band
- Gastrocnemius
- Gluteus minimus
- Peroneus longus
- Peroneus brevis
- Vastus lateralis

Back of calf (posterior leg)
- Soleus
- Gluteus minimus
- Gastrocnemius
- Semitendinosus
- Semimembranosus
- Soleus
- Flexor digitorum longus
- Tibialis posterior
- Plantaris

Front of (anterior) ankle
- Tibialis anterior
- Peroneus tertius
- Extensor digitorum longus
- Extensor hallucis longus

Outside of (lateral) ankle
- Peroneus longus
- Peroneus brevis
- Peroneus tertius

Inner (medial) ankle
- Abductor hallucis
- Flexor digitorum longus

Back of (posterior) ankle
- Soleus
- Tibialis posterior

Heel
- Soleus
- Quadratus plantae
- Abductor hallucis
- Tibialis posterior

Back of (dorsal) forefoot
- Extensor digitorum brevis
- Extensor hallucis brevis
- Extensor digitorum longus
- Flexor hallucis brevis
- Interossei of foot
- Tibialis anterior

Bottom surface of (plantar) midfoot
- Gastrocnemius
- Flexor digitorum longus
- Adductor hallucis
- Soleus
- Interossei of foot
- Abductor hallucis
- Tibialis posterior

Ball of the foot (metatarsal head)
- Flexor hallucis brevis
- Flexor digitorum brevis
- Adductor hallucis
- Flexor hallucis longus

- Interossei of foot
- Abductor digiti minimi
- Flexor digitorum longus
- Tibialis posterior

Back of (dorsal) great toe
- Tibialis anterior
- Extensor hallucis longus
- Flexor hallucis brevis

Back of (dorsal) lesser toe
- Interossei of foot
- Extensor digitorum longus

Bottom surface of (plantar) great toe
- Flexor hallucis longus
- Flexor hallucis brevis
- Tibialis posterior

Bottom surface of (plantar) lesser toe
- Flexor digitorum longus
- Tibialis posterior

APPENDIX D

Suggested Readings

Archer P, Nelson L. *Applied Anatomy & Physiology for Manual Therapists*. Philadelphia, PA: Lippincott Williams & Wilkins; 2012.

Bucci C. *Condition-Specific Massage Therapy*. Philadelphia, PA: Lippincott Williams & Wilkins; 2011.

Clemente C. *Anatomy: A Regional Atlas of the Human Body*. 6th ed. Baltimore, MD: Lippincott Williams & Wilkins; 2010.

Granger J. *Neuromuscular Therapy Manual*. Baltimore, MD: Lippincott Williams & Wilkins; 2010.

Kendall FP, McCreary EK, Provance PG, et al. *Muscles: Testing and Function, with Posture and Pain*. Baltimore, MD: Lippincott Williams & Wilkins; 2005.

Lieber RL. *Skeletal Muscle Structure and Function: Implications for Rehabilitation and Sports Medicine*. 3rd ed. Philadelphia, PA: Lippincott Williams & Wilkins; 2010.

Muscolino J. *Advanced Treatment Techniques for the Manual Therapist: Neck*. Baltimore, MD: Lippincott Williams & Wilkins; 2012.

Muscolino J. *Manual Therapy for the Low Back and Pelvis: A Clinical Orthopedic Approach*. Baltimore, MD: Lippincott Williams & Wilkins; 2014.

Travell JG, Simons, DG. *Travell & Simons' Myofascial Pain and Dysfunction: The Trigger Point Manual*. Vol. 1. Baltimore, MD: Lippincott Williams & Wilkins; 1998a.

Travell JG, Simons, DG. *Travell & Simons' Myofascial Pain and Dysfunction: The Trigger Point Manual*. Vol. 2. Baltimore, MD: Lippincott Williams & Wilkins; 1998b.

Walton T. *Medical Conditions and Massage Therapy: A Decision Tree Approach*. Baltimore, MD: Lippincott Williams & Wilkins; 2010.

Glossary

Actin filament The protein filament in a sarcomere that is pulled inward by the heads on the myosin filament to effect contraction

Active trigger point A trigger point that actively causes referred pain without being directly stimulated

Agonist A muscle that is contracting to perform an action, opposed by an antagonist

Antagonist A muscle that opposes the action of an agonist

Articular process A small flat projection found on the surfaces of the arches on either side of the vertebrae that articulate with adjoining vertebrae

Articular facet A small articular surface of a bone, especially a vertebra

Atlas First cervical vertebra, articulating with the occipital bone and rotating around the odontoid process of the axis (Greek *Atlas*, in Greek mythology a Titan who supported the earth on his shoulders)

Axis The second cervical vertebra

Bindegewebsmassage German for *connective tissue massage,* a therapeutic approach developed by Elisabeth Dicke

Biopsychosocial Of, relating to, or concerned with the biological, psychological, and social aspects in contrast to the strictly biomedical aspects of disease

Bipennate Muscle architecture in which fibers lie at two angles to the force-generating axis

Body mechanics The use of the therapist's body to perform effective work with minimum strain or injury

Bodywork Any holistic approach to examination and manual manipulation of the soft tissues of the body for therapeutic purposes

Cartilaginous joint A joint in which two bony surfaces are united by cartilage. The two types of cartilaginous joints are **synchondroses** and **symphyses**

Caudad Toward the tail (coccyx)

Cephalad Toward the head

Chiropractic A health discipline focused on treatment of the joints, particularly those of the vertebrae. These practitioners attribute pain and other health problems to misalignments of the vertebral joints that impinge on nerve roots, resulting in abnormal functions of the nervous system

Clinical massage therapy Manual manipulation of the soft tissues to resolve specific problems of pain or dysfunction

Compression The application of pressure to the body using the hand, fist, elbow, knuckles, fingertips, or thumb

Concentric contraction Muscular contraction that results in shortening of the muscle

Condyle A rounded articular surface at the extremity of a bone

Connective tissue The supportive tissues of the body, made of a ground substance and fibrous tissues, taking a wide variety of forms. Although bone, blood, and lymph are technically connective tissues, the term is normally used in massage therapy and bodywork to refer to fascia, tendons, and ligaments

Convergent Type of muscle architecture in which muscle fibers from a broad attachment converge to a narrow attachment, forming a fan shape

Core™ Myofascial Therapy A systematic approach of applying slow, deep pressure to the myofascial tissue following Langer's lines

Coronal A vertical plane perpendicular to the sagittal plane dividing the body into anterior and posterior portions, also called the frontal plane

Cross-bridge theory The theory that actin combines with myosin and ATP (adenosine triphosphate) to produce muscle contractions

Cross-fiber friction Deep stroking perpendicular to the fiber of a muscle, tendon, or ligament with the fingertips, thumb, or elbow

Deep Away from the surface of the body; the opposite of superficial (e.g., pectoralis minor lies deep to pectoralis major)
Distal Away from the center of the body or from the origin
Dorsal Relating to the back; posterior
Dorsiflexion Backward flexion or bending, as of the hand or the foot; turning the hand or foot upward towards the body

Eccentric contraction Muscular contraction during lengthening of the muscle, helping to control movement
Exhaustion The state of muscle cells in which the energy source, ATP, is temporarily depleted

Facet A small surface, especially of bone. A facet joint is a joint comprised of two surfaces in contact
Fascia Fibrous connective tissue continuously enveloping the whole body, including the viscera, individual muscles, and parts of muscles
Fascicle A bundle of muscle fibers
Fossa A hollow or depressed area, trench, or channel
Frontal A vertical plane perpendicular to the sagittal plane dividing the body into anterior and posterior portions; also called the coronal plane

Gate control theory The theory that physical pain is not a direct result of activation of pain receptor neurons, but rather its perception is modulated by interaction between different neurons

Hellerwork™ A type of structural bodywork emphasizing fascial manipulation developed by Joseph Heller, MD, based on the work of Ida Rolf
HIPAA Health Insurance Portability Accountability Act Laws meant to protect personal identifying information related to their health care
Horizontal A plane perpendicular to the gravitational force

Idiopathic scoliosis A type of scoliosis of unknown origin that may commence in infancy (infantile scoliosis), childhood (juvenile scoliosis), or adolescence (adolescent scoliosis)
Ischemic compression Compression of a point in muscle tissue, usually of a trigger point, that obstructs the flow of blood in the tissue

Kyphosis Excessive flexion (convex curvature) of the spine

Langer's lines (lines of cleavage) Lines indicating the principal axis of orientation of the subcutaneous connective tissue fibers; these lines vary in direction with the region of the body surface
Latent trigger point A trigger point that refers pain or other sensations only when compressed; however, it may limit lengthening of the muscle in which it resides, or cause muscle shortening in its referral zone
Lateral Away from the sagittal midline of the body; the opposite of medial
Lordosis Excessive extension (concave curvature) of the spine

Mandible The lower jaw bone, which articulates with the temporal bone on either side
Massage therapy Manual manipulation of the soft tissues for relaxation, pain relief, or other healthful purposes
Medial Toward the sagittal midline of the body; the opposite of lateral
Motor unit A single motor neuron and the group of muscle fibers that it innervates
Multipennate Muscle architecture in which fibers lie at multiple angles to the force-generating axis
Muscle architecture The structure of a muscle in terms of the directions of its fibers
Muscle cell, skeletal A single cell of muscle tissue, containing several nuclei and many myofibrils, innervated along with other cells in the same motor unit by a single neuron
Muscle fiber Synonym for *muscle cell*
Myofascial release A system of myofascial work intended to influence the fascia
Myofibril A sequential strand of sarcomeres within a muscle cell
Myofilament A filament of either myosin or actin, which together form the contractile element of muscle tissue

Myosin The protein filament in a sarcomere from which molecular "heads" extend to pull the actin filament inward to effect contraction

National Certification Board for Therapeutic Massage and Bodywork A national organization that tests and certifies qualified massage therapists and bodyworkers

Neuromatrix theory a theory of pain that states that the perception of painful stimuli does not result from the brain's passive registration of tissue trauma, but from its active generation of subjective experiences through a network of neurons

Neuromuscular junction The synaptic connection of the axon of the motor neuron with a muscle fiber

Neuromuscular therapy A systematic approach to myofascial treatment that attempts to interrupt the neuromuscular feedback that maintains pain or dysfunction. The two main traditions are British (Leon Chaitow) and American (Judith Walker Delaney, Paul St. John)

Occipital condyle An elongated oval facet on the undersurface of the occipital bone on either side of the foramen magnum, which articulates with the atlas vertebra

Odontoid process A process projecting upward from the body of the axis vertebra around which the atlas rotates

Osteopathy A type of medicine that combines conventional medical diagnostic and treatment techniques with physical manipulation

Palmar Relating to the palm, the anterior surface of the hand in anatomical position

Parallel (longitudinal) Muscle architecture in which muscle fibers are parallel to the force-generating axis

Passive shortening Reduction in the length of a muscle without contraction

Passive stretching Stretching or lengthening of a muscle by another person

Pennate Any muscle architecture in which the fibers lie at angles to the force-generating axis

Physical therapy A type of medical therapy in which passive movement and exercise are the primary means of treatment

Primary trigger point The original trigger point from trauma or injury, which may generate other satellite trigger points

Process A projection or outgrowth from a bone

Proximal Nearer to the center of the body or origin

Reciprocal inhibition The relaxation of a muscle in response to the contraction of its antagonist

Recruitment The activation of motor units by motor neurons

Release Palpable relaxation and softening of myofascial tissue. In myofascial stretching, the therapist experiences release as a lengthening of the tissue. In compression of tender or trigger points, the therapist feels a softening in the tissue, and the client reports a lessening or cessation of pain

Rib hump A symptomatic elevation of the posterior ribs on one side during forward bending in idiopathic scoliosis

Rolfing™ A type of structural bodywork, originally called structural integration, developed by Ida Rolf, PhD, which focuses on manipulation of the fascia

Sagittal plane A vertical plane perpendicular to the frontal (coronal) plane, dividing the body into left and right sides (Latin *sagitta*, arrow)

Sarcomere A group of myofilaments forming the unit of contraction in a muscle

Sarcoplasmic reticulum The complex of vesicles and tubules that form a continuous structure around myofibrils and carry the chemical trigger, calcium, necessary to initiate muscle contraction at the molecular level

Satellite trigger point A secondary trigger point activated by a primary trigger point. Satellite trigger points will not respond to treatment without resolution of the primary trigger point

Scoliosis Any lateral curvature of the spine. The most common types are postural, idiopathic, neuromuscular, and congenital

Skin rolling A fascial treatment technique in which the therapist picks up folds of skin and superficial fascia with the fingertips using alternating hands

Stripping, stripping massage Moving pressure, usually along the fiber of a muscle from origin to insertion, using thumb(s), fingertips, the heel of the hand, the knuckles, the elbow, or the forearm

Superficial Nearer to the surface of the body; the opposite of deep (e.g., pectoralis major is superficial to pectoralis minor)

Swedish massage A general term for relaxation massage, derived from the type of massage taught by Pehr Henrik Ling. The strokes of effleurage, petrissage, friction, tapotement, vibration, and nerve strokes are usually applied systematically

Synapse The point of contact of a nerve cell with another nerve cell, a muscle or gland cell, or a sensory receptor cell, across which chemical neurotransmitters move to transmit nerve impulses

Synchondrosis A union between two bones formed either by hyaline cartilage or fibrocartilage

Symphysis A union between two bones formed by fibrocartilage

Tender point Any point on the body that is tender only at its location; tender points do not refer pain to other areas

Traditional Western medicine The anatomically and physiologically based approach to diagnosing and treating disease and injury that predominates health care in Western cultures; also known as allopathic medicine

Transverse tubules Microscopic tubes surrounding and penetrating myofibrils that connect the sarcoplasmic reticulum to the muscle cell membrane

Trigger point A point in muscle or connective tissue that is painful in response to pressure and that refers or radiates pain to some other area of the body. Trigger points in muscle are found in taut bands in the tissue

Unipennate Type of muscle architecture in which fibers lie at a single angle to the force-generating axis

Ventral A synonym for anterior, usually applied to the torso, from Latin *venter*, belly

Volar Referring to the palm of the hand (or, less often, the sole of the foot), usually used in reference to the anterior forearm

References

Chapter 1

1. Quintner JL, Bove GM, Cohen ML. A critical evaluation of the trigger point phenomenon. *Rheumatology (Oxford)*. 2015. http://www.ncbi.nlm.nih.gov/pubmed/25477053. Accessed January 5, 2015.
2. Cherkin D, Sherman K, Kahn J, et al. A comparison of the effects of 2 types of massage and usual care on chronic low back pain: a randomized controlled trial. *Ann Intern Med*. 2011;155(1):1–9.
3. IASP Task Force on Taxonomy. Part III: pain terms, a current list with definitions and notes on usage. In: Merskey H, Bogduk N, eds. *Classification of Chronic Pain*. 2nd ed. Seattle, WA: IASP Press; 1994:209–214.
4. Engel GL. (1977). The need for a new medical model: a challenge for biomedicine. *Science*. 1977;196:129–136. doi:10.1126/science.847460.
5. Melzack R. Pain and the neuromatrix in the brain. *J Dent Educ*. 2001;65(12). http://www.jdentaled.org/content/65/12/1378.full.pdf. Accessed January 3, 2015.
6. Melzack R, Wall PD. Pain mechanisms: a new theory. *Science*. 1965;150(3699):971–979.
7. Melzack R. Evolution of the neuromatrix theory of pain. *Pain Pract*. 2005;5(2):85–94. http://neuromodulation.wordpress.com/2007/06/06/neuromatrix-theory-of-pain/. Accessed January 4, 2015.
8. Roberts AS. Central sensitization: clinical implications for chronic head and neck pain. *Clin Med Diagn*.2011;1(1):1–7. doi:10.5923/j.cmd.20110101.01.
9. Transcript of Ida Rolf lecture, Tape A5 1970, Side 1. Guild for Structural Integration Web site.www.rolfguild.org. Accessed January 4, 2015.
10. Schleip R. Fascial plasticity: a new neurobiological explanation. *J Bodyw Mov Ther*. 2003;7(1):11–19.
11. Guimberteau JC. *Strolling Under the Skin* [Video]. http://www.guimberteau-jc-md.com/en/videos.php. Accessed May 28, 2015.
12. Cheng JW, Tsai WC, Yu TY, Huang KY. Reproducibility of sonographic measurement of thickness and echogenicity of the plantar fascia. *J Clin Ultrasound*. 2012; 40(1):14–19. http://www.ncbi.nlm.nih.gov/pubmed/22109854. Accessed May 28, 2015.
13. Langevin H, Stevens-Tuttle D, Fox J, et al. Ultrasound evidence of altered lumbar connective tissue structure in human subjects with chronic low back pain. *BMC Musculoskelet Disord*. 2009;10:151. http://www.ncbi.nlm.nih.gov/pmc/articles/PMC2796643/. Accessed May 28, 2015.
14. Chaudhry H, Schleip R, Ji Z, et al. Three-dimensional mathematical model for deformation of human fasciae in manual therapy. *J Am Osteopath Assoc*. 2008;108(8):379–390. http://www.ncbi.nlm.nih.gov/pubmed/18723456. Accessed January 4, 2015.

Chapter 3

1. Centers for Disease Control and Prevention. Table 47. Severe headache or migraine, low back pain, and neck pain among adults aged 18 and over, by selected characteristics: United States, selected years 1997–2012. http://www.cdc.gov/nchs/data/hus/2012/047.pdf. Accessed February 2, 2015.
2. http://www.daltonarticles.com/public_html/42PoundHead.html.
3. Sun A, Yeo HG, Kim TU, et al. Radiologic assessment of forward head posture and its relation to myofascial pain syndrome. *Ann Rehabil Med*. 2014;38(6):821–826.

Chapter 4

1. Shultz SJ, Houglum PA, Perrin DH. Examine injuries of the shoulder joint. Human Kinetics Web site. http://www.humankinetics.com/excerpts/excerpts/examine-injuries-of-the-shoulder-joint.

2. Gaskill TR, Braun S, Millett PJ. Multimedia article. The rotator interval: pathology and management. *Arthroscopy.* 2011;27(4):556–567. http://www.ncbi.nlm.nih.gov/pubmed/21295939.

Chapter 6

1. Simons DG, Travell JG, Simons LS. *Travell & Simons' Myofascial Pain and Dysfunction: The Trigger Point Manual.* Vol. 1. 2nd ed. Baltimore, MD: Lippincott Williams & Wilkins; 1999:261–263, 354, 436, 809–8122.

Index

Note: Page numbers in *italics* refer to figures.

N

O

P

Q

R

S

T

U

V

W

X

Z